PSYCHOPATHOLOGY

FOUNDATIONS FOR A
CONTEMPORARY UNDERSTANDING

PSYCHOPATHOLOGY

FOUNDATIONS FOR A
CONTEMPORARY UNDERSTANDING

Edited by

James E. Maddux
George Mason University

Barbara A. Winstead
Old Dominion University

LEA LAWRENCE ERLBAUM ASSOCIATES, PUBLISHERS
2005 Mahwah, New Jersey   London

Senior Consulting Editor:	Susan Milmoe
Editorial Assistant:	Kristen Depken
Cover Design:	Kathryn Houghtaling Lacey
Textbook Production Manager:	Paul Smolenski
Full-Service Compositor:	TechBooks
Text and Cover Printer:	Hamilton Printing Company

This book was typeset in 10/12 pt. Times New Roman, Bold, and Italic.
The heads were typeset in Sabon Bold, and Bold Italic.

Lawrence Erlbaum Associates, Inc., Publishers
10 Industrial Avenue
Mahwah, New Jersey 07430
www.erlbaum.com

Library of Congress Cataloging-in-Publication Data

Psychopathology : foundations for a contemporary understanding / edited by
James E. Maddux, Barbara A. Winstead.
    p. cm.
   Includes bibliographical references and index.
   ISBN 0-8058-4077-X (alk. paper)
  1. Psychology, Pathological. I. Maddux, James E. II. Winstead, Barbara A.
   RC454.P786 2004
   616.89—dc22   2004011703

Printed in the United States of America
10 9 8 7 6 5 4 3

"To the students and clients who have inspired us and taught us so much."

Contents

Preface

Since 1990, more than thirty textbooks for undergraduate abnormal psychology courses have been published. This count does not include revised editions of existing books. The same period has seen the publication of numerous "handbooks" in psychopathology and psychiatry, which are conceived primarily as reference books for clinical practitioners and researchers. What has been missing is a true textbook of psychopathology for first-year graduate students in clinical psychology, counseling psychology, and related fields. Our goal in creating this book was to provide the "missing link" in the continuum. We designed content and coverage for a first-level graduate course (or an advanced-level undergraduate course for exceptional students or those who have already taken an entry-level undergraduate course in abnormal psychology). This book was designed and written with *students* in mind. The length, organization, content, and level and style of writing reflect this intention. We, the editors, are clinical psychologists with a combined forty-five years of experience teaching doctoral students in clinical psychology. The chapter authors are among the most distinguished researchers in the fields of clinical psychology and psychopathology.

We had two primary goals for the book:

1. *To provide up-to-date information about theory and research on the etiology and treatment of the most important psychological disorders.* Toward this end, we chose well-known authors who are not only familiar with the cutting-edge research in their areas of specialization but are also actively contributing to it.

2. *To challenge students to think critically about psychopathology, not just memorize information.* We tried to accomplish this goal in two ways. First, we encouraged authors to challenge traditional assumptions and theories about the problems they were addressing. Second, and more important, we commissioned chapters that dealt directly and in depth with such crucial and controversial issues as the definition of psychopathology, the influences of culture and gender, the validity of psychological testing, clinical judgment and decision making, the validity and utility of traditional psychiatric diagnosis, and the role of biological factors in the cause of psychological problems.

We believe strongly that a sophisticated understanding of psychopathology in general and of specific psychological problems requires much more than the memorization of a list of diagnostic criteria (as in the DSM) or the findings of numerous studies. Instead, it requires the mastery of *ideas* and *concepts* and how to use them to be critical consumers of research and critical readers of the DSM. For the most part, current books pay too little attention to these ideas, concepts, and issues. In Part I, we devote six chapters to these issues. The major reason for placing these general chapters before the chapters on disorders is to give students a set of conceptual tools that will help them read more thoughtfully and critically the material on specific disorders.

This textbook is divided into two main parts. Part I is devoted to discussions of the ideas, concepts, and issues noted previously. Part II is devoted to discussions of the most common problems and disorders. We asked authors to follow, to the extent possible, a common format consisting of:

1. A definition and description of the disorder or disorders.
2. A brief history of the study of the disorder.
3. Theory and research on etiology.
4. Research on empirically validated treatments.
5. A discussion of the issues covered in Part I where appropriate.

Editors always must make choices regarding what should be included in a textbook and what should not. A book that devoted a chapter to each and every disorder described in the DSM would be unwieldy and impossible to cover in a single semester. Our choices regarding what to include and what to exclude were guided primarily by our experiences with the kinds of psychological problems clinical students typically encounter in their training and subsequent clinical careers. For these reasons, we included three chapters on the psychological and cognitive problems of children and adolescents.

We hope that both instructors and students will find our approach to psychopathology challenging and useful. We have learned much from our contributing authors in the process of editing their chapters, and we hope that students will learn much from reading what the authors have produced.

James E. Maddux
George Mason University
Fairfax, VA
Barbara A. Winstead
Old Dominion University
Norfolk, VA

April 26, 2004

Contributors

Michele Boivin, University of Toronto
Annie Bollini, Emory University
Linda Anne Coker, University of Kentucky
Georg H. Eifert, Chapman University
William Fals-Stewart, University at Buffalo, The State University of New York
Katherine A. Fowler, Emory University
Paul J. Frick, University of New Orleans
Dolores Gallagher-Thompson, Stanford University School of Medicine
Howard N. Garb, University of Pittsburgh
Jennifer T. Gosselin, Pepperdine University
Peter J. Guarnaccia, Rutgers, The State University of New Jersey
C. Peter Herman, University of Toronto
Karen Hochman, Emory University
Robert H. Howland, University of Pittsburgh School of Medicine
Rick Ingram, University of Kansas
Lisa Kestler, Emory University
Eva R. Kimonis, University of New Orleans
Lisa M. Kinoshita, Stanford University School of Medicine
Scott O. Lilienfeld, Emory University
Steven Regeser López, University of California, Los Angeles
James E. Maddux, George Mason University
Nathaniel McConaghy, University of New South Wales
Jack Naglieri, George Mason University
Thomas H. Ollendick, Virginia Polytechnic Institute and State University
Janet Polivy, University of Toronto
Johannes Rojahn, George Mason University
Claudia Salter, George Mason University
Janis Sanchez, Old Dominion University
Janay B. Sander, Virginia Polytechnic Institute and State University
Alison L. Shortt, Virginia Polytechnic Institute and State University

Kristen H. Sorocco, University of Oklahoma Health Sciences Center
Lucy Trenary, University of Colorado
Elaine Walker, Emory University
Thomas A. Widiger, University of Kentucky
S. Lloyd Williams, Stuttgart, Germany
Barbara A. Winstead, Old Dominion University
Michael J. Zvolensky, The University of Vermont

THINKING ABOUT
PSYCHOPATHOLOGY

1

Conceptions of Psychopathology: A Social Constructionist Perspective

James E. Maddux
George Mason University

Jennifer T. Gosselin
Pepperdine University

Barbara A. Winstead
Old Dominion University

A textbook about a subject should begin with a clear definition of the subject. Unfortunately, in the case of a textbook on psychopathology, definition is difficult if not impossible. The definitions or conceptions of *psychopathology* and related terms such as *mental disorder* have been the focus of heated debate throughout the history of psychology and psychiatry, and the debate is far from over (e.g, Gorenstein, 1984: Horwitz, 2002; Widiger, 1997). Despite many variations, the debate has centered on a single overriding question—are psychopathology and related terms such as mental disorder and mental illness scientific terms that can be defined objectively and by scientific criteria or are they social constructions (Gergen, 1985) that are defined entirely by societal and cultural values? The goal of this chapter is to address this question. Addressing it early is important because readers' views of everything they read in the rest of this book will be influenced by their views on this question.

A conception of psychopathology is not a theory of psychopathology (Wakefield, 1992a). A conception of psychopathology provides one definition of the term—it delineates which human experiences are considered psychopathological and which are not. A conception of psychopathology does not try to explain the psychological phenomena that are considered pathological but instead tells us what psychological phenomena are considered pathological and thus need to be explained. A theory of psychopathology, however, provides an explanation of those psychological phenomena and experiences that have been identified by the conception as pathological. This chapter deals with conceptions of psychopathology. Theories and explanations can be found in a number of other chapters, including all of those in part II.

Understanding various conceptions of psychopathology is important for many reasons. As medical philosopher Lawrie Reznek (1987) said, "Concepts carry consequences—classifying things one way rather than another has important implications for the way we behave towards such things" (p. 1). In speaking of the importance of the conception of disease, Reznek wrote:

The classification of a condition as a disease carries many important consequences. We inform medical scientists that they should try to discover a cure for the condition. We inform benefactors that they should support such research. We direct medical care towards the condition, making it appropriate to treat the condition by medical means such as drug therapy, surgery, and so on. We inform our courts that it is inappropriate to hold people responsible for the manifestations of the condition. We set up early warning detection services aimed at detecting the condition in its early stages when it is still amenable to successful treatment. We serve notice to health insurance companies and national health services that they are liable to pay for the treatment of such a condition. Classifying a condition as a disease is no idle matter. (p. 1)

If we substitute the term psychopathology or mental disorder for the word *disease* in this paragraph, Reznek's message still holds true. How we conceive of psychopathology and related terms has wide-ranging implications for individuals, medical and mental health professionals, government agencies and programs, and society at large.

TRADITIONAL CONCEPTIONS OF PSYCHOPATHOLOGY

Various conceptions of psychopathology have been offered over the years. Each has its merits and its deficiencies, but none suffices as a truly scientific definition.

Psychopathology as Statistical Deviance

A common and common sense conception of psychopathology is that pathological psychological phenomena are those that are abnormal or statistically deviant or infrequent. *Abnormal* literally means away from the norm. The word *norm* refers to what is typical or average. Thus, in this conception, psychopathology is viewed as deviation from psychological normality.

One of the merits of this conception is its commonsense appeal. It makes sense to most people to use terms such as psychopathology and mental disorder to refer only to behaviors or experiences that are infrequent (e.g., paranoid delusions, hearing voices) and not to those that are relatively common (e.g., shyness, sadness following the death of a loved one).

A second benefit of this conception is that it lends itself to accepted methods of measurement that give it at least a semblance of scientific respectability. The first step in using this conception scientifically is to determine what is statistically normal (typical, average). The second step is to determine how far a particular psychological phenomenon or condition deviates from statistical normality. This step is often accomplished by developing an instrument or measure that attempts to quantify the phenomenon and then assigns numbers or scores to people's experiences or manifestations of the phenomenon. Once the measure is developed, norms are typically established so that an individual's score can be compared to the mean or average score of some group of people. Scores that are sufficiently far from average are considered to be indicative of abnormal or pathological psychological phenomena. This process describes most tests of intelligence and cognitive ability and many commonly used measures of personality and emotion (e.g., the Minnesota Multiphasic Personality Inventory).

Despite its commonsense appeal and its scientific merits, this conception presents problems. It sounds relatively objective and scientific because it relies on well-established psychometric methods for developing measures of psychological phenomena and developing norms. Yet, this approach leaves much room for subjectivity.

Subjectivity first comes into play in the conceptual definition of the construct for which a measure is developed. A measure of any psychological construct, such as intelligence, must begin with a conceptual definition. We have to ask ourselves, "What is intelligence?" Of course, different people (including different psychologists) will offer different answers to this question. How then can we scientifically and objectively determine which definition or conception is true or correct? The answer is that we cannot. Although we have proven methods for developing a reliable and valid (i.e., it predicts what we want to predict) measure of a psychological construct once we have agreed on its conception or definition, we cannot use these same methods to determine which conception or definition is true or correct. There is no one true definition of intelligence and no objective, scientific way of determining one. Intelligence is not a thing that exists inside of people and makes them behave in certain ways and that awaits our discovery of its true nature. Instead, it is an abstract idea that is defined by people as they use the words *intelligence* and *intelligent* to describe certain kinds of human behavior and the covert mental processes that supposedly precede or are concurrent with the behavior.

We usually can observe and describe patterns in the way most people use the words intelligence and intelligent to describe their own behavior and that of others. The descriptions of the patterns then comprise the definitions of the words. If we examine the patterns of the use of intelligence and intelligent, we find that at the most basic level, they describe a variety of specific behaviors and abilities that society values and thus encourages; unintelligent behavior is a variety of behaviors that society does not value and thus discourages. The fact that the definition of intelligence is grounded in societal values explains the recent expansion of the concept to include good interpersonal skills, self-regulatory skills, artistic and musical abilities, and other abilities not measured by traditional tests of intelligence. The meaning of intelligence has broadened because society has come to place increasing value on these other attributes and abilities, and that change in values is the result of a dialogue or discourse among the people in society, both professionals and laypersons. One measure of intelligence may be more reliable than and more useful than another measure in predicting what we want to predict (e.g., academic achievement, income), but what we want to predict reflects what we value, and values are not scientifically derived.

Subjectivity also influences the determination of how deviant a psychological phenomenon must be from the norm to be considered abnormal or pathological. We can use objective, scientific methods to construct a measure such as an intelligence test and develop norms for the measure, but we are still left with the question of how far from normal an individual's score must be to be considered abnormal. This question cannot be answered by the science of psychometrics because the distance from the average that a person's score must be to be considered abnormal is a matter of debate, not a matter of fact. It is true that we often answer this question by relying on statistical conventions such as using one or two standard deviations from the average score as the line of division between normal and abnormal (see the chapter on cognitive abilities in childhood). Yet the decision to use that convention is itself subjective. Why should one standard deviation from the norm designate abnormality? Why not two standard deviations? Why not half a standard deviation? Why not use percentages? The lines between normal and abnormal can be drawn at many different points using many different strategies. Each line of demarcation may be more or less useful for certain purposes, such as determining the criteria for eligibility for limited services and resources. Where the line is set also determines the prevalence of abnormality or mental disorder among the general population (Kutchens & Kirk, 1997), so it has great practical significance. But no such line is more or less true than the others, even when based on statistical conventions.

We cannot use the procedures and methods of science to draw a definitive line of demarcation between normal and abnormal psychological functioning, just as we cannot use them to draw lines of demarcation between short and tall people or hot and cold on a thermometer. No such lines exist in nature awaiting our discovery.

Psychopathology as Maladaptive (Dysfunctional) Behavior

Most of us think of psychopathology as behavior and experience that are not just statistically abnormal but also maladaptive (dysfunctional). *Normal* and *abnormal* are statistical terms, but *adaptive* and *maladaptive* refer not to statistical norms and deviations but to the effectiveness or ineffectiveness of a person's behavior. If a behavior is effective for the person—if the behavior helps the person deal with challenge, cope with stress, and accomplish his or her goals—then we say the behavior is more or less adaptive. If the behavior does not help in these ways, or if the behavior makes the problem or situation worse, we say it is more or less maladaptive.

Like the statistical deviance conception, this conception has commonsense appeal and is consistent with the way most laypersons use words such as pathology, disorder, and illness. Most people would find it odd to use these words to describe statistically infrequent high levels of intelligence, happiness, or psychological well being. To say that someone is pathologically intelligent or pathologically well-adjusted seems contradictory because it flies in the face of the commonsense use of these words.

The major problem with the conception of psychopathology as maladaptive behavior is its inherent subjectivity. The distinction between adaptive and maladaptive, like the distinction between normal and abnormal, is fuzzy and often arbitrary. We have no objective, scientific way of making a clear distinction. Very few human behaviors are in and of themselves either adaptive or maladaptive; their adaptiveness and maladapativeness depends on the situations in which they are enacted and on the judgment and values of the observer. Even behaviors that are statistically rare and therefore abnormal are more or less adaptive under different conditions and more or less adaptive in the opinion of different observers. The extent to which a behavior or behavior pattern is viewed as more or less adaptive or maladaptive depends on a number of factors, such as the goals the person is trying to accomplish and the social norms and expectations of a given situation. What works in one situation might not work in another. What appears adaptive to one person might not appear so to another. What is usually adaptive in one culture might not be so in another. Even so-called normal personality involves a good deal of occasionally maladaptive behavior, for which you can find evidence in your own life and the lives of friends and relatives. In addition, people given personality disorder diagnoses by clinical psychologists and psychiatrists often can manage their lives effectively and do not always behave in disordered ways.

Another problem with the psychopathological-equals-maladaptive conception is that determinations of adaptiveness and maladaptiveness are logically unrelated to measures of statistical deviation. Of course, often we do find a strong relationship between the statistical abnormality of a behavior and its maladaptiveness. Many of the problems described in the *Diagnostic and Statistical Manual of Mental Disorders* (DSM; American Psychiatric Association [APA], 2000) and in this textbook are both maladaptive and statistically rare. There are, however, major exceptions to this relationship. First, psychological phenomena that deviate from normal or average are not all maladaptive. In fact, sometimes deviation from normal is adaptive and healthy. For example, IQ scores of 130 and 70 are equally deviant from normal, but abnormally high intelligence is much more adaptive than abnormally low intelligence. Likewise, people who consistently score abnormally low on measures of anxiety and depression are probably happier and better adjusted than people who consistently score equally abnormally high on such measures.

Second, maladaptive psychological phenomena are not all statistically infrequent and vice versa. For example, shyness is very common and therefore is statistically frequent, but shyness is almost always maladaptive to some extent, because it almost always interferes with a person's ability to accomplish what he or she wants to accomplish in life and relationships. This is not to say that shyness is pathological but only that it makes it difficult for some people to live full and happy lives. The same is true of many of the problems with sexual functioning that are included in the DSM as mental disorders.

Psychopathology as Distress and Disability

Some conceptions of psychopathology invoke the notions of subjective distress and disability. Subjective distress refers to unpleasant and unwanted feelings such as anxiety, sadness, and anger. Disability refers to a restriction in ability (Ossorio, 1985). People who seek mental health treatment are not getting what they want out of life, and many feel that they are unable to do what they would like to do. They may feel inhibited or restricted by their situation, their fears or emotional turmoil, or by physical or other limitations. The individual may lack the necessary self-efficacy beliefs (beliefs about personal abilities), physiological or biological components, and/or situational opportunities to make positive changes (Bergner, 1997).

Subjective distress and disability are simply two different but related ways of thinking about adaptiveness and maladaptiveness rather than alternative conceptions of psychopathology. Although the notions of subjective distress and disability may help refine our notion of maladaptiveness, they do nothing to resolve the subjectivity problem. Different people define personal distress and personal disability in vastly different ways, as do different mental health professionals and those in different cultures. Likewise, people differ in how much distress or disability they can tolerate. Thus, we are still left with the problem of how to determine normal and abnormal levels of distress and disability. As noted previously, the question "How much is too much?" cannot be answered using the objective methods of science.

Another problem is that some conditions or patterns of behavior (e.g., sexual fetishisms, antisocial personality disorder) that are considered psychopathological (at least officially, according to the DSM) are not characterized by subjective distress, other than the temporary distress that might result from social condemnation or conflicts with the law.

Psychopathology as Social Deviance

Another conception views psychopathology as behavior that deviates from social or cultural norms. This conception is simply a variation of the conception of psychopathology as abnormality, except that in this case judgments about deviations from normality are made informally by people rather than formally according to psychological tests or measures.

This conception also is consistent to some extent with common sense and common parlance. We tend to view psychopathological or mentally disordered people as thinking, feeling, and doing things that most other people do not do and that are inconsistent with socially accepted and culturally sanctioned ways of thinking, feeling, and behaving.

The problem with this conception, as with the others, is its subjectivity. Norms for socially normal or acceptable behavior are not scientifically derived but instead are based on the values, beliefs, and historical practices of the culture, which determine who is accepted or rejected by a society or culture. Cultural values develop not through the implementation of scientific methods but through numerous informal conversations and negotiations among the people and institutions of that culture. Social norms differ from one culture to another, and therefore what is psychologically abnormal in one culture may not be so in another (See López & Guarnaccia, this book). Also, norms of a given culture change over time; therefore, conceptions of psychopathology also change over time, often very dramatically, as evidenced by American society's changes over the past several decades in attitudes toward sex, race, and gender. For example, psychiatrists in the 1800s classified masturbation, especially in children and women, as a disease, and it was treated in some cases by clitoridectomy (removal of the clitoris), which

Western society today would consider barbaric (Reznek, 1987). Homosexuality was an official mental disorder in the DSM until 1973.

In addition, the conception of psychopathology as social norm violations is at times in conflict with the conception of psychopathology as maladaptive behavior. Sometimes violating social norms is healthy and adaptive for the individual and beneficial to society. In the 19th century, women and African-Americans in the United States who sought the right to vote were trying to change well-established social norms. Their actions were uncommon and therefore abnormal, but these people were far from psychologically unhealthy, at least by today's standards. Earlier in the 19th century, slaves who desired to escape from their owners were said to have "drapetomania." Today slavery itself, although still practiced in some parts of the world, is seen as socially deviant and pathological, and the desire to escape enslavement is considered to be as normal and healthy as the desire to live and breathe.

CONTEMPORARY CONCEPTIONS: PSYCHOPATHOLOGY AS HARMFUL DYSFUNCTION

A more recent attempt at defining psychopathology is Wakefield's (1992a, 1992b, 1993, 1997, 1999) harmful dysfunction (HD) conception. Presumably grounded in evolutionary psychology (e.g., Cosmides, Tooby, & Barkow, 1992), the HD conception acknowledges that the conception of mental disorder is influenced strongly by social and cultural values. It also proposes, however, a supposedly scientific, factual, and objective core that is not dependent on social and cultural values. In Wakefield's (1992a) words:

> A [mental] disorder is a harmful dysfunction wherein harmful is a value term based on social norms, and dysfunction is a scientific term referring to the failure of a mental mechanism to perform a natural function for which it was designed by evolution... a disorder exists when the failure of a person's internal mechanisms to perform their function as designed by nature impinges harmfully on the person's well-being as defined by social values and meanings. (p. 373)

One of the merits of this approach is that it acknowledges that the conception of mental disorders must include a reference to social norms; however, this conception also tries to ground the concept of mental disorder in a scientific theory—that is, the theory of evolution.

Wakefield (1999) recently has reiterated this definition in writing that "a disorder attribution requires both a scientific judgment that there exists a failure of designed function and a value judgment that the design failure harms the individual" (p. 374). However, the claim that identifying a failure of a designed function is a scientific judgment and not a value judgment is open to question. Wakefield's claim that dysfunction can be defined in "purely factual scientific" (Wakefield, 1992a, p. 383) terms rests on the assumption that the designed functions of human mental mechanisms have an objective and observable reality and, thus, that failure of the mechanism to execute its designed function can be objectively assessed. A basic problem with this notion is that although the physical inner workings of the body and brain can be observed and measured, mental mechanisms have no objective reality and thus cannot be observed directly—no more so than the unconscious forces that provide the foundation for Freudian psychoanalysis.

Evolutionary theory provides a basis for explaining human behavior in terms of its contribution to reproductive fitness. A behavior is considered more functional if it increases the survival of those who share your genes in the next generation and the next and less functional if it does not. Evolutionary psychology cannot, however, provide a catalogue of mental mechanisms and their natural functions. Wakefield states that "discovering what in fact is natural or dysfunctional may be extraordinarily difficult" (1992b, p. 236). The problem with this statement is that, when applied to human behavior, natural and dysfunctional are not properties that can be discovered; they are value judgments. The judgment that a behavior represents a dysfunction relies on the observation that the behavior is excessive and/or inappropriate under certain conditions. Arguing that these behaviors represent failures of an evolutionarily designed mental mechanisms (itself an untestable hypothesis because of the occult nature of mental mechanisms) does not relieve us of the need to make value judgments about what is excessive or inappropriate in what circumstances. These value judgments are based on social norms, not on scientific facts, an issue that we will explore in greater detail later in this chapter.

Another problem with the HD conception is that it is a moving target. Recently, Wakefield modified the HD conception by saying that it refers not to what a mental disorder is but only to what most scientists think it is. For example, he states that "My comments were intended to argue, not that PTSD [posttraumatic stress disorder] is a disorder, but that the HD analysis is capable of explaining why the symptom picture in PTSD is commonly judged to be a disorder" (1999, p. 390).

According to Sadler (1999), Wakefield's original goal was to "define mental disorders prescriptively [and to] help us decide whether someone is mentally disordered or not. [However, his current view] avoids making any prescriptive claims, instead focusing on explaining the conventional clinical use of the disorder concept [and he] has abandoned his original task to be prescriptive and has now settled for being descriptive only, for example, telling us why a disorder is judged to be one" (pp. 433–434).

Describing how people have agreed to define a concept is not the same as defining the concept in scientific terms, even if those people are scientists. Thus, Wakefield's revised HD conception simply offers another criterion that people (clinicians, scientists, and laypersons) might use to judge whether or not something is a mental disorder. But consensus of opinion, even among scientists, is not scientific evidence. Therefore, no matter how accurately this criterion might describe how some or most people define mental disorder, it is no more or no less scientific than other conceptions that also are based on how some people agree to define mental disorder. It is no more scientific than the conceptions involving statistical infrequency, maladaptiveness, or social norm violations. (See also Widiger, this book.)

CONTEMPORARY CONCEPTIONS: THE DSM DEFINITION OF MENTAL DISORDER

Any discussion of conceptions of psychopathology has to include a discussion of the most influential conception of all—that of the DSM. The DSM documents "what is currently understood by most scientists, theorists, researchers, and clinicians to be the predominant forms of psychopathology" (Widiger, this book). First published in 1952 and revised and expanded five times since, the DSM provides the organizational structure for virtually every textbook (including this one) on abnormal psychology and psychopathology, as well as almost every professional book on the assessment and treatment of psychological problems. (See Widiger, this book, for a more detailed history of psychiatric classification and the DSM.)

Just as a textbook on psychopathology should begin by defining its key term, so should a taxonomy of mental disorders. To their credit, the authors of the DSM attempted to do that. The difficulties inherent in attempting to define psychopathology and related terms is clearly illustrated by the definition of mental disorder found in the latest edition of the DSM, the DSM–IV–TR (APA, 2000):

> ... a clinically significant behavioral or psychological syndrome or pattern that occurs in an individual and that is associated with present distress (e.g., a painful symptom) or disability (i.e., impairment in one or more important areas of functioning) or with a significantly increased risk of suffering death, pain, disability, or an important loss of freedom. In addition, this syndrome or pattern must not be merely an expectable and culturally sanctioned response to a particular event, for example, the death of a loved one. Whatever its original cause, it must currently be considered a manifestation of a behavioral, psychological, or biological dysfunction in the individual. Neither deviant behavior (e.g., political, religious, or sexual) nor conflicts that are primarily between the individual and society are mental disorders unless the deviance or conflict is a symptom of a dysfunction in the individual, as described above. (p. xxxi)

All of the conceptions of psychopathology described previously can be found to some extent in this definition—statistical deviation (i.e., not expectable); maladaptiveness, including distress and disability; social norms violations; and some elements of the harmful dysfunction conception (a dysfunction in the individual), although without the flavor of evolutionary theory. For this reason, it is a comprehensive, inclusive, and sophisticated conception and probably as good as, if not better than, any proposed so far. Nonetheless, it contains the same problems with subjectivity as other conceptions. For example, what is the meaning of clinically significant and how should clinical significance be measured? Does clinical significance refer to statistical infrequency, maladaptiveness, or both? How much distress must people experience or how much disability must people exhibit before they are said to have a mental disorder? Who judges a person's degree of distress or disability? How do we determine whether a particular response to an event is expectable or culturally sanctioned? Who determines this? How does one determine whether deviant behavior or conflicts are primarily between the individual and society? What exactly does this mean? What does it mean for a dysfunction to exist or occur in the individual? Certainly a biological dysfunction might be said to be literally in the individual, but does it make sense to say the same of psychological and behavioral dysfunctions? Is it possible to say that a psychological or behavioral dysfunction can occur in the individual apart from the sociocultural and interpersonal milieu in which the person is acting? Clearly, the DSM's conception of mental disorder raises as many questions as do the conceptions it was meant to supplant.

CATEGORIES VERSUS DIMENSIONS

The difficulty inherent in the DSM conception of psychopathology and other attempts to distinguish between normal and abnormal or adaptive and maladaptive is that they are categorical models in which individuals are determined either to have or not have a disorder. An alternative model, overwhelmingly supported by research, is the dimensional model. In the dimensional model, normality and abnormality, as well as effective and ineffective psychological functioning, lie along a continuum; so-called psychological disorders are simply extreme variants of normal psychological phenomena and ordinary problems in living (Keyes & Lopez, 2002; Widiger, this book). The dimensional model is concerned not with classifying people or disorders but with identifying and measuring individual differences in psychological phenomena such as emotion, mood, intelligence, and personal styles (e.g., Lubinski, 2000). Great differences among individuals on the dimensions of interest are expected, such as the differences we find on formal tests of intelligence. As with intelligence, divisions made between normality and abnormality may be demarcated for convenience or efficiency but are not to be viewed as indicative of true discontinuity among types of phenomena or types of people. Also, statistical deviation is not viewed as necessarily pathological, although extreme variants on either end of a dimension (e.g., introversion–extraversion, neuroticism, intelligence) may be maladaptive if they lead to inflexibility in functioning.

Empirical evidence for the validity of a dimensional approach to psychological adjustment is strongest in the area of personality and personality disorders (Coker & Widiger, this book; Costello, 1996; Maddux & Mundell, 2005). Factor analytic studies of personality problems among the general population and clinical populations with personality disorders demonstrate striking similarity between the two groups. In addition, these factor structures are not consistent with the DSM's system of classifying disorders of personality into categories (Maddux & Mundell, 2005). The dimensional view of personality disorders also is supported by cross-cultural research (Alarcon, Foulks, & Vakkur, 1998).

Research on other problems supports the dimensional view. Studies of the varieties of normal emotional experiences (e.g., Oatley & Jenkins, 1992) indicates that clinical emotional disorders are not discrete classes of emotional experience that are discontinuous from everyday emotional upsets and problems. Research on adult attachment patterns in relationships strongly suggests that dimensions are more useful descriptions of such patterns than are categories (Fraley & Waller, 1998). Research on self-defeating behaviors has shown that they are extremely common and are not by themselves signs of abnormality or symptoms of disorders (Baumeister & Scher, 1988). Research on children's reading problems indicates that dyslexia is not an all-or-none condition that children either have or do not have, but rather, the condition occurs in degrees without a natural break between dyslexic and nondyslexic children (Shaywitz, Escobar, Shaywitz, Fletcher, & Makuch, 1992). Research on attention deficit/hyperactivity (Barkley, 1997) and posttraumatic stress disorder (Anthony, Lonigan, & Hecht, 1999) demonstrates this same dimensionality. Research on depression and schizophrenia indicates that these disorders are best viewed as loosely related clusters of dimensions of individual differences, not as disease-like syndromes (Claridge, 1995; Costello, 1993a, 1993b; Persons, 1986). The coiner of the term *schizophrenia*, Eugen Bleuler, viewed so-called pathological conditions as continuous with so-called normal conditions and noted the occurrence of schizophrenic symptoms among normal individuals (Gilman, 1988). In fact, Bleuler referred to the major symptom of schizophrenia (thought disorder) as simply ungewöhnlich, which in German means unusual, not bizarre, as it was translated in the first English version of Bleuler's classic monograph (Gilman, 1988). Essentially, the creation of schizophrenia was "an artifact of the ideologies implicit in nineteenth century European and American medical nosologies" (Gilman, p. 204). (See also Walker, Bollini, Hochman, & Kestler, this book.) Finally, biological researchers continue to discover continuities between so-called normal and abnormal (or pathological) psychological conditions (Claridge, 1995; Livesley, Jang, & Vernon, 1998).

SOCIAL CONSTRUCTIONISM AND CONCEPTIONS OF PSYCHOPATHOLOGY

If we cannot derive an objective and scientific conception of psychopathology and mental disorder, then what way is left to us to understand these terms? How then are we to conceive of psychopathology? The solution to this problem is not to develop yet another definition of psychopathology. The solution, instead, is to accept the fact that the problem has no solution— at least not a solution that can be arrived at by scientific means. We have to give up the goal of developing a scientific definition and accept the idea that psychopathology and related terms cannot be defined through the processes that we usually think of as scientific. We have to stop struggling to develop a scientific conception of psychopathology and attempt instead to try to understand the struggle itself—why it occurs and what it means. We need to better understand how people go about trying to conceive of and define psychopathology and how and why these conceptions are the topic of continual debate and undergo continual revision.

We start by accepting the idea that psychopathology and related concepts are abstract ideas that are not scientifically constructed but instead are socially constructed. To do this is to engage in social constructionism, which involves "elucidating the process by which people come to describe, explain, or otherwise account for the world in which they live" (Gergen, 1985, pp. 3–4). Social constructionism is concerned with "examining ways in which people understand the world, the social and political processes that influence how people define words and explain events, and the implications of these definitions and explanations—who benefits and who loses because of how we describe and understand the world" (Gergen, 1985, pp. 3–4). From this point of view, words and concepts such as *psychopathology* and *mental disorder* "are products of particular historical and cultural understandings rather than . . . universal and immutable categories of human experience" (Bohan, 1996, p. xvi). Universal or true definitions of concepts do not exist because these definitions depend on who does the defining. The people who define them are usually people with power, and so these definitions reflect and promote their interests and values (Muehlenhard & Kimes, 1999, p. 234). Therefore, "When less powerful people attempt to challenge existing power relationships and to promote social change, an initial battleground is often the words used to discuss these problems" (Muehlenhard & Kimes, 1999, p. 234). Because the interests of people and institutions are based on their values, debates over the definition of concepts often become clashes between deeply and implicitly held beliefs about the way the world works or should work and about the difference between right and wrong. Such clashes are evident in the debates over the definitions of *domestic violence* (Muehlenhard & Kimes, 1999), *child sexual abuse* (Holmes & Slapp, 1998; Rind, Tromovich, & Bauserman, 1998), and other such terms.

The social constructionist perspective can be contrasted with the essentialist perspective. Essentialism assumes that there are natural categories and that all members of a given category share important characteristics (Rosenblum & Travis, 1996). For example, the essentialist perspective views our categories of race, sexual orientation, and social class as objective categories that are independent of social or cultural processes. It views these categories as representing "empirically verifiable similarities among and differences between people" (Rosenblum & Travis, 1996, p. 2). In the social constructionist view, however, "reality cannot be separated from the way that a culture makes sense of it" (Rosenblum & Travis, 1996, p. 3). In social constructionism, such categories represent not what people *are* but rather the ways that people think about and attempt to make sense of differences among people. Social processes also determine what differences among people are more important than other differences (Rosenblum & Travis, 1996).

Thus, from the essentialist perspective, psychopathologies and mental disorders are natural entities whose true nature can be discovered and described. From the social constructionist perspective, however, they are but abstract ideas that are defined by people and thus reflect their values—cultural, professional, and personal. The meanings of these and other concepts are not revealed by the methods of science but are negotiated among the people and institutions of society who have an interest in their definitions. In fact, we typically refer to psychological terms as constructs for this very reason—that their meanings are constructed and negotiated rather than discovered or revealed. The ways in which conceptions of such basic psychological constructs as the self (Baumeister, 1987) and self-esteem (Hewitt, 2002) have changed over time and the different ways they are conceived by different cultures (e.g., Cross & Markus, 1999; Cushman, 1995; Hewitt, 2002) provide an example of this process at work. Thus "all categories of disorder, even physical disorder categories convincingly explored scientifically, are the product of human beings constructing meaningful systems for understanding their world" (Raskin & Lewandowski, 2000, p. 21). In addition, because "what it means to be a person is determined by cultural ways of talking about and conceptualizing personhood . . . identity and disorder are socially constructed, and there are as many disorder constructions as there are cultures." (Neimeyer & Raskin, 2000, p. 6–7). Finally, "if people cannot reach the objective truth about what disorder really is, then viable constructions of disorder must compete with one another on the basis of their use and meaningfulness in particular clinical situations" (Raskin & Lewandowski, 2000, p. 26).

From the social constructionist perspective, sociocultural, political, professional, and economic forces influence professional and lay conceptions of psychopathology. Our conceptions of psychological normality and abnormality are not facts about people but abstract ideas that are constructed through the implicit and explicit collaborations of theorists, researchers, professionals, their clients, and the culture in which all are embedded and that represent a shared view of the world and human nature. For this reason, mental disorders and the numerous diagnostic categories of the DSM were not discovered in the same manner that an archeologist discovers a buried artifact or a medical researcher discovers a virus. Instead, they were invented (see Raskin & Lewandowski, 2000, in Neimeyer & Raskin). By saying that mental disorders are invented, however, we do not mean that they are myths (Szasz, 1974) or that the distress of people who are labeled as mentally disordered is not real. Instead, we mean that these disorders do not exist and have properties in the same manner that artifacts and viruses do. Therefore, a conception of psychopathology "does not simply describe and classify characteristics of groups of individuals, but . . . actively constructs a version of both normal and abnormal . . . which is then applied to individuals who end up being classified as normal or abnormal" (Parker, Georgaca, Harper, McLaughlin, & Stowell-Smith, 1995, p. 93).

Conceptions of psychopathology and the various categories of psychopathology are not mappings of psychological facts about people. Instead, they are social artifacts that serve the same sociocultural goals as do our conceptions of race, gender, social class, and sexual orientation—those of maintaining and expanding the power of certain individuals and institutions and maintaining social order, as defined by those in power (Beall, 1993; Parker et al., 1995; Rosenblum & Travis, 1996). As are these other social constructions, our concepts of psychological normality and abnormality are tied ultimately to social values—in particular, the values of society's most powerful individuals, groups, and institutions—and the contextual rules for behavior derived from these values (Becker, 1963; Parker et al., 1995; Rosenblum & Travis, 1996). As McNamee and Gergen (1992) state: "The mental health profession is not politically, morally, or valuationally neutral. Their practices typically operate to sustain certain values, political arrangements, and hierarchies of privilege" (p. 2). Thus, the debate over the definition of psychopathology, the struggle over who defines it, and the continual revisions of the DSM are not aspects of a search for truth. Rather, they are debates over the definition of socially constructed abstractions and struggles for the personal, political, and economic power that derives from the authority to define these abstractions and thus to determine what and whom society views as normal and abnormal.

These debates and struggles are described in detail by Allan Horwitz in *Creating Mental Illness* (2002). According to Horwitz:

The emergence and persistence of an overly expansive disease model of mental illness was not accidental or arbitrary. The widespread creation of distinct mental diseases developed in specific historical circumstances and because of the interests of specific social groups... By the time the DSM-III was developed in 1980, thinking of mental illnesses as discrete disease entities ... offered mental health professionals many social, economic, and political advantages. In addition, applying disease frameworks to a wide variety of behaviors and to a large number of people benefited a number of specific social groups including not only clinicians but also research scientists, advocacy groups, and pharmaceutical companies, among others. The disease entities of diagnostic psychiatry arose because they were useful for the social practices of various groups, not because they provided a more accurate way of viewing mental disorders. (p. 16)

Psychiatrist Mitchell Wilson (1993) has offered a similar position. He has argued that the dimensional/continuity view of psychological wellness and illness posed a basic problem for psychiatry because it "did not demarcate clearly the well from the sick" (p. 402) and that "if conceived of psychosocially, psychiatric illness is not the province of medicine, because psychiatric problems are not truly medical but social, political, and legal" (p. 402). The purpose of DMS-III, according to Wilson, was to allow psychiatry a means of marking out its professional territory. Kirk and Kutchins (1992) reached the same conclusion following their thorough review of the papers, letters, and memos of the various DSM working groups.

The social construction of psychopathology works something like this. Someone observes a pattern of behaving, thinking, feeling, or desiring that deviates from some social norm or ideal or identifies a human weakness or imperfection that, as expected, is displayed with greater frequency or severity by some people than others. A group with influence and power decides that control, prevention, or treatment of this problem is desirable or profitable. The pattern is then given a scientific-sounding name, preferably of Greek or Latin origin. The new scientific name is capitalized. Eventually, the new term may be reduced to an acronym, such as OCD (Obsessive-Compulsive Disorder), ADHD (Attention-Deficit/Hyperactivity Disorder), and BDD (Body Dysmorphic Disorder). The new disorder then takes on an existence all its own and becomes a disease-like entity. As news about the disorder spreads, people begin thinking they have it; medical and mental health professionals begin diagnosing and treating it; and clinicians and clients begin demanding that health insurance policies cover the treatment of it. Once the disorder has been socially constructed and defined, the methods of science can be used to study it, but the construction itself is a social process, not a scientific one. In fact, the more "it" is studied, the more everyone becomes convinced that "it" is a valid "something."

Medical philosopher Lawrie Reznek (1987) has demonstrated that even our definition of physical disease is socially constructed. He writes:

Judging that some condition is a disease is to judge that the person with that condition is less able to lead a good or worthwhile life. And since this latter judgment is a normative one, to judge that some condition is a disease is to make a normative judgment... This normative view of the concept of disease explains why cultures holding different values disagree over what are diseases (p. 211)... Whether some condition is a disease depends on where we choose to draw the line of normality, and this is not a line that we can discover. (p. 212)... disease judgments, like moral judgments, are not factual ones.

Likewise, Sedgwick (1982) points out that human diseases are natural processes. They may harm humans, but they actually promote the life of other organisms. For example, a virus's reproductive strategy may include spreading from human to human. Sedgwick writes:

There are no illnesses or diseases in nature. The fracture of a septuagenarian's femur has, within the world of nature, no more significance than the snapping of an autumn leaf from its twig; and the invasion of a human organism by cholera germs carries with it no more the stamp of "illness" than does the souring of milk by other forms of bacteria. Out of his anthropocentric self-interest, man has chosen to consider as "illnesses" or "diseases" those natural circumstances which precipitate death (or the failure to function according to certain values). (p. 30)

If these statements are true of physical disease, they are certainly true of psychological disease or psychopathology. Like our conception of physical disease, our conceptions of psychopathology are social constructions that are grounded in sociocultural goals and values, particularly our assumptions about how people should live their lives and about what makes life worth living. (See also López & Guarnaccia, this book, and Widiger, this book.) This truth is illustrated clearly in the American Psychiatric Association's 1952 decision to include homosexuality in the first edition of the DSM and its 1973 decision to revoke its disease status (Kutchins & Kirk, 1997; Shorter, 1997). As stated by Wilson (1993), "The homosexuality controversy seemed to show that psychiatric diagnoses were clearly wrapped up in social constructions of deviance" (p. 404). This issue also was in the forefront of the debates over post-traumatic stress disorder, paraphilic rapism, and masochistic personality disorder (Kutchins & Kirk, 1997), as well as caffeine dependence, sexual compulsivity, low intensity orgasm, sibling rivalry, self-defeating personality, jet lag, pathological spending, and impaired sleep-related painful erections, all of which were proposed for inclusion in DSM-IV (Widiger & Trull, 1991). Others have argued convincingly that schizophrenia (Gilman, 1988), addiction (Peele, 1995), personality disorder (Alarcon et al., 1998), and dissociative identity disorder (formerly multiple personality disorder) (Spanos, 1996) also are socially constructed categories rather than disease entities.

With each revision, our most powerful professional conception of psychopathology, the DSM, has had more and more to say about how people should live their lives and about what makes life worth living. The number of pages increased from 86 in 1952 to almost 900 in 1994, and the number of mental disorders increased from 106 to 297. As the scope of mental disorder has expanded with each DSM revision, life has become increasingly pathologized, and the sheer number of people with diagnosable mental disorders has continued to grow. Moreover, mental health professionals have not been content to label only obviously and blatantly dysfunctional patterns of behaving, thinking, and feeling as mental disorders. Instead, we have defined the scope of psychopathology to include many common problems in living.

Consider some of the mental disorders found in the DSM-IV. Cigarette smokers have Nicotine Dependence. If you drink large quantities of coffee, you may develop Caffeine Intoxication or Caffeine-Induced Sleep Disorder. If you have "a preoccupation with a defect in appearance" that causes "significant distress or impairment in . . . functioning" (p. 466), you have a Body Dysmorphic Disorder. A child whose academic achievement is "substantially below that expected for age, schooling, and level of intelligence" (p. 46) has a Learning Disorder. Toddlers who throw tantrums have Oppositional Defiant Disorder. Not wanting sex often enough is Hypoactive Sexual Desire Disorder. Not wanting sex at all is Sexual Aversion Disorder. Having sex but not having orgasms or having them too late or too soon is an Orgasmic Disorder. Failure (for men) to maintain "an adequate erection . . . that causes marked distress or interpersonal difficulty" (p. 504) is Male Erectile Disorder. Failure (for women) to attain or maintain "an adequate lubrication or swelling response of sexual excitement" (p. 502) accompanied by distress is Female Sexual Arousal Disorder.

The past few years have witnessed media reports of epidemics of internet addiction, road rage, pathological stock market day trading, and "shopaholism." Discussions of these new disorders have turned up at scientific meetings and in courtrooms. They are likely to find a home in the next revision of the DSM if the media, mental health professions, and society at large continue to collaborate in their construction and if treating them and writing books about them become lucrative.

Those adopting the social constructionist perspective do not deny that human beings experience behavioral and emotional difficulties, sometimes very serious ones. They insist, however, that such experiences are not evidence for the existence of entities called mental disorders that then explain those behavioral and emotional difficulties. The belief in the existence of these entities is the product of the all-too-human tendency to socially construct categories in an attempt to make sense of a confusing world.

SUMMARY AND CONCLUSIONS

The debate over the conception or definition of psychopathology and related terms has been going on for decades and will continue, just as we will always have debates over the definitions of truth, beauty, justice, and art. Our position is that psychopathology and mental disorder are not the kinds of terms whose true meanings can be discovered or defined objectively by using the methods of science. They are social constructions—abstract ideas whose meanings are negotiated among the people and institutions of a culture and that reflect the values and power structure of that culture at a given time. Thus, the conception and definition of psychopathology always has been and always will be debated and always has been and always will be changing. It is not a static and concrete thing whose true nature can be discovered and described once and for all.

By saying that conceptions of psychopathology are socially constructed rather than scientifically derived, we are not proposing, however, that human psychological distress and suffering are not real or that the patterns of thinking, feeling, and behaving that society decides to label psychopathological cannot be studied objectively and scientifically. Instead, we are saying that it is time to acknowledge that science can no more determine the proper or correct conception of psychopathology and mental disorder than it can determine the proper and correct conception of other social constructions such as beauty, justice, race, and social class. We can nonetheless use science to study the phenomena that our culture refers to as psychopathological. We can use the methods of science to understand a culture's conception of mental or psychological health and disorder, how this conception has evolved, and how it affects individuals and society. We also can use the methods of science to understand the origins of the patterns of thinking, feeling, and behaving that a culture considers psychopathological and to develop and test ways of modifying those patterns.

Psychology and psychiatry will not be diminished by acknowledging that their basic concepts are socially and not scientifically constructed—any more than medicine is diminished by acknowledging that the notions of health and illness are socially constructed (Reznek, 1987), nor economics by acknowledging that the notions of poverty and wealth are socially constructed. Science cannot provide us with purely factual scientific definitions of these concepts. They are fluid and negotiated matters of value, not fixed matters of fact.

As Lilienfeld and Marino (1995) have said:

> *Removing the imprimatur of science . . . would simply make the value judgments underlying these decisions more explicit and open to criticism . . . heated disputes would almost surely arise concerning which conditions are deserving of attention from mental health professionals. Such disputes, however, would at least be settled on the legitimate basis of social values and exigencies, rather than on the basis of ill-defined criteria of doubtful scientific status. (pp. 418–419)*

REFERENCES

Alarcon, R. D., Foulks, E. F., & Vakkur, M. (1998). *Personality disorders and culture: Clinical and conceptual interactions.* New York: Wiley.

American Psychiatric Association. (2000). *Diagnostic and statistical manual of mental disorders* (4th ed., text rev.). Washington, DC: Author.

Anthony, J. L., Lonigan, C. J., & Hecht, S. A. (1999). Dimensionality of post-traumatic stress disorder symptoms in children exposed to disaster: Results from a confirmatory factor analysis. *Journal of Abnormal Psychology, 108,* 315–325.

Barkley, R. A. (1997). *ADHD and the nature of self-control.* New York: Guilford.

Baumeister, R. F. (1987). How the self became a problem: A psychological review of historical research. *Journal of Personality and Social Psychology, 52,* 163–176.

Baumeister, R. F., & Scher, S. J. (1988). Self-defeating behavior patterns among normal individuals: Review and analysis of common self-destructive tendencies. *Psychological Bulletin, 104*(1), 3–22.

Beall, A. E. (1993). A social constructionist view of gender. In A. E. Beall & R. J. Sternberg (Eds.), *The psychology of gender* (pp. 127–147). New York: Guilford.

Becker, H. S. (1963). *Outsiders.* New York: Free Press.

Bergner, R. M. (1997). What is psychopathology? And so what? *Clinical Psychology: Science and Practice, 4,* 235–248.

Bohan, J. (1996). *The psychology of sexual orientation: Coming to terms.* New York: Routledge.

Claridge, G. (1995). *Origins of mental illness.* Cambridge, MA: Malor Books/ISHK.

Cosmides, L., Tooby, J., & Barkow, J. H. (1992). Introduction: Evolutionary psychology and conceptual integration. In J. H. Barkow, L. Cosmides, and J. Tooby (Eds.), *The adapted mind: Evolutionary psychology and the generation of culture* (pp. 3–17). New York: Oxford University Press.

Costello, C. G. (1993a). *Symptoms of depression.* New York: Wiley.

Costello, C. G. (1993b). *Symptoms of schizophrenia.* New York: Wiley.

Costello, C. G. (1996). *Personality characteristics of the personality disordered.* New York: Wiley.

Cross, S. E., & Markus, H. R. (1999). The cultural constitution of personality. In L. A. Pervin & O. P. John (Eds.), *Handbook of personality: Theory and Research* (2nd ed.) (pp. 378–396). New York: Guilford.

Cushman, P. (1995). *Constructing the self, constructing America.* New York: Addison-Wesley.

Fraley, R. C., & Waller, N. G. (1998). Adult attachment patterns: A test of the typological model. In J. A. Simpson & W. S. Rholes (Eds.), *Attachment theory and close relationships* (pp. 77–114). New York: Guilford.

Gergen, K. J. (1985). The social constructi nist movement in modern psychology. *American Psychologist, 40*(3), 266–275.

Gilman, S. L. (1988). *Disease and representation: Images of illness from madness to AIDS.* Ithaca, NY: Cornell University Press.

Gorenstein, E. E. (1984). Debating mental illness: Implications for science, medicine, and social policy. *American Psychologist, 39,* 50–56.

Hewitt, J. P. (2002). The social construction of self-esteem. In C. R. Snyder & S. J. Lopez (Eds.), *Handbook of positive psychology* (pp. 135–147). New York: University Press.

Holmes, W. C., & Slapp, G. B. (1998). Sexual abuse of boys: Definition, prevalence, correlates, sequelae, and managament. *Journal of the American Medical Association, 280,* 1855–1862.

Horwitz, A. V. (2002). *Creating mental illness.* Chicago: University of Chicago Press.

Keyes, C. L., & Lopez, S. J. (2002). Toward a science of mental health: Positive directions in diagnosis and interventions. In C. R. Snyder & S. J. Lopez (Eds.), *Handbook of positive psychology* (pp. 45–59). London: Oxford University Press.

Kirk, S. A., & Kutchins, H. (1992). *The selling of DSM: The rhetoric of science in psychiatry.* New York: Aldine de Gruyter.

Kutchins, H., & Kirk, S. A. (1997). *Making us crazy: DSM: The psychiatric bible and the creation of mental disorder.* New York: Free Press.

Lilienfeld, S. O., & Marino, L. (1995). Mental disorder as a Roschian concept: A critique of Wakefield's "harmful dysfunction" analysis. *Journal of Abnormal Psychology, 104*(3), 411–420.

Livesley, W. J., Jang, K. L., & Vernon, P. A. (1998). Phenotypic and genotypic structure of traits delineating personality disorder. *Archives of General Psychiatry, 55,* 941–948.

Lubinski, D. (2000). Scientific and social significance of assessing individual differences: "Sinking shafts at a few critical points." *Annual Review of Psychology, 51,* 405–444.

Maddux, J. E., & Mundell, C. E. (2005). Disorders of personality: Diseases or individual differences? In V. J. Derlega, B. A. Winstead, & W. H. Jones (Eds.), *Personality: Contemporary theory and research* (3rd ed.) (pp. 541–571). Chicago: Nelson-Hall.

McNamee, S., & Gergen, K. J. (1992). *Therapy as social construction.* Thousand Oaks, CA: Sage.

Muehlehard, C. L., & Kimes, L. A. (1999). The social construction of violence: The case of sexual and domestic violence. *Personality and Social Psychology Review, 3,* 234–245.

Neimeyer, R. A., & Raskin, J. D. (2000). On practicing postmodern therapy in modern times. In R. A. Neimeyer & J. D. Raskin (Eds.), *Constructions of disorder: Meaning-making frameworks for psychotherapy* (pp. 3–14). Washington, DC: American Psychological Association.

Oatley, K., & Jenkins, J. M. (1992). Human emotions: Function and dysfunction. *Annual Review of Psychology, 43,* 55–85.

Ossorio, P. G. (1985). Pathology. *Advances in Descriptive Psychology, 4,* 151–201.

Parker, I., Georgaca, E., Harper, D., McLaughlin, T., & Stowell-Smith, M. (1995). *Deconstructing psychopathology.* London: Sage.

Peele, S. (1995). *Diseasing of America: How we allowed recovery zealots and the treatment industry to convince us we are out of control.* San Francisco: Lexington Books.

Persons, J. (1986). The advantages of studying psychological phenomena rather than psychiatric diagnosis. *American Psychologist, 41,* 1252–1260.

Raskin, J. D., & Lewandowski, A. M. (2000). The construction of disorder as human enterprise. In R. A. Neimeyer & J. D. Raskin (Eds.), *Constructions of disorder: Meaning-making frameworks for psychotherapy* (pp. 15–40). Washington, DC: American Psychological Association.

Reznek, L. (1987). *The nature of disease.* London: Routledge & Kegan Paul.

Rind, B., Tromovich, P., & Bauserman, R. (1998). A meta-analytic examination of assumed properties of child sexual abuse using college samples. *Psychological Bulletin, 124,* 22–53.

Rosenblum, K. E., & Travis, T. C. (1996). Constructing categories of difference: Framework essay. In K. E. Rosenblum & T. C. Travis (Eds.), *The meaning of difference: American constructions of race, sex and gender, social class, and sexual orientation* (pp. 1–34). New York: McGraw-Hill.

Sadler, J. Z. (1999). Horsefeathers: A commentary on "Evolutionary versus prototype analyses of the concept of disorder." *Journal of Abnormal Psychology, 108,* 433–437.

Sedgwick, P. (1982). *Psycho politics: Laing, Foucault, Goffman, Szasz, and the future of mass psychiatry.* New York: Harper & Row.

Shaywitz, S. E., Escobar, M. D., Shaywitz, B. A., Fletcher, J. M., & Makuch, R. (1992). Evidence that dyslexia may represent the lower tail of a normal distribution of reading ability. *New England Journal of Medicine, 326*(3), 145–150.

Shorter, E. (1997). *A history of psychiatry: From the era of the asylum to the age of Prozac.* New York: Wiley.

Spanos, N. P. (1996). *Multiple identities and false memories: A sociocognitive perspective.* Washington, DC: American Psychological Association.

Szasz, T. S. (1974). *The myth of mental illness.* New York: Harper & Row.

Wakefield, J. C. (1992a). The concept of mental disorder: On the boundary between biological facts and social values. *American Psychologist, 47*(3), 373–388.

Wakefield, J. C. (1992b). Disorder as harmful dysfunction: A conceptual critique of DSM-III-R's definition of mental disorder. *Psychological Review, 99,* 232–247.

Wakefield, J. C. (1993). Limits of operationalization: A critique of Spitzer and Endicott's (1978) proposed operational criteria for mental disorder. *Journal of Abnormal Psychology, 102,* 160–172.

Wakefield, J. C. (1997). Normal inability versus pathological inability: Why Ossorio's definition of mental disorder is not sufficient. *Clinical Psychology: Science and Practice, 4,* 249–258.

Wakefield, J. C. (1999). Evolutionary versus prototype analyses of the concept of disorder. *Journal of Abnormal Psychology, 108,* 374–399.

Widiger, T. A. (1997). The construct of mental disorder. *Clinical Psychology: Science and Practice, 4,* 262–266.

Widiger, T. A., & Trull, T. J. (1991). Diagnosis and clinical assessment. *Annual Review of Psychology, 42,* 109–134.

Wilson, M. (1993). DSM-III and the transformation of American psychiatry: A history. *American Journal of Psychiatry, 150,* 399–410.

2

Cultural Dimensions of Psychopathology: The Social World's Impact on Mental Illness

Steven Regeser López
University of California

Peter J. Guarnaccia
Rutgers, The State University of New Jersey

Over the past several decades, researchers have increasingly examined cultural influences in psychopathology. However, for much of this period, the study of culture and mental disorders was a marginal field of inquiry. As we demonstrate in this chapter, cultural issues have moved to the fore in the study of psychopathology. A landmark event marking this transition came in 1977 when Kleinman heralded the beginning of a "new cross-cultural psychiatry," an interdisciplinary research approach integrating anthropological methods and conceptualizations with traditional psychiatric and psychological approaches. Mental health researchers were encouraged to respect indigenous illness categories and to recognize the limitations of traditional illness categories, such as depression and schizophrenia. Also, the new cross-cultural psychiatry distinguished between disease, a "malfunctioning or maladaptation of biological or psychological processes," and illness, "the personal, interpersonal, and cultural reaction to disease" (p. 9). The perspective that Kleinman and others (Fabrega, 1975; Kleinman, Eisenberg, & Good, 1978) articulated in the seventies reflected an important direction for the study of culture and psychopathology—to understand the social world within mental illness. (See also Draguns, 1980, and Marsella, 1980).

Many advances were made during the first decade of the new cross-cultural psychiatry. One was the establishment of the interdisciplinary journal *Culture, Medicine, and Psychiatry*. This newly founded journal, in conjunction with *Transcultural Psychiatry* in Canada (formerly *Transcultural Psychiatric Research Review*), provided and continues to provide an important forum for cultural research. Also, during the eighties, large-scale epidemiological studies were carried out. The second multinational World Health Organization (WHO) study of schizophrenia was launched and preliminary findings were reported (Sartorius et al., 1986). The Epidemiological Catchment Area (ECA) studies were conducted as well (Regier et al., 1984). Some may question how culturally informed these classic studies were (Edgerton & Cohen, 1994; Fabrega, 1990; Guarnaccia, Kleinman, & Good, 1990). However, most reviews of culture, ethnicity, and mental disorders today refer to the findings from the WHO and ECA studies to address how social, ethnic, and cultural factors are related to the distribution of psychopathology. Also during this time, the National Institute of Mental Health (NIMH) funded research centers with the sole purpose of conducting research on and for specific ethnic minority groups (African Americans, American Indians, Latino Americans, and Asian Americans). Some of the research from these centers contributed to the growing cultural psychopathology database (e.g., Cervantes, Padilla, & Salgado de Snyder, 1991; King, 1978; Manson, Shore, & Bloom, 1985; Neighbors, Jackson, Campbell, & Wilson, 1989; Rogler, Malgady, & Rodriguez, 1989).

Dialogues across disciplines were also initiated during this time. For example, Kleinman and Good's (1985) influential book, *Culture and Depression*, brought together the research not only of anthropologists, but also of psychologists and psychiatrists. Another significant indicator of the field's development was and continues to be its success in attracting new investigators, as suggested by Harvard's long-standing cultural anthropology and mental health training grant (for a summary see Kleinman, 1988). Indeed, these first ten years can be characterized as an exciting and fertile time for the study of cultural psychopathology.

Despite the many advances, the field's main concepts were not reaching larger audiences. Investigators were communicating primarily among themselves in their specialty journals and books. Those findings that were published in widely distributed mainstream journals were scattered among a broad array of journals. Thus, from the perspective of mainstream investigators, the developments of the new cross-cultural psychiatry went largely unnoticed. On a rare occasion, one would find a special issue on cultural research in a mainstream journal (e.g., *Journal of Consulting and Clinical Psychology*, 1987).

In an effort to bring the field's concepts to a broader audience (general psychiatry and other mental health fields), Kleinman (1988) provided a comprehensive review of culture, psychopathology, and related research. Drawing on empirical data and theory, Kleinman argued that culture matters for the study and treatment of mental disorders. This book serves as a significant marker in the development of the new cross-cultural psychiatry, which we refer to here as the study of cultural psychopathology.

KEY DEVELOPMENTS

Conceptual Contributions

Definition of Culture.   Central to the study of cultural psychopathology is the definition of *culture*. Much of the past and even current research relies on a definition of culture that is outdated. In fact, Betancourt and López (1993) wrote a critical review of culture and psychological research in which culture was defined as the values, beliefs, and practices that pertain to a given ethnocultural group. The strength of this definition is that it begins to unpack culture. Instead of arguing that a given expression of distress pertains to a given ethnocultural group, for example, researchers argue that the expression of distress is related to a specific value or belief orientation. We see this change as a significant advancement. It helps researchers begin to operationalize what about culture matters in the specific context. Furthermore, it recognizes the heterogeneity within specific ethnocultural groups. Knowing that someone belongs to a specific ethnic group provides guidelines to potential cultural issues in psychopathology, but it does not imply that that person adheres to all the cultural values and practices of that group.

The definition of culture as values, beliefs, and practices has important limitations (Lewis-Fernandez & Kleinman, 1995). One is that it depicts culture as residing largely within individuals. The emphasis on values and beliefs points out the psychological nature of culture.

We argue that culture is manifested in the interaction between people and is highly social in nature. Situating practices (customs and rituals) with values and beliefs gives the impression that the practices in the social world are a function of values and beliefs. For example, people are thought to rely on their family in times of crisis because they are high in familism or family orientation. Investigators rarely examine what about the social world facilitates or fosters reliance on family members. Perhaps harsh environmental conditions contribute to families coming together to overcome adversity. When applying the values and beliefs definition of culture, the social world is subjugated to the psychological world of the individual. Contrary to this perspective, we argue that it is action in the social and physical world that produces culture as much as people's ideas about the world. In our view, the social world interacts equally with the psychological world in producing human behavior.

A second limitation of this frequently used definition of culture is that it depicts culture as a static phenomenon. We believe that culture is a process. Culture is a dynamic and creative process (Garro, 2001; Greenfield, 1997), some aspects of which are shared by large groups of individuals resulting from particular life circumstances and histories. Given the changing nature of our social world and given the efforts of individuals to adapt to such changes, culture can best be viewed as an ongoing process, a system or set of systems in flux. Therefor, attempts to freeze culture into a set of generalized value orientations or behaviors will continually misrepresent culture.

A related limitation of the values-based definition of culture is that it depicts people as recipients of culture from a generalized society with little recognition of individuals' roles in negotiating their cultural worlds. More recent approaches to culture in anthropology, while not discarding the importance of a person's cultural inheritance of ideas, values, and ways of relating, have focused equally on the emergence of culture from the life experiences of individuals and small groups. People can change, add to, or reject cultural elements through social processes such as migration and acculturation. A viable definition of culture acknowledges the agency of individuals in establishing their social worlds.

In sum, current views of culture attend much more to people's social world than did past views of culture that emphasized the individual. Of particular interest are people's daily routines and how such activities are tied to families, neighborhoods, villages, and social networks. By examining people's daily routines, one can identify what matters most to people (Gallimore, Goldenberg, & Weisner, 1993) or what is most at stake for people (Ware & Kleinman, 1992). Furthermore, this perspective captures the dynamic nature of culture as a product of group values, norms, and experiences, as well as of individual innovations and life histories. The use of this broader definition of culture should help guide investigators away from flat, unidimensional notions of culture, to discover the richness of a cultural analysis for the study of psychopathology. An important component of this perspective is the examination of intracultural diversity. In particular, social class, poverty, and gender continue to affect different levels of mental health both within cultural groups and across cultural groups.

Goals of Cultural Research. Culture is important in a number of domains within psychopathology research. It is important in the expression and measurement of disorder and distress; a cultural analysis can point out the variability in the manner in which mental illness is manifested. Social and cultural factors can also affect the prevalence of disorder by differentially placing some at more risk than others for developing psychopathology. In addition, the course of disorder, as reflected in the degree of disability or in the number of clinical relapses, is also related to important cultural factors. We encourage all of these lines of inquiry.

Regardless of the specific domain of research, there are two metagoals of cultural research. Some writers imply that cultural research should test the generality of given theoretical notions.

For example, in a thoughtful analysis of cultural research, Clark (1987) noted: "Conceptual progress in psychology requires a unified base for investigating psychological phenomena, with culture-relevant variables included as part of the matrix" (p. 465). From Clark's point of view, cross-cultural work can serve to enhance the generality of given conceptual models by adding, when necessary, cultural variables to an existing theoretical model to explain between group and within group variance. Although Clark acknowledges the possibility that a construct developed in one country may not have a counterpart in another country, at no time does she discuss the value of deriving models of distinct clinical entities found in only one country, ethnocultural group or one group marked by specific social or historical factors. This approach suggests that for Clark, the main purpose of studying culture is to enhance the validity of existing psychological models by attending to cross-cultural variations.

In contrast, both Fabrega (1990) and Rogler (1989) criticize researchers for paying little attention to the cultural specificity of mental illness and mental health. Fabrega examines researchers' use of mainstream instruments and conceptualizations in studying mental disorders among Latinos and challenges such researchers to be bold in their critiques of "establishment psychiatry." Rogler recommends a framework for mainstream psychiatric researchers that attends more fully to culture. For both Fabrega and Rogler, the risk of overlooking cultural variations is much greater in current psychopathology research than the risk of overlooking cultural similarities. Focusing on culture-specific phenomena at this time is of central importance to Fabrega and Rogler.

An important conceptual advancement is the recognition of both positions, that is, studying culture to identify general processes and studying culture to identify culture-specific processes. By focusing only on generalities, we overlook the importance of culture-specific phenomena. On the other hand, by emphasizing culture-specific phenomena we overlook the possibility of generalities. The overall purpose of cultural research, then, is to advance our understanding of general processes, culture-specific processes, and the manner in which they interact in specific contexts (see also Draguns, 1990). Our aim is to identify culture's mark amidst the ubiquity of human suffering.

Major Advances: DSM–IV, the World Mental Health Report, and the Surgeon General's Report on Mental Health: Culture, Race, and Ethnicity

We now turn to selected recent developments in the study of culture and psychopathology. We begin with a discussion of three of the most important projects that were carried out since 1988: the incorporation of cultural factors in the *Diagnostic and Statistical Manual of Mental Disorders*, 4th ed., (DSM–IV; American Psychiatric Association, 1994); the publication of the *World Mental Health Report* (Desjarlais, Eisenberg, Good, & Kleinman, 1996); and the release of the *U.S. Surgeon General's Report on Mental Health: Culture, Race, and Ethnicity* (U.S. Department of Health and Human Services, DHHS, 2001).

The NIMH funded the establishment of a culture and diagnosis task force to inform the development of the DSM–IV. The task force's efforts resulted in three main contributions to DSM–IV: (a) inclusion of some discussion of how cultural factors can influence the expression, assessment, and prevalence of specific disorders; (b) an outline of a cultural formulation of clinical diagnosis to complement the multiaxial assessment; and (c) a glossary of relevant culture-bound syndromes from around the world. A more complete documentation of the task force's findings is available in the DSM–IV Sourcebook (Mezzich et al., 1997) and in other publications (e.g., Alarcon, 1995; Kirmayer, 1998; Kleinman, Mezzich, Fabrega, & Parron,

1996). Without a doubt the attention given to culture in DSM–IV is a major achievement in the history of classifications of mental disorders. Never before had classification schemas or related diagnostic interviews addressed to this degree the role of culture in psychopathology (López & Núñez, 1987; Rogler 1996). (See Kirmayer, 1998 for a discussion of the limitations of how DSM–IV referred to culture).

A second major development within the last decade was the publication of the World Mental Health Report (Desjarlais et al., 1996). Desjarlais and colleagues compiled research from around the world to identify the range of mental health and behavioral problems (e.g., mental disorders, violence, suicide), particularly among low-income countries in Africa, Latin America, Asia, and the Pacific. The authors derived several conclusions. Perhaps the most significant was that mental illness and related problems exact a significant toll on the health and well-being of people worldwide and produce a greater burden based on a "disability-adjusted life years" index than that from tuberculosis, cancer, or heart disease (see Murray and Lopez, 1996). Depressive disorders alone were found to produce the fifth greatest burden for women and seventh greatest burden for men across all physical and mental illnesses.

A second important observation was that mental illness and behavioral problems are intricately tied to the social world. For example, the authors identified the social roots of the poor mental health of women. Among the many factors include hunger—undernourishment afflicts more than 60% of women in developing countries; work—women are poorly paid for dangerous, labor intensive jobs; and domestic violence—surveys in some low-income communities worldwide report up to 60% of women having been beaten. The research on women's mental health illustrates that psychopathology is as much pathology of the social world as pathology of the mind or body.

Based on their findings, Desjarlais and associates make specific recommendations to advance both mental health policy and research to help reduce the significant burden of mental illness across the world. Their consideration of the social world leads easily to recommending specific interventions to address not only the clinical problem but also the social conditions with which they are associated. In addressing the poor mental health of women, for example, they call for coordinated efforts both to empower women economically and to reduce violence against women in all its forms. In addition, women's mental health is identified as one of the top five research priorities worldwide. They call for research to examine the social factors that influence women's health in specific cultural contexts and to identify effective community-based interventions in improving their health status.

The most recent development since 1988 was the Surgeon General's Supplemental Report on Mental Health concerning culture, race, and ethnicity (U.S. Department of Health and Human Services, DHHS, 2001). The surgeon general first published a landmark report on the status of the nation's mental health (U.S. DHHS, 1999). Some observers were concerned that insufficient attention was given to the mental health of the country's ethnic and racial minority groups (López, 2003). In response to this concern and under the leadership of the Substance Abuse and Mental Health Services Administration, the surgeon general published a report on the mental health of the nation's four main minority groups: American Indians/Alaska Natives, African Americans, Asian Americans/Pacific Islanders, and Latino Americans. Although the report's focus was on mental health care, considerable attention was given to our current understanding of the psychopathology of these groups, based largely on epidemiological and clinical research.

The main message of the Surgeon General's report is that "culture counts." "The cultures from which people hail affect all aspects of mental health and illness, including the types of stresses they confront, whether they seek help, what types of help they seek, what symptoms and concerns they bring to clinical attention, and what types of coping styles and social supports they possess" (p. ii). The Surgeon General's report compiles the best available research that culture matters in these domains. For example, evidence is reviewed regarding the relationship between racism and mental health (e.g., Kessler, Mickelson, & Williams, 1999) and ethnicity and psychopharmacology (e.g., Lin, Poland, & Anderson, 1995). In addition, the report outlines future directions to address the mental health needs of these underserved communities, including expanding the science base and training mental health scientists and practitioners. In all, this report has served two important functions. It has brought together the best available mental health research regarding the main U.S. minority groups. Also, because of the status and visibility of the Office of the Surgeon General, the report has alerted the nation to the mental health needs of the four main ethnic and racial minority groups.

Together the DSM–IV, the World Mental Health Report, and the Surgeon General's Supplemental Report on Mental Health make major contributions to the study of culture and psychopathology. Furthermore, they illustrate the range of conceptualizations of culture and the importance of the social domain. For DSM–IV, culture tends to be depicted as exotic, through its influence on symptom expression, the noted culture-bound syndromes, and its reference to persons from "culturally different" groups. There is little attention to culture being part of every clinical encounter, influencing the client, provider, and the broader community context, regardless of the patient's ethnic or racial background.

The World Mental Health Report, on the other hand, recognizes the dynamic, social processes linked to culture. Hunger, work, and education, for example, are integrally related to how people adapt or fail to adapt. Clinical phenomena are recognized, but so are behavioral problems not traditionally considered in psychiatric classification systems, such as domestic violence and sexual violence. Throughout, the authors recognize cultural variability but their stance is not extreme cultural relativism, as they recognize the moral and health implications for controversial practices, such as female circumcision.

The surgeon general's report falls between the two perspectives. It recognizes the importance of culture in specific clinical entities (both culture-bound syndromes and mainstream mental disorder categories). It also acknowledges the importance of the broader social world though the emphasis tends to be more disorder-based and less contextually based than the World Mental Health Report. Despite the differences in the treatment of culture, these three publications indicate that culture as a subject matter is no longer solely within the purview of cultural psychologists, psychiatrists, and anthropologists. It is now the subject matter of all users of DSM–IV, worldwide policy makers, national health policy makers, and mental health researchers.

Disorder-Related Research

We now turn to the examination of selected psychopathology research. We selected the study of anxiety, schizophrenia, and childhood psychopathology because within each of these areas systematic studies examine the cultural basis of the expression of these disorders as well as the social and cultural processes that underlie the development and course of illness.

Anxiety. We chose to focus our attention on one line of research, the study of *ataques de nervios*. This is an important line of research because it focuses on a culture-specific phenomenon for which the triangulation of ethnography, epidemiology, and clinical research has made important contributions. Thus, we will be able to examine some ways ethnography informs mainstream research.

Ataque de nervios is an idiom of distress particularly prominent among Latinos from the Caribbean, but also recognized among other Latino groups. Symptoms commonly associated with *ataques de nervios* include trembling, attacks of crying, screaming uncontrollably, and becoming verbally or physically aggressive. Other symptoms that are prominent in some *ataques* but not others are seizure-like or fainting episodes, dissociative experiences, and suicidal gestures. A general feature experienced by most sufferers of *ataques de nervios* is feeling out of control. Most episodes occur as a direct result of a stressful life event related to family or significant others (e.g., death or divorce). After the *ataque*, people often experience amnesia of what occurred, but then quickly return to their usual level of functioning.

Guarnaccia initiated a program of research by first carrying out open-ended, descriptive interviews with people who had experienced *ataques de nervios* in clinical settings (De La Cancela, Guarnaccia, & Carillo, 1986, Guarnaccia, De La Cancela, & Carillo, 1989a). Drawing from the rich description of clinical cases and an understanding of the social history of Puerto Ricans living in the United States, these investigators pointed out an association between social disruptions (family and immediate social networks) and the experience of *ataques*. To build on the ethnographic base, Guarnaccia and colleagues turned to epidemiological research to examine its prevalence in Puerto Rico. After preliminary epidemiological research in which a somatic symptom scale index was used as a proxy measure of *ataques* (Guarnaccia, Rubio-Stipec, & Canino, 1989b), a subsequent study was carried out in which respondents were directly queried as to whether they had suffered an *ataque de nervios* and what the experience was like (Guarnaccia, Canino, Rubio-Stipec, & Bravo, 1993). The prevalence rate was found to be high, from 16% to 23% of large community samples ($Ns = 912$ and 1513), and *ataques de nervios* were found to be associated with a wide range of mental disorders, particularly anxiety and mood disorders. The social context continued to be important. *Ataques* were found to be more prevalent among women, persons older than 45, those from lower socioeconomic background, and those from disrupted marital relations. More recently, Guarnaccia, Rivera, Franco, and Neighbors (1996) returned to the ethnographic mode to explicate the experience of *ataques* from those persons who had reported suffering an *ataque de nervios* in the epidemiological study. Through in-depth interviewing, the full range of symptoms and the specific social contexts were identified. This "experience-near" or ethnographic research approach enabled Guarnaccia and associates to examine carefully how the social world can become part of the physical self as reflected in *ataques de nervios*.

Clinical research has broadened the examination of *ataques de nervios*. Liebowitz and colleagues (1994) carried out clinical diagnostic interviews of 156 Latino patients from an urban psychiatric clinic that specializes in the treatment of anxiety. They examined the relationship between patients having an *ataque de nervios* and meeting criteria for panic disorder, other anxiety disorders, or an affective disorder. Their fine-grained analysis suggests that the different expressions of *ataque de nervios* are affected by their relationship to different coexisitng psychiatric disorders. Persons with an *ataques de nervios* who also suffer from panic disorder present largely panic-like symptoms. However, in those with an affective disorder, *ataques de nervios* are characterized by emotional lability, especially anger (Salmán et al., 1998). Thus, in addition to the social factors previously noted, these findings suggest that the clinical context may also play a role in understanding *ataque de nervios*.

The study of *ataque de nervios* is exemplary for many reasons. What is most striking is the systematic ongoing dialogue among ethnographic, epidemiological, and now clinical researchers which advances our understanding of *ataques of nervios* and how the social world interacts with psychological and physical processes in the individual. With the multiple approaches, one observes the shifting of the researchers' lenses (Kleinman & Kleinman, 1991). In the early ethnographic work, Guarnaccia and colleagues drew from a small number of clinical cases and interpreted their findings with broad strokes focusing on the broader social contexts of the individuals, particularly their migration experience and experiences of marginal social status. In the epidemiological research, the investigators used large, representative samples to identify people with *ataques* and the social correlates of that experience. In this research, the social context is reduced to single questions concerning gender, age, educational level, and marital status, which provides some basis for interpretation but certainly lacks the richness of ethnographic material. The clinical studies provide an in-depth profile of patients' symptomatology and the symptom patterns of those with and without an *ataque*, but they provide less information about the social world of the sufferer. Each approach has its strengths and limitations. What matters, though, is not the strengths or limitations of a given study but the weaving of multiple studies with multiple approaches to understand the given phenomenon in some depth.

In addition to the ongoing dialogue between research approaches, the research is exemplary by placing *ataque de nervios* and related mental disorders in their social context. In almost all studies, *ataque de nervios* is presented not as a popular illness (that is, an illness defined by the community) or clinical entity (that is, a psychologically or biologically defined disorder) that resides within individuals, but as a popular illness that reflects the lived experience of women with little power and disrupted social relations. In adopting multiple approaches, the emphasis given to the social domain is likely to shift. Nevertheless, over the several studies Guarnaccia and his colleagues have maintained considerable attention to the social context. In so doing, they have demonstrated how to include the social in epidemiological (e.g., Guarnaccia et al., 1993), clinical (Salmán et al., 1998), and ethnographic studies. Overall, the study of *ataque de nervios* provides a model for the investigation of culture and psychopathology, particularly for research that begins with a culture-specific form of distress.

Schizophrenia. The cultural conception of the self can influence the manner in which disorders are expressed and understood by others. This belief is articulated in Fabrega's (1989) thoughtful overview of how past anthropologically informed research contributed to the study of psychosis and how future studies can advance our understanding of the interrelations of culture and schizophrenia. According to Fabrega, the effect of schizophrenia on individuals and communities depends on whether they conceive of the self as autonomous and separate from others or as connected and bound to others (Markus & Kitayama, 1991; Shweder & Bourne, 1984). The research that most directly addresses this notion is that which examines the role of social factors in the course of schizophrenia. Two prominent lines of inquiry include the WHO cross-national study of schizophrenia and a series of studies examining the relationship of families' emotional climate to the course of illness. (For an examination of culture and symptom expression in schizophrenia, see Brekke and Barrio, 1997, and Weisman et al., 2000)

The WHO's International Pilot Study on Schizophrenia (IPSS) and the follow-up study Determinants of Outcomes of Severe Mental Disorder (DOSMD) represent the largest multinational study of schizophrenia to date (IPSS: 9 countries and 1202 patients; DOSMD: 10 countries and 1379 patients; Jablensky et al., 1992; WHO, 1979). These investigations have made many contributions, including finding evidence of the comparability of schizophrenia's core symptoms across several countries (for a critique, see Kleinman, 1988). The finding that has received the most attention by cultural researchers is that schizophrenia in developing countries has a more favorable course than in developed countries (Weisman, 1997). Some investigators have referred to this basic finding as "arguably the single most important finding of cultural differences in cross-cultural research on mental illness" (Lin & Kleinman, 1988, p. 563). Others have been most critical of the studies' methods and interpretations (see Cohen, 1992; Edgerton & Cohen, 1994; Hopper, 1991). For example, Edgerton and Cohen point out that the distinction between developed and developing countries is unclear. Moreover, they argue that the cultural explanation for the differences in course is poorly substantiated. They also suggest that such research could be more culturally informed through the direct measure of specific cultural factors in conjunction with observations of people's daily lives (see also Hopper 1991). What is clear is that the WHO findings have provided the basis for an important discussion of method and theory in the context of schizophrenia and the social world.

Another line of research addressing culture's role in the course of schizophrenia focuses on families' emotional climates. Based on the early work of George Brown and associates (e.g., Brown, Birley, & Wing, 1972), research has found that patients who return to households marked by criticism, hostility, and emotional involvement (together this pattern is referred to as high expressed emotion, EE) are more likely to relapse than those who return to households that are not so characterized (Bebbington & Kuipers, 1994; Butzlaff & Hooley, 1998; Leff & Vaughn, 1985). This line of investigation is important to the study of culture because it points out the importance of the social world. More specifically, cross-national and cross-ethnic studies have uncovered interesting differences in the level and nature of expressed emotion (Jenkins & Karno 1992). These studies show that cultural factors in the definitions and experiences of schizophrenia affect the emotional climate of families where ill individuals live. Furthermore, these cultural differences have important effects on mental health outcomes.

The most systematic cultural analysis of families' roles in schizophrenia has been carried out by Jenkins and her colleagues. In using both clinical research methods based on the prototypic contemporary study of expressed emotion (Vaughn & Leff, 1976) and ethnographic methods based on in-depth interviews, Jenkins and associates extended this line of study to Mexican American families in Los Angeles. In the first major report, Karno et al. (1987) replicated the general finding that patients who return to high EE families are more likely to relapse than patients who return to low EE families. Jenkins (1988a) then carried out an in-depth examination of Mexican American families' conceptualizations of schizophrenia, specifically *nervios,* and how this differed from a comparable sample of Anglo American families who viewed schizophrenia largely as a mental illness (see also Guarnaccia, Parra, Deschamps, Milstein, & Argiles, 1992). Based on both quantitative (coded responses to open-ended questions) and qualitative data, Jenkins (1988b) suggested that Mexican Americans' preference for *nervios* is tied to the family members' efforts to decrease the stigma associated with the illness and also to promote family support and cohesiveness. In subsequent papers, Jenkins (1991, 1993) critiqued the cultural basis of the expressed emotion construct in general and its components, criticism and emotional overinvolvement, in particular. A most important theoretical contribution to the study of the course of schizophrenia is that Jenkins situates families' expressed emotion, not in the family members' attitudes, beliefs, or even feelings, which is the approach taken by most investigators, but in the patient–family social interaction. Overall, Jenkins' work has brought much needed attention to how serious mental illness is embedded in specific social and cultural contexts.

Building on Jenkins' work, López and colleagues have further critiqued the notion of expressed emotion with its focus on negative family functioning (López, Nelson, Snyder, & Mintz, 1999). They point out that at an early juncture in the study of families and relapse, investigators (i.e., Brown et al., 1972) opted to focus on aspects of family conflict that predict relapse rather than the prosocial aspects of family functioning that buffer relapse. In a reanalysis and extension of the Mexican American sample (Karno et al., 1987) and a comparable Anglo American sample (Vaughn, Snyder, Jones, Freeman, & Falloon, 1984), López et al. (2004) found that a lack of family warmth predicted relapse for Mexican Americans whereas criticism predicted relapse for Anglo Americans. In other words, Mexican American patients who returned to families marked by low warmth were much more likely to relapse than those who returned to families characterized by high warmth. For Anglo Americans, warmth was unrelated to relapse. López and colleagues did not attribute this ethnic difference to a set of presumed cultural beliefs associated with the Mexican culture or a collectivist culture. Instead, they noted that most of the Mexican origin families and patients were immigrants, and that maintaining family ties may be crucial to the survival of low-income immigrants living in a foreign and at times hostile environment. The latter interpretation is consistent with a socially defined view of culture rather than a value or belief perspective.

These findings in conjunction with two other international studies (Italy: Bertrando et al., 1992; Yugoslavia: Ivanovi, Vuleti, & Bebbington, 1994) are consistent with the hypothesis that culture plays a role in the manner in which families respond to relatives with schizophrenia, which in turn relates to the course of illness. A limitation of these findings is that there was no direct measure of cultural processes. Nevertheless, the importance of this study is that the exploration of possible cultural variability led to the beginning of a line of inquiry that examines what families do to prevent relapse. Such research has the potential to add a much needed balance to family research by focusing on both positive and negative aspects of families' behaviors (see also Weisman, Gomes, & López, 2003). The study of caregiving (e.g., Guarnaccia, 1998; Lefley, 1998) and families' day to day interactions with ill family members will likely shed further light on the importance of families' prosocial functioning.

Childhood Disorders. The study of child psychopathology is a rich field of inquiry for those interested in culture. As noted by Weisz, McCarty, Eastman, Chaiyasit, & Suwanlert, (1997), child psychopathology requires attention to the behavior of children as well as the views of adults—parents, teachers, and mental health practitioners—for it is the adults who usually decide whether a problem exists. The fact that others determine whether children's behavior is problematic indicates the importance of the social world in defining mental illness and disorders of children and adolescents.

John Weisz and his colleagues have carried out the most systematic research on culture and childhood psychopathology (for a review, see Weisz et al., 1997). In the first study, conducted in Thailand and the United States, Weisz, Suwanlert, Chaiyasit, Weiss, and Walter (1987a) found that Thai children and adolescents who were referred to mental health clinics reported more internalizing problems than U.S. children and adolescents. In contrast, U.S. children and adolescents reported more externalizing problems than Thai children and adolescents. In follow-up community studies, where the mental health referral process was not a factor in the identification of problem behaviors, the cross-national differences were confirmed for internalizing problems but not for externalizing problems (Weisz et al., 1987b; Weisz et al., 1993b). U.S. and Thai children and adolescents identified in their respective communities did not differ in terms of acting-out problems. Weisz and colleagues argue that the findings with regard to internalizing problems are consistent with the idea that culture shapes the manner in which children and adolescents express psychological distress. Because they come from a largely Buddhist religious and cultural background that values self-control and emotional restraint, Thai children may be more likely than U.S. children to express psychological distress in a manner that does not violate cultural norms.

Aside from the intriguing findings, two other factors stand out in Weisz and colleagues' research: the systematic nature of the research, and the care with which the research has been conducted. Weisz began this line of investigation in mental health clinics, then went to a community survey to rule out the possibility of referral factors (Weisz et al., 1987b). Based on these findings, Weisz and Weiss (1991) derived a referability index for specific problem behaviors (e.g., vandalism and poor school work) that indexes the likelihood that a given problem will be referred for treatment, taking into account the problem's prevalence in a given community. In this study, they demonstrated how gender and nationality influence whether a problem is brought to the attention of mental health professionals. Subsequently, Weisz and colleagues examined teachers' reports of actual children (Weisz et al., 1989) and both parents' and teachers' ratings of hypothetical cases (Weisz, Suwanlert, Chaiyasit, Weiss, & Jackson, 1991). In a more recent study of teachers' reports of problem behaviors, Weisz, Chaiyasit, Weiss, Eastman, & Jackson (1995) found that Thai teachers report more internalizing and externalizing problem behaviors in Thai children than U.S. teachers report in U.S. children. Each of Weisz and colleagues' studies systematically builds on their previous work in advancing an understanding of how adults with differing social roles define children's problem behaviors. Multiple cross-cultural studies using different methods with different research participants provide a rich network of findings to advance our understanding of how the social context shapes the identification of youths' mental health problems.

The care Weisz and colleagues take with their research is best illustrated in the study of teachers' ratings of problem behaviors (Weisz et al., 1995). They found that Thai teachers rate more internalizing and externalizing problem behaviors for Thai students than U.S. teachers rate for their own students. Given that this finding runs counter to the previous clinical and community studies, which found differences only for internalizing problems, they devised an innovative observational methodology to assess whether something about the children or the teachers contributed to this contradictory finding. Weisz and associates (1995) used independent observers of both children's school behavior and teachers to rate the same children who were observed in Thailand and in the United States. One of the independent raters was a bilingual Thai psychologist who had received graduate training in the United States. His being part of both teams of independent observers was critical to assessing the reliability of the Thai and U.S. observers. The relationship between his ratings and those of the other U.S. and Thai raters were equally high, suggesting that the ratings were reliable across both national sites. Interestingly, the observers rated Thai children as having less than half as many problem and off-task behaviors as U.S. children, yet Thai teachers rated the observed students as having many more problem behaviors than U.S. teachers rated their students. These data suggest that Thai teachers have a much lower threshold than U.S. teachers for identifying problem behaviors in their students. Findings in cross-cultural research are often open to multiple interpretations. By using careful methodology across multiple studies, Weiz and collaborators were able to pin down the specific meaning of their complex set of findings. In doing so, they highlight the importance of contextual factors in the assessment of child psychopathology and demonstrate that it is untenable to view the assessment of child psychopathology as culture-free.

Developmental researchers are examining more closely the influence of culture on the type and degree of problem behaviors of children and adolescents. Weisz and associates extended their Thai–U.S. research to Jamaica and Kenya (Lambert, Weisz, & Knight, 1989; Weisz, Sigman, Weiss, & Mosk, 1993a). Other investigators have compared rates of internalizing and externalizing problems in other parts of the world (e.g., Denmark: Arnett & Balle-Jensen, 1993; and Puerto Rico: Achenbach et al., 1990). Still other researchers have examined specifically internalizing type problem behaviors (Greenberger & Chen,1996) or externalizing type problem behaviors (e.g., Weine, Phillips, & Achenbach, 1995) in cross-national or cross-ethnic samples. An important trend in this research is that epidemiological research that compares groups cross-nationally and suggests possible cultural explanations is now being complemented by research that examines the psychosocial processes associated with children's and adolescents' adjustment or psychopathology. For example, Chen, Greenberger, Lester, Dong, and Guo (1998) examined risk factors (parent–adolescent conflict and perceived peer approval of misconduct) and protective factors (parental warmth and parental monitoring) associated with acting-out problems across four groups of adolescents: European Americans, Chinese Americans, Taipei Chinese, and Beijing Chinese. They found that although there were similar levels of reported misconduct across the four groups, peer approval/disapproval accounted for more of the misconduct for the two groups of Americans adolescents than for the two groups of the Chinese adolescents.

The strength of the more recent studies is that they examine processes that may underlie potential cross-national differences and similarities, including social (family and peers) and psychological (values) processes. Thus, an important step has been taken to understand why differences and similarities may occur in behavior problems cross-nationally. Although the conceptual models used to frame such research are rich, include social processes, and have a strong empirical tradition in psychological research, they are not well informed by cultural specific processes (for an exception see Polo, 2002). Investigators apply models developed largely in the United States. Ethnographic research that examines what about the social and cultural world might play a role in the expression of distress and disorder among children would be especially welcome. This research could then lead to testing directly those culture-specific factors that are thought to affect psychopathology within a given conceptual framework as evidenced in the work of some developmental researchers (e.g., Fuligni, 1998), and as advocated by others (e.g., Schneider, 1998). The growing interest of researchers in studying internalizing and externalizing problem behaviors cross-nationally and cross-ethnically attests to the utility of this approach for enhancing our understanding of culture and childhood psychopathology.

Emerging Trends

Immigration.   A number of recent findings highlight the importance of immigration in understanding mental health and mental illness. The Los Angeles Epidemiologic Catchment Area study reported that Mexican-born Mexican Americans had significantly lower prevalence rates across a wide range of disorders than U.S.-born Mexican Americans (Burnam, Hough, Karno, Escobar, & Telles, 1987). This finding was replicated in a more recent epidemiologic study comparing the prevalence rates of rural and urban Mexican-origin adults in Fresno and nearby communities (Vega et al., 1998). An important contribution of the Fresno study is that evidence was provided from a Mexico City sample indicating that Mexico City residents had comparable rates to the Mexican immigrant sample, thus countering the hardy immigrant hypothesis. These and other studies (Ortega, Rosenheck, Alegria, & Desai, 2000) have been interpreted as suggesting that acculturation to the American culture may be harmful to Latinos' mental health. Marshall and Orlando (2002) provide a counterpoint that acculturation can serve as a protective factor rather than a risk factor, particularly in the domain of dissociation associated with trauma among young Latinos. The social and psychological mechanisms that are responsible for the differing prevalence rates for the immigrant groups at this time are unknown. Nevertheless, available studies indicate that research on immigration and acculturation can contribute much to our understanding of how the social world and psychopathology interrelate (see also Rogler, 1994). A particularly wide-open area of study is the examination of immigration and mental health and illness among children and adolescents (see Guarnaccia & López, 1998; Polo, 2002). Not only will immigration/acculturation research be able to address important conceptual and methodological issues in the study of culture, but it will also have important policy implications for the delivery of mental health services to underserved communities (e.g., Salgado de Snyder, Diaz-Perez, & Bautista, 1998).

U.S. Ethnic Minority Groups.   We are encouraged by the growing interest in the study of psychopathology among U.S. ethnic minority groups. With regard to African Americans, there has been an increase in the study of anxiety disorders since Neal and Turner's (1991) call for research. The most recent studies include clinical studies (e.g., Friedman, Paradis, & Hatch, 1994), epidemiologic studies (Horwath, Johnson, & Hornig, 1993), a combined ethnographic and epidemiological study (Heurtin-Roberts, Snowden, & Miller, 1997), and a study of childhood fears (Neal, Lilly, & Zakis, 1993). Although these studies are largely descriptive, there is some attention to the differential social world of African American and White patients. For example, Friedman and associates found that, relative to White patients with panic disorder and agoraphobia, African American patients reported a greater likelihood of having been separated as children from their parents and of having experienced their parent's divorce.

A systematic series of studies has examined the mental health problems of American Indian children (e.g., Beiser, Sack, Manson, Redshirt, & Dion, 1998; Dion, Gotowiec, & Beiser, 1998) and adults (Maser & Dinges, 1992/1993). Although many of these studies use mainstream models of disorder and distress (see O'Nell's 1989 critique), there are growing efforts to contextualize the mental health problems within these communities. In one study, Ducos and colleagues (1998) found that nearly half of the Indian adolescents detained in the juvenile justice system met criteria for mental disorders ranging from substance abuse/dependence (38%) to major depression (10%). These rates were much higher than community surveys of Indian youth and non-Indian youth. These researchers argue that the juvenile justice system has the potential to serve as an important site to treating these high-risk youth, many of whom would otherwise go untreated. In another study, O'Nell and Mitchell (1996) found that the line between normal and pathological drinking among adolescent Indians is contextually based. Their ethnographic findings suggest that a rigid model of alcohol abuse defined by biology (frequency and amount of alcohol) or psychology (distress) without significant attention to the sociocultural context (e.g., when and with whom one drinks) is limited in distinguishing between normative and pathological drinking. Overall, we are impressed by recent systematic efforts of psychopathology researchers of American Indians to assess the interrelations of distress and disorder to the social world. This emphasis is continuing as reflected in Spero Manson and colleagues' major research endeavor entitled "American Indian Services Utilization, Psychiatric Epidemiology, Risk and Protective Factors Project." This project is the largest study of American Indian groups to use state-of-the-art measures to assess the level of psychopathology and service utilization patterns and gaps in services for these communities.

With regard to Asian American research, Sue, Fujino, Hu, Takeuchi, & Zane (1991) have had a long-standing interest in treatment issues. Most recently, Sue and colleagues have broadened their interests to include psychopathology (Sue, Sue, Sue, & Takeuchi, 1995). Of particular importance is the epidemiological survey of depressive disorders among Chinese Americans residing in the Los Angeles area (Takeuchi et al., 1998). Researchers have been able to examine prevalence rates of traditional depressive and related disorders, as well as neurasthenia (Zheng et al., 1997), a concept that was retired in the classification of mental disorders in the United States but is still in use in China and other parts of Asia. *Neurasthenia* usually refers to weakness or fatigue, often accompanied by a variety of psychological (e.g., poor concentration) and physical symptoms (e.g., diffuse aches and pains). Of particular interest is the finding that neurasthenia had the highest one-year prevalence rate (6.4%) of any disorder in the Chinese American epidemiologic survey. This was the case even after removing those persons with both neurasthenia and another disorder such as anxiety or depression (pure neurasthenia rate = 3.6%). The study of neurasthenia is another example of how culture can contribute to shaping the expression of disorder.

Most of the research with Latinos has involved adults. Vega, Khoury, Zimmerman, Gil, & Warheit (1995), however, conducted an important study regarding Latino adolescents in Miami, Florida. A significant contribution of this research is that it points out that the relationship between specific acculturative stressors (e.g., language conflicts, perceived discrimination) and problem behaviors varies by immigration status. In addition, in their prevalence study of adolescents in the Houston metropolitan area, Roberts, Roberts, & Chen (1997) found that of nine ethnic groups, Mexican Americans reported the highest rates of major depression. Both studies are characterized by rigor in sampling schools, multiethnic samples, and large sample sizes. Additional studies are currently being carried out by Canino and colleagues among children and adolescents in both the community and service system in Puerto Rico, and by Landsverk, Hough, and colleagues in the youth service systems in San Diego. When these studies are published, they will add to the limited attention addressing Latino youth.

CONCLUSIONS

Cultural psychopathology, the study of culture and the definition, experience, distribution, and course of psychological disorders, is now on the map. Articles are being published in culture-focused journals as well as mainstream journals (e.g., *American Journal of Psychiatry*, *Journal of Abnormal Psychology*, *Child Development*). Substantive areas of psychopathology research are being shaped by cultural research. Efforts to integrate idioms of distress with mainstream constructs, for example, are well underway (*ataques de nervios* and anxiety and affective disorders, *nervios* and families' conceptualizations of serious mental illness; see Guarnaccia and Rogler, 1999). In 1988, it was important for Kleinman to get the message out that culture matters. The message has been received; cultural research is providing an innovative and fresh perspective to our understanding of several important aspects of psychopathology.

For cultural researchers to build on the empirical and conceptual foundation that has been established, it is important at this juncture for us to continue to be critical of how culture is conceptualized and how such conceptualizations guide our research. It is clear from this review that culture can no longer be treated solely as an independent variable or as a factor to be controlled for. Rather, culture infuses the full social context of mental health research. Culture is important in all aspects of psychopathology research—from the design and translation of instruments, to the conceptual models that guide the research, to the interpersonal interaction between researcher and research participants, to the definition and interpretation of symptom and syndromes, to the structure of the social world that surrounds a person's mental health problems. Cultural psychopathology research requires a framework that incorporates culture in multifaceted ways. Accordingly, it is most important that cultural research not obscure the importance of other social forces such as class, poverty, and marginality that work in conjunction with culture to shape people's everyday lives. The examination of both social and cultural processes is one way to help guard against superficial cultural analyses that ignore or minimize the powerful political economic inequalities that coexist with culture.

A corollary of the need for a broad framework for research is the need for approaches that integrate qualitative and quantitative methods. Cultural psychopathology research can serve as an important site for integrating ethnographic, observational, clinical, and epidemiological research approaches. Mental health problems cannot be fully understood through one lens. Ethnographic research provides insights into the meaning of mental health problems and how they are experienced in their sociocultural context. Observational research captures people's functioning in their daily lives. Clinical research can provide detailed phenomenologies of psychopathological processes and can contribute to developing treatments to alleviate suffering at the individual as well as social levels. Epidemiological research can broaden perspectives to more generalized processes and populations. It is the integration of these perspectives, both in methodologies and in the composition of research teams, that will make the cultural agenda succeed.

The ultimate goal of cultural psychopathology research is to alleviate suffering and improve people's lives. This requires attention to the multiple levels of individual, family, community, and the broader social system. Our enhanced notion of culture leads to analysis of the expression and sources of psychopathology at all of these levels. Our commitment to making a difference in peoples' everyday lives argues for the development of treatment and prevention interventions at these multiple levels as well. The increasing cultural diversity of the United States and the massive movements of people around the globe provide both an opportunity and imperative for cultural psychopathology research.

REFERENCES

Achenbach, T. M., Bird, H. R., Canino, G., Phares, V., Gould, M. S., & Rubio-Stipec, M. (1990). Epidemiological comparisons of Puerto Rican and U.S. mainland children: Parent, teacher and self-reports. *Journal of the American Academy of Child & Adolescent Psychiatry, 29*(1), 84–93.

Alarcon, R. D. (1995). Culture and psychiatric diagnosis: Impact on DSM-IV and ICD-10. *Psychiatric Clinics of North America, 18*, 449–465.

American Psychiatric Association. (1994). *Diagnostic and statistical manual of mental disorders* (4th ed.). Washington, DC: Author.

Arnett, J., & Balle-Jensen, L. (1993). Cultural bases of risk behavior: Danish adolescents. *Child Development, 64*, 1842–1855.

Bebbington, P., & Kuipers, L. (1994). The predictive utility of expressed emotion in schizophrenia: An aggregate analysis. *Psychological Medicine, 24*, 707–718.

Beiser, M., Sack, W., Manson, S., Redshirt, R., & Dion, R. (1998). Mental health and the academic performance of First Nations and majority-culture children. *American Journal of Orthopsychiatry, 68*, 455–467.

Bertrando, P., Beltz, J., Bressi, C., Clerici, M., Farma, T., Invernizzi, G., & Cazzullo, C. L. (1992). Expressed emotion and schizophrenia in Italy: A study of an urban population. *British Journal of Psychiatry, 161*, 223–229.

Betancourt, H., & López, S. R. (1993). The study of culture, race and ethnicity in American psychology. *American Psychologist, 48*, 629–637.

Brekke, J. S., & Barrio, C. (1997). Cross-ethnic symptom differences in schizophrenia: The influence of culture and minority status. *Schizophrenia Bulletin, 23*, 305–316.

Brown, G. W., Birley, J. L. T., & Wing, J. K. (1972). Influence of family life on the course of schizophrenic disorders: A replication. *British Journal of Psychiatry, 21*, 241–258.

Burnam, A., Hough, R. L., Karno, M., Escobar, J. I., & Telles, C. (1987). Acculturation and lifetime prevalence of psychiatric disorders among Mexican Americans in Los Angeles. *Journal of Health and Social Behavior, 28*, 89–102.

Butzlaff, R. L., & Hooley, J. M. (1998). Expressed emotion and psychiatric relapse: A meta-analysis. *Archives of General Psychiatry, 55*, 547–552.

Cervantes, R. C., Padilla, A. M., & Salgado de Zinder, V. N. (1991). The Hispanic Stress Inventory: A culturally relevant approach to psychological assessment. *Psychological Assessment, 3*, 438–447.

Chen, C., Greenberger, E., Lester, J., Dong, Q., & Guo, M. (1998). A cross-cultural study of family and peer correlates of adolescent misconduct. *Developmental Psychology, 34*, 770–781.

Clark, L. A. (1987). Mutual relevance of mainstream and cross-cultural psychology. *Journal of Consulting and Clinical Psychology, 55*, 41–70.

Cohen, A. (1992). Prognosis for schizophrenia in the Third World: A reevaluation of cross-cultural research. *Culture, Medicine, and Psychiatry, 16*, 53–75.

De La Cancela, V., Guarnaccia, P., & Carrillo, E. (1986). Psychosocial distress among Latinos. *Humanity Society, 10*, 431–447.

Desjarlais, R., Eisenberg, L., Good, B., & Kleinman, A. (1996). *World mental health: Problems priorities in low-income countries.* Oxford: Oxford University Press.

Dion, R., Gotowiec, A., & Beiser, M. (1998). Depression and conduct disorder in Native and non-Native children. *Journal of the American Academy of Child & Adolescent Psychiatry, 37*, 736–742.

Draguns, J. G. (1980). Disorders of clinical severity. In H. C. Triandis & J. G. Draguns (Eds.), *Handbook of cross-cultural psychology: Vol. 6. Psychopathology* (pp. 99–174). Boston: Allyn & Bacon.

Draguns, J. G. (1990). Culture and psychopathology: Toward specifying the nature of the relationship. In J. Berman (Ed.), *Nebraska Symposium on Motivation. 1989: Cross-Cultural Perspectives* (pp. 235–277). Lincoln: University of Nebraska.

Duclos, C. W., Beals, J., Novins, D. K., Martin, C., Jewett, C. S., & Manson, S. M. (1998). Prevalence of common psychiatric disorders among American Indian adolescent detainees. *Journal of the American Academy of Child & Adolescent Psychiatry, 37*, 866–873.

Edgerton, R., & Cohen, A. (1994). Culture and schizophrenia: The DOSMD challenge. *British Journal of Psychiatry, 164*, 222–231.

Fabrega, H. (1975). The need for an ethnomedical science. *Science, 189*, 969–975.

Fabrega, H. (1989). On the significance of an anthropological approach to schizophrenia. *Psychiatry, 52*, 45–65.

Fabrega H. (1990). Hispanic mental health research: A case for cultural psychiatry. *Hispanic Journal of Behavioral Science, 12*, 339–365.

Friedman, S., Paradis, C. M., Hatch, M. (1994). Characteristics of African-American and White patients with panic disorder and agoraphobia. *Hospital and Community Psychiatry, 45*, 798–803.

Fuligni, A. (1998). Authority, autonomy, and parent-adolescent conflict and cohesion: A study of adolescents from Mexican, Chinese, Filipino, and European backgrounds. *Developmental Psychology, 34*, 782–792.

Gallimore, R., Goldenberg, C. N., & Weisner, T. S. (1993). The social construction and subjective reality of activity settings: Implications for community psychology. *American Journal of Community Psychology, 21*, 537–559.

Garro, L. (2001). The remembered past in a culturally meaningful life: Remembering as cultural, social and cognitive process. In C. Moore & H. Mathews (Eds.), *The Psychology of Cultural Experience* (pp. 105–147). Cambridge: Cambridge University Press.

Greenberger, E., & Chen, C. (1996). Perceived family relationships and depressed mood in early and late adolescence: A comparison of European and Asian Americans. *Developmental Psychology, 32*, 707–716.

Greenfield, P. M. (1997). Culture as process: Empirical methods for cultural psychology. In J. W. Berry, Y. H. Poortinga, & J. Pandey (Eds.), *Handbook of Cross-Cultural Psychology: Vol. 1. Theory and Method* (pp. 301–346). Needham Heights, MA: Allyn & Bacon.

Guarnaccia, P. J. (1998). Multicultural experiences of family caregiving: A study of African American, European American and Hispanic American families. In H. Lefley (Ed.), *Families coping with illness: The cultural context* (pp. 45–61). San Francisco: Jossey-Bass.

Guarnaccia, P. J., Canino, G., Rubio-Stipec, M., & Bravo, M. (1993). The prevalence of *ataques de nervios* in the Puerto Rico study: The role of culture in psychiatric epidemiology. *Journal of Nervous and Mental Disease, 181*, 157–165.

Guarnaccia, P. J., De La Cancela, V., & Carrillo, E. (1989a). The multiple meanings of ataques de nervios in the Latino community. *Medical Anthropology, 11*, 47–62.

Guarnaccia, P. J., Kleinman, A., & Good, B. J. (1990). A critical review of epidemiological studies of Puerto Rican mental health. *American Journal of Psychiatry, 147*, 449–456.

Guarnaccia, P. J., & López S. (1998). The mental health and adjustment of immigrant and refugee children. *Child & Adolescent Psychiatric Clinics of North America, 7*, 537–553.

Guarnaccia, P. J., Parra, P., Deschamps, A., Milstein, G., & Argiles, N. (1992). Si Dios quiere: Hispanic families' experiences of caring for a seriously mentally ill family member. *Culture, Medicine, and Psychiatry, 16*, 187–215.

Guarnaccia, P. J., Rivera, M., Franco, F., & Neighbors, C. (1996). The experiences of ataques de nervios: Towards an anthropology of emotions in Puerto Rico. *Culture, Medicine, and Psychiatry, 20*, 343–367.

Guarnaccia, P. J., & Rogler, L. H. (1999). Research on culture-bound syndromes: New directions. *American Journal of Psychiatry, 156*, 1322–1327.

Guarnaccia, P. J., Rubio-Stipec, M., & Canino, G. (1989b). *Ataques de nervios* in the Puerto Rican Diagnostic Interview Schedule: The impact of cultural categories on psychiatric epidemiology. *Culture, Medicine, and Psychiatry, 13*, 275–295.

Heurtin-Roberts, S., Snowden, L., & Miller, L. (1997). Expressions of anxiety in African Americans: Ethnography and the Epidemiological Catchment Area studies. *Culture, Medicine, and Psychiatry, 21*, 337–363.

Hopper, K. (1991). Some old questions for the new cross-cultural psychiatry. *Medical Anthropology Quarterly, 5*, 299–330.

Horwath, E., Johnson, J., & Hornig, C. D. (1993). Epidemiology of panic disorder in African-Americans. *American Journal of Psychiatry, 150*, 465–469.

Ivanovi, M., Vuleti, Z., & Bebbington, P. (1994). Expressed emotion in the families of patients with schizophrenia and its influence on the course of illness. *Social psychiatry and psychiatric epidemiology, 29*, 61–65.

Jablensky, A., Sartorius, N., Ernberg, G., Ankar, M., & Korten, A., Cooper, J. E., Day, R., & Bertelsen, A. (1992). Schizophrenia: Manifestations, incidence and course in different cultures. *Psychological Medicine, 20*(Suppl.), 1–97.

Jenkins, J. H. (1988a). Conceptions of schizophrenia as a problem of nerves: A cross-cultural comparison of Mexican-Americans and Anglo-Americans. *Social Science & Medicine, 26*, 1233–1243.

Jenkins, J. H. (1988b). Ethnopsychiatric interpretations of schizophrenic illness: The problem of *nervios* within Mexican-American families. *Culture, Medicine, and Psychiatry, 12*, 303–331.

Jenkins, J. H. (1991). Anthropology, expressed emotion, and schizophrenia. *Ethos, 19*, 387–431.

Jenkins, J. H. (1993). Too close for comfort: Schizophrenia and emotional overinvolvement among Mexicano families. In A. D. Gaines (Ed.), *Ethnopsychiatry* (pp. 203–221). Albany: State University of New York Press.

Jenkins, J., & Karno, M. (1992). The meaning of expressed emotion: Theoretical issues raised by cross-cultural research. *American Journal of Psychiatry, 149*, 9–21.

Karno, M., Jenkins, J. H., de la Selva, A., Santana, F., Telles, C., Lopez, S., & Mintz, J. (1987). Expressed emotion and schizophrenic outcome among Mexican-American families. *Journal of Nervous and Mental Disease, 175*, 143–151.

Kessler, R. C., Mickelson, K. D., & Williams, D. R. (1999). The prevalence, distribution, and mental health correlates of perceived discrimination in the United States. *Journal of Health and Social Behavior, 40*, 208–230.

King, L. M. (1978). Social and cultural influences on psychopathology. *Annual Review of Psychology, 29*, 405–433.

Kirmayer, L. J. (1998). Editorial: The fate of culture in DSM-IV. *Transcultural Psychiatry, 35*, 339–342.

Kleinman, A. (1988). *Rethinking Psychiatry: From cultural category to personal experience.* New York: Free Press.

Kleinman, A., Eisenberg, L., & Good, B. (1978). Culture, illness, and care: Clinical lessons from anthropologic and cross-cultural research. *Annals of Internal Medicine, 88*, 251–258.

Kleinman, A., & Good, B. J. (Eds.). (1985). *Culture and Depression.* Berkeley: University of California Press.

Kleinman, A., & Kleinman, J. (1991). Suffering and its professional transformations: Toward an ethnography of experience. *Culture, Medicine, and Psychiatry, 15*, 275–301.

Kleinman, A. M. (1977). Depression, somatization and the "New Cross-Cultural Psychiatry." *Social Science and Medicine, 11*, 3–10.

Lambert, M. C., Weisz, J. R., & Knight, F. (1989). Over- and undercontrolled clinic referral problems of Jamaican and American children and adolescents: The culture-general and the culture-specific. *Journal of Consulting and Clinical Psychology, 57*, 467–472.

Leff, J. P., & Vaughn, C. E. (1985). *Expressed emotion in families.* NY: Guilford.

Lefley, H. (Ed.). (1998). *Families coping with illness: The cultural context.* San Francisco: Jossey-Bass.

Lewis-Fernandez, R., & Kleinman, A. (1995). Cultural psychiatry: Theoretical, clinical and research issues. *Psychiatric Clinics of North America, 18*, 433–448.

Liebowitz, M. R., Salmán, E., Jusino, C. M., Garfinkel, R., Street, L., Cardenas, D. L., Silvestre, J., Fyer, A., Carrasco, J. L., Davies, S., Guarnaccia, P., & Klein, D. F. (1994). Ataque de nervios and panic disorder. *American Journal of Psychiatry, 151*, 871–875.

Lin, K. M., & Kleinman, A. M. (1988). Psychopathology and clinical course of schizophrenia: A cross-cultural perspective. *Schizophrenia Bulletin, 14*, 555–567.

Lin, K. M., Poland, R. E., & Anderson, D. (1995). Psychopharmacology, ethnicity and culture. *Transcultural Psychiatric Research Review, 32*, 3–40.

López, S. R. (2003). Reflections on the Surgeon General's report on mental health, culture, race, and ethnicity. *Culture, Medicine and Psychiatry, 27*, 419–443.

López, S. R., Nelson, K., Polo, A., Jenkins, J. H., Karno, M., Vaughn, C., & Snyder, K. (2004). Ethnicity, expressed emotion, attributions and course of schizophrenia: Family warmth matters. *Journal of Abnormal Psychology, 113*.

López, S. R., Nelson, K., Snyder, K., & Mintz, J. (1999). Attributions and affective reactions of family members and course of schizophrenia. *Journal of Abnormal Psychology, 108*(2), 307–314.

López, S., & Núñez, J. A. (1987). The consideration of cultural factors in selected diagnostic criteria and interview schedules. *Journal of Abnormal Psychology, 96*, 270–272.

Manson, S. M., Shore, J. H., & Bloom, J. D. (1985). The depressive experience in American Indian communities: A challenge for psychiatric theory and diagnosis. In A. Kleinman & B. J. Good (Eds.), *Culture and depression* (pp. 331–368). Berkeley: University of California Press.

Markus, H. R., & Kitayama, S. (1991). Culture and the self: Implications for cognition, emotion, and motivation. *Psychological Review, 98*, 224–253.

Marsella, A. J. (1980). Depressive experience and disorder across cultures. In H. Triandis & J. Draguns (Eds.), *Handbook of cross-cultural psychology: Vol. 6. Psychopathology* (pp. 237–289). Boston: Allyn and Bacon.

Marshall, G. N., & Orlando, M. (2002). Acculturation and peritraumatic dissociation in young adult Latino survivors of community violence. *Journal of Abnormal Psychology, 111*, 166–174.

Maser, J. D., & Dinges, N. (1992/93). The co-morbidity of depression, anxiety and substance abuse among American Indians and Alaska natives. *Culture, Medicine, and Psychiatry, 16*, 409–577.

Mezzich, J. E, Kleinman, A., Fabrega, H., & Parron, D. L. (Eds.). (1996). *Culture and psychiatric diagnosis: A DSM-IV perspective.* Washington, DC: American Psychiatric Association.

Mezzich, J. E., Kleinman, A., Fabrega, H., Parron, D. L., Good, B. J., Lin, K., & Manson, S. M. (1997). Cultural issues for DSM-IV. In T. A. Widiger, A. J. Frances, H. A. Pincus, R. Ross, M. B. First, W. Davis (Eds.). *DSM-IV sourcebook:* Vol. 3 (pp. 861–1016). Washington, DC: American Psychiatric Association.

Murray, C. J. L., & Lopez, A. D. (1996). *The global burden of disease: A comprehensive assessment of mortality and disability from diseases, injuries, and risk factors in 1990 and projected to 2020.* Cambridge, MA: Harvard University Press.

Neal, A. M., Lilly, R. S., & Zakis, S. (1993). What are African American children afraid of? *Journal of Anxiety Disorders, 7,* 129–139.

Neal, A. M., & Turner, S. M. (1991). Anxiety disorders research with African Americans: Current status. *Psychological Bulletin, 109,* 400–410.

Neighbors, H. W., Jackson, J. S., Campbell, L., & Williams, D. (1989). The influence of racial factors on psychiatric diagnosis: A review and suggestions for research. *Community Mental Health Journal, 25,* 301–310.

O'Nell, T. (1989). Psychiatric investigations among American Indians and Alaska Natives: A critical review. *Culture, Medicine, and Psychiatry, 13,* 51–87.

O'Nell, T., & Mitchell, C. M. (1996). Alcohol use among American Indian adolescents: The role of culture in pathological drinking. *Social Science and Medicine, 42,* 565–578.

Ortega, A., N., Rosenheck, R., Alegria, M., & Desai, R. A. (2000). Acculturation and the lifetime risk of psychiatric and substance use disorders among Hispanics. *Journal of Nervous and Mental Disease, 188,* 728–735.

Polo, A. J. (2002). *Mental health problems among Mexican American youth: Socio-cultural and family correlates.* Doctoral dissertation, University of California, Los Angeles.

Regier, D. A., Myers, J. K., Kramer, M., Robins, L. N., Blazer, D. G., Hough, R. L., Eaton, W. W., & Locke, B. Z. (1984). The NIMH Epidemiologic Catchment Area program. *Archives of General Psychiatry, 41,* 934–941.

Roberts, R. E., Roberts, C. R., & Chen, Y. R. (1997). Ethnocultural differences in prevalence of adolescent depression. *American Journal of Community Psychology, 25,* 95–110.

Rogler, L. H. (1989). The meaning of culturally sensitive research in mental health. *American Journal of Psychiatry, 146,* 296–303.

Rogler, L. H. (1994). International migrations: A framework for directing research. *American Psychologist, 49,* 701–708.

Rogler, L. H. (1996). Framing research on culture in psychiatric diagnosis: The case of the DSM-IV. *Psychiatry: Interpersonal & Biological Processes, 59,* 145–155.

Rogler, L. H., Malgady, R. G., & Rodríguez, O. (1989). *Hispanics and mental health: A framework for research.* Malabar, FL: Krieger.

Salgado de Snyder, V. N., Diaz-Perez, M., & Bautista, E. (1998). Pathways to mental health services among inhabitants of a Mexican village with high migratory tradition to the United States. *Health and Social Work, 23,* 249–261.

Salmán E., Liebowitz, M., Guarnaccia, P. J., Jusino, C. M., Garfinkel, R., L. Street, et al. (1998). Subtypes of ataques de nervios: The influence of coexisting psychiatric diagnosis. *Culture, Medicine, and Psychiatry, 22,* 231–44.

Sartorius, N., Jablensky, A., Korten, A., Ernberg, G., Anker, M., Cooper, J. E., & Day, R. (1986). Early manifestations and first-contact incidence of schizophrenia in different cultures. *Psychological Medicine, 16,* 909–928.

Schneider, B. H. (1998). Cross-cultural comparison as doorkeeper in research on social and emotional adjustment of children and adolescents. *Developmental Psychology, 34,* 793–797.

Shweder, R. A., & Bourne, E. J. (1984). Does the concept of the person vary cross-culturally? In R. A. Shweder & R. A. LeVine (Eds.). *Culture theory: Essays on mind, self and emotion* (pp. 158–199). Cambridge: Cambridge University Press.

Sue S., Fujino D. C., Hu, L., Takeuchi, D., & Zane, N. (1991). Community mental health services for ethnic minority groups: A test of the cultural responsiveness hypothesis. *Journal of Consulting and Clinical Psychology, 59,* 533–540.

Sue, S., Sue, D., Sue, L., & Takeuchi D. (1995.) Asian American psychopathology. *Cultural Diversity and Mental Health, 1,* 39–51.

Takeuchi, D. T., Chung, R. C. Y., Lin, K. M., Shen, H., Kurasaki K., Chung, C. A., & Sue, S. (1998). Lifetime and twelve-month prevalence rates of major depressive episodes and dysthymia among Chinese Americans in Los Angeles. *American Journal of Psychiatry, 155,* 1407–1414.

U.S. Department of Health and Human Services (1999). *Mental health: A report of the Surgeon General.* Rockville, MD: Author.

U.S. Department of Health and Human Services (2001). *Mental health: Culture, race, and ethnicity—A supplement to mental health: A report of the Surgeon General.* Rockville, MD: Author.

Vaughn, C. E., & Leff, J. P. (1976). The influence of family and social factors on the course of psychiatric illness. *British Journal of Psychiatry, 129,* 125–137.

Vaughn, C. E., Snyder, K. S., Jones, S., Freeman, W. B., & Falloon, I. R. (1984). Family factors in schizophrenic relapse: Replication in California of British research on expressed emotion. *Archives of General Psychiatry, 41,* 1169–1177.

Vega, W., Khoury, E. L., Zimmerman, R. S., Gil, A. G., & Warheit, G. J. (1995). Cultural conflicts and problem behaviors of Latino adolescents in home and school environments. *Journal of Community Psychology, 23,* 167–179.

Vega, W. A., Kolody, B., Aguilar-Gaxiola, S., Aldrete, E., Catalana, R., Caraveo-Anduaga, J. (1998). Lifetime prevalence of DSM-III-R psychiatric disorders among urban and rural Mexican Americans in California. *Archives of General Psychiatry, 55*, 771–778.

Ware, N., & Kleinman A. (1992). Culture and somatic experience: The social course of illness in neurasthenia and chronic fatigue syndrome. *Psychosomatic Medicine, 54*, 546–560.

Weine, A. M., Phillips, J. S., & Achenbach, T. M. (1995). Behavioral and emotional problems among Chinese and American children: Parent and teacher reports for ages 6 to 13. *Journal of Abnormal Child Psychology, 23*, 619–639.

Weisman, A. (1997). Understanding cross-cultural prognostic variability for schizophrenia. *Cultural Diversity and Mental Health, 3*, 3–35.

Weisman, A. G., Gomes, L., & López, S. R. (2003). Shifting blame away from ill relatives: Latino families' reactions to schizophrenia. *Journal of Nervous and Mental Disease, 191*, 574–581.

Weisman, A. G., Lopez, S. R., Ventura, J., Nuechterlein, K. H., Goldstein, M. J., & Hwang, S. (2000). A comparison of psychiatric symptoms between Anglo-Americans and Mexican-Americans with schizophrenia. *Schizophrenia Bulletin, 26*, 817–824.

Weisz, J. R., Chaiyasit, W., Weiss, B., Eastman, K. L., & Jackson, E. W. (1995). A multimethod study of problem behavior among Thai and American children in school: Teacher reports versus direct observation. *Child Development, 66*, 402–415.

Weisz, J. R., McCarty, C. A., Eastman, K. L., Chaiyasit, W., & Suwanlert, S. (1997). Developmental psychopathology and culture: Ten lessons from Thailand. In S. S. Luthar, J. A. Burack, D. Cicchetti, & J. R. Weisz (Eds.). *Developmental psychopathology: Perspectives on adjustment, risk, and disorder* (pp. 568–592). Cambridge: Cambridge University Press.

Weisz, J. R., Sigman, M., Weiss, B., Mosk J. (1993a). Parent reports of behavioral and emotional problems among children in Kenya, Thailand, and the United States. *Child Development, 64*, 98–109.

Weisz, J. R., Suwanlert, S., Chaiyasit, W., Weiss, B., Achenbach, T. M., & Eastman, K. L. (1993b). Behavioral and emotional problems among Thai and American adolescents: Parent reports for ages 12–16. *Journal of Abnormal Psychology, 102*, 395–403.

Weisz, J. R., Suwanlert, S., Chaiyasit, W., Weiss, B., Achenbach, T.M., & Trevathan D. (1989). Epidemiology behavioral and emotional problems among Thai and American children: Teacher reports for ages 6–11. *Journal of Child Psychology and Psychiatry & Allied Disciplines, 30*, 471–484.

Weisz, J. R., Suwanlert, S., Chaiyasit, W., Weiss, B., Achenbach, T. M., & Walter, B. R. (1987b). Epidemiology of behavioral and emotional problems among Thai and American children: Parent reports for ages 6 to 11. *Journal of the American Academy of Child & Adolescent Psychiatry, 26*, 890–897.

Weisz, J. R., Suwanlert, S., Chaiyasit, W., Weiss, B., & Jackson, E. W. (1991). Adult attitudes toward over- and undercontrolled child problems: Urban and rural parents and teachers from Thailand and the United States. *Journal of Child Psychology and Psychiatry & Allied Disciplines, 32*, 645–654.

Weisz, J. R., Suwanlert, S., Chaiyasit, W., Weiss, B., & Walter, B. (1987a). Over- and undercontrolled referral problems among children and adolescents from Thailand and the United States: The *wat* and *wai* of cultural differences. *Journal of Consulting & Clinical Psychology, 55*, 719–726.

Weisz, J. R., & Weiss, B. (1991). Studying the "referability" of child clinical problems. *Journal of Consulting & Clinical Psychology, 59*, 266–273.

World Health Organization. (1979). *Schizophrenia: An international follow-up study.* New York: Wiley.

Zheng, Y. P., Lin, K. M, Takeuchi, D., Kurasaki, K. S., Wang, Y., & Cheung, F. (1997). An epidemiological study of neurasthenia in Chinese-Americans in Los Angeles. *Comprehensive Psychiatry, 38*, 249–259.

3

Gender and Psychopathology

Barbara A. Winstead and Janis Sanchez
Old Dominion University

What role does gender play in psychopathology? Do women and men, girls and boys experience different types of psychological disorders? Do they experience the same disorder in different ways? Are they treated differently by the mental health system? Do recommended treatments work equally well for males and females? Should treatments take the sex of the client into account? Does it matter whether the therapist is female or male? What difference does gender make? And, if gender makes a difference, why? Do biological and/or sociocultural factors account for these differences? This chapter tackles these questions. In the end we will discover that these questions raise more questions. Clear-cut answers are scarce, but the questions themselves shed light on the process of psychological diagnosis and treatment of psychological disorders. Finally, although this chapter focuses on gender, gender interacts with culture, race/ethnicity, Socioeconomic Status, ability, age, and other variables to form unique experiences for individuals. Hence, gender must be understood as a potentially multidimensional as opposed to a unidimensional variable.

The first half of the chapter discusses information and issues involving gender differences in diagnosis and treatment. In the second part of the chapter, two specific disorders—depression, an adult disorder that women suffer more often than men, and conduct disorder, a childhood disorder diagnosed more often in boys than girls—are used to illustrate the ways in which researchers and clinicians struggle with the issue of gender and psychopathology.

DIAGNOSIS

To understand and treat a psychological disorder requires accurate diagnosis. The process of diagnosis and treatment is less than perfect, but the goal can be clearly stated: We wish to identify the problem, treat it, and thereby permit the client to lead a more productive and rewarding life. But how do we identify the problem? With physical symptoms, physicians are aided by diagnostic tests that identify abnormalities in biochemistry, histology, or anatomy that signal specific disease processes. With psychological problems, there are rarely physical signs such as an abnormal cell count. We may use diagnostic tests, but these are likely to be based on the self-reports of clients, not blood chemistry or cell cultures. Often psychological diagnosis is accomplished through interviews in which clinicians learn about symptoms directly from the client or through observation of symptoms. What the *Diagnostic and Statistical Manual of Mental Disorders* (DSM–IV–TR: American Psychiatric Association, 2000) provides is a set of agreed-on criteria that help clinicians make diagnoses based on sets of symptoms. Psychological diagnosis, following the medical model, leads to present/absent decisions, although many have argued that a continuous rather than a categorical model is better for understanding psychological disorders (Maddux, 2002). With either model, we want to be able to make an accurate assessment of the individual and to this end we assess the reliability and validity of clinical tests, clinical interviews, and systems for identifying mental disorders (See Widiger, chap. 4; Garb, Lilienfeld, & Fowler, chap. 5). With a perfectly reliable and valid system we could easily discover if men and women have similar or different psychological disorders, if the etiologies or disease courses of these illnesses are similar or different, and ultimately if men and women benefit from similar or different treatments. But with less than perfect diagnostic systems our questions about gender become more difficult to answer.

An official nomenclature for identifying mental illnesses was first established in part to create a common language for mental health professionals and researchers (see Widiger, chap. 4). Beginning in 1980, with DSM–III, this goal was largely accomplished in the United States, and researchers of psychological disorders and treatments adopted this system of diagnosis. Efforts to improve the reliability and validity of the DSM have led to revised and updated editions, DSM–III–R (1987) and the current DSM–IV–TR (2000). The purpose of a carefully articulated diagnostic system is to provide clinicians and researchers with an objective-as-possible basis for making decisions about the presence or absence of specific psychopathology. But the question of gender bias in the diagnostic categories themselves was raised almost immediately (Kaplan, 1983). Furthermore, to the extent that information relies on the interviewing and interpersonal skills of a diagnostician (as opposed to a standardized survey or interview), the gathering of pertinent information to make this determination may be biased. Even items on standardized scales may introduce gender or sex bias. Finally, although DSM guidelines are in black and white, putting all the symptoms together to arrive at a diagnosis may be influenced by clinician expectations and beliefs about gender and sex differences in prevalence rates.

A fundamental issue, for example, is whether or not the prevalence rates of disorders are different for females and males. Hartung and Widiger (1998) conclude that "Most of the mental disorders diagnosed with the DSM–IV do appear to have significant differential sex prevalence rates" (p. 280). According to their analysis, the DSM–IV provides information on differential sex prevalence for 101 of its 125 described psychological disorders. Excluding disorders that are, by definition, specific to one sex or the other (e.g., female orgasmic disorder, male erectile disorder), 84% of the DSM–IV disorders, for which information on prevalence by sex is available, are reported to occur at different rates in females and males. A general summary of these differences indicates that males are more likely to be diagnosed with the infancy, childhood, and adolescent disorders and with substance-related, sexual, gender identity, and impulsive disorders. Females are more likely to be diagnosed with depression, anxiety, somatization, dissociative, and eating disorders. Diagnoses of personality disorders tend to parallel expected sex differences in personality traits or even gender stereotypes: Females are reported to have higher rates of borderline, histrionic, and dependent personality disorders; males are reported to have higher rates of paranoid, schizoid, schizotypal, antisocial, and compulsive personality disorders.

The DSM–IV–TR (2000) relies on the best available data for making its estimates of sex differences in prevalence rates; but how good are these data? How do we know how many individual girls, boys, women, or men actually experience a certain psychological disorder? Widiger (1998) cites six ways in which diagnoses may reflect a sex bias: "(1) biased diagnostic constructs, (2) biased diagnostic thresholds, (3) biased application of the diagnostic criteria, (4) biased sampling of persons with the disorder, (5) biased instruments of assessment, and/or (6) biased diagnostic criteria" (p. 96). Using these categories as a basis for understanding gender bias in diagnosis, we will discuss biases in diagnostic standards (e.g., constructs, criteria, and thresholds), biased applications of these diagnostic standards, including assessment instruments, and biased sampling.

Biased Diagnostic Standards

Critics of DSM–III (1980) and DSM–III–R (1987) argued that the diagnostic constructs themselves were sexist and that women are pathologized by DSM diagnostic criteria (Brown, 1992; Caplan, 1991, 1995; Kaplan, 1983; Walker, 1994). This point was argued most often in reference to the personality disorders. Histrionic personality disorder and dependent personality disorder have been cited as the most egregious examples of gendered, in this case feminine, traits being used to establish the presence of psychopathology (Kaplan, 1983). Kaplan (1983) proposed "independent personality disorder" and "restricted personality disorder," and Pantony and Caplan (1991) suggested "delusional dominating personality disorder" as comparable, but masculine stereotyped, disorders. Others, however, argued that DSM–III already includes personality disorders that captured maladaptive masculine traits, specifically, antisocial personality disorder and compulsive personality disorder (Williams & Spitzer, 1983).

Ross, Frances, and Widiger (1995) suggest: "The DSM–III/DSM–III–R personality disorder criteria were constructed, for the most part, by males with little input from systematic empirical research. It would not be surprising to find that male clinicians would have a lower threshold for the attribution of maladaptive feminine traits than for the attribution of maladaptive masculine traits" (p. 212). They describe how the DSM–IV Personality Disorders Work Group addressed this problem both by extensive reviews of existing empirical research and by creating more gender-neutral criteria. For example, the histrionic personality disorder item "inappropriately sexually seductive in appearance or behavior" (DSM–III–R, 1987) was changed to "interaction with others is often characterized by inappropriate sexually seductive or provocative behavior." Removing the reference to "appearance" was intended to reduce the possibility that the normal female response to social pressure to appear physically attractive might be viewed as "inappropriately sexually seductive."

DSM–III–R (1987) also introduced an appendix titled "Proposed Diagnostic Categories Needing Further Study." All three proposed categories—late luteal phase dysphoric disorder, sadistic personality disorder, and self-defeating personality disorder—were controversial (Ross, Frances, & Widiger, 1995). Critics argued that the term *late luteal phase disorder* might stigmatize women by making behavioral reactions related to the menstrual cycle a mental disorder. Questions about the empirical base for including this category as a DSM disorder were also raised. Based on extensive reviews of the research literature and data reanalyses, the work group suggested renaming the disorder premenstrual dysphoric disorder and continuing to include it in an appendix that for DSM–IV is titled "Criteria Sets and Axes Provided for Further Study." The term *self-defeating personality disorder* was particularly disturbing to some because of its potential for being used to pathologize victims of abuse. The proposed criteria make an abusive environment an exclusion criterion, but it was unclear how this approach might be used in practice. A concern with the term *sadistic personality disorder* was that criminal behavior (e.g., assault, abuse) might be labeled a mental illness. In the end neither self-defeating personality disorder nor sadistic personality disorder was retained in DSM–IV, based primarily on their having been the focus of very little research (Ross, Frances, & Widiger, 1995). This brief description of a lengthy process indicates the ways in which the establishment of constructs that comprise a diagnostic system such as the DSM is a very human process, influenced inevitably by both subjective and objective judgments (as noted in chap. 1).

Other diagnostic categories also represent a challenge for gender neutrality. Somatization disorder is a disorder reported to range from "0.2% to 2% among women and less than 0.2% in men" (DSM–IV, 1994, p. 447). Although substantial revisions were made to make criteria less sex biased, DSM–IV retains criteria that make a diagnosis in men unlikely. Clients must meet all of the four criteria, and the symptoms reported must be found to be not fully explained by a medical condition. Set 3 is "one sexual or reproductive symptom other than pain." The examples given include four symptoms that apply exclusively to women (irregular menses, excessive menstrual bleeding, vomiting throughout pregnancy), one that applies to men (erectile or ejaculatory dysfunction), and one that may apply more often to women (sexual indifference) (DSM–IV, p. 449). These symptoms may be the most valid criteria for somatization disorder, especially for women, but they also tend to exclude men. Hartung and Widiger (1998) make this point and conclude: "Research on the epidemiology of the disorder therefore continues to use a criteria set that is biased against making the diagnosis in males, complicating any identification of the disorder in males" (p. 269). They further point out that the World Health Organization criteria for this disorder, although still including menstrual symptoms, also list gastrointestinal symptoms, abnormal skin sensations, and blotchiness as common symptoms, resulting in this disorder being reported more frequently in males within other cultures.

The question of criterion bias is further complicated by the issue of the diagnostic validity of specific symptoms for females and males. The purpose of gathering information about a client's feelings, thoughts, and behaviors is to identify a psychological disorder. It may be the case that certain symptoms are predictive of a diagnostic category, future symptoms, or responsiveness to treatment for males but not for females or vice versa. An example from the arena of physical illness illustrates this problem. Although heart disease is the #1 killer of both women and men in the United States and more women than men have died from heart disease every year since 1984 (Giardina, 2000), heart disease is still generally regarded as a greater problem for men than for women. Symptoms of a heart attack (e.g., tightness or discomfort in the chest, spreading pain in the arms, back, jaw, or stomach) are widely advertised because seeking medical treatment quickly is critical to preventing or limiting the damage caused by a heart attack. It is estimated, however, that 35% of heart attacks in women are unreported. Women having heart attacks are as likely as men to experience chest pain, but they are somewhat more likely to experience other symptoms, such as breathlessness, perspiration, nausea, and a sensation of fluttering in the heart (Giardina, 2000). An unfamiliar constellation of symptoms may prevent women or health professionals from suspecting the presence of heart disease. In the case of heart attacks, although the underlying condition is the same, the presenting symptoms for women and men are somewhat different. It is likely that for some psychological disorders a similar process occurs. Being able to identify a criterion that is differentially valid for females or males requires a diagnostic system that is independent of this criterion. In the case of heart disease, whatever the presenting symptoms, the presence or absence of a myocardial infarction can be assessed independently. For psychological disorders, there is no similar confirmation. In reference to establishing criteria for personality disorders, Robins and Guze (1970) advocated for validation studies that would "assess the extent to which the criteria select persons who have a history, present, and/or future consistent with the construct of a (particular) personality disorder" (p. 17). One might also suggest a validity test that considers the effectiveness of standard interventions for persons with and without a particular diagnostic criterion.

Widiger (chap. 4) recognizes that a challenge for DSM–V, the next edition of DSM, will be addressing the problem of making diagnostic criteria more gender neutral (i.e., criteria that apply equally to females and males) or developing separate sets of criteria, at least for some disorders, for females and males. This debate has been particularly salient to the diagnosis of conduct disorder and will be explored further in that section.

According to DSM–IV (1994), "The definition of *mental disorder* . . . requires that there be clinically significant impairment or distress" (p. 7). Thresholds for diagnoses should represent the point at which the accumulation of symptoms reaches this level of impairment or distress. But where is it? The issue of thresholds is one of the arguments for a continuous rather than categorical view of psychopathology (Maddux, 2002), but it remains the case that clinicians and clinical researchers are regularly faced with the task of a present/absent decision in regard to the diagnosis of pathology. Prevalence of a disorder among women and men will be affected by the setting of this threshold; and for disorders more often diagnosed in women or in men the setting of this threshold will affect overall rates of psychopathology for the sexes. It is important to note that, for the most part, the number of criteria needed to reach threshold for a DSM–IV diagnosis is established by committee rather than by empirical research that would justify that particular number.

In an effort to determine the relative pathology represented by female-typed and male-typed personality disorders, Funtowicz and Widiger (1995) identified college student participants at the threshold of the disorders and then examined their levels of social and occupational dysfunction. They found lower levels of dysfunction for male-typed disorders, suggesting that "it might be relatively easier to obtain a male-typed personality disorder diagnosis than some female-typed personality disorder diagnoses" (Funtowicz & Widiger, 1995, p. 157). Whether males or females are more in danger of biased diagnoses, without thresholds established through research, the DSM is vulnerable to the criticism of gender bias in diagnostic thresholds.

Biased Application of the Diagnostic Criteria

Diagnosis may also involve objective tests or structured or semistructured interviews. Although bias often suggests subjectivity in judgment, standardized tests can also contain sex or gender bias. Lindsay and Widiger (1995) have argued that any self-report or interview response that does not reflect dysfunction but does apply to one sex more than the other represents a sex-biased item. A gender-biased item is related to gender (femininity or masculinity) but not to psychopathology. A biased item occurs when men or women (sex bias) or masculine or feminine persons (gender bias) are more likely to endorse the item. The item itself is not a symptom, nor is it related to general psychopathology, but it does contribute to a scale that measures a personality disorder. Using college students, Lindsay and Widiger (1995) determined that 13% to 31% of the items from three standardized measures of personality disorder showed some evidence of sex or gender bias according to these criteria. In a follow-up study Lindsay, Sankis, and Widiger (2000) used outpatients from mental health clinics and updated versions of the instruments: Millon Clinical Multiaxial Inventory–III (MMCI–III), Minnesota Multiphasic Personality Inventory–II (MMPI–II), and Personality Diagnostic Questionnaire–Revised (PDQ–R). Four personality disorder scales (histrionic, dependent, antisocial, and narcissistic) from these instruments were analyzed for sex or gender bias. None of the scale scores from any of the inventories was related to biological sex. Only three scale items showed sex bias (women or men were more likely to endorse them but the item was unrelated to a measure of psychopathology, the Personality Assessment Inventory), whereas 36 items suggested gender bias—that is, the item correlated with a measure of femininity or masculinity but not with the measure of psychopathology. An example of an item that demonstrated sex bias and gender bias was "It's very easy for me to make many friends" from the MCMI–III Histrionic scale. This item is not indicative of a psychological problem, but it does contribute to a higher score for histrionic personality disorder. It is also more frequently endorsed by women than men and it correlates positively with measures of femininity. This item, then, would tend to give women and feminine individuals higher scores for histrionic personality disorder while endorsing an item that does not represent a maladaptive trait or behavior. Although the few items (three) demonstrating sex bias were all from the Histrionic scales, more examples of gender bias were from the Narcissistic scale, suggesting that masculine individuals may receive a higher score by endorsing items that reflect adaptive, rather than pathological, characteristics.

Regardless of the care taken to establish reliable and valid diagnostic tools, the clinicians using the tools may be affected by their own gender stereotypes in applying them, as has been shown to occur in numerous analogue studies. In analogue studies clinicians are presented with case histories that are identical except for the sex of the patient. Half of the clinicians in the research diagnose the "female patient," and half diagnose the "male patient." Given the same information, will clinicians come to the same or different conclusions about the presence of psychological disorders? Warner (1978) gave clinicians ambiguous patient profiles, with a mixture of hysterical and antisocial symptoms (e.g., suicide attempts, no close relationships, self-centered, shoplifting with no remorse for crime, flirtatious). Female profiles were more likely than male profiles to be labeled hysterical (76% vs. 49%), and male profiles were more likely than female to be labeled antisocial (41% vs. 22%). It can be argued that with ambiguous information, clinicians rely on base rates (women are more likely to be hysterical; men are more likely to be antisocial). The base rates themselves, however, may also represent a biased accumulation of data on women and men. If clinicians use stereotyped perceptions of women and men in their diagnoses (as these studies indicate), then the data based on their clinical judgments will be biased.

To circumvent the issue of base rates, many studies have presented clinicians with cases that meet the DSM criteria for one or more disorders. Ford and Widiger (1989) created cases based on DSM–III criteria for histrionic and antisocial personality disorders: One case met diagnostic criteria for antisocial personality disorder, one met criteria for histrionic personality disorder, and one failed to reach diagnostic criteria for either. Histrionic personality disorder was more frequently diagnosed in women, even when the case contained more antisocial than histrionic criteria; and antisocial personality disorder was less often diagnosed in women. Adler, Drake, and Teague (1990) developed one case history that met the explicit criteria of four diagnoses: histrionic, narcissistic, borderline, and dependent. Men were more likely to receive a diagnosis of narcissistic personality disorder; women, histrionic personality disorder. There were no differences for borderline or dependent (which was rarely used) personality disorder. In research using a case that met the criteria of borderline personality disorder (BPD) and posttraumatic stress disorder, however, women did receive higher ratings for BPD (Becker & Lamb, 1994). Fernbach, Winstead, and Derlega (1989) created separate cases for antisocial and somatization disorders and found that there were no sex-of-vignette differences for somatization disorder; but for antisocial personality disorder, although most cases were accurately diagnosed, men (73%) were more likely than women (53%) to receive the diagnosis. Loring and Powell (1988) included both personality disordered (dependent) and psychotic (undifferentiated schizophrenia) symptoms in the cases to be diagnosed and race (Black vs. White) as well as gender as demographic characteristics of the case. They also examined gender and race of the diagnosing psychiatrists as influences on the diagnostic process. They found that similarity in race and gender between clinician and client produced the most accurate diagnoses, that male clinicians overdiagnosed depression and histrionic personality disorder in women, and that all clinicians overdiagnosed paranoia in Black clients. This study reinforces the conclusion that gender has a powerful influence on diagnosis, but complicates the picture by indicating that race also matters and that the demographic characteristics of the diagnosing clinician may interact with client characteristics to affect diagnosis.

If the diagnostic criteria for a disorder are built into a description of the client, then the presence of clinician bias represents a failure to adhere to the DSM diagnostic criteria. Clinicians are coming up with the "wrong" answer when they indicate a diagnostic category other than the one intended. Ford and Widiger (1989) demonstrated that at the level of individual criteria, there is no sex bias. Specific behaviors were rated as indicative of histrionic personality disorders and antisocial personality disorder with equal frequency for men and women. But they did find sex bias when assigning clients to one of these diagnostic categories. Ford and Widiger (1989) concluded that histrionic personality disorder was overdiagnosed in women and underdiagnosed in men. Blashfield and Herkov (1996) and Morey and Ochoa (1989) looked at clinicians' ratings of DSM criteria for their own patients and compared ratings on individual criteria with actual diagnoses of these patients. They found weak associations between clinicians' ratings of the criteria and the clinicians' diagnoses, suggesting that giving a diagnosis does not necessarily involve an objective formula based on the presence or absence or the total number of certain criteria. Morey and Ochoa (1989) found that clinicians overdiagnose antisocial personality disorder in men and BPD in women, although Blashfield and Herkov (1996) did not replicate these findings. The absence of sex bias for specific criteria in contrast to the presence of sex bias in assigning DSM-based diagnosis suggests that dimensional approaches to diagnosis may be less prone to bias than categorical labels, as judgments in the dimensional approach remain at the level of behavioral indicators rather than a summary diagnostic decision.

These studies indicate that clinicians do use sex of patient as information that affects their judgment about the diagnosis of a case. Some diagnoses are more prone to this bias than others, and the bias may be primarily at the level of categorization rather than at the level of judging if a particular trait or behavior is present. Although analogue studies allow the researcher to present clinicians with identical information while varying sex of patient, the responses of clinicians to paper-and-pencil or even audio or video versions of a patient cannot completely capture the more interactive process that actually occurs during diagnosis, a process that may be even more susceptible to bias.

Gender bias in the application of criteria is a reality in the practice of mental health care. Furthermore, to the degree that accurate diagnosis leads to more effective treatment of disorders, these biases that lead to inaccurate diagnoses are particularly troublesome.

Biased Sampling

The most convenient data for analysis of prevalence rates are data obtained in clinical settings. When individuals come into a clinical setting (either by their own volition or by the actions of others (e.g., parent, courts)), they generally receive a diagnosis. Assuming diagnoses are accurately obtained, these data would appear to be a good source of information. But do all individuals with a particular disorder show up in a clinical setting? Factors bringing adults into a clinical setting include willingness to acknowledge the symptoms, willingness to seek treatment, or the persuasive or coercive influence of others. Factors bringing children into a clinical setting include parents' and teachers' perceptions of the severity of the problem and of the possibilities for treatment. These factors are likely to be influenced by the sex of the affected individual. Women may be more likely to recognize and less resistant to acknowledging that symptoms are indicative of an emotional problem that needs treatment (Yoder, Shute, & Tryban, 1990). For children the diagnostic categories that appear in the DSM are likely influenced by what parents and teachers consider problematic. Although internalizing (e.g., anxiety, depression) and externalizing (e.g., conduct disorder; attention deficit hyperactivity disorder, ADHD) problems are recognized by experts in childhood psychopathology, externalizing disorders are more likely to cause problems in the school setting as well as at home, creating additional pressures on the family to seek some intervention. To the extent that gender ratios in clinical populations are the result of gender differences in help seeking, problem recognition, tolerance/intolerance for symptoms by self or others, or attitude toward mental health care, then gender differences in prevalence rates in clinical settings will reflect these differences and not just true differences in the occurrence of the psychological disorder.

The solution to this dilemma is epidemiological studies with community samples. In these studies, interviewers contact individuals in representative samples and acquire information about symptoms. Diagnosis is accomplished independently of the participants' acknowledgement or concern about the disorder. Whereas gender differences in clinical populations reflect gender differences in the psychological disorders plus gender differences in various nondisordered behaviors such as help seeking, gender differences in community samples will not have this problem. For numerous disorders, DSM–IV–TR (2000) cites discrepancies in community versus clinical samples or suggests that clinical data may over- or underrepresent females or males because of disorder-specific factors that encourage or discourage treatment seeking. For example, trichotillomania (compulsive hair pulling) is seen more often in women in clinical settings, but women may be more inclined to seek treatment for such an appearance-altering problem. More men than women seek help for gambling, but female gamblers may feel stigmatized and unwilling to seek treatment (see Hartung and Widiger, 1998). Ideally, every disorder would have an adequate and current base of epidemiological data from community samples. This is not the case, and often statements about gender differences in prevalence rates are based on potentially biased clinical samples.

TREATMENT

During the 1970s and 1980s the discipline of clinical psychology, like other areas of research and practice, was strongly influenced by the feminist movement. In the review of the impact of gender on diagnosis, the voices of female (and male) critics of the potentially male-biased creators of the DSM were heard again and again. These critics raised important questions that led to research, reviews of research, and careful scrutiny of the criteria and diagnoses that make up DSM–IV–TR (2000). It is unlikely that gender bias has been completely removed from the manual or from the subjective processes that lead to diagnostic decisions in clinics and clinicians' offices, but awareness of these issues is an important step in the right direction. At the same time, clinicians and researchers began to focus on another area where gender may matter, that is, therapeutic outcomes. Are women or men, girls or boys, more likely to benefit from therapy? While the examination of sex and gender bias in diagnosis turns out to be fairly complicated, the search for the answer to this seemingly simple question about therapy outcomes is even more complex. In their "gold standard" *Handbook of Psychotherapy and Behavior Change*, Bergin and Garfield (1994) include lengthy chapters dealing with client variables, therapist variables, process variables, four different therapeutic approaches, and seven chapters on special groups and settings. In order to answer the question "Does sex affect treatment?," we need to consider at minimum the sex of the therapist, the type of therapy (e.g., cognitive, behavioral, family, psychopharmacological), the length of therapy, the therapy setting, and the type of problem being treated (e.g., depression, substance abuse). Many studies do not have the methodological controls that allow for random assignment of clients to therapists and therapists to clients, making therapist or client sex nonexperimental variables. A further complexity is that sex may interact with other important variables (e.g., ethnicity, client motivation, therapist training or years of experience).

Influence of Sex of Therapist on Therapy Outcomes

Perhaps in part as the result of the influx of women into the mental health professions, there was a strong interest in the 70s and 80s in the impact of therapist sex on therapeutic outcomes. In a substantial review article of the effective ingredients in psychotherapy, Gomes-Schwartz, Hadley, and Strupp (1978) concluded that there was no evidence that therapist sex per se is related to therapist effectiveness.

Beutler, Marchado, and Neufeldt (1994) reviewed several studies and concluded that there are "weak and largely negative conclusions" (p. 233) concerning the influence of sex of therapist on outcomes. Jones and Zoppel (1982), however, obtained self-reports from clients and therapists regarding the results of therapy. Female clients paired with female therapists were perceived by both clients and therapists as having experienced the most positive outcomes, suggesting that sex matching made the difference. This study did not randomly assign clients to therapists nor did it provide any external or objective assessment of therapy results. Jones, Krupnick, and Kerig (1987), however, in research that did randomly assign 60 women to 11 male or 14 female therapists found greater symptomatic improvement at the end of treatment and at follow-up for the clients assigned to female therapists. Because there were no male clients in this study, the relative advantage of having a female therapist may be a sex-of-therapist effect or a sex-matching effect.

In a recent study, Zlotnick, Elkin, and Shea (1998) took advantage of an exceptional opportunity to investigate sex-of-therapist effects in a well-controlled study, the National Institute of Mental Health Treatment of Depression Collaborative Research Program (TDCRP). In this research all clients were experiencing major depression and were assigned randomly to different treatment conditions, but also to either a female or male therapist. Attrition, treatment outcome (based on the Hamilton Rating Scale for Depression), and client-reported therapist empathy were assessed. Analyses revealed that "among depressed patients, a male or female therapist, or same- versus opposite-gender pairing, was not significantly related to level of depression at termination, to attrition rates, or to the patient's perceptions of the therapist's degree of empathy early in treatment and at termination" (Zlotnick et al., 1998. p. 657). Clients' beliefs about whether a female or male therapist would be more helpful were also assessed before therapy, but these beliefs had no impact on outcomes whether they were assigned to the person they believed would be more helpful or not.

Another study considered sex- and race-matching factors in the treatment of substance abuse. Sterling, Gottheil, Weinstein, and Serota (2001) found no effects for either race- or sex-matching in terms of retention or outcome in a study of African American cocaine-dependent persons.

Together these studies demonstrate no overall difference in outcomes for male or female therapists, but suggest the possibility that female therapist–female client pairs have in some cases better therapeutic results than male therapist–female client pairs.

Influence of Sex of Client on Therapy Outcomes

Garfield (1994) reviewed studies concerning the impact of sex of client on therapy outcomes and concluded that "one cannot make much of a case for sex of client as a significant variable related to outcome in psychotherapy" (p. 208). Examining various demographic variables as predictors of outcome or differential treatment effects in the TDCRP, Elkin (1994) found no evidence that sex of client had a significant effect. A review of the literature since 1994 shows that questions regarding the influence of sex of client on therapy has generated relatively little research. Thase et al. (1994) examined men and women in a study of the efficacy of cognitive therapy for outpatients with major depression. Men and women had similar outcomes; however, clients with higher pretreatment depression scores had poorer outcomes, and among this subset of severely depressed clients, women had significantly poorer outcomes than men.

A 1992 general review of treatment outcomes for abusers of alcohol, drugs, and nicotine found that women and men most often had equal therapeutic results, with women's sometimes being better than men's (Toneatto, Sobel, & Sobel, 1992). More recent studies confirm these findings. Triffleman (2001) tested two treatment protocols on individuals with coexisting substance dependence and posttraumatic stress disorder (PTSD). Although women showed signs of greater severity at the beginning of treatment, there were no sex differences at the end of treatment or follow-up in either PTSD or substance abuse. Similarly, in an outpatient addiction treatment center Galen, Brower, Gillespie, and Zucker (2000) found that women had greater psychiatric severity than did men at the beginning of treatment but that there were no sex differences in outcomes. Another study compared treatment funding (fee-for-service vs. managed care) and treatment outcomes for cocaine- or alcohol-dependent men and women. Neither funding type nor sex of client was related to treatment outcome (Alterman, Randall, & McLellan, 2000). Finally, a randomized clinical trial evaluating pharmacotherapies for cocaine abuse found more severe drug problems for women at intake, but no sex differences at trial's end and more positive outcomes for women at the six-month follow-up (Kosten, Gawin, Kosten, & Rounsaville, 1993). Although these studies found no sex differences in therapy outcome, the higher level of problem severity for women at the beginning of the studies suggests that women made greater gains during therapy than did men.

Issues about women's special needs in substance abuse treatment have been discussed (Wilke, 1994). Treatments included in the studies reviewed previously were all outpatient programs. Many interventions for substance abuse or addiction rely, however, on inpatient treatment. Some women may be unable to participate in inpatient treatment or need to terminate treatment prematurely because of child-care issues. Although the extent of this problem is not known, some women in need of inpatient treatment may be the sole caregiver for their children (Wilke, 1994). Questions have also been raised about differences in the effectiveness of single-sex versus mixed-sex treatment groups. Dahlgren and Willander (1989) found that women in a single-sex group reported better social adjustment and lower alcohol consumption at a two-year follow-up than did women in a mixed-sex group.

Studies of smoking interventions also have found few effects for sex of client. In a study of 1,978 smokers receiving clinician advice and nurse-assisted intervention, women and men did not differ in participation in each step of the intervention nor in reported quit attempts and cessation at three and twelve months nor in relapse twelve months later. Women did, however, use a greater number and variety of smoking-cessation strategies (Whitlock, Vogt, Hollis, & Lichtenstein, 1997). In a study of sustained smoking cessation (after three years), men had a higher rate of quitting than women. These gender differences were, however, largely explained by gender differences in demographics and smoking history (Bjornson, Rand, Connett, & Lindgren, 1995).

Possible Exceptions to No Effects for Sex of Client or Therapist

Although most studies have found that sex of client and sex of therapist have relatively little impact on the outcome of psychotherapy, there are particular circumstances in which differences may occur. Liddle (1996) examined therapist sex and sexual orientation as predictors of gay and lesbian clients' reports of therapist practices. She found that gay or bisexual male therapists and gay, bisexual, or heterosexual female therapists were rated as equally helpful but more helpful than heterosexual male therapists. The fact that men generally have less positive attitudes toward homosexuality than women may help explain why heterosexual male therapists were perceived as least helpful (Liddle, 1996). The therapist's attitude toward client sexual orientation may be a better predictor of outcome than sex or sexual orientation per se.

Certain deleterious effects of psychotherapy are also more likely to occur in some sex-of-therapist–sex-of-client combinations. For example, data suggest that sexual relationships occur between therapist and client in 5% to 6% of therapy relationships with 85% of these involving a male therapist with a female client (Lamb & Catanzaro, 1998). This particular negative therapeutic experience is clearly more likely to affect women.

Sex differences in the presentation and course of a mental disorder can represent a challenge for achieving sex equality in therapy outcomes. For example, although bipolar disorder (with depressive and manic episodes) occurs with equal frequency in women and men (DSM–IV–TR, 2000), women are more likely than men to experience rapid cycling, more frequent depressive episodes, and the type of bipolar disorder that includes depressive and hypomanic (vs. manic) episodes (DSM–IV, 1994; Leibenluft, 1997). Rapid cycling is particularly difficult to treat, suggesting that women will be overrepresented in the group of clients who do not respond positively to treatment (Leibenluft, 1997). The assumption, however, that women might be less responsive to lithium maintenance is challenged by a recent study that found that women showed better (albeit not statistically significantly different) responses to lithium treatment and a significantly longer median time than did men before a first recurrence of illness (Viguera, Baldessarini, & Tondo, 2001). Women in this study, however, did not show a greater episode frequency and so did not represent the rapid cycling subgroup of concern to clinicians.

Studies have also found reliable sex differences in schizophrenia. Although there are no established sex differences in presenting symptoms in acute phases of the disorder, men experience more negative symptoms (e.g., flat affect, social withdrawal) and women are more likely to be diagnosed as paranoid, to experience later onset of the disorder and better premorbid adjustment, and to maintain a higher level of functioning during the course of the illness and be less aggressive and self-destructive ((DSM–IV–TR, 2000; Tamminga, 1997). Female schizophrenics also respond better and more rapidly to pharmacological treatment and require lower doses than men in both acute episodes (Szymanski, Lieberman, Alvir, & Mayerhoff, 1995) and ongoing treatment (Tamminga, 1997).

Sex Differences for Psychopharmacology

In previous decades, the exclusion of women from clinical drug trials and the failure to analyze data for sex differences led to a lack of information about the differential responses of women and men to psychopharmacological treatment. In the 1990s the federal government issued guidelines intended to make women's health, mental health, and treatment issues a greater priority in federally funded research (Blumenthal, 1995).

Effects of sex differences in drug treatment may include absorption, distribution, metabolism, and elimination, all of which affect the bioavailability of the therapeutic substance. Women tend to have more fat tissue than men, which affects the metabolism and storage of drugs. Women's endogenous (e.g., menstrual cycle, pregnancy, postpartum, menopause) and exogenous (e.g., birth control pills; hormone replacement therapy, HRT) hormone levels also affect drug response (Yonkers & Hamilton, 1995). Estrogens, for example, tend to increase the effectiveness of some antipsychotic drugs (Seeman, 1995), meaning that women may be treated with lower doses; but, they may also experience more side effects or toxicity from doses that are safe in men (Yonkers & Hamilton, 1995). Research suggests that estrogen affects metabolic processes and drug response, and estrogen has been tried with mixed to positive results, alone and combined with antidepressants, in treatment for women with refractory depression and for postmenopausal women (Casper, 1998; Kornstein, 1997). Research also suggests that women respond more poorly than men to some medications (e.g., triclyclics) and better than men to others (e.g., SSRIs). Women are also more likely than men to be exposed to more than one psychoactive drug because of a greater incidence of comorbidity (see below), and so drug interaction effects must be considered (Casper, 1998).

Finally, psychological disorders, especially depression, frequently occur in women twenty to forty-five years of age, years when women are likely to bear children. The effects of psychopharmacological agents on maternal health, the health of the developing fetus, and lactation must be understood. To date research suggests that benzodiazepines (antianxiety drugs) lead to craniofacial abnormalities and, when taken in late pregnancy, floppy infant syndrome; lithium (used in treating bipolar disorder) has been associated with cardiovascular, central nervous system, and mental and physical abnormalities; antidepressant medications have shown no adverse effects in some investigations, but small increased risks of miscarriage or deformities in others; research on the effects of antipsychotics is also mixed (Casper, 1998). Clearly research clarifying the effects of medication during various stages of pregnancy and during lactation is critical.

Gender and Comorbidity

Another issue facing therapists in their efforts to provide effective treatment to both women and men is gender differences in comorbidity, that is, the assignment of more than one diagnostic category to a client. Clients presenting with a primary disorder frequently have other symptoms that need treatment. Epidemiological studies suggest that comorbidity is particularly evident in women (Kessler et al., 1994; Marsh & Casper, 1998). For example, the relatively common co-occurrence of anxiety and depression affects women perhaps twice as often as men (Marsh & Casper, 1998). Women with substance abuse disorders are found to have more affective disorders, especially major depression, than men with substance abuse disorders (Benishek, Bieschke, Stoffelmayr, Mavis, & Humphries, 1992). Other studies have found that women with substance abuse also report more family, social, employment, and other psychiatric problems than men (Alterman et al., 2000; Brown, Alterman, Rutherford, Cacciola, & Zabalero, 1993). Also, although both substance abuse and antisocial personality disorder occur at higher rates in men than women, their comorbidity appears to be higher for women. In other words, the likelihood of a diagnosis of antisocial personality disorder given the presence of alcohol dependence has been found to be greater for women than for men (Kessler, Crum, Warner, Nelson, Schulenberg, & Anthony, 1997; Lewis & Bucholz, 1991). Furthermore, the presence of antisocial personality disorder may lead to less positive change during treatment (Galen et al., 2000). In addition, women with schizophrenia, compared to schizophrenic men, are more likely to have depressive symptoms, in addition to psychotic symptoms, that also require treatment (Seeman, 1995). Finally, certain distressing life events linked to mental disorders, such as incest, sexual abuse, and rape, occur more frequently in the lives of women. PTSD, linked to traumatic events, occurs more often in women than men; and a higher rate of comorbidity is associated with PTSD (Wong & Yehuda, 2002). Increased comorbidity generally leads to a higher level of personal distress, disability, and chronicity (Marsh & Casper, 1998). Clients presenting with multiple problems may be less responsive to treatment. Studies of treatment outcomes, however, often control for diagnosis by selecting participants with just one diagnosis. To the extent that women are more likely than men to be given more than one diagnosis, these studies will be less representative of women. Furthermore, therapies considered efficacious based on this research may not be effective for women (and men) with multiple diagnoses.

SPECIFIC DISORDERS: DEPRESSION

Evidence suggests that some disorders are diagnosed more often in one sex than the other. If this is so, why? Given the presence of a diagnosis, we also want to know if standard treatments for the disorders are equally effective for both sexes and if sex is taken into account when applying and assessing these treatments.

Sex Differences in the Diagnosis of Depression

Women are more likely to experience depression than men (Burt, 2002; Culbertson, 1997; Kornstein, 1997; Nolen-Hoeksema, Larson, & Grayson, 1999; Sprock & Yoder, 1997; Wolk & Weissman, 1995). Epidemiological studies in the United States and other developed countries consistently find that women are more likely to experience major depression, and dysthymia, but not bipolar affective disorder, than men (Culbertson, 1997; Sprock & Yoder, 1997; Wolk & Weissman, 1995). Data from less developed countries are inconsistent, sometimes finding no sex difference in depression (Culbertson, 1997). In the United States, not only do women seek treatment for depression more often than men, but, according to interview studies conducted in the community among those who never seek treatment, women are more likely to meet diagnostic criteria for these depressive disorders. The consensus is that the female-to-male ratio for depression is 2:1 and for major depression it may be 3:1 or 4:1 (Culbertson, 1997). This sex difference has been found across ethnic groups (African American, Caucasian, Hispanic). Women also experience more chronic and recurring depressive episodes and more seasonal affective disorder (Burt, 2002; Kornstein, 1997). Finally, women experience more comorbidity than men. Disorders that may be present at the same time as depression include anxiety, phobias, eating disorders, PTSD, as well as medical conditions such as migraine or chronic fatigue syndrome (Burt, 2002).

There are reliable and valid standardized assessment tools for depression—for example, the Beck Depression Inventory (BDI) and Hamilton Rating Scale for Depression. Item analyses for gender bias of the BDI with a large sample of depressed outpatients and nonpatients found little evidence for gender item bias. The only problematic item was an item assessing distortion of body image, an item endorsed more often by women (Santor, Ramsay, & Zuroff, 1994). On the other hand, Sprock and Yoder (1997) reviewed studies that suggest that circumstances and age may affect the validity of these instruments. When scales were described as measures of depression, items were endorsed less often by men than by women; but there was no sex difference when the instruments were described as hassles scales (Page & Bennesch, 1993). In a sample of geriatric patients hospitalized for major unipolar depression, Allen-Burge, Storandt, Kincherf, & Rubin (1994) found that the BDI and the Geriatric Depression Scale were more likely to detect depression in elderly women than in elderly men. In addition, depressed women report more symptoms of depression than do depressed men, even when clinicians' judgments of severity of depression do not differ, leading Sprock and Yoder (1997) to suggest that the number of criteria for diagnosis of depression should perhaps be greater for women than for men. Clinician bias also remains a problem. Potts, Burnam, and Wells (1991) compared clinicians' judgments to diagnoses made with a standardized interview assessment and found that there were discrepancies between standardized assessment and clinician judgments in that medical practitioners were less likely to diagnose depression in men and mental health practitioners were more likely to diagnose depression in women. Clearly in the real world of persons interacting with health and mental health practitioners, diagnosis of depression, as with other disorders, is not free of sex bias.

Explaining the Sex Difference in Depression

The repeated confirmation of the finding that women are twice as likely as men to suffer from depression has led to studies that attempt to explain this sex difference in depression. Most explanations of sex differences are biological, sociocultural, or some combination of each. "Women have a particularly increased vulnerability to depressive disorders during the childbearing years [when]... women shoulder myriad role responsibilities, are more likely to experience sexual and domestic violence, and are frequently disadvantaged in terms of both social and financial status. Also, during these years, many women experience both pregnancy and the postpartum" (Burt, 2002, pp. 101–102). That these reproductive years include both environmental and biological stressors makes identifying causal factors difficult.

Biological explanations of sex differences in depression have been sought primarily in hormonal and neurophysiological differences between women and men. Some markers that distinguish the depressed from the nondepressed—greater global and regional cerebral metabolic rate of glucose utilization, response to the dexamethasone suppression test, lower levels of natural killer cells—also demonstrate sex differences, with women responding more like depressed persons (Sprock & Yoder, 1997). The influence of hormones on women's depression is suggested by the fact that rates of depression are similar in girls and boys before puberty (see chap. 16, "Internalizing Disorders") and that the sex difference is less pronounced in the elderly (Sprock & Yoder; 1997; Wolk & Weissman, 1995). A direct connection between hormone levels and depression, however, has not been demonstrated. Nor has an association between menopause and depression been supported by empirical research (Wolk & Weissman, 1995). On the other hand, women are at increased risk for psychiatric illness immediately following childbirth. Levels of estrogen and progesterone drop dramatically with the expulsion of the placenta following childbirth. However, direct correlations between hormone levels and postpartum blues, postpartum depression, or postpartum psychosis have not been found. It is true that a history of depression or psychiatric illness is a risk factor in postpartum psychosis or depression; and a history of one postpartum illness predicts subsequent ones (30% to 50% for postpartum depression; 20% to 33% for postpartum psychosis) (Kornstein, 1997; Wolk & Weissman, 1995).

Sociocultural explanations of depression are concerned with life events, social roles, and cognitive and coping styles. For example, stressful life events and marital problems are risk factors for postpartum depression (Wolk & Weissman, 1995). Women are also more likely than men to cite a stressful life event in the six months before the onset of a major depressive episode, and they are not only more reactive to stress in their own lives but also in the lives of those with whom they have relationships (Kornstein, 1997). Even having supportive family networks can be less rather than more helpful for some women. Veiel (1993) found that women who were homemakers and reported having a supportive family were less likely than men or working women to recover from major depression. For these women the demands of family relationships may have done more harm than the support a family can provide.

Some psychologists have proposed that gender socialization of women leads them to have an experience of learned helplessness which predisposes them to depression, although direct links between learned helplessness and higher rates of depression have not been demonstrated (Wolk & Weissman, 1995). In many cases the association between relationship or cognitive variables and depression may not reflect a causal influence of the former variables, but rather an effect of depression on how people think or interact with others. In a longitudinal study (one year) of adults across the age span, Nolen-Hoeksema et al. (1999) were able to demonstrate that women experience more chronic strain, lower sense of mastery, and more rumination than men and that these factors mediated the sex differences in depression; that is, sex was no longer a significant predictor of depression at time two (one year later) when the influence of these variables was removed. Chronic strain, low mastery, and rumination interacted in complex ways to predict depression, and depressive symptoms also contributed to more rumination and less mastery. In this study, rumination and low sense of mastery were particularly strong predictors of depression and, assuming they also contribute to the sex difference in depression, we are nevertheless left with the question of how sex differences in rumination and sense of mastery come about.

Sex Differences in the Treatment of Depression

As reported previously, outcome studies of treatment for depression suggest that women and men both benefit from the standard therapies. Components of the psychotherapeutic process that make it effective, however, have rarely been studied. Gender differences in personality, relationships, and coping styles suggest that a finer tuned look at the components of therapy may find sex differences in the relative effectiveness of different therapy components or therapist styles. A major review of treatments for depression failed to address the question of sex difference at all, except to acknowledge that because women are prone to depression in the childbearing years, the relative success of psychotherapy without medication is encouraging (Hollon, Thase, & Markowitz, 2002). Research on the effectiveness of antidepressant medication, however, suggests that women respond more poorly than men to tricyclics and better than men to serotonin reuptake inhibitors (SSRIs) and monoamine oxidase inhibitors (Kornstein, 1997). Women may respond more slowly to pharmacotherapy and hormonal state will affect optimal doses. Reducing doses of tricyclics for women taking oral contraceptives and increasing doses in the second half of pregnancy may be beneficial (Sramek & Frackiewicz, 2002).

Summary

The challenge posed by including gender in understanding and treating depression is at least threefold. First, we must be certain that we are not underdiagnosing depression in men. Men may be less willing than women to identify negative emotional states or to admit that they are symptoms of depression. Clinicians hearing about negative emotions from men may be less likely to see them as signs of depression. Second, we must be careful not to overdiagnose depression in women. In seeking causal factors and discovering that certain psychological characteristics or experiences that differ for women and men contribute to depression, we need to look further to understand why women and men differ in these characteristics or experiences. Third, although moderate success for psychological and psychopharmacological treatments for depression are well documented and seem to provide women and men with comparable relief, the data indicate that there are sex differences in some drug responses and certain conditions, such as severity of symptoms or comorbidity. The impact of these differences on the effect of sex on therapy outcomes deserves further investigation.

SPECIFIC DISORDERS: CONDUCT DISORDER

Another disorder that has a significant sex difference in diagnosis is conduct disorder, described in DSM–IV (1994) as "a repetitive and persistent pattern of behavior in which the basic rights of others or major age-appropriate societal norms or rules are violated" (p. 85). Although this is a disorder of childhood or adolescence, it can be used for persons over 18 if they do not meet the criteria for antisocial personality disorder. We are not surprised to learn that it is more often diagnosed in boys (two to three times more often) than in girls (DSM–IV, 1994; Kann & Hanna, 2000).

Sex Differences in the Diagnosis of Conduct Disorder

A look at the history of conduct disorder in the DSM reveals that the basic definition as quoted in the previous paragraph appears with very minor differences in all three versions under review (DSM–III, DSM–III–R, DSM–IV); but other diagnostic criteria change. Starting with DSM–III, conduct disorder must be diagnosed by meeting criteria to one of four subtypes: undersocialized, aggressive; undersocialized, nonaggressive; socialized, aggressive; or socialized, nonaggressive. The undersocialized versus socialized portion of this diagnosis was made based on the child's degree of affection, empathy, or bond with others. The essential characteristic of conduct disorder, however, is either one of the nonaggressive criteria—chronic violations of important home or school rules, repeated running away overnight, persistent serious lying, or stealing without confrontation—or one of the aggressive criteria—physical violence against persons or property (not in self-defense) or thefts outside the home involving confrontation. According to DSM–III conduct disorder is more common among boys with sex ratios of 4:1 to 12:1, except the undersocialized, nonaggressive type "which may be equally common in both sexes" (p. 47).

The four subtypes were dropped in DSM–III–R in favor of diagnoses involving antisocial behavior perpetrated by a child alone (solitary aggressive type) versus antisocial behavior perpetrated by a child in a group and an undifferentiated type for children that do not fit the solitary versus gang distinction. But these are types, not different diagnoses, and the basic diagnosis rests on the presence, lasting at least six months, of three of a list of thirteen behaviors: stole without confrontation; ran away overnight at least twice; often lies; set fires; often truant; broke into house, building, car; destroyed property (other than by fire); physically cruel to animals; forced someone into sexual activity; used a weapon in more than one fight; often initiates physical fights; stole with confrontation; physically cruel to people. These changes made the diagnosis difficult to make unless the child or adolescent engaged in physically violent behavior, a change that would tend to make the diagnosis "rarer and more restricted to males" (Zoccolillo, Tremblay, & Vitaro, 1996, p. 462). Estimates of prevalence were stated as 9% for males and 2% for females.

DSM–IV (1994) includes a "modification [that] is based on the field-trial results and provides a definition that includes behaviors characteristic of females with Conduct Disorder" (p. 775). Items from the DSM–III–R list are included. Two items are added: "often bullies, threatens, or intimidates others" and "often stays out at night despite parental prohibitions, beginning before age 13 years" (p. 90). Estimates of prevalence are somewhat higher than in DSM–III–R, but the sex ratio is less extreme: "for males . . . rates range from 6% to 16%; for females, rates range from 2% to 9%" (p. 88). The list of criteria still favors aggression and destruction of property (nine of the fifteen criteria), although it is possible to meet the threshold for diagnosis (three of the fifteen) based on deceitfulness, theft without confrontation, or serious rules violations. DSM–IV emphasizes gender differences in the pattern of symptoms: "Males . . . exhibit fighting, stealing, vandalism, and school discipline problems. Females . . . are more likely to exhibit lying, truancy, running away, substance use, and prostitution" (DSM–IV, p. 88). Curiously, the behaviors characteristic of males are all criteria for diagnosis of conduct disorder, but some behaviors cited as characteristic of females, substance use and prostitution, are not included.

Based on his concerns about DSM–III–R, Zoccolillo (1993) recommended that separate criteria be used for diagnosing conduct disorder in girls because of clear sex differences in behavioral problems. He and others (Robins, 1986) find that "Adolescent girls with conduct disorder have a poor outcome including early and violent death, arrest, substance abuse and dependence, antisocial personality disorder, failing to finish high school, and teenage pregnancy" (Zoccolillo et al., 1996, p. 462). Early identification and intervention for these girls could perhaps ameliorate these negative outcomes (Webster-Stratton, 1996). On the other hand, Zahn-Waxler (1993) has pointed out that different criteria for girls and boys could lead to pathologizing a behavior, such as substance use or rules violations, in girls that might be considered more acceptable in boys. Accordingly, this perspective holds that, if boys are more likely to be diagnosed with conduct disorder, it is because they do in fact engage in the aggressive and violent behavior characteristic of this disorder more often than girls do. Missing from these arguments is the possibility that particular behaviors are differentially predictive for women and men of the dire outcomes cited by Zoccolillo et al. (1996). Research examining the predictive power of aggressive or destructive behavior versus lying or rules violations versus prostitution or substance abuse in childhood or early adolescence on various negative outcomes (criminal conduct, early parenthood, interrupted education, chronic substance abuse, death) for women and men would be more instructive perhaps than debates on the criteria for DSM diagnoses.

Another issue for diagnosis of conduct disorder in girls and boys is that it relies on behaviors that are considered problematic by others, that is, parents, teachers, peers, but generally not by the child herself or himself. Thus, the symptomatic behaviors must come to the attention of these others (especially adults). Because girls' behaviors are less often overtly aggressive and may, in fact, be covert, they are less likely to come to the attention of caretakers. Also noncompliance and verbal aggression may be less likely than physical aggression to cause teachers to recommend or parents to seek treatment (Kann & Hanna, 2000; Webster-Stratton, 1996). To the extent that girls engage in behaviors not noticed by or successfully hidden from parents and teachers, they may not receive a diagnosis and intervention. To the extent that early intervention yields positive outcomes, failure to identify the problem is troublesome. Finally, as with other psychological disorders, girls with conduct disorder are more likely than boys to be given another diagnosis, including attention deficit disorder, substance abuse, and learning disorders (McMahon & Wells, 1998).

Explaining the Sex Difference in Conduct Disorder

Whichever diagnostic system is used, however, and despite these caveats, it is likely that boys engage in disruptive and aggressive behaviors characteristic of conduct disorder more often than girls. In an attempt to understand more about this sex difference, Cote, Tremblay, Nagin, Zoccolillo, and Vitaro (2002) examined the risk trajectories of a large sample of girls and boys from kindergarten to grade six. They focused on three behavioral dimensions: hyperactive, fearful, and unhelpful. The only profile that predicted conduct disorder (using DSM–III–R criteria) for girls was hyperactive plus unhelpful. Three profiles predicted for boys: hyperactive (only), hyperactive plus unhelpful, and hyperactive plus fearless plus unhelpful. The last profile, a combination of all three predictive dimensions, did not occur in the female sample. Almost eight times more boys than girls had a risk profile in kindergarten and almost three times more boys had a conduct disorder diagnosis in adolescence. "Thus a higher proportion of boys were on highly stable risk trajectories from kindergarten on" (Cote et al., 2002, p. 1092).

Keenan and Shaw (1997) have also examined early childhood influences on problem behaviors. They found that beginning around age four, girls show a decline in difficult temperament, whereas boys show an increase or a smaller decline. Thus, boys persist in problem behaviors, whereas girls show improvement. They suggest two hypotheses that might explain this sex

difference: socialization that channels girls into internalizing behaviors and girls' development of adaptive skills. A review of socializing influences reveals several that may contribute
to the sex difference. Girls may receive less physical punishment than boys (Lytton & Romney,
1991). Boys' aggressive behavior, rather than being extinguished by physical punishment, may
be modeled on it (Kann & Hanna, 2000). With very young children (one year), mothers make
a continued effort to teach difficult girls but tend to withdraw from difficult boys (Maccoby,
Snow, & Jacklin, 1984). In a sample of $3\frac{1}{2}$ -year-olds, girls' assertions were more often
ignored by parents than boys' assertions, whereas girls' compliant behaviors received more
positive responses from fathers than did boys' compliant behaviors (Kerig, Cowan, & Cowan,
1993). Mothers of two-year-old daughters were more likely to point out the consequences
of rule breaking on others than mothers of sons (Smetana, 1989). Parents supervising their
toddlers' play with a same-sex peer tend to encourage relinquishing a toy to the peer, but
they do so more with daughters than with sons (Ross, Tesla, Kenyon, & Lollis, 1990). Peers
also treat girls and boys differently. Fagot and Hagan (1985) found that among toddlers, girls'
aggression was more likely to be ignored by peers and that this was effective in ending the
aggression. Together these studies indicate that girls are being taught to be compliant, perspective taking, and prosocial, all behaviors that may serve to reduce the behaviors associated with
conduct disorder. One wonders what the impact would be if these behaviors were stressed for
boys as well.

Keenan and Shaw (1997) also consider sex differences in rate of maturation as a possible
explanation for sex differences in problem behaviors. Research generally finds that girls develop
language more rapidly than boys. Language can provide children with nonphysical means for
resolving disputes and getting their way without aggression. An early development of these
abilities may facilitate declines in conduct problems in childhood. Girls also develop empathic
responding and prosocial behaviors earlier than boys (Kennan & Shaw, 1997). To the extent that
any of these abilities are a result of faster neurological development, this difference provides
a more biological explanation for the sex difference in conduct disorder.

Hastings, Zahn-Waxler, Robinson, Usher, and Bridges (2000) investigated the development
of concern for others in a longitudinal study of children five to ten. They concluded that "One
of the most salient results of this investigation was the demonstration of the protective role that
concern for others may play in the development of children's externalizing behavior problems"
(p. 542). Children displaying concern at five years showed a decline in externalizing problems
from five to seven years. Mothers' socialization behaviors also played a role. They found that
strict, harshly punitive mothers who display anger or disappointment and fail to reason with
their children or establish consistent rules interfere with their children's prosocial development.
In this study girls at all ages showed more concern for others than boys.

Whether acquired through socialization or maturation or both, the emergence of prosocial
or helpful behaviors in girls at an earlier age than in boys may explain the later sex difference in
the prevalence of conduct disorder. The data from Cote et al. (2002) indicate that risk profiles
including "unhelpful" (vs. "helpful") are more predictive of conduct disorder (CD) for boys
(% with CD: 12.13 vs. 9.97) but especially for girls (% with CD: 7.57 vs. 3.87), suggesting
that helpfulness is protective against developing CD.

Sex Differences in Treatment of Conduct Disorder

Recommended interventions for children and adolescents with CD include parent management
training, problem-solving skills training, and multisystemic therapy (Kazdin, 2003). Unfortunately, many studies of therapy effectiveness do not include girls or do not examine sex
differences when both girls and boys are included (Kann & Hanna, 2000; Webster-Stratton,
1996). Webster-Stratton (1996) did examine sex differences in the effects of parent training on

four- to seven-year-olds with conduct problems. At baseline, mothers reported more external-izing problems for boys than for girls whereas fathers reported more internalizing problems for girls than for boys. Teachers reported more behavior problems, hostile–aggressive prob-lems and hyperactive behaviors for boys than for girls. Mothers, fathers, and teachers reported significant reductions in externalizing behavior problems from pre- to postintervention, but no change from postintervention to follow-up for boys and girls. The effects were the same for both boys and girls. Even following the intervention, teachers perceived boys as more hostile–aggressive and hyperactive than girls.

Webster-Stratton (1996) also investigated child, parenting, and family variables as predic-tors of outcomes. Girls and boys did not initially differ on the parenting and family variables, except mothers used more physically negative behavior with boys. At follow-up boys' exter-nalizing problems were predicted primarily by prior externalizing behavior and nothing else except father negativity. On the other hand, girls' externalizing problems had more significant parenting predictors (mother inappropriate discipline, mother and father negativity, mother depression, father life stress) suggesting that girls' conduct problems are more influenced by parent variables than boys'. This finding further suggests that additional therapeutic focus on parenting and family variables may be differentially beneficial to girls. We can also speculate that the different symptom profiles presented by girls and boys (e.g., boys engaging in more hostile–aggressive behaviors) might lead to sex differences in the efficacy of different therapies or different components of a therapy. Girls, because of their higher rate of comorbidity, may also pose more challenging and complex problems for the therapist.

Summary

Diagnostic criteria for conduct disorder raise the issue of the relative validity of using the same, preferably gender neutral, symptoms for both boys and girls versus different sets of criteria for the two sexes. Identifying child and adolescent behaviors that predict adult problems for females and for males appears to be the direction research in this area should take. The focus on boys to the exclusion of girls in understanding this disorder or evaluating therapy outcomes needs to change. Studies that include both sexes and compare predictors of adolescent CD and predictors of therapy outcome suggest that the developmental trajectory for CDs and the impact of interventions may differ for girls and boys and are in need of further investigation.

SUMMARY AND CONCLUSIONS

Identifying and explaining the role played by sex or gender in psychopathology and its treatment are ongoing challenges for clinical scientists. A difficult issue for diagnosis of psychological disorders is how to make diagnostic criteria equally valid for women and men, girls and boys. Even when criteria are made as objective as possible, clinicians may apply them differentially based on the sex of the client and, as has been demonstrated, may more readily assign diagnostic labels that conform to gender stereotypes. Dimensional descriptions rather than categorical labels may alleviate some of these problems. But standardized tests designed to measure diagnostic categories are not always free of sex or gender bias. Efforts to use the diagnostic system to determine prevalence rates are further biased by using clinical samples rather than community samples. A challenge for DSM–V will be determining if the same criteria ought to be used for males and females or if some psychological disorders will require different sets of criteria to be optimally accurate. Research on the effects of sex on therapy outcomes has produced mixed results, but much data suggest that neither sex of therapist nor sex of client has a predictable or sizable effect on therapy outcome. Sex of client or therapist may play an important role, however, in particular circumstances (e.g., inpatient treatment for single mothers, therapy for gays and lesbians, sexual misconduct by therapists). Comorbidity may also be a greater issue in the treatment of women. Depression and conduct disorder serve as concrete examples of clinical researchers' efforts to understand the effects of sex on diagnosis, etiology, and treatment for specific disorders.

REFERENCES

Adler, D., Drake, R., & Teague, G. (1990). Clinicians' practices in personality assessment: Does gender influence the use of DAM-III Axis II? *Comprehensive Psychiatry, 31*, 125–133.

Allen-Burge, R., Storandt, M., Kinscherf, D. A., & Rubin, E. H. (1994). Sex differences in the sensitivity of two self-report depression scales in older depressed inpatients. *Psychology and Aging, 9*, 443–445.

Alterman, A. I., Randall, M., & McLellan, A. T. (2000). Comparisons of outcomes by gender and for fee-for-service versus managed care: A study of nine community programs. *Journal of Substance Abuse Treatment, 19*, 127–134.

American Psychiatric Association (1980). *Diagnostic and statistical manual of mental disorders* (3rd ed.). Washington, DC: Author.

American Psychiatric Association (1987). *Diagnostic and statistical manual of mental disorders* (3rd ed., rev.). Washington, DC: Author.

American Psychiatric Association (1994). *Diagnostic and statistical manual of mental disorders* (4th ed.). Washington, DC: Author.

American Psychiatric Association (2000). *Diagnostic and statistical manual of mental disorders* (4th ed., *text rev.*). Washington, DC: Author.

Becker, D., & Lamb, S. (1994). Sex bias in the diagnosis of borderline personality disorder and posttraumatic stress disorder. *Professional Psychology: Research and Practice, 25*, 55–61.

Benishek, L. A., Bieschke, J., Stoffelmayr, B., Mavis, B., & Humphries, K. A. (1992). Gender differences in depression and anxiety among alcoholics. *Journal of Substance Abuse, 4*, 235–245.

Bergin, A. E., & Garfield, S. L. (Eds.) (1994). *Handbook of psychotherapy and behavior change.* NY: Wiley.

Beutler, L. E., Machado, P. P. P., & Neufeldt, S. A. (1994). Therapist variables. In A. E. Bergin & S. I. Garfield (Eds.), *Handbook of psychotherapy and behavior change* (pp. 229–269). New York, NY: John Wiley.

Bjornson, W., Rand, C., Connett, J. E., & Lindgren, P. (1995). Gender differences in smoking cessation after 3 years in the Lung Health Study. *American Journal of Public Health, 85*, 223–230.

Blashfield, R. K., & Herkov, M. J. (1996). Investigating clinician adherence to diagnosis by criteria: A replication of Morey and Ochoa (1989). *Journal of Personality Disorders, 10*, 219–228.

Blumenthal, S. J. (1995). Improving women's mental and physical health: Federal initiative and programs. In J. M. Oldham & M. B. Riba (Eds.), *Review of Psychiatry* (Vol. 14, pp. 195–204). Washington, DC: American Psychiatric Press.

Brown, L. S. (1992). A feminist critique of personality disorders. In L. S. Brown & M. Ballou (Eds.), *Personality and psychopathology: Feminist reappraisals* (pp. 206–228). New York: Guilford.

Brown, L. S., Alterman, A. I., Rutherford, M. J., Cacciola, J. S., & Zabalero, A. (1993). ASI scores of four racial/gender groups of MM patients. *Journal of Substance Abuse, 5*, 269–279.

Burt, V. K. (2002). Women and depression: Special considerations in assessment and management. In F. Lewis-Hall, T. S. Williams, J. A. Panetta, & J. M. Herrera (Eds.), *Psychiatric illness in women*. Washington, DC: American Psychiatric Publishing.

Caplan, P. J. (1991). How do they decide who is normal? The bizarre, but true, tale of the DSM process. *Canadian Psychology, 32*, 162–170.

Caplan, P. J. (1995). *They say you're crazy. How the world's most powerful psychiatrists decide who's normal.* Reading, MA: Addison-Wesley.

Casper, R. (1998). The psychopharmacology of women. In R. C. Casper (Ed.), *Women's health: Hormones, emotions and behavior* (pp. 192–218). Cambridge: Cambridge University Press.

Cote, S., Tremblay, R. E., Nagin, D. S., Zoccolillo, M., Vitaro, F. (2002). Childhood behavioral profiles leading to adolescent conduct disorder: Risk trajectories for boys and girls. *Journal of the American Academy of Child and Adolescent Psychiatry, 41*, 1086–1094.

Culbertson, F. (1997). Depression and gender: An international review. *American Psychologist, 52*, 25–31.

Dahlgren, L., & Willander, A. (1989). Are special treatment facilities for female alcoholics needed? A controlled 2-year follow-up study from a specialized female unit (EWA) versus a missed male-female treatment facility. *Alcoholism: Clinical and Experimental Research, 13*, 499–504.

Elkin, I. (1994). The NIMH treatment of depression collaborative research program: Where we began and where we are. In A. E. Bergin & S. I. Garfield (Eds.), *Handbook of psychotherapy and behavior change* (pp. 114–139). New York: John Wiley.

Fagot, B. I., & Hagan, R. (1985). Aggression in toddlers: Responses to the assertive acts of boys and girls. *Sex Roles, 12*, 341–351.

Fernbach, B. E., Winstead, B. A., & Derlega, V. J. (1989). Sex differences in diagnosis and treatment recommendations for antisocial personality and somatization disorders. *Journal of Social and Clinical Psychology, 8*, 238–255.

Ford, M., & Widiger, T. A. (1989). Sex bias in the diagnosis of histrionic and antisocial personality disorders. *Journal of Consulting and Clinical Psychology, 57*, 301–305.

Funtowicz, M. N., & Widiger, T. A. (1995). Sex bias in the diagnosis of personality disorders: A different approach. *Journal of Psychopathology and Behavioral Assessment, 17*, 145–165.

Galen, L. W. Brower, K. J., Gillespie, B. W., & Zucker, R. A. (2000). Sociopathy, gender, and treatment outcome among outpatient substance abusers. *Drug & Alcohol Dependence, 61*, 23–33.

Garfield, S. L. (1994). Research on client variables in psychotherapy. In A. E. Bergin & S. I. Garfield (Eds.), *Handbook of psychotherapy and behavior change* (pp. 190–228). New York: John Wiley.

Giardina, E. G. (2000). Heart disease in women. *International Journal of Fertility and Women's Medicine, 45*, 350–357.

Gomes-Schwartz, B., Hadley, W. W., & Strupp, H. H. (1978). Individual psychotherapy and behavior therapy. *Annual Review of Psychology, 29*, 435–471.

Hartung, C. A., & Widiger, T. A. (1998). Gender differences in the diagnosis of mental disorders: Conclusions and controversies of the DSM-IV. *Psychological Bulletin, 123*, 260–278.

Hastings, P. D., Zahn-Waxler, C., Robinson, J., Usher, B., & Bridges, D. (2000). The development of concern for others in children with behavior problems. *Developmental Psychology, 36*, 531–546.

Hollon, S. D., Thase, M. E., & Markowitz, J. C. (2002). Treatment and prevention of depression. *Psychological Science in the Public Interest, 3*, 39–77.

Jones, E. E., Krupnick, J. L., & Kerig, P. K. (1987). Some gender effects in brief psychotherapy. *Psychotherapy, 24*, 336–352.

Jones, E. E., & Zoppel, C. L. (1982). Impact of client and therapist gender on psychotherapy process and outcome. *Journal of Consulting and Clinical Psychology, 50*, 259–272.

Kann, T., & Hanna, F. J. (2000). Disruptive behavior disorders in children and adolescents: How do girls differ from boys? *Journal of Counseling and Development, 78*, 267–274.

Kazdin, A. E. (2003). Psychotherapy for children and adolescents. *Annual Review of Psychology, 54*, 253–276.

Kaplan, M. (1983). A woman's view of DSM-III. *American Psychologist, 38*, 786–792.

Keenan, K., & Shaw, D. (1997). Developmental and social influences on young girls' early problem behavior. *Psychological Bulletin, 12*, 95–113.

Kerig, P. K., Cowan, P. A., & Cowan, C. P. (1993). Marital quality and gender differences in parent-child interaction. *Developmental Psychology, 29*, 931–939.

Kessler, R. C., Crum, R. M., Warner, L. A., Nelson, C. B., Schulenberg, J., & Anthony, J. C. (1997). Lifetime co-occurrence of DSM-III-R alcohol Abuse and dependence with other psychiatric disorders in the National Comorbidity Survey. *Archives of General Psychiatry, 54*, 313–321.

Kessler, R. C., McGonagle, K. A., Zhao, S., Nelson, C. B., Hughes, M., Eshleman, S., Wittchen, H. V., & Kendler, K. S. (1994). Lifetime and 12-month prevalence of DSM-III-R psychiatric disorders in the United States: Results from the National Comorbidity Survey. *Archives of General Psychiatry, 51*, 8–19.

Kornstein, S. G. (1997). Gender differences in depression: Implications for treatment. *Journal of Clinical Psychiatry, 58*(Suppl. 15), 12–18.

Kosten, T. A., Gawin, F. H., Kosten, T. R., & Rounsaville, B. J. (1993). Gender differences in cocaine use and treatment response. *Journal of Substance Abuse Treatment, 10*, 63–66.

Lamb, D. H., & Catanzaro, S. J. (1998). Sexual and nonsexual boundary violations involving psychologists, clients, supervisees, and students: Implication for professional practice. *Professional Psychology: Research and Practice, 29*, 498–503.

Leibenluft, E. (1997). Issues in the treatment of women with bipolar illness. *Journal of Clinical Psychiatry, 58*(Suppl. 15), 5–11.

Lewis, C., & Bucholz, K. (1991). Alcoholism, antisocial behavior and family history. *British Journal of Addiction, 86*, 177–194.

Liddle, B. J. (1996). Therapist sexual orientation, gender, and counseling practices as they related to ratings of helpfulness by gay and lesbian clients. *Journal of Counseling Psychology, 43*, 394–402.

Lindsay, K. A., Sankis, L. M., & Widiger, T. A. (2000). Gender bias in self-report personality disorder inventories. *Journal of Personality Disorders, 14*, 218–232.

Lindsay, K. A., & Widiger, T. A. (1995). Sex and gender bias in self-report personality disorder inventories: Items analyses of the MCMI-II, MMPI, and PDQ-R. *Journal of Personality Assessment, 65*, 1–20.

Loring, M., & Powell, B. (1988). Gender, race and DSM-III: A study of the objectivity of psychiatric diagnostic behavior. *Journal of Health and Social Behavior, 29*, 1–22.

Lytton, H., & Romney, D. M. (1991). Parents' differential socialization of boys and girls: A meta-analysis. *Psychological Bulletin, 109*, 267–296.

Maccoby, E. E., Snow, M. E., & Jacklin, C. N. (1984). Children's dispositions and mother-child interaction at 12 and 18 months: A short-term longitudinal study. *Developmental Psychology, 20*, 459–472.

Maddux, J. E. (2002). Stopping the "madness": Positive psychology and the deconstruction of the illness ideology and the *DSM*. In C. R. Snyder & S. J. Lopez (Eds.), *Handbook of positive psychology* (pp. 13–25). NY: Oxford.

Marsh, L., & Casper, R. (1998). Gender differences in brain morphology and in psychiatric disorders. In R. C. Casper (Ed.), *Women's health: Hormones, emotions and behavior* (pp. 53–82). Cambridge: Cambridge University Press.

McMahon, R. J., & Wells, K. C. (1998). Conduct problems. In E. J. Mash & R. A. Barkley (Eds.), *Treatment of childhood disorders* (pp. 111–207). NY: Guilford.

Morey, L. C., & Ochoa, E. (1989). An investigation of adherence to diagnostic criteria: Clinical diagnosis of the DSM-III personality disorders. *Journal of Personality Disorders, 3*, 180–192.

Nolen-Hoeksema, S., Larson, J., & Grayson, C. (1999). Explaining the gender difference in depressive symptoms. *Journal of Personality and Social Psychology, 77*, 1061–1072.

Page, S., & Bennesch, S. (1993). Gender and reporting differences in measures of depression. *Canadian Journal of Behavioural Science, 25*, 579–589.

Pantony, K. L., & Caplan, P. J. (1991). Delusional dominating personality disorder: A modest proposal for identifying some consequences of rigid masculine socialization. *Canadian Psychology, 32*, 120–133.

Potts, M. K., Burnam, M. A., & Wells, K. B. (1991). Gender differences in depression detection: A comparison of clinician diagnosis and standardized assessment. *Psychological Assessment, 3*, 609–615.

Robins, E., & Guze, S. B. (1970). Establishment of diagnostic validity of psychiatric illness: Its application to schizophrenia. *American Journal of Psychiatry, 126*, 983–986.

Robins, L. N. (1986). The consequences of conduct disorder in girls. In D. Olweus, J. Block, & M. Radke-Yarrow (Eds.), *Development of antisocial and prosocial behavior.* Orlando, FL: Academic Press.

Ross, H., Tesla, C., Kenyon, B., & Lollis, S. (1990). Maternal intervention in toddler peer conflict: The socialization of principles of justice. *Developmental Psychology, 26*, 994–1003.

Ross, R., Frances, A. J., & Widiger, T. A. (1995). Gender issues in DSM-IV. In J. M. Oldham & M. B. Riba (Eds.), *Review of psychiatry* (Vol. 14, pp. 205–226). Washington, DC: American Psychiatric Press.

Santor, D. A., Ramsay, J. O., & Zuroff, D. C. (1994). Nonparametric item analyses of the Beck Depression Inventory: Evaluating gender item bias and response option weights. *Psychological Assessment, 6*, 255–270.

Seeman, M. V. (1995). Gender differences in treatment response in schizophrenia. In M. V. Seeman (Ed.), *Gender and psychopathology.* Washington, DC: American Psychiatric Press.

Smetana, J. G. (1989). Toddlers' social interactions in the context of moral and conventional transgressions in the home. *Developmental Psychology, 25*, 499–508.

Sprock, J., & Yoder, C. Y. (1997). Women and depression: An update on the report of the APA task force. *Sex Roles, 36*, 269–303.

Sramek, J. J., & Frackiewicz, E. J. (2002). Effect of sex on psychopharmacology of antidepressants. In F. Lewis-Hall, T. S. Williams, J. A., Panetta, & J. M. Herrera (Eds.), *Psychiatric illness in women* (pp. 113–131). Washington, DC: American Psychiatric Publishing.

Sterling, R. C., Gottheil, E., Weinstein, S. P., & Serota, R. (2001). The effect of therapist/patient race- and sex-matching in individual treatment. *Addiction, 96*, 1015–1022.

Szymanski, S., Lieberman, J. A., Alvir, J. M., Mayerhoff, D., (1995). Gender differences in onset of illness, treatment response, course and biologic indexes in first-episode schizophrenic patients, *American Journal of Psychiatry, 152*, 698–703.

Tamminga, C. A. (1997). Gender and schizophrenia, *Journal of Clinical Psychiatry, 58*(Suppl. 15), 33–37.

Thase, M. E., Reynolds, C. F., Frank, E., Simons, A. D., McGeary, J., Fasiczka, A. L., Garamoni,G. G., Jennings, R., & Kupfer, D. J. (1994). Do depressed men and women respond similarly to cognitive behavior therapy? *American Journal of Psychiatry, 151*, 500–505.

Toneatto, A., Sobell, L. C., & Sobell, M. B. (1992). Gender issues in the treatment of abusers of alcohol, nicotine, and other drugs. *Journal of Substance Abuse, 4*, 209–218.

Triffleman, E. (2001). Gender differences in a controlled pilot study of psychosocial treatments in substance dependent patients with post-traumatic stress disorder: Design considerations and outcomes. *Alcoholism Treatment Quarterly, 18*, 113–126.

Veiel, H. O. F. (1993). Detrimental effects of kin support networks on the course of depression. *Journal of Abnormal Psychology, 102*, 419–429.

Viguera, A. D., Baldessarini, R. J., Tondo, L. (2001). Response to lithium maintenance treatment in bipolar disorders: Comparison of women and men. *Bipolar Disorders, 3*, 245–252.

Walker. L. E. A. (1994). Are personality disorders gender biased? In S. A. Kirk & S. D. Einbinder (Eds.), *Controversial issues in mental health* (pp. 22–29). New York: Allyn & Bacon.

Warner, R. (1978). The diagnosis of antisocial and hysterical personality disorders. *Journal of Nervous and Mental Disease, 166*, 839–845.

Webster-Stratton, C. (1996). Early-onset conduct problems: Does gender make a difference? *Journal of Consulting and Clinical Psychology, 64*, 540–551.

Whitlock, E. P., Vogt, T. M., Hollis, J. R., & Lichtenstein, E. (1997). Does gender affect response to a brief clinic-based smoking intervention? *American Journal of Preventive Medicine, 13*, 159–166.

Widiger, T. A. (1998). Invited essay: Sex biases in the diagnoses of personality disorders. *Journal of Personality Disorders, 12*, 95–118.

Wilke, D. (1994). Women and alcoholism: How a male-as-norm bias affects research, assessment, and treatment. *Health and Social Work, 19*, 29–35.

Williams, J. B. W., & Spitzer, R. L. (1983). The issue of sex bias in DSM-III. Critique of "A woman's view of DSM-III" by Marcie Kaplan. *American Psychologist, 38*, 793–798.

Wolk, S. I., & Weissman, M. M. (1995). Women and depression: An update. *Review of Psychiatry, 14*, 227–259.

Wong, C. M., & Yehuda, R. (2002). Sex differences in posttraumatic stress disorder. In F. Lewis-Hall & T. S. Williams, (Eds.), *Psychiatric illness in women: Emerging treatments and research* (pp. 57–96).

Yoder, C. Y., Shute, G. E., & Tryban, G. M. (1990). Community recognition of objective and subjective characteristics of depression. *American Journal of Community Psychology, 18*, 547–566.

Yonkers, K. A., & Hamilton, J. A. (1995). Psychotropic medications. In J. M. Oldham & M. B. Riba (Eds.), *Review of psychiatry* (Vol. 14, pp. 307–332). Washington, DC: American Psychiatric Press.

Zahn-Waxler, C. (1993). Warriors and worriers: Gender and psychopathology. *Development and Psychopathology, 5*, 79–89.

Zlotnick, C., Elkin, I., & Shea M. T. (1998). Does the gender of a patient or the gender of a therapist affect the treatment of patients with major depression? *Journal of Consulting and Clinical Psychology, 66*, 655–659.

Zoccolillo, M. (1993). Gender and the development of conduct disorder. *Development and Psychopathology, 5*, 65–78.

Zoccolillo, M., Tremblay, R., & Vitaro, F. (1996). DSM-III-R and DSM-III criteria for conduct disorder in preadolescent girls: Specific but insensitive. *Journal of the American Academy of Child and Adolescent Psychiatry, 35*, 461–470.

4

Classification and Diagnosis: Historical Development and Contemporary Issues

Thomas A. Widiger
University of Kentucky

Aberrant, dysfunctional, and maladaptive thinking, feeling, behaving, and relating are of substantial concern to many different professions, the members of which will hold an equally diverse array of beliefs regarding etiology, pathology, and intervention. It is imperative that these persons be able to communicate meaningfully with one another. The primary purpose of an official diagnostic nomenclature is to provide this common language of communication (Kendell, 1975; Sartorius et al., 1993).

Official diagnostic nomenclatures, however, can be exceedingly powerful, impacting significantly many important social, forensic, clinical, and other professional decisions (Schwartz & Wiggins, 2002). Persons think in terms of their language, and the predominant languages of psychopathology are the fourth edition of the American Psychiatric Association's (1994, 2000) *Diagnostic and Statistical Manual of Mental Disorders* (DSM–IV) and the tenth edition of the World Health Organization's *International Classification of Diseases* (ICD–10; 1992). As such, these nomenclatures have a substantial impact on how clinicians, social agencies, and the general public conceptualize psychopathology.

These two languages, however, are not the final word. Interpreting DSM–IV or ICD–10 as conclusively validated nomenclatures exaggerates the extent of their empirical support (Frances, Pincus, Widiger, Davis, & First, 1990). On the other hand, DSM–IV and ICD–10 are not lacking in credible or compelling empirical support. DSM–IV and ICD–10 contain many flaws but they are also well-reasoned, scientifically researched, and well-documented nomenclatures that describe what is currently understood by most scientists, theorists, researchers, and clinicians to be the predominant variants of psychopathology (Nathan & Langenbucher, 1999; Widiger & Trull, 1993). This chapter will overview the DSM–IV diagnostic nomenclature, beginning with historical background, followed by a discussion of major issues facing future revisions.

HISTORICAL BACKGROUND

The impetus for the development of an official diagnostic nomenclature was the crippling confusion generated by its absence (Widiger, 2001). "For a long time confusion reigned. Every self-respecting alienist [the 19th century term for a psychiatrist], and certainly every professor, had his own classification" (Kendell, 1975, p. 87). The production of a new system for classifying psychopathology became a right of passage in the nineteenth century for the young, aspiring professor.

> To produce a well-ordered classification almost seems to have become the unspoken ambition of every psychiatrist of industry and promise, as it is the ambition of a good tenor to strike a high C. This classificatory ambition was so conspicuous that the composer Berlioz was prompted to remark that after their studies have been completed a rhetorician writes a tragedy and a psychiatrist a classification. (Zilboorg, 1941, p. 450)

In 1908 the American Bureau of the Census asked the American Medico-Psychological Association (which subsequently altered its title in 1921 to the American Psychiatric Association) to develop a standard nosology to facilitate the obtainment of national statistics. This committee affirmed the need for a uniform system.

> The present condition with respect to the classification of mental diseases is chaotic. Some states use no well-defined classification. In others the classifications used are similar in many respects but differ enough to prevent accurate comparisons. Some states have adopted a uniform system, while others leave the matter entirely to the individual hospitals. This condition of affairs discredits the science. (Salmon, Copp, May, Abbot, & Cotton, 1917, pp. 255–256)

The American Medico-Psychological Association, in collaboration with the National Committee for Mental Hygiene, issued a nosology in 1918, titled *Statistical Manual for the Use of Institutions for the Insane* (Grob, 1991; Menninger, 1963). This nomenclature, however, failed to gain wide acceptance. It included only 22 diagnoses, which were confined largely to psychoses with a presumably neurochemical pathology. "In the late twenties, each large teaching center employed a system of its own origination, no one of which met more than the immediate needs of the local institution" (American Psychiatric Association [APA], 1952, p. v). A conference was held at the New York Academy of Medicine in 1928 to develop a more authoritative and uniformly accepted manual. The resulting nomenclature was modeled after the *Statistical Manual* but it was distributed to hospitals within the American Medical Association's *Standard Classified Nomenclature of Disease*. Many hospitals used this system, but it eventually proved to be inadequate when the attention of the profession expanded well beyond psychotic disorders during World War II.

ICD–6 and DSM–I

The Navy, Army, and Veterans Administration developed their own, largely independent nomenclatures during World War II mainly because of the inadequacies of the *Standard Classified*. "Military psychiatrists, induction station psychiatrists, and Veterans Administration psychiatrists, found themselves operating within the limits of a nomenclature specifically not designed for 90% of the cases handled" (APA, 1952, p. vi). The World Health Organization (WHO) accepted the authority in 1948 to produce the 6th edition of the *International Statistical Classification of Diseases, Injuries, and Causes of Death* (ICD). ICD–6 was the first to include a section devoted to mental disorders (Kendell, 1975; Kramer, Sartorius, Jablensky, & Gulbinat, 1979), perhaps in recognition of the many psychological casualties of World War II and the increasing impact of mental health professions. The United States Public Health Service commissioned a committee, chaired by George Raines (with representations from a variety of professions and public health agencies), to develop a variant of the mental disorders section of ICD–6 for use within the United States. The United States, as a member of the WHO, was obliged to use ICD–6, but modifications could be made to maximize its acceptance and utility for use within the United States. The resulting nomenclature resembled closely the Veterans Administration system developed by Brigadier General William Menninger (brother to Karl Menninger, 1963). Responsibility for publishing and distributing this nosology was given to the American Psychiatric Association (1952) under the title *Diagnostic and Statistical Manual. Mental Disorders* (hereafter referred to as DSM–I).

DSM–I was generally successful in obtaining acceptance, mainly because of its expanded coverage, including somatoform disorders, stress reactions, and personality disorders. However, the New York State Department of Mental Hygiene, which had been influential in the development of the *Standard Nomenclature*, continued for some time to use its own classification. DSM–I also included narrative descriptions of each disorder to facilitate understanding and more consistent applications. Nevertheless, fundamental criticisms regarding the reliability and validity of psychiatric diagnoses were also raised (e.g., Zigler & Phillips, 1961). For example, a widely cited reliability study by Ward, Beck, Mendelson, Mock, and Erbaugh (1962) concluded that most of the poor agreement among psychiatrists' diagnoses was due largely to inadequacies of DSM–I.

ICD–6 was less successful. The "mental disorders section [of ICD–6] failed to gain [international] acceptance and eleven years later was found to be in official use only in Finland, New Zealand, Peru, Thailand, and the United Kingdom" (Kendell, 1975, p. 91). The WHO therefore commissioned a review by the English psychiatrist Erwin Stengel. Stengel (1959) reiterated the importance of establishing an official nomenclature:

> A ... serious obstacle to progress in psychiatry is difficulty of communication. Everybody who has followed the literature and listened to discussions concerning mental illness soon discovers that psychiatrists, even those apparently sharing the same basic orientation, often do not speak the same language. They either use different terms for the same concepts, or the same term for different concepts, usually without being aware of it. It is sometimes argued that this is inevitable in the present state of psychiatric knowledge, but it is doubtful whether this is a valid excuse. (Stengel, 1959, p. 601)

Stengel attributed the failure of clinicians to accept the mental disorders section of ICD–6 to the presence of theoretical biases, cynicism regarding any psychiatric diagnoses (some theoretical perspectives opposed the use of any diagnostic terms), and the presence of abstract, highly inferential diagnostic criteria that hindered consistent, uniform applications by different clinicians.

ICD–8 and DSM–II

Work began on ICD–8 soon after Stengel's (1959) report (ICD–6 had been revised to ICD–7 in 1955, but there were no revisions to the mental disorders). Considerable effort was made to develop a system that would be used by all of the member countries of the WHO. The final edition of ICD–8 was approved by the WHO in 1966 and became effective in 1968. A companion glossary, in the spirit of Stengel's (1959) recommendations, was to be published conjointly, but work did not begin on the glossary until 1967 and it was not completed until 1972. "This delay greatly reduced [its] usefulness, and also [its] authority" (Kendell, 1975, p. 95). In 1965, the American Psychiatric Association appointed a committee, chaired by Ernest M. Gruenberg, to revise DSM–I to be compatible with ICD–8 and yet also be suitable for use within the United States. The final version was approved in 1967, with publication in 1968.

The diagnosis of mental disorders, however, was receiving substantial criticism during this time (e.g., Rosenhan, 1973; Szasz, 1961). A fundamental problem continued to be the absence of empirical support for the reliability, let alone the validity, of its diagnoses (e.g., Blashfield & Draguns, 1976). Researchers, however, took to heart the recommendations of Stengel (1959) by developing more specific and explicit criterion sets (Blashfield, 1984). The most influential of these efforts was produced by a group of neurobiologically oriented psychiatrists at Washington University in St. Louis. Their criterion sets generated so much interest that they were published separately in what has become one of the most widely cited papers in psychiatry (i.e., Feighner et al., 1972). Research has since indicated that mental disorders can be diagnosed reliably and do provide valid information regarding etiology, pathology, course, and treatment (Nathan & Langenbucher, 1999).

ICD–9 and DSM–III

By the time Feighner et al. (1972) was published, work was nearing completion on the ninth edition of the ICD. The authors of ICD–9 had decided to include a glossary that would provide more precise descriptions of each disorder, but it was apparent that ICD–9 would not include the more specific and explicit criterion sets used in research (Kendell, 1975). In 1974, the American Psychiatric Association appointed a task force, chaired by Robert Spitzer, to revise DSM–II in a manner that would be compatible with ICD–9 but would also incorporate many of the current innovations in diagnosis. DSM–III was published in 1980 and was remarkably innovative, including (a) a multiaxial diagnostic system (most mental disorders were diagnosed on Axis I, personality and specific developmental disorders were diagnosed on Axis II, medical disorders on Axis III, psychosocial stressors on Axis IV, and level of functioning on Axis V), (b) specific and explicit criterion sets for all but one of the disorders (schizoaffective), (c) a substantially expanded text discussion of each disorder to facilitate diagnosis (e.g., age at onset, course, complications, sex ratio, and familial pattern), and (d) removal of terms (e.g., neurosis) that appeared to favor a particular theoretical model for the disorder's etiology or pathology (Spitzer, Williams, & Skodol, 1980).

DSM–III–R

A disadvantage of DSM–III was that errors in criterion sets were as specific and explicit as the diagnostic criterion sets, and a number of such errors were soon apparent (e.g., panic disorder could not be diagnosed in the presence of a major depression). "Criteria were not entirely clear, were inconsistent across categories, or were even contradictory" (APA, 1987, p. xvii). The American Psychiatric Association therefore authorized the development of a revision to DSM–III to correct these errors. Fundamental revisions were to be tabled until work began on ICD–10. However, it might have been unrealistic to expect the authors of DSM–III–R to confine their efforts to refinement and clarification, given the impact, success, and importance of DSM–III.

The impact of DSM–III has been remarkable. Soon after its publication, it became widely accepted in the United States as the common language of mental health clinicians and researchers for communicating about the disorders for which they have professional responsibility. Recent major textbooks of psychiatry and other textbooks that discuss psychopathology have either made extensive reference to DSM–III or largely adopted its terminology and concepts. (APA, 1987, p. xviii)

It was not difficult to find persons who wanted to be involved in the development of DSM–III–R, and most persons who were (or were not) involved wanted to have a significant impact. More persons were involved in making corrections to DSM–III than were used in its original construction, and, not surprisingly, there were many proposals for additions, revisions, and deletions. Four of the diagnoses approved for inclusion by the authors of DSM–III–R (i.e., sadistic personality disorder, self-defeating personality disorder, late luteal phase dysphoric disorder, and paraphiliac rapism) generated so much controversy that a special ad hoc committee was appointed by the Board of Trustees of the American Psychiatric Association to reconsider their inclusion. A concern common to all four was that their inclusion might result in harm to women. For example, paraphiliac rapism might be used to mitigate criminal responsibility for rape and self-defeating personality disorder might be used to blame female victims for having been abused. Another concern was the lack of sufficient empirical support to address or offset these concerns. A compromise was eventually reached in which the two personality disorders and late luteal phase dysphoric disorder were included in an appendix (Endicott, 2000; Widiger, 1995); paraphiliac rapism was deleted entirely.

ICD–10 and DSM–IV

By the time work was completed on DSM–III–R, work had already begun on ICD–10. The decision of the authors of DSM–III to develop an alternative to ICD–9 was instrumental in developing a highly innovative manual (Kendell, 1991; Spitzer et al., 1980). However, its innovations were also at the cost of decreasing compatibility with the ICD–9 nomenclature that was used throughout the rest of the world, which is problematic to the stated purpose of providing a common language of communication. In May of 1988 the American Psychiatric Association appointed a DSM–IV task force, chaired by Allen Frances (Frances, Widiger, & Pincus, 1989). Mandates for DSM–IV included better coordination with ICD–10 and improved documentation of empirical support.

The DSM–IV committee aspired to use a more conservative threshold for the inclusion of new diagnoses and to have decisions that were guided more explicitly by the scientific literature (Nathan & Langenbucher, 1999). Frances et al. (1989) suggested that "the major innovation of DSM–IV will not be in its having surprising new content but rather will reside in the systematic and explicit method by which DSM–IV will be constructed and documented" (p. 375). Proposals for additions, deletions, or revisions were guided by 175 literature reviews that used a specific format that maximized the potential for critical review, containing (for example) a method section that documented explicitly the criteria for including and excluding studies and the process by which the literature had been reviewed. Each of these reviews has since been published in three volumes of a DSM–IV Sourcebook (Widiger et al., 1994, 1996, 1997). Testable questions that could be addressed with existing data sets were also explored in thirty-six studies, which emphasized the aggregation of multiple data sets from independent researchers, and twelve field trials were conducted to provide reliability and validity data on proposed revisions. The results of the thirty-six studies and twelve field trials were published in the fourth volume of the DSM–IV Sourcebook (Widiger et al., 1998). Critical reviews of these 223 projects were obtained by sending initial drafts to advisors or consultants to a respective work group, by presenting drafts at relevant conferences, and by submitting drafts to peer-reviewed journals (Widiger, Frances, Pincus, Davis, & First, 1991).

DSM–IV-TR

One of the innovations of DSM–III was the inclusion of a relatively detailed text discussion of each disorder, including information on age of onset, gender, course, and familial pattern (Spitzer et al., 1980). This text was expanded in DSM–IV to include cultural and ethnic group variation, variation across age, and laboratory and physical exam findings (Frances, First, & Pincus, 1995). Largely excluded from the text is information concerning etiology, pathology, and treatment as this material was considered to be too theoretically specific and more suitable for academic texts. Nevertheless, it had also become apparent that DSM–IV was being used as a textbook, and the material on age, course, prevalence, and family history was quickly becoming outdated as new information was being gathered.

Therefore, in 1997, the American Psychiatric Association appointed a DSM–IV Text Revision work group, chaired by Michael First (editor of the text and criterion sets for DSM–IV) and Harold Pincus (Vice-Chair for DSM–IV) to update the text material. No substantive changes in the criterion sets were considered, nor were any new additions, subtypes, deletions, or other changes in the status of any diagnoses implemented. In addition, each of the proposed revisions to the text had to be supported by a systematic literature review that was critiqued by a considerable number of advisors. The DSM–IV Text Revision (DSM–IV–TR) was published in 2000 (APA, 2000).

ICD–11 and DSM–V

DSM–I, DSM–II, DSM–III, and DSM–IV were each coordinated, at least in timing, with an edition of the ICD (ICD–6, ICD–8, ICD–9, and ICD–10, respectively). If this coordination were to continue, DSM–V would begin in tandem with the development of ICD–11. However, the WHO experienced substantial difficulty completing all of the sections of the ICD (Kendell, 1991). The mental disorders section of ICD–10 was published in 1992, but to this day has still not been implemented officially within the United States. The WHO is unlikely to attempt again to revise the entire ICD. Future revisions will be confined to individual sections of the manual, each being revised on its own schedule. Revisions to the mental disorders section of the ICD may in fact be coordinated with the development of DSM–V (rather than vice versa) partly because of the recognized success of the recent editions of the DSM.

In 1999, a conference jointly sponsored by the National Institute of Mental Health (NIMH) and the American Psychiatric Association was held to identify the research that would most likely be informative for the authors of DSM–V (McQueen, 2000). Substantive issues emphasized by research planning work groups developed from this conference included (but were not limited to) cross-cultural issues, gender differences, developmental differences, the distinction between Axis I and Axis II, the definition of mental disorder, the threshold for diagnosis, the use of laboratory findings in diagnosis, the impact of neuroscience, and dimensional models of psychopathology (e.g., Alarcon et al., 2002; First et al., 2002; Lehman et al., 2002, Rounsaville et al., 2002). A series of more specific international conferences are likely to follow, leading up to a DSM–V task force that may not be formed until approximately 2005, with an anticipated publication of DSM–V in approximately 2010.

CONTINUING ISSUES FOR DSM–V

The issues considered by the DSM–V research planning work groups (McQueen, 2002) will not necessarily be new or unique to DSM–V. In fact, some of them concern fundamental issues that have been raised throughout the history of the diagnosis of mental disorders (Blashfield, 1984; Kendell, 1975; Zilboorg, 1941). Six issues worth highlighting in particular are (1) the definition of mental disorder and threshold for diagnosis, (2) multiple diagnoses (i.e., excessive diagnostic co-occurrence), (3) categorical versus dimensional models of classification, (4) culture and values, (5) gender, and (6) the inclusion of laboratory tests within diagnostic criterion sets. Each of these issues will be discussed briefly in turn.

Definition of Mental Disorder and Threshold for Diagnosis

The boundaries of the diagnostic manual have been increasing with each edition, and there has been vocal concern that much of this expansion represents an encroachment into normal problems of living (Caplan, 1995; Folette & Houts, 1996). Diagnoses proposed for DSM–IV were ultimately included within an appendix primarily because they might be below an appropriate threshold for diagnosis, such as mixed anxiety–depressive disorder, age-related cognitive decline, and minor depressive disorder (Widiger & Coker, 2003). A difficult task facing the authors of DSM–V will be establishing a meaningful boundary between abnormal and normal psychological functioning. (See Maddux, Gosselin, & Winstead, this book, for a more detailed discussion of this issue.)

The extract that follows provides the definition of mental disorder presented in DSM–IV–TR (APA, 2000).

> In DSM–IV, each of the mental disorders is conceptualized as a clinically significant behavioral or psychological syndrome or pattern that occurs in an individual and that is associated with present distress (e.g., a painful symptom) or disability (i.e., impairment in one or more important areas of functioning) or with a significantly increased risk of suffering death, pain, disability, or an important loss of freedom. In addition, this syndrome or pattern must not be merely an expectable and culturally sanctioned response to a particular event, for example, the death of a loved one. Whatever its original cause, it must currently be considered a manifestation of a behavioral, psychological, or biological dysfunction in the individual. Neither deviant behavior (e.g., political, religious, or sexual) nor conflicts that are primarily between the individual and society are mental disorders unless the deviance or conflict is a symptom of a dysfunction in the individual, as described above. (American Psychiatric Association, 2000, p. xxxi)

This definition was the result of an effort by the authors of DSM–III to develop specific and explicit criteria for deciding whether a behavior pattern (homosexuality in particular) should be classified as a mental disorder (Spitzer & Williams, 1982). The intense controversy over homosexuality has largely abated, but the issues raised in this historical debate continue to apply.

For example, in order to be diagnosed with pedophilia, DSM–III–R (APA, 1987) required only that an adult have recurrent intense urges and fantasies involving sexual activity with a prepubescent child over a period of at least six months and have acted on them (or be markedly distressed by them). Every adult who engaged in a sexual activity with a child for longer than six months would meet these diagnostic criteria. The authors of DSM–IV were therefore concerned that DSM–III–R was not providing adequate guidance for determining when deviant sexual behavior is the result of a mental disorder. Deviant behavior alone has not traditionally been considered sufficient for a diagnosis (Gorenstein, 1984). Presumably, some persons can engage in deviant, aberrant, and even heinous activities without being compelled to do so by the presence of psychopathology. The authors of DSM–IV, therefore, added the requirement that "the behavior, sexual urges, or fantasies cause clinically significant distress or impairment in social, occupational, or other important areas of functioning" (APA, 1994, p. 523).

Require Presence of Pathology? Spitzer and Wakefield (1999), however, have argued that the impairment criteria included in DSM–IV are inadequate. They concurred with a
concern raised by the National Law Center for Children and Families that DSM–IV might contribute to a normalization of pedophilic and other paraphilic behavior by allowing the diagnoses
not to be applied if the persons who have engaged in these acts are not themselves distressed
by their behavior or do not otherwise experience impairment. In response, Frances et al. (1995)
had argued that pedophilic sexual "behaviors are inherently problematic because they involve
a nonconsenting person (exhibitionism, voyeurism, frotteurism) or a child (pedophilia) and
may lead to arrest and incarceration" (p. 319). Therefore, any person who engaged in an illegal
sexual act (for longer than six months) would be exhibiting a clinically significant social impairment and would therefore meet the DSM–IV threshold for diagnosis. However, using the
illegality of an act as a diagnostic criterion presents three problems. First, it undermines the
original rationale for the inclusion of the impairment criterion (i.e., to distinguish immoral or
illegal acts from abnormal or disordered acts). Second, it provides no meaningful basis for determining when deviant sexual acts or fantasies are or are not due to a mental disorder. Third, it
is inconsistent with the stated definition of a mental disorder that indicates that neither deviance
nor conflicts with the law are sufficient to warrant a diagnosis (see previous APA definition).
Spitzer and Wakefield argued that the distinction between disordered and nondisordered abuse
of children requires an assessment for the presence an underlying, internal pathology (e.g.,
irrational cognitive schema or neurochemical dysregulation).

Wakefield (1997) has provided examples of other criterion sets from DSM–IV less politically
or socially controversial than pedophilia, which he has argued have also failed to make a
necessary distinction between maladaptive problems in living and true psychopathology due
to the reliance within the criterion sets on indicators of distress or impairment rather than
references to pathology. For example, the DSM–IV criterion set for major depressive disorder
currently excludes most instances of depressive reactions to the loss of a loved one (i.e.,
uncomplicated bereavement). Depression after the loss of a loved one can be considered a
mental disorder, though, if "the symptoms persist for longer than two months" (APA, 1994,
p. 327). Allowing two months to grieve before one is diagnosed with a mental disorder might
be as arbitrary and meaningless as allowing a person to engage in a sexually deviant act
only for six months before the behavior is diagnosed as a paraphilia. Similar concerns have
been raised by Regier et al. (1998) regarding the diagnosis of common anxiety and mood
disorders. They suggested that the prevalence rates for many of the anxiety, mood, and other
mental disorders obtained by the NIMH Epidemiologic Catchment Area program (ECA) and
the National Comorbidity Survey (NCS) were excessive. "Based on the high prevalence rates
identified in both the ECA and NCS, it is reasonable to hypothesize that some syndromes in
the community represent transient homeostatic responses to internal or external stimuli that
do not represent true psychopathologic disorders" (Regier et al., 1998, p. 114).

The inclusion of pathology within diagnostic criterion sets (e.g., irrational cognitive
schemas, unconscious defense mechanisms, or neurochemical dysregulations) would be consistent with the definition of mental disorder provided in DSM–IV, which states that the syndrome
"must currently be considered a manifestation of a behavioral, psychological, or biological
dysfunction in the individual" (APA, 2000, p. xxxi; see previous APA definition). However, a
limitation of this proposal is that there is currently little agreement over the specific pathology
that should be required for any particular disorder. There is insufficient empirical support to
give preference to one particular cognitive, interpersonal, neurochemical, psychodynamic, or
other theoretical model of pathology. The precise nature of this pathology could be left unde-
fined or characterized simply as an "internal dysfunction" (Wakefield, Pottick, & Kirk, 2002),
but an assessment of an unspecified pathology is unlikely to be reliable. Clinicians will have

very different opinions concerning the nature of the internal dysfunction and quite different thresholds for its attribution.

The assumption that the expansion of the nomenclature is subsuming normal problems in living is itself questionable. Persons critical of the nomenclature have decried the substantial expansion of the diagnostic manual over the past 50 years (e.g., Caplan, 1995; Follette & Houts, 1996; Kutchins & Kirk, 1997). It would have been more surprising, however, to find that scientific research and increased knowledge have failed to lead to the recognition of more instances of psychopathology (Wakefield, 1998). In fact, the current manual might still be inadequate in its coverage despite the expansion. Quite often, the most common diagnosis in general clinical practice is not-otherwise-specified (NOS; Clark, Watson, & Reynolds, 1995). The NOS diagnosis is provided when a clinician has determined that psychopathology is present but the symptomatology fails to meet criteria for any one of the existing disorders. Clinicians providing the diagnosis of NOS for anxiety, mood, personality, and other disorders is a testament to the inadequate coverage currently provided (although perhaps one could argue as well that this is a testament to a tendency of clinicians to diagnose normal problems in living as being instances of mental disorder).

The inclusion of pathology within diagnostic criterion sets may even fail to result in a more conservative threshold for diagnosis. Irrational cognitive schemas and neurochemical dysregulations (Prigerson et al., 1999) might be found in the ostensibly normal cases of bereavement described by Regier et al. (1998) and Wakefield (1997). Pathology might also be present in the absence of any impairment or distress (Lehman et al., 2002). Optimal psychological functioning, as in the case of optimal physical functioning, might represent an ideal that is achieved by only a small minority of the population. The rejection of a high prevalence rate of psychopathology may reflect the best of intentions, such as concerns regarding the stigmatization of mental disorder diagnoses (Kutchins & Kirk, 1997) or the potential impact on funding for treatment (Regier et al., 1998). These social and political concerns, however, could also hinder a more dispassionate and accurate recognition of the true rate of a broad range of psychopathology within the population (Widiger & Sankis, 2000).

Harmful Dysfunction or Dyscontrolled Maladaptivity?

Harmful Dysfunction or Dyscontrolled Maladaptivity? Wakefield (1992) has developed an alternative harmful dysfunction definition of mental disorder where dysfunction is a failure of an internal mechanism to perform a naturally selected function (e.g., the capacity to experience feelings of guilt in a person with antisocial personality disorder) and harm is a value judgment that the design failure is harmful to the individual (e.g., failure to learn from mistakes results in repeated punishments, arrests, loss of employment, and eventual impoverishment). Wakefield's model has received substantial attention and is being considered for inclusion in DSM–V (Rounsaville et al., 2002). However, the model has also received compelling criticism (e.g., Bergner, 1997; Kirmayer & Young, 1999; Lilienfeld & Marino, 1999). A fundamental limitation is its girding within evolutionary theory, thereby limiting its relevance and usefulness to alternative models of etiology and pathology (Bergner, 1997). Wakefield's model might even be inconsistent with some sociobiological models of psychopathology. Cultural evolution may at times outstrip the pace of biological evolution, rendering some designed functions that were originally adaptive within earlier time periods maladaptive in many current environments (Lilienfeld & Marino, 1999; Widiger & Sankis, 2000). For example, "the existence in humans of a preparedness mechanism for developing a fear of snakes may be a relic not well designed to deal with urban living, which currently contains hostile forces far more dangerous to human survival (e.g., cars, electrical outlets) but for which humans lack evolved mechanisms of fear preparedness" (Buss, Haselton, Shackelford, Bleske, & Wakefield, 1998, p. 538).

Missing from Wakefield's (1992) definition of mental disorder is any reference to dyscontrol. Harm within Wakefield's conceptualization of mental disorder is concerned with the presence of impairment, dysfunction with the presence of pathology. Mental disorders, however, are perhaps better understood as dyscontrolled impairments in psychological functioning (Kirmayer & Young, 1999; Klein, 1999; Widiger & Trull, 1991). "Involuntary impairment remains the key inference" (Klein, 1999, p. 424). Dyscontrol is one of the fundamental features of mental disorder emphasized in Bergner's (1997) significant restriction and Widiger and Sankis' (2000) dyscontrolled maladaptivity definitions of mental disorder.

Fundamental to the concept of a mental disorder is the presence of impairments to feelings, thoughts, or behaviors over which a normal (healthy) person is believed to have adequate control. To the extent that a person willfully, intentionally, freely, or voluntarily engages in harmful sexual acts, drug usage, gambling, or child abuse, the person is not considered to have a mental disorder. Persons seek professional intervention in large part to obtain the insights, techniques, skills, or other tools (e.g., medications) that increase their ability to better control their mood, thoughts, or behavior. In sum, impairment and dyscontrol might provide the optimal means with which to identify a meaningful boundary between, or an important parameter for quantifying, normal and abnormal psychological functioning, if these constructs are more precisely defined, calibrated, and assessed. (See also Maddux, Gosselin, & Winstead, this book.)

Multiple Diagnoses

The difficulty in delineating a point of demarcation between normal and abnormal psychological functioning is paralleled by an equally fundamental problem of differentiating individual mental disorders from one another. "DSM–IV is a categorical classification that divides mental disorders into types based on criterion sets with defining features" (APA, 2000, p. xxxi). The intention of the diagnostic manual is to help the clinician determine which particular disorder is present, the diagnosis of which would purportedly indicate the presence of a specific pathology that would explain the occurrence of the symptoms and suggest a specific treatment that would ameliorate the patient's suffering (Kendell, 1975; Frances et al., 1995).

It is evident, however, that DSM–IV routinely fails in the goal of guiding the clinician to the presence of one specific disorder. Despite the best efforts of those who have been the primary authors of each revision, multiple diagnoses are the norm (Clark et al., 1995). It is rare for a patient to meet the DSM–IV–TR diagnostic criteria for just one mental disorder. The number of multiple diagnoses is even higher when one includes lifetime as well as current functioning and it might be remarkably high if all of the disorders within DSM–IV–TR are in fact considered. Excluded from prior epidemiologic studies have been many disorders (e.g., personality disorders and specific substance abuse disorders) that might increase even further the occurrence of multiple diagnoses (Widiger & Sankis, 2000).

In general medicine, the presence of multiple diagnoses would logically suggest the presence of multiple disorders (i.e., comorbidity). However, the frequency with which psychiatric patients routinely meet diagnostic criteria for three, four, five, and even more mental disorders has raised questions concerning the validity of this straightforward understanding. "The greatest challenge that the extensive comorbidity data pose to the current nosological system concerns the validity of the diagnostic categories themselves—do these disorders constitute distinct clinical entities?" (Mineka, Watson, & Clark, 1998, p. 380). Diagnostic comorbidity has become so prevalent that some argue for an abandonment of the term *comorbidity* in favor of a term (e.g., co-occurrence) that does not imply the presence of distinct clinical entities (Lilienfeld, Waldman, & Israel, 1994). There are instances in which the presence of multiple diagnoses do suggest the presence of distinct yet comorbid psychopathologies, but in many instances the presence of co-occurring diagnoses does appear to suggest the presence of an etiology or pathology that is shared by the purportedly distinct disorders (Widiger & Clark, 2000).

Categorical and Dimensional Models of Classification

There has been substantial interest in identifying a specific gene (or other form of specific etiology) for each mental disorder, modeled after the success obtained with some physical disorders. "As the rare Mendelian disorders such as cystic fibrosis and Huntington's disease are solved, the entire genetics community is, with great excitement, turning its attention to complex disorders . . . [and] psychiatric illnesses are fully and unquestionably viewed as part of the next challenge in mainstream genetics" (Hyman, 1998, p. 38). However, the complex disorders of psychopathology appear unlikely to have specific etiologies or even specific genetic etiologies (McGue & Bouchard, 1998), and initial successes in identifying specific genes have typically failed to replicate (Portin & Alanen, 1997). For example, up to 85% of the susceptibility to schizophrenia appears to be attributable to genetic contributions, but the extensive genome scan studies of schizophrenia currently "do not support the hypothesis that a single gene causes a large increase in the risk of schizophrenia" (Levinson et al., 1998, p. 741).

"Categorical disease models are being challenged . . . by the recent data indicating that individuals may carry a genetic risk factor to develop a disorder that can be measured premorbidly . . . and that may or may not ultimately be expressed as the full form of the disorder, depending on the occurrence of a variety of factors" (Andreasen, 1997, p. 1587). There continues to be a hope of demarcating "a clear-cut, natural, qualitative subgroup" of psychopathology (Lenzenweger, 1999, p. 186), but it might be unrealistic to expect maladaptive cognitions, affects, and behaviors, or any particular constellation of symptoms, to have a specific etiology. Not only would this etiology have to have provided a uniquely and specifically important contribution to their development (Meehl, 1977), but the phenomenology of the disorder would also have to have been largely resilient to the potential impact of other genetic and environmental influences. The symptomatology of most mental disorders appears to be, in contrast, responsive to a wide variety of neurochemical, interpersonal, cognitive, and other mediating variables. Mental disorders are most likely the result of polygenetic dispositions and multiple, interacting etiologies (Rutter, 1997).

Many researchers are now turning their attention to the identification of underlying spectra of dysfunction that cut across the existing diagnostic categories. For example, Brown, Chorpita, and Barlow (1998) conducted a series of confirmatory factor analyses of the symptomatology evident among 350 anxiety and mood disorder patients. Their results confirmed the presence of latent dimensions of pathology (e.g., abnormal levels of positive affectivity and arousal), some of which cut across the mood and anxiety disorders (e.g., negative affectivity or neuroticism). In an extensive longitudinal epidemiological study, Krueger, Caspi, Moffitt, and Silva (1998) assessed a range of symptomatology in a large, unselected birth cohort in New Zealand at ages 18 and 21. Using structural equation modeling to examine cross-sectional and longitudinal co-occurrence patterns, they identified the presence of "stable, underlying 'core psychopathological processes' " (Krueger et al., 1998, p. 216). More specifically, Krueger et al. suggested that a broad domain of internalization (neuroticism or negative affectivity) underlies the mood and anxiety disorder diagnostic categories and a complementary factor of externalization (low constraint, disinhibition) underlies the disruptive behavior and substance use disorder diagnostic categories. Krueger (1999) obtained similar results in a confirmatory factor analysis of the patterns of co-occurrence among the diagnoses included within the NCS and concluded that "comorbidity results from common, underlying core psychopathological processes" (p. 921).

Lynam and Widiger (2001) aggregated the diagnostic co-occurrence among the personality disorder diagnoses obtained in fifteen previous studies. "Although high comorbidity presents a fundamental challenge to the validity of the categorical approach , it is easily accommodated within a dimensional model that views the categories as configurations of basic dimensions of personality" (Lynam & Widiger, 2001, p. 403). They indicated that when personality disorders are understood in terms of the domains and facets of the dimensional Five-Factor Model of general personality functioning, the apparent comorbidity is readily explained. A Five-Factor Model understanding of the personality disorders is presented in Coker and Widiger (this book).

A model for the future diagnosis of all mental disorders might be provided by one of the oldest and best validated diagnoses, mental retardation, a disorder for which much is known of its etiology, pathology, and classification. The point of demarcation for its diagnosis is an arbitrary, quantitative distinction along the normally distributed levels of the multivariate domain of intelligence. Mental retardation is diagnosed primarily on the basis of having an intelligence quotient (IQ) of 70 or below (APA, 2000). There are persons with an IQ less than 70 for whom a qualitatively distinct disorder is evident. However, this disorder is not mental retardation, it is a physical disorder (e.g., Down syndrome) that can be traced to a specific biological event (i.e., trisomy 21). Intelligence is itself distributed as a continuous variable. In addition, "in approximately 30%–40% of individuals seen in clinical settings, no clear etiology for the Mental Retardation can be determined despite extensive evaluation efforts" (APA, 2000, p. 45). Intelligence is the result of a complex array of multiple genetic, fetal and infant development, and environmental influences (Neisser et al., 1996). There are no discrete breaks in the distribution of intelligence that would provide an absolute distinction between normal intelligence and abnormal intelligence.

Culture and Values

It is the intention of the authors of ICD–10 to provide a universal diagnostic system, but diagnostic criteria and constructs can have quite different implications and meanings across different cultures. DSM–IV addresses cultural issues in three ways. First, the text of DSM–IV provides a discussion of how each disorder is known to vary in its presentation across different cultures. Second, an appendix of culture-bound syndromes describes disorders that are currently thought to be specific to a particular culture. Third, an additional appendix provides a culturally informed diagnostic formulation that considers the cultural identity of the individual and the culture-specific explanations of the person's presenting complaints (Mezzich et al., 1997).

There is both a strong and a weak cross-cultural critique of current scientific understanding of psychopathology. The weak critique does not question the validity of a concept of mental disorder but does argue that social and cultural processes affect and potentially bias the "science of psychopathology and diagnosis: a) by determining the selection of persons and behaviors as suitable material for analysis; b) by emphasizing what aspects of this material will be handled as relevant from a [clinical] standpoint; c) by shaping the language of diagnosis, including that of descriptive psychopathology; d) by masking the symptoms of any putative 'universal' disorder; e) by biasing the observer and would-be diagnostician; and f) by determining the goals and endpoints of treatment" (Fabrega, 1994, p. 262). These concerns are not weak in the sense that they are trivial or inconsequential but they are relatively weak in that they do not necessarily dispute the fundamental validity of a concept of a mental disorder or the science of psychopathology. The strong critique, in contrast, is that the construct of mental disorder is itself a culture-bound belief that reflects the local biases of western society, and that the science of psychopathology is valid only in the sense that it is an accepted belief system of a particular culture (Lewis-Fernandez & Kleinman, 1995).

The concept of mental disorder does include a value judgment that there should be necessary, adequate, or optimal psychological functioning (Wakefield, 1992). However, this value judgment is also a fundamental component of the construct of physical disorder (Widiger, 2002). In a world in which there were no impairments or threats to physical functioning, the construct of a physical disorder would have no meaning except as an interesting thought experiment. Meaningful and valid scientific research on the etiology, pathology, and treatment of physical disorders occurs because in the world as it currently exists there are impairments and threats to physical functioning. It is provocative and intriguing to conceive of a world in which physical health and survival would or should not be valued or preferred over illness, suffering, and death, but this form of existence is unlikely to emerge anytime in the near future. Placing a value on adequate or optimal physical functioning might be a natural result of evolution within a world in which there are threats to functioning and survival. Likewise, in the world as it currently exists, there are impairments and threats to adequate psychological functioning. It is provocative and intriguing to conceive of a society (or world) in which psychological health would or should not be valued or preferred, but this form of existence is also unlikely to emerge anytime in the near future. Placing a value on adequate, necessary, or optimal psychological functioning might be inherent to and a natural result of existing in this world. Any particular definition of what would constitute adequate, necessary, or optimal psychological functioning would likely be biased to some extent by local cultural values, but this situation is perhaps best understood as only the failing of one particular conceptualization of mental disorder (i.e., a weak rather than a strong critique). Valuing adequate, necessary, or optimal psychological functioning could itself still be a logical and natural result of existing in a world in which there are threats to psychological functioning, just as placing a value on adequate, necessary, or optimal physical functioning would be a logical and natural result of existing in a world in which there are threats to physical functioning (Widiger, 2002).

Different societies, cultures, and even persons within a particular culture will disagree as to what constitutes optimal or pathological biological and psychological functioning (Lopez & Guarnaccia, 2000; this book). An important and difficult issue is how best to understand the differences between cultures with respect to what constitutes dysfunction and pathology (Alarcon et al., 2002). For example, simply because diagnostic criterion sets are applied reliably across different cultures does not necessarily indicate that the constructs themselves are valid or meaningful within these cultures (Lewis-Fernandez & Kleinman, 1995). A reliably diagnosed criterion set can be developed for an entirely illusory diagnostic construct. On the other hand, it is perhaps equally unclear why it would be necessary for the establishment of a disorder's construct validity to obtain cross-cultural (i.e., universal) acceptance. Lewis-Fernandez and Kleinman argue that it is necessary "to produce a comprehensive nosology that is both internationally and locally valid" (p. 435). A universally accepted diagnostic system will have an international social utility and consensus validity (Kessler, 1999), but it is also apparent that belief systems vary in their veridicality. Recognition of and appreciation for alternative belief systems is important for adequate functioning within an international community, but respect for alternative belief systems does not necessarily imply that all belief systems are equally valid (Widiger, 2002).

Kirmayer, Young, and Hayton (1995) illustrate well many of the complexities of cross-cultural research. For example, a woman's housebound behavior might be diagnosed as agoraphobic within western cultures but considered normative (or even virtuous) within a Muslim culture; submissive behavior that is diagnosed as pathologic dependency within western societies might be considered normative within the Japanese culture. However, simply because a behavior pattern is valued, accepted, encouraged, or even statistically normative within a particular culture does not necessarily mean it is conducive to healthy psychological functioning.

"In societies where ritual plays an important role in religious life . . . such societies may pre-dispose individuals to obsessive-compulsive symptoms and mask the disorder when present" (Kirmayer et al., 1995, p. 507). "The congruence between religious belief and practice and obsessive-compulsive symptoms also probably contributes to relatively low rates of insight into the irrationality of the symptoms" (Kirmayer et al., p. 508). Behaviors diagnosed as dis-ordered within one culture might be normative within another, but what is accepted, allowed, encouraged, or even statistically normative within a culture might still be pathological. On the other hand, it is equally important not to assume that what is believed to be associated with maladaptive (or adaptive) functioning in one culture should also be considered to be maladaptive (or adaptive) within all other cultures (Alarcon et al., 2002). "This possible ten-sion between cultural styles and health consequences is in urgent need of further research" (Kirmayer et al., p. 517), and it is important for this research to go beyond simply identifying differences in behaviors, belief systems, and values across different cultures. This research also needs to address the fundamental question of whether differences in beliefs actually question the validity of any universal conceptualization of psychopathology or suggest instead simply different perspectives on a common, universal issue. (See Lopez & Guarnaccia, this book, for a more detailed discussion of culture and psychopathology.)

Gender

Differential sex prevalence rates can be highly controversial as gender differences can reflect wider social, political controversies (Eagly, 1995). The diagnoses that generated the most controversy in the development of the recent editions of the DSM were problematic largely because of their questionable application to women (Ross, Frances, & Widiger, 1995). The basic charge was that the DSM is fundamentally flawed through its imposition of patriarchal or masculine biases of what does or should constitute psychopathology (e.g., Caplan, 1991, 1995). In perhaps one of the more widely cited critiques, Kaplan (1983) argued that "our diagnostic system, like the society it serves, is male centered" (p. 791) and that "masculine-biased assumptions about what behaviors are healthy and what behaviors are crazy are codified in diagnostic criteria" (p. 786). Pantony and Caplan (1991) characterized DSM–IV as "sex discrimination in one of its most damaging and dangerous forms" (p. 120).

The premenstrual dysphoric disorder diagnosis has been particularly controversial (Caplan, 1991; Ross et al., 1995). A majority of women may suffer from some form of premenstrual dysphoria. Only 3% to 5% of women would meet the DSM–IV diagnostic criteria for premen-strual dysphoric disorder, but the reliability of the distinction between normal premenstrual dysphoria and premenstrual dysphoric disorder in general clinical practice is questionable. DSM–IV requires daily ratings of mood for at least two months before the diagnosis is made, and it is unlikely that practicing clinicians or patients would actually adhere to this requirement. The pharmaceutical industry might also market treatments to women who are well below the threshold for the diagnosis, and attributions concerning the harm, pathology, and impairments of premenstrual dysphoria are often exaggerated and can be highly stigmatizing.

Histrionic personality disorder has been criticized for being too closely associated with stereotypic traits of femininity (Kaplan, 1983). Kaplan (1983) went so far as to argue that by virtue of being feminine "a healthy woman automatically earns the diagnosis of Histrionic Personality Disorder" (p. 789). There is no research to support the claim that normal, healthy women meet diagnostic criteria for histrionic personality disorder. Studies have indicated that the diagnostic criteria for this disorder include maladaptive variants of stereotypic feminine traits, but it is unclear whether this association is inappropriate for a personality disorder diagnosis. The inclusion of gender-related traits, however, does appear to contribute to the occurrence of gender-biased applications of the diagnostic criteria and gender-biased assessment instruments (Widiger, 1998).

There may not be a disorder in DSM–IV for which gender differences have not been problematic and even controversial (Kaplan, 1983). Concerns about gender bias have been raised for almost every diagnosis, either with respect to the diagnostic criteria, the applications of these diagnostic criteria by clinicians, the assessment instruments used in research and clinical practice, or the populations that have been sampled (Hartung & Widiger, 1998). An issue for the authors of DSM–V is whether to revise diagnostic criteria to improve their gender neutrality or to develop different criterion sets for males and females. Currently, the same diagnostic criteria are used for males and females for all but a few of the disorders (the exceptions being gender-identity disorder and sexual dysfunctions), but the text of DSM–IV indicates how each respective disorder appears differently in males and females (Frances et al., 1995). Achieving gender-neutral diagnostic criteria for many of these disorders might be difficult (Sprock, Crosby, & Nielsen, 2001). On the other hand, separate diagnostic criteria could result in the creation of different disorders for each sex that might have even more problematic implications of gender bias (Wakefield, 1987; Zahn-Waxler, 1993). For example, Zoccolillo (1993) suggested that the diagnostic criteria for conduct disorder were gender biased because they described a masculine way in which the disorder is expressed. She suggested placing relatively more emphasis for girls on rule violations, substance abuse, prostitution, chronic lying, running away from home, and poor school performance and less emphasis on vandalism, fire setting, burglary, use of a weapon in fights, and rape. However, placing more emphasis on rule violations, rebelliousness, and deceitfulness for girls, and violent and aggressive behavior for boys, could have the effect of diagnosing (and stigmatizing) girls at a level of dysfunction that is much lower than is used to diagnose the disorder in boys (Zahn-Waxler, 1993). Zahn-Waxler suggested alternatively that the criterion set appropriately includes gender-related behaviors (e.g., rape) because the disorder is itself related to gender in its etiology and pathology. (See Winstead & Sanchez, this book, for a more detailed discuss of gender and psychopathology.)

Laboratory Measures, Diagnostic Criteria, and Clinical Diagnosis

"Diagnoses in the rest of medicine are often heavily influenced by laboratory tests" (Frances et al., 1995, p. 22). Laboratory tests within medical practice go beyond the assessment of symptoms. They provide a more direct and objective assessment of an underlying physical pathology. A hope is that laboratory tests could do the same for psychiatry as they have done for other domains of medicine (Nemeroff, Kilts, & Berns, 1999; Rounsaville et al., 2002). "The increasing use of laboratory tests in psychiatric research raises the question of whether and when these tests should be included within the diagnostic criteria sets" (Frances et al., 1995, p. 22).

Substantial attention is being given to structural and functional brain imaging with the expectation that these instruments could be used eventually to diagnose neurophysiological pathology (Drevets, 2002; Epstein, Isenberg, Stern, & Silbersweig, 2002). However, clearly limiting these and other neurophysiological measures' potential for incorporation within diagnostic criterion sets is the virtual absence of research indicating their ability to provide independent, blind diagnoses. Despite the enthusiasm for their potential diagnostic value, there are currently no studies that have assessed the sensitivity and specificity of neuroimaging techniques for the diagnosis or differential diagnosis of specific mental disorders (Rounsaville et al., 2002; Steffens & Krishnan, 1998).

The inclusion of laboratory data in the diagnosis of a disorder has been particularly controversial for the sleep disorders. Most sleep disorder specialists use the International Classification of Sleep Disorders (ICSD) developed by the American Sleep Disorders Association (1990). The twelve DSM–IV sleep disorder diagnoses are coordinated with the ICSD, but differ significantly in failing to include polysomnographic diagnostic criteria (e.g., time of onset of rapid-eye-movement sleep). Detailed references are made to polysomnographic findings within the text of DSM–IV, and it was acknowledged by its authors that "for sleep disorders other than insomnia, such as narcolepsy and sleep apnea, the utility of sleep laboratory testing is widely accepted" (Buysse, Reynolds, & Kupfer, 1998, pp. 1104–1105). Nevertheless, polysomography findings were not required because of the extensive cost of the technology and their lack of availability within many clinical settings (Buysse et al., 1998; Frances et al., 1995).

There is, however, a precedent in DSM–IV for the requirement of laboratory test findings obtained by a specialist. Laboratory tests are fundamental components of the diagnostic criteria for learning disorders and mental retardation. For example, "the essential feature of Mental Retardation is significantly subaverage general intellectual functioning ... [and] general intellectual functioning is defined by the intelligence quotient (IQ or IQ-equivalent) obtained by assessment with one or more of the standardized, individually administered intelligence tests (e.g., Wechsler Intelligence Scales for Children, 3rd Edition; Stanford-Binet, 4th Edition; Kaufman Assessment Battery for Children)" (APA, 2000, p. 41). Psychological tests administered by a trained specialist using standardized equipment are essentially equivalent to the provision of laboratory testing. There are compelling concerns regarding the precise accuracy of IQ tests (Neisser et al., 1996), but routine diagnoses of mental retardation by practicing clinicians without the input of individually administered IQ tests would be substantially more problematic and controversial.

The precedent established by mental retardation and learning disorders should perhaps be extended to other disorders (Widiger & Clark, 2000). "Although diagnostic criteria are the framework for any clinical or epidemiological assessment, no assessment of clinical status is independent of the reliability and validity of the methods used to determine the presence of a diagnosis" (Regier et al., 1998, p. 114). The DSM–III innovation of providing relatively specific and explicit diagnostic criteria is not realized if clinicians do not in fact adhere to the criterion sets and assess them in a comprehensive, systematic, and consistent fashion (Rogers, 2001). Researchers would be hard pressed to get their findings published if they failed to document that their diagnoses were based on a systematic, replicable, and objective method, yet no such requirements are provided for clinical diagnoses, with the exception of mental retardation and learning disorders. Clinicians generally prefer to rely on their own experience, expertise, and subjective impressions obtained through unstructured interviews (Westen, 1997), but it is precisely this reliance on subjective and idiosyncratic clinical interviewing that often undermines the reliability and ultimately the validity of clinical diagnoses (Garb, 1998; Rogers, 2001).

One of the new additions to the text of DSM–IV was a section devoted to laboratory and physical exam findings. This material was intended to provide the initial step toward the eventual inclusion of laboratory tests within diagnostic criterion sets (Frances et al., 1995). A noteworthy exclusion from this text are references to psychological tests and instruments (Rounsaville et al., 2002; Widiger & Clark, 2000). It is ironic that psychological tests are included already within the criterion sets for mental retardation and learning disorders, yet virtually no reference is made to any psychological tests within the sections devoted to laboratory test findings.

The discussion of laboratory instruments is confined in DSM–IV to measures of neurophysiology (e.g., functional brain imaging and the dexamethasone suppression test). Semistructured interviews and self-report inventories that assess cognitive, behavioral, affective, or other components of psychological functioning that comprise explicitly the diagnostic criterion sets for these disorders, and for which substantial research already provides specificity and sensitivity rates not obtained by the neurophysiological instruments, should at least be acknowledged along with the neurophysiological measures. The inclusion of additional psychological tests within diagnostic criterion sets might have professional implications for the necessary qualifications to render a clinical diagnosis. For example, it is unclear whether many psychiatrists and even some psychologists are sufficiently trained in the administration and interpretation of the most informative and valid psychological tests. In any case, the American Psychiatric Association has already developed an authoritative manual for the best "psychiatric" instruments for the assessment of each disorder included within DSM–IV (Rush et al., 2000).

CONCLUSIONS

Nobody is fully satisfied with, or lacks valid criticisms of, DSM–IV and ICD–10. Zilboorg's (1941) suggestion that budding 19th century theorists and researchers cut their first teeth by providing a new classification of mental disorders still applies, although perhaps the right of passage today is to provide a critique of the ICD and/or DSM.

None, however, appear to be suggesting that all official diagnostic nomenclatures be abandoned. The benefits do appear to outweigh the costs (Salmon et al., 1917; Stengel, 1959; Regier et al., 1998). Everybody finds fault with this language, but there is at least the ability to communicate disagreement. Communication among researchers, theorists, and clinicians would be much worse in the absence of a common language.

Clinicians, theorists, and researchers will at times experience the frustration of being required to use the DSM or the ICD. It can be difficult to obtain a grant, publish a study, or receive insurance reimbursement without reference to a DSM–IV diagnosis. However, DSM–IV also provides a useful point of comparison that ultimately facilitates the development and understanding of a new way of conceptualizing psychopathology. Viable alternatives to particular sections of DSM–IV are being developed, some of which will eventually be incorporated within future revisions of the diagnostic manual. Their effective development will have been due in part to the existence of and empirical support for DSM–IV. DSM–IV and ICD–10 are the official diagnostic systems because of their substantial empirical support, theoretical cogency, and clinical utility. They provide a common language of communication and a well-validated foil for future contenders to overcome.

REFERENCES

Alarcon, R. D., Bell, C. C., Kirmayer, L., Lin, K-H, Ustun, B., & Wisner, K. (2002). Beyond the fun-house mirrors: Research agenda on culture and psychiatric diagnosis. In D. J. Kupfer, M. B. First, & D. A. Regier (Eds.), A research agenda for DSM-V (pp. 219–281). Washington, DC: American Psychiatric Press.

American Psychiatric Association. (1952). *Diagnostic and statistical manual. Mental Disorders*. Washington, DC: Author.

American Psychiatric Association. (1968). *Diagnostic and statistical manual of mental disorders* (2nd ed.). Washington, DC: Author.

American Psychiatric Association. (1980). *Diagnostic and statistical manual of mental disorders* (3rd ed.). Washington, DC: Author.

American Psychiatric Association. (1987). *Diagnostic and statistical manual of mental disorders* (3rd ed., rev.). Washington, DC: Author.

American Psychiatric Association. (1994). *Diagnostic and statistical manual of mental disorders* (4th ed.). Washington, DC: Author.

American Psychiatric Association. (2000). *Diagnostic and statistical manual of mental disorders* (4th ed., text rev.). Washington, DC: Author.

American Sleep Disorders Association. (1990). *International classification of sleep disorders: Diagnostic and coding manual*. Rochester, Minnesota: Author.

Andreasen, N. C. (1997). Linking mind and brain in the study of mental illnesses: A project for a scientific psychopathology. *Science, 275*, 1586–1593.

Bergner, R. M. (1997). What is psychopathology? And so what? *Clinical Psychology: Science and Practice, 4*, 235–248.

Blashfield, R. K. (1984). *The classification of psychopathology. Neo-Kraepelinian and quantitative approaches*. NY: Plenum.

Blashfield, R. K., & Draguns, J. G. (1976). Evaluative criteria for psychiatric classification. *Journal of Abnormal Psychology, 85*, 140–150.

Brown, T. A., Chorpita, B. F., & Barlow, B. F. (1998). Structural relationships among dimensions of the DSM-IV anxiety and mood disorders and dimensions of negative affect, positive affect, and autonomic arousal. *Journal of Abnormal Psychology, 107*, 179–192.

Buss, D. M., Haselton, M. G., Shackelford, T. K., Bleske, A. L., & Wakefield, J. C. (1998). Adaptations, exaptations, and spandrels. *American Psychologist, 53*, 533–548.

Buysse, D. J., Reynolds, C. F., & Kupfer, D. J. (1998). DSM-IV sleep disorders: Final overview. In T. A. Widiger, A. J. Frances, H. A. Pincus, R. Ross, M. B. First, W. Davis, & M. Kline (Eds.), *DSM-IV sourcebook* (Vol. 4, pp. 1103–1122). Washington, DC: American Psychiatric Association.

Caplan, P. J. (1991). How do they decide who is normal? The bizarre, but true, tale of the DSM process. *Canadian Psychology, 32*, 162–170.

Caplan, P. J. (1995). *They say you're crazy. How the world's most powerful psychiatrists decide who's normal*. Reading, MA: Addison-Wesley.

Clark, L. A., Watson, D., & Reynolds, S. (1995). Diagnosis and classification of psychopathology: challenges to the current system and future directions. *Annual Review of Psychology, 46*, 121–153.

Drevets, W. C. (2002). Neuroimaging studies of mood disorders. In J. E. Helzer & J. J. Hudziak (Eds.), *Defining psychopathology in the 21st century* (pp. 71–105). Washington, DC: American Psychiatric Press.

Eagly, A. H. (1995). The science and politics of comparing women and men. *American Psychologist, 50*, 145–158.

Endicott, J. (2000). History, evolution, and diagnosis of premenstrual dysphoric disorder. *Journal of Clinical Psychiatry, 62*, (Suppl. 24), 5–8.

Epstein, J., Isenberg, N., Stern, E., & Silbersweig, D. (2002). Toward a neuroanatomical understanding of psychiatric illness: The role of functional imaging. In J. E. Helzer & J. J. Hudziak (Eds.), *Defining psychopathology in the 21st century* (pp. 57–69). Washington, DC: American Psychiatric Press.

Fabrega, H. (1994). International systems of diagnosis in psychiatry. *Journal of Nervous and Mental Disease, 182*, 256–263.

Feighner, J. P., Robins, E., Guze, S. B., Woodruff, R. A., Winokur, G., & Munoz, R. (1972). Diagnostic criteria for use in psychiatric research. *Archives of General Psychiatry, 26*, 57–63.

First, M. B., Bell, C. B., Krystal, J. H., Reiss, D., Shea, M. T., Widiger, T. A., & Wisner, K. L. (2002). Gaps in the current system: Recommendations. In D. J. Kupfer, M. B. First, & D. A. Regier (Eds.), *A research agenda for DSM-V* (pp. 123–199). Washington, DC: American Psychiatric Press.

Folette, W. C., & Houts, A. C. (1996). Models of scientific progress and the role of theory in taxonomy development: A case study of the DSM. *Journal of Consulting and Clinical Psychology, 64*, 1120–1132.

Frances, A. J., First, M. B., & Pincus, H. A. (1995). *DSM-IV guidebook*. Washington, DC: American Psychiatric Press.

Frances, A. J., Pincus, H. A., Widiger, T. A., Davis, W. W., & First, M. B. (1990). DSM-IV: Work in progress. *American Journal of Psychiatry, 147*, 1439–1448.

Frances, A. J., Widiger, T. A., & Pincus, H. A. (1989). The development of DSM-IV. *Archives of General Psychiatry, 46*, 373–375.

Garb, H. N. (1998). *Studying the clinician. Judgment research and psychological assessment*. Washington, DC: American Psychological Association.

Gorenstein, E. (1984). Debating mental illness. *American Psychologist, 39*, 50–56.

Grob, G.N. (1991). Origins of DSM-I: A study in appearance and reality. *American Journal of Psychiatry, 148*, 421–431.

Hartung, C. M., & Widiger, T. A. (1998). Gender differences in the diagnosis of mental disorders: Conclusions and controversies of DSM-IV. *Psychological Bulletin, 123*, 260–278.

Hyman, S. E. (1998). NIMH during the tenure of Director Steven E. Hyman, M.D. (1996-present): the now and future of NIMH. *American Journal of Psychiatry, 155* (Suppl.), 36–40.

Kaplan, M. (1983). A woman's view of DSM-III. *American Psychologist, 38*, 786–792.

Kendell, R. E. (1975). *The role of diagnosis in psychiatry*. London: Blackwell Scientific Publications.

Kendell, R. E. (1991). Relationship between the DSM-IV and the ICD-10. *Journal of Abnormal Psychology, 100*, 297–301.

Kessler, R. C. (1999). The World Health Organization International Consortium in Psychiatric Epidemiology: Initial work and future directions - the NAPE lecture. *Acta Psychiatrica Scandinavica, 99*, 2–9.

Kirmayer, L. J., & Young, A. (1999). Culture and context in the evolutionary concept of mental disorder. *Journal of Abnormal Psychology, 108*, 446–452.

Kirmayer, L. J., Young, A., & Hayton, B. C. (1995). The cultural context of anxiety disorders. *Psychiatric Clinics of North America, 18*, 503–521.

Klein, D. F. (1999). Harmful dysfunction, disorder, disease, illness, and evolution. *Journal of Abnormal Psychology, 108*, 421–429.

Kramer, M., Sartorius, N., Jablensky, A., & Gulbinat, W. (1979). The ICD-9 classification of mental disorders. A review of its development and contents. *Acta Psychiatrica Scandinavika, 59*, 241–262.

Krueger, R. F. (1999). The structure of common mental disorders. *Archives of General Psychiatry, 56*, 921–926.

Krueger, R. F., Caspi, A., Moffitt, T. E., & Silva, P. A. (1998). The structure and stability of common mental disorders (DSM-III-R): A longitudinal-epidemiological study. *Journal of Abnormal Psychology*, 107, 216–227.

Kutchins, H., & Kirk, S. A. (1997). *Making us crazy. DSM: the psychiatric bible and the creation of mental disorders.* New York: The Free Press.

Lehman, A. F., Alexopoulos, G. S., Goldman, H. H., Jeste, D. V., Offord, D., & Ustun, T. B. (2002). Disability and impairment recommendations. In D. J. Kupfer, M. B. First, & D. A. Regier (Eds.), *A research agenda for DSM-V* (pp. 201–218). Washington, DC: American Psychiatric Press.

Lenzenweger, M. F. (1999). Deeper into the schizotypy taxon: On the robust nature of maximum covariance analysis. *Journal of Abnormal Psychology, 108*, 182–187.

Levinson, D. F., Mahtani, M. M., Nancarrow, D. J., Brown, D. M., Kruglyak L, Kirby, A., Hayward, N. K., Crowe, R. R., Andreasen, N. C., Black, D. W., Silverman, J. M., Endicott, J., Sharpe, L., Mohs, R. C., Siever, L. J., Walters, M. K., Lennon, D. P., Jones, H. L., Nertney, D. A., Daly, M. J., Gladis, M., & Mowry, B. J. (1998). Genome scan of schizophrenia. *American Journal of Psychiatry, 155*, 741–750.

Lewis-Fernandez, R., & Kleinman, A. (1995). Cultural psychiatry. Theoretical, clinical, and research issues. *Psychiatric Clinics of North America, 18*, 433–446.

Lilienfeld, S. O., & Marino, L. (1999). Essentialism revisited: Evolutionary theory and the concept of mental disorder. *Journal of Abnormal Psychology, 108*, 400–411.

Lilienfeld, S. O., Waldman, I. D., & Israel, A. C. (1994). A critical examination of the use of the term "comorbidity" in psychopathology research. *Clinical Psychology: Science and Practice, 1*, 71–83.

Lopez, S. R., & Guarnaccia, J. J. (2000). Cultural psychopathology: Uncovering the social world of mental illness. *Annual Review of Psychology, 51*, 571–598.

Lynam, D. R., & Widiger, T. A. (2001). Using the five factor model to represent the DSM-IV personality disorders: An expert consensus approach. *Journal of Abnormal Psychology, 110*, 401–412.

McGue, M., & Bouchard, T. J. (1998). Genetic and environmental influences on human behavioral differences. *Annual Review of Neuroscience, 21*, 1–24.

McQueen, L. (2000). Committee on Psychiatric Diagnosis and Assessment update on publications and activities. *Psychiatric Research Report, 16*(2), 3.

Meehl, P. E. (1977). Specific etiology and other forms of strong influence. Some quantitative meanings. *Journal of Medicine and Philosophy, 2*, 33–53.

Menninger, K. (1963). *The vital balance.* NY: Viking.

Mezzich, J. E., Kleinman, A., Fabrega, H., Parron, D. L., Good, B. J., Lin, K-H., & Manson, S. M. (1997). Cultural issues for DSM-IV. In T. A. Widiger, A. J. Frances, H. A. Pincus, R. Ross, M. B. First, & W. Davis (Eds.), *DSM-IV sourcebook* (Vol. 3, pp. 861–866). Washington, DC: American Psychiatric Association.

Mineka, S., Watson, D., & Clark, L. A. (1998). Comorbidity of anxiety and unipolar mood disorders. *Annual Review of Psychology, 49*, 377–412.

Nathan, P., & Langenbucher, J. W. (1999). Psychopathology: Description and classification. *Annual Review of Psychology, 50*, 79–107.

Neisser, U., Boodoo, G., Bouchard, T. J., Boykin, A. W., Brody, N., Ceci, S. J., Halpern, D. F., Loehlin, J. C., Perloff, R., Sternberg, R. J., & Urbina, S. (1996). Intelligence: Knowns and unknowns. *American Psychologist, 51*, 77–101.

Nemeroff, C. B., Kilts, C. D., & Berns, G. S. (1999). Functional brain imaging: Twenty-first century phrenology or psychobiological advance for the millennium? *American Journal of Psychiatry, 156*, 671–673.

Pantony, K-L., & Caplan, P. J. (1991). Delusional dominating personality disorder: A modest proposal for identifying some consequences of rigid masculine socialization. *Canadian Psychology, 32*, 120–133.

Portin, P., & Alanen, Y. O. (1997). A critical review of genetic studies of schizophrenia. II. Molecular genetic studies. *Acta Psychiatrica Scandinavica, 95*, 73–80.

Prigerson, H. G., Shear, M. K., Jacobs, S. C., Reynolds, C. F., Maciejewski, P. K., Davidson, J. R. T., Rosenheck, R. A., Pilkonis, P. A., Wortman, C. B., Williams, J. B. W., Widiger, T. A., Frank, E., Kupfer, D. J., & Zisook, S. (1999). Consensus criteria for traumatic grief: A preliminary empirical test. *British Journal of Psychiatry, 174*, 67–73.

Regier, D. A., Kaelber, C. T., Rae, D. S., Farmer, M. E., Knauper, B., Kessler, R. C., & Norquist, G. S. (1998). Limitations of diagnostic criteria and assessment instruments for mental disorders. Implications for research and policy. *Archives of General Psychiatry, 55*, 109–15.

Rogers, R. (2001). *Handbook of diagnostic and structured interviewing*. NY: Guilford.

Rosenhan, D. L. (1973). On being sane in insane places. *Science, 179*, 250–258.

Ross, R., Frances, A. J., & Widiger, T. A. (1995). Gender issues in DSM-IV. In J. M. Oldham & M. B. Riba (Eds.), *Review of psychiatry* (Vol. 14, pp. 205–226). Washington, DC: American Psychiatric Press.

Rounsaville, B. J., Alarcon, R. D., Andrews, G., Jackson, J. S., Kendell, R. E., Kendler, K. S., & Kirmayer, L. J. (2002). Toward DSM-V: Basic nomenclature issues. In D. J. Kupfer, M. B. First, & D. A. Regier (Eds.), *A research agenda for DSM-V* (pp. 1–29). Washington, DC: American Psychiatric Press.

Rush, A. J., Pincus, H. A., First, M. B., Blacker, D., Endicott, J., Keith, S. J., Phillips, K. A., Ryan, N. D., Smith, G. R., Tsuang, M. T., Widiger, T. A., & Zarin, D. A. (Eds.). (2000). *Handbook of psychiatric measures*. Washington, DC: American Psychiatric Association.

Rutter, M. L. (1997). Nature-nurture integration. The example of antisocial behavior. *American Psychologist, 52*, 390–398.

Salmon, T. W., Copp, O., May, J. V., Abbot, E. S., & Cotton, H. A. (1917). Report of the committee on statistics of the American Medico-Psychological Association. *American Journal of Insanity, 74*, 255–260.

Sartorius, N., Kaelber, C. T., Cooper, J. E., Roper, M., Rae, D. S., Gulbinat, W., Ustun, T. B., & Regier, D. A. (1993). Progress toward achieving a common language in psychiatry. *Archives of General Psychiatry, 50*, 115–124.

Schwartz, M. A., & Wiggins, O. P. (2002). The hegemony of the DSMs. In J. Sadler (Ed.), *Descriptions and prescriptions: Values, mental disorders, and the DSM* (pp. 199–209). Baltimore: Johns Hopkins University Press.

Spitzer, R. L., & Wakefield, J. C. (1999). DSM-IV diagnostic criterion for clinical significance: Does it help solve the false positives problem? *American Journal of Psychiatry, 156*, 1856–1864.

Spitzer, R. L., & Williams, J. B. W. (1982). The definition and diagnosis of mental disorder. In W. R. Gove (Ed.), *Deviance and mental illness* (pp. 15–32). Beverly Hills, CA: Sage.

Spitzer, R. L., Williams, J. B. W., & Skodol, A. E. (1980). DSM-III: The major achievements and an overview. *American Journal of Psychiatry, 137*, 151–164.

Sprock, J., Crosby, J. P., & Nielsen, B. A. (2001). Effects of sex and sex roles on the perceived maladaptiveness of DSM-IV personality disorder symptoms. *Journal of Personality Disorders, 15*, 41–59.

Steffens, D. C., & Krishnan, K. R. R. (1998). Structural neuroimaging and mood disorders: recent findings, implications for classification, and future directions. *Biological Psychiatry, 43*, 705–712.

Stengel, E. (1959). Classification of mental disorders. *Bulletin of the World Health Organization, 21*, 601–663.

Szasz, T. S. (1961). *The myth of mental illness*. NY: Hoeber-Harper.

Wakefield, J. C. (1987). Sex bias in the diagnosis of primary orgasmic dysfunction. *American Psychologist, 42*, 464–471.

Wakefield, J. C. (1992). The concept of mental disorder: On the boundary between biological facts and social values. *American Psychologist, 47*, 373–88.

Wakefield, J. C. (1997). Diagnosing DSM-IV–Part I: DSM-IV and the concept of disorder. *Behavioral Research and Therapy, 35*, 633–649.

Wakefield, J. C. (1998). The DSM's theory-neutral nosology is scientifically progressive: Response to Follette and Houts (1996). *Journal of Consulting and Clinical Psychology, 66*, 846–852.

Wakefield, J. C., Pottick, K. J., & Kirk, S. A. (2002). Should the DSM-IV diagnostic criteria for conduct disorder consider social context? *American Journal of Psychiatry, 159*, 380–386.

Ward, C. H., Beck, A. T., Mendelson, M., Mock, J. E., & Erbaugh, J. K. (1962). The psychiatric nomenclature. Reasons for diagnostic disagreement. *Archives of General Psychiatry, 7*, 198–205.

Westen, D. (1997). Divergences between clinical and research methods for assessing personality disorders: Implications for research and the evolution of Axis II. *American Journal of Psychiatry, 154*, 895–903.

Widiger, T. A. (1995). Deletion of the self-defeating and sadistic personality disorder diagnoses. In W. J. Livesley (Ed.), *The DSM-IV personality disorders* (pp. 359–373). New York: Guilford.

Widiger, T. A. (1998). Sex biases in the diagnosis of personality disorders. *Journal of Personality Disorders, 12*, 95–118.

Widiger, T. A. (2001). Official classification systems. In W. J. Livesley (Ed.), *Handbook of personality disorders* (pp. 60–83). NY: Guilford.

Widiger, T. A. (2002). Values, politics, and science in the construction of the DSM. In J. Sadler (Ed.), *Descriptions and prescriptions: Values, mental disorders, and the DSM* (pp. 25–41). Baltimore: Johns Hopkins University Press.

Widiger, T. A., & Clark, L. A. (2000). Toward DSM-V and the classification of psychopathology. *Psychological Bulletin, 126*, 946–963.

Widiger, T. A., & Coker, L. A. (2003). Mental disorders as discrete clinical conditions: Dimensional versus categorical classification. In S. M. Turner & M. Hersen (Eds.), *Adult psychopathology and diagnosis* (4th ed. pp. 3–35). NY: John Wiley.

Widiger, T., Frances, A., Pincus, H., Davis, W., & First, M. (1991). Toward an empirical classification for DSM-IV. *Journal of Abnormal Psychology, 100*, 280–288.

Widiger, T. A. Frances, A. J., Pincus, H. A., First, M. B., Ross, R. R., & Davis, W. W. (Eds.) (1994). *DSM-IV sourcebook* (Vol. 1). Washington, DC: American Psychiatric Association.

Widiger, T. A., Frances, A. J., Pincus, H. A., First, M. B., Ross, R. R., & Davis, W. W. (Eds.). (1996). *DSM-IV sourcebook* (Vol. 2). Washington, DC: American Psychiatric Association.

Widiger, T. A., Frances, A. J., Pincus, H. A., Ross, R. R., First, M. B., & Davis, W. W. (Eds.). (1997). *DSM-IV sourcebook* (Vol. 3). Washington, DC: American Psychiatric Association.

Widiger, T. A., Frances, A. J., Pincus, H. A., Ross, R., First, M. B., Davis, W. W., & Kline, M. (Eds.). (1998). *DSM-IV Sourcebook* (Vol. 4). Washington, DC: American Psychiatric Association.

Widiger, T. A., & Sankis, L. M. (2000). Adult psychopathology: Issues and controversies. *Annual Review of Psychology, 51*, 377–404.

Widiger, T. A., & Trull, T. J. (1991). Diagnosis and clinical assessment. *Annual Review of Psychology, 42*, 109–133.

Widiger, T. A., & Trull, T. J. (1993). The scholarly development of DSM-IV. In J. A. Costa e Silva & C. C. Nadelson (Eds.), *International review of psychiatry* (Vol. 1, pp. 59–78). Washington, DC: American Psychiatric Press.

World Health Organization. (1992). *The ICD-10 classification of mental and behavioural disorders. Clinical descriptions and diagnostic guidelines*. Geneva, Switzerland: Author.

Zahn-Waxler, C. (1993). Warriors and worriers: gender and psychopathology. *Development and Psychopathology, 5*, 79–89.

Zigler, E., & Phillips, L. (1961). Psychiatric diagnosis: A critique. *Journal of Abnormal and Social Psychology, 63*, 607–618.

Zilboorg, G. (1941). *A history of medical psychology*. NY: Norton.

Zoccolillo, M. (1993). Gender and the development of conduct disorder. *Development and Psychopathology, 5*, 65–78.

5

Psychological Assessment and Clinical Judgment

Howard N. Garb
University of Pittsburgh

Scott O. Lilienfeld and
Katherine A. Fowler
Emory University

What major advances have occurred in the assessment of psychopathology over the past 25 years? Many psychologists would argue that the most important breakthroughs include the development of explicit diagnostic criteria, the growing popularity of structured interviews, and the proliferation of brief measures tailored for use by mental health professionals conducting empirically supported treatments (e.g., Antony & Barlow, 2002). Others would disagree. Even an advance that most mental health professionals have embraced, the use of explicit criteria for making psychiatric diagnoses, has been challenged (Beutler & Malik, 2002). For example, Weiner (2000) referred to the current *Diagnostic and Statistical Manual of Mental Disorders* (DSM–IV, American Psychiatric Association, 1994) as "a psychometrically shaky, inferential nosological scheme involving criteria and definitions that change from one revision to the next" (p. 436). (See also Widiger, this book.) Controversies abound in the domain of assessment, and most beginning readers of this literature are left with little guidance regarding how to navigate the murky scientific waters.

In this chapter, we intend to provide such guidance. Specifically, we discuss fundamental conceptual and methodological issues in the assessment of psychopathology, with a particular focus on recent developments and advances. We compare different types of assessment instruments, including structured interviews, brief self-rated and clinician-rated measures, projective techniques, self-report personality inventories, and behavioral assessment and psychophysiological methods. We also review research on the validity of assessment instruments and research on clinical judgment and decision making.

Our principal goal in this chapter is to assist readers with the task of becoming well-informed and discerning consumers of the clinical assessment literature. In particular, we intend to provide readers with the tools necessary to distinguish scientifically supported from unsupported assessment instruments and to make valid judgments on the basis of the former instruments.

PSYCHOMETRIC PRINCIPLES

Before describing the validity of assessment instruments and research on clinical judgment and decision making, we must first clarify the meaning of several key terms. Specifically, we will define and discuss reliability, validity, and treatment utility [see also the *Standards for Educational and Psychological Testing*, American Educational Research Association, American Psychological Association, & National Council on Measurement in Education (AERA, APA, & NCME), 1999].

Reliability refers to consistency of measurement. It is evaluated in several ways. If all of the items of a test are believed to measure the same trait, we want the test to possess good internal consistency: Test items should be positively intercorrelated. If a test is believed to measure a stable trait, then the test should possess test–retest reliability: on separate administrations of the test, clients should obtain similar scores. Finally, when two or more psychologists make diagnoses or other judgments for the same clients, interrater reliability should be high: Their ratings should tend to agree.

Traditionally, interrater reliability was evaluated by calculating the percentage of cases on which raters agree. For example, two psychologists might agree on diagnoses for 80% of the patients on a unit. However, percentage agreement is unduly affected by base rates. In this context, a *base rate* refers to the prevalence of a disorder. When the base rates of a disorder are high, raters may agree on a large number of cases because of chance. For example, if 80% of the patients on a chronic psychiatric inpatient unit suffer from schizophrenia, then two clinicians who randomly make diagnoses of schizophrenia for 80% of the patients will agree on the diagnosis of schizophrenia for about 64% of the cases ($.8 \times .8 = .64$). Thus, a moderately high level of agreement is obtained even though diagnoses are made arbitrarily. By calculating kappa or an intraclass correlation coefficient (ICC), one can calculate the level of agreement beyond the chance level of agreement. This calculation is accomplished by taking into account the base rates of the disorder being rated.

When interpreting kappa and ICC, one generally uses the following criteria: Interrater reliability is poor for values below .40, fair for values between .40 and .59, good for values between .60 and .74, and excellent for values above .75 (Fleiss, 1981, p. 218). However, these criteria are typically used for making judgments (e.g., diagnoses or predictions of behavior), not for scoring test protocols. For scoring protocols, a reliability coefficient of at least .90 is desirable (Nunnally, 1978, pp. 245–246). Reliability should be higher for scoring tests than for making clinical judgments because if a test cannot be scored reliably, judgments based on those test scores will necessarily have poor reliability.

According to the *Standards for Educational and Psychological Testing* (AERA et al., 1999), *validity* refers to "the degree to which evidence and theory support the interpretations of test scores" (p. 9). Put another way, validity is good if the use of a test allows us to draw accurate inferences about clients (e.g., if the use of test scores helps us to provide correct descriptions of traits, psychopathology, and diagnoses).

Reliability and validity differ in important ways. Reliability refers to the consistency of test scores and judgments; validity refers to the accuracy of interpretations and judgments. When reliability is good, validity can be good or poor. For example, two psychologists can agree on a client's diagnosis, yet both can be wrong. Or a client can obtain the same scores on two administrations of a test, yet inferences made using the test scores may be invalid. In contrast, when reliability is poor, validity is necessarily also poor. For example, if two psychologists cannot agree on a client's diagnosis, at least one of them is not making a valid diagnosis.

Different types of evidence can be obtained to evaluate validity. First, evidence can be based on test content (*content validity*). For example, a measure of a specific anxiety disorder, such as obsessive-compulsive disorder, should include an adequate representation of items to assess the principal features of this disorder, in this case obsessions and compulsions. To ensure content validity, many structured interviews contain questions that inquire comprehensively about the DSM criteria for anxiety disorders and other conditions (e.g., Anxiety Disorders Interview Schedule–IV, ADIS–IV; Brown, Di Nardo, & Barlow, 1994). Second, evidence can be based on the relation between test scores (or inferences based on test scores) and other variables (*convergent validity*). For example, test scores can be used to predict behavioral outcomes (e.g., suicide), or they can be related to independent ratings of a trait (e.g., anxiety). When test scores are used to forecast future outcomes, psychologists refer to *predictive validity*; when these scores are correlated with indices measured at approximately the same time, psychologists refer to *concurrent validity*. The validity of an assessment instrument can also be evaluated by examining its internal structure (*structural validity*; see Loevinger, 1957). If a test generates many scores that do not intercorrelate as expected, this result may suggest that inferences based on those test scores are wrong. For example, one problem with the Rorschach Inkblot Test is that scores that are purported to reflect psychopathology are highly correlated with the number of responses produced by clients (Lilienfeld, Wood, & Garb, 2000, p. 34). That is, the more responses a client produces on the Rorschach, the greater the likelihood the client will generate responses that ostensibly indicate the presence of psychopathology. For example, a single Rorschach food response is purportedly indicative of dependent personality traits, but the more overall responses a client produces, the greater the likelihood of the client making a food response.

When we describe the content validity, convergent validity, or structural validity of an assessment instrument, we are also describing its construct validity. A construct is a theoretical variable that cannot be measured perfectly. More specifically, constructs are hypothesized attributes of individuals that cannot be observed directly, such as extraversion or schizophrenia (Cronbach & Meehl, 1955). Construct validity is a broad concept that subsumes content validity, convergent validity, and structural validity.

A number of statistics can be used to evaluate the validity of assessment instruments. Researchers commonly calculate correlations between a test and other measures, including scores on related tests. Other statistics can yield even more useful information. For example, results on sensitivity and specificity are presented routinely in the medical literature, but only infrequently in the literature on psychological assessment (Antony & Barlow, 2002). *Sensitivity* is the likelihood that one will test positive given that one has a specified mental disorder. *Specificity* is the likelihood one will test negative given that one does not have the specified disorder. Ideally, one attempts to maximize both sensitivity and specificity, although there may be cases in which one elects to emphasize one statistic over the other. For example, if one were attempting to predict suicide in a large group of patients, one would presumably be more concerned with sensitivity than specificity. Other important statistics are positive and negative predictive power. *Positive predictive power* describes the likelihood of a disorder given the presence of a particular result on an assessment instrument. *Negative predictive power* describes the likelihood of the absence of a disorder given the absence of the particular result on the assessment instrument.

The concepts of sensitivity, specificity, positive predictive power, and negative predictive power are illustrated in Table 5.1. In this scenario, provisional diagnoses of a mood disorder are made when the T-score for Scale 2 (Depression) of the MMPI–2 is ≥ 65 (the standard cutoff for psychopathology on the MMPI–2)[1]. In the sample with a base rate of 50% (50% of the clients are depressed), 500 clients are depressed and 500 clients are not depressed. For the 500 clients who are depressed, 425 have a T-score ≥ 65. Thus, sensitivity is equal to $425/500 = 85.0\%$.

---

[1] We use the term "provisional diagnoses" because formal diagnoses of psychiatric disorders should not be made on the basis of the MMPI–2 alone.

TABLE 5.1

Effect of Base Rate on Positive Predictive Power (PPP), Negative Predictive Power (NPP),
Sensitivity, and Specificity

Base Rate = 50%

	Depressed						
Scale 2(D)	Yes	No	Total	PPP	=	425/575	=	73.9%
T ≥ 65	425	150	575	NPP	=	350/425	=	82.4%
T < 65	75	350	425	Sensitivity	=	425/500	=	85.0%
Total	500	500	1000	Specificity	=	350/500	=	70.0%

Base Rate = 2%

	Depressed						
Scale 2(D)	Yes	No	Total	PPP	=	17/311	=	5.0%
T ≥ 65	17	294	311	NPP	=	686/689	=	99.6%
T < 65	3	686	689	Sensitivity	=	17/20	=	85.0%
Total	20	980	1000	Specificity	=	686/980	=	70.0%

Computations for specificity, positive predictive power, and negative predictive power are also presented in the table.

Depending on the statistic used to evaluate validity, accuracy can vary with the base rate of the behavior being predicted (Meehl & Rosen, 1955; also see Greene, 2000, pp. 365–366). As can be seen from Table 1, when percentage correct, positive predictive power, and negative predictive power are used to describe validity, accuracy varies with the base rate. For example, percentage correct is 425 + 350 divided by 1000 = 77.5% when the base rate is 50%, and 17 + 686 divided by 1000 = 70.3% when the base rate is 2%. In contrast, when sensitivity and specificity are used to describe validity, accuracy does not vary with the base rate. Put another way, when percentage correct, positive predictive power, and negative predictive power are used to describe accuracy, the same test will be described as having varying levels of accuracy depending on the base rates in different samples. In general, positive predictive power tends to decrease when base rates decrease, whereas negative predictive power tends to increase when base rates decrease. Thus, statistically rare events (e.g., suicide) are difficult to predict, whereas common events (e.g., no suicide) are relatively easy to predict.

When reading about positive findings for a test score, psychologists should be aware that the score may not work well in their work setting if the base rate in their work setting differs widely from the base rate in the study. If the base rate for a disorder is .5 in a study but .01 in a clinic, one can expect results for positive predictive power to be much less favorable in the clinic. Nevertheless, a large body of psychological research indicates that psychologists tend to (a) neglect or greatly underuse base rates when making judgments and predictions and (b) focus too heavily on whether a client falls above or below a test's cutoff score (Finn & Kamphuis, 1995). As a consequence, clinicians' judgments can sometimes be grossly inaccurate when the base rates of the phenomenon in question are extreme (e.g., very low).

Signal detection theory (SDT) often provides the most useful information regarding the validity of an assessment instrument. SDT is a statistical approach that is used when the task is to detect a signal, such as the presence of major depression in a client. By using SDT, we can describe the validity of an assessment instrument across all base rates and across all cutoff scores (the signal is said to be present when a client's score exceeds the cutoff score). Different clinicians may set different cutoff scores for the same test; it is important that our estimate of the validity of a test not be influenced by the placement of the cutoff score. As observed by McFall and Treat (1999): "There is no longer any excuse for continuing to conduct business as usual, now that SDT-based indices represent a clear and significant advance over traditional accuracy indices such as sensitivity, specificity, and predictive power" (p. 227). Although such indices as sensitivity, specificity, and predictive power are informative, we agree with McFall and Treat that in many cases the use of SDT is more appropriate and comprehensive.

Other important psychometric concepts are norms, incremental validity, and treatment utility. *Norms* are scores that provide a frame of reference for interpreting a client's results. For the assessment of psychopathology, normative data can be collected by administering a test to a representative sample of individuals in the community. If a client's responses are similar to the normative data, psychologists should be very cautious about inferring the presence of psychopathology. *Incremental validity* describes the extent to which an instrument contributes information above and beyond already available information (e.g., other measures). For example, the use of a psychological test may allow clinicians to make judgments at a level better than chance, but judgments made using interview and test information may not be more accurate than judgments based on interview information only. One major criticism of the Rorschach Inkblot Test has been the paucity of evidence for its incremental validity beyond more easily administered instruments, such as questionnaires (Lilienfeld et al., 2000). *Treatment utility* describes the extent to which an assessment instrument contributes to enhanced treatment outcome. An assessment instrument could have good validity and good incremental validity, yet not lead to improved treatment outcome. Surprisingly, few researchers have examined the treatment utility of assessment instruments (Harkness & Lilienfeld, 1997).

ASSESSMENT INSTRUMENTS

Interviews

Unstructured interviews are used predominantly in clinical practice, whereas structured and semistructured interviews are used predominantly in research. One exception is that structured and semistructured interviews are used for clinical care in a growing number of university-based clinics. When conducting an *unstructured interview*, a psychologist is responsible for deciding what questions to ask. In contrast, when conducting a *structured interview*, questions are standardized. As one might surmise, *semistructured interviews* represent a balance between structured and unstructured interviews, providing guidance for interviewers but affording them some flexibility.

Reliability.   Interrater reliability has generally been good when clinicians conduct unstructured interviews as long as they attend to diagnostic criteria (Garb, 1998, pp. 41–42). For example, acceptable levels of interrater reliability were obtained for many, but not all, diagnostic categories in the DSM–III field trials and in the field trials for the tenth revision of the *International Classification of Diseases* (ICD–10; American Psychiatric Association, 1980, pp. 470–471; Sartorius et al., 1993). However, clinicians who participated in the DSM–III and ICD–10 field trials were familiar with, and presumably adhered to, the diagnostic criteria. Other studies indicate that many mental health professionals do not attend to criteria when making diagnoses, but instead make diagnoses by comparing patients with their concept of the typical person with a given mental disorder (e.g., Blashfield & Herkov, 1996; Garb, 1996; Morey & Ochoa, 1989). When psychologists do not adhere to diagnostic criteria, interrater reliability is often poor.

The use of semistructured and structured interviews tends to lead to good (a) adherence to diagnostic criteria and (b) interrater reliability (Antony & Barlow, 2002; Rogers, 1995). For example, the ADIS–IV (Brown et al., 1994) requires interviewers to inquire about the DSM–IV criteria for anxiety disorders. Favorable reliability results have been found for this instrument: kappa values have ranged from .67 to .86 for diagnoses of the DSM–IV anxiety disorders (Brown, Di Nardo, Lehman, & Campbell, 2001).

Validity. Some psychologists have argued that diagnoses should not be made using the DSM criteria. For example, as already noted, Weiner (2000) argued that the DSM criteria are questionable, in part because they are inconsistent across editions of the manual. However, virtually all mental disorders are open concepts. As noted by Meehl (1986), *open concepts* are marked by (a) intrinsically fuzzy boundaries, (b) an indicator list that is potentially infinite, and (c) an unclear inner nature. One can expect the working definition of a mental disorder to change as more is learned about that disorder. For example, we may eventually learn that certain individuals who meet the DSM–IV criteria for schizophrenia actually have disorders that have not yet been identified. Still, the construct of schizophrenia can be useful even though we are aware that the meaning of the term is somewhat imprecise and will change as more research is conducted. DSM diagnoses can be valid and useful even when we possess an incomplete understanding of their nature, etiology, course, and treatment.

As already noted, structured and semistructured interviews are used routinely in research studies. When important discoveries are made about the nature, etiology, course, and/or treatment of a disorder, they support the validity of the instruments used in the studies. For example, if a structured interview is used to select participants for a study on treatment outcome and the treatment intervention is found to be effective, one can infer that a client who obtains a specific diagnosis on the structured interview is likely to respond to the treatment. Thus, the bulk of the evidence on validity that supports structured and semistructured interviews derives from studies on psychopathology and treatment outcome. Similarly, evidence that supports the validity of the DSM criteria supports the validity of assessment instruments that help to determine if a participant satisfies those criteria. Because there is no "gold standard" for evaluating the validity of structured interviews (Faraone & Tsuang, 1994) or other assessment measures in psychopathology research, validity is established by evaluating "the degree to which evidence and theory support the interpretations of test scores" (AERA et al., 1999, p. 9).

There are several reasons to believe that structured interviews are more valid than unstructured interviews, at least when clinicians conducting unstructured interviews do not adhere to diagnostic criteria. First, interrater reliability tends to be better for structured and semistructured interviews, so all things being equal they are more likely to be valid. Second, many structured interviews are designed to inquire comprehensively about the DSM criteria. To the extent that the DSM criteria have been validated, the validity of these structured and semistructured interviews will be supported. Third, when interviews and self-report instruments are used to diagnose personality disorders, clinicians using unstructured interviews typically show the lowest agreement with other assessment instruments. In his review of the literature, Widiger (2002) noted that "the worst median convergent validity coefficient was obtained in the only study to have used unstructured interviews by practicing clinicians" (p. 463).

Additional evidence raises questions about the validity of diagnoses made by many practicing clinicians. Agreement between structured interview diagnoses and diagnoses made in clinical practice is generally poor (e.g., Brockington, Kendell, & Leff, 1978; Molinari, Ames, & Essa, 1994; Steiner, Tebes, Sledge, & Walker, 1995). For example, in one study (Steiner et al., 1995), clinical diagnoses made for 100 patients were compared with diagnoses made by research investigators using a structured interview. An overall weighted kappa coefficient indicated that agreement between the two interview methods was poor (kappa = .25). Values for kappa are typically higher when one structured interview is compared with another, although to a surprising degree this issue has not been studied for some widely used interviews (Rogers, 1995). Thus, based on the available evidence, one cannot argue that it makes little difference whether one conducts an unstructured or structured interview.

Although structured interviews generally appear to be more valid than unstructured interviews, their limitations need to be recognized. Because these limitations are shared with unstructured interviews, they do not indicate that unstructured interviews possess advantages over structured interviews. First, it is relatively easy for respondents to consciously underreport or overreport psychopathology on structured interviews (Alterman et al., 1996). Second, because memory is fallible, reports in interviews are often inaccurate or incomplete, even when clients are not intentionally trying to appear healthier or sicker than they really are (Henry, Moffitt, Caspi, Langley, & Silva, 1994). Third, when clinicians are instructed to make use of medical records and other information in addition to structured interviews, considerable clinical judgment is required because information from different sources may conflict. This requirement is a potential limitation because clinical judgment is fallible.

Finally, an important methodological advance in evaluating the validity of interviews is the LEAD standard. LEAD is an acronym for *longitudinal, expert*, and *all data*. When using the LEAD standard (Spitzer, 1983), diagnoses made by using interviews are compared with diagnoses made by collecting longitudinal data. Using this approach, clients are followed over time to provide longitudinal data for making diagnoses, and diagnoses are made by expert clinicians using all relevant data. Although the LEAD standard can help us learn about the validity of diagnoses, it has rarely been used. Using this approach, one can more accurately evaluate the validity of unstructured, structured, and semistructured interviews.

Brief Self-Rated and Clinician-Rated Measures

Brief self-rated and clinician-rated measures have been constructed to provide information necessary to deliver standardized, evidence-based interventions. For example, the Beck Depression Inventory–II, the Beck Anxiety Scale, and other scales are frequently used to assess depression and anxiety (Beck & Steer, 1990; Beck, Steer, & Brown, 1996). As another example, psychologists who use cognitive behavioral techniques to treat panic disorder frequently use self-rated and clinician-rated measures to describe (a) the severity and frequency of panic-related symptoms, (b) cognitions or beliefs that are frequently associated with panic disorder, (c) clients' perceptions of their control over threatening internal situations, and (d) panic-related avoidance behaviors (e.g., Baker, Patterson, & Barlow, 2002). Because psychologists who use cognitive behavioral techniques are not usually concerned with measuring broad areas of psychopathology and personality, brief self-rated and clinician-rated measures are typically best suited for their needs.

The reliability and validity of many of these measures appears to be adequate. For example, the Panic Disorder Severity Scale (PDSS; Shear et al., 1997) is a seven-item scale that can be completed by either clients or clinicians to describe key features of panic disorder with agoraphobia. When completed by a clinician, the ratings are based on information that has been gathered in interview and therapy sessions. Ratings are made for frequency of panic, anxiety about future panic attacks, magnitude of distress during panic, interference in social functioning, interference in work functioning, and avoidance behaviors. The PDSS possesses excellent interrater reliability (kappa = .87; Shear et al., 1997). In addition, PDSS ratings are correlated significantly with other measures of features of panic disorder. For example, Shear et al. (1997) obtained a correlation of $r = .55$ for the relation between total scores on the PDSS and severity ratings for panic disorder on the ADIS–IV. Equally important is evidence related to the content of the scale items: The PDSS was designed to assess problems that are important for treatment planning. In fact, a reason that brief self-rated and clinician-rated measures are popular is that they evaluate dimensions believed to be important for treatment planning. That is, they are designed to (a) evaluate problems that need to be addressed in treatment and (b) provide information that is required to implement empirically-based treatment interventions. Finally, the PDSS can be used to track a client's progress. This use bears important implications for treatment use. For example, if the measure is administered during the course of treatment and indicates that a client is not improving, one should consider trying a different intervention. In one study (Shear et al., 1997), clients were classified as treatment responders and nonresponders on the basis of ratings made by independent evaluators. A different group of evaluators made PDSS ratings for all clients before and after treatment. In contrast to nonresponders, responders showed statistically significant improvement on the PDSS.

In general, the incremental validity of brief self-rated and clinician-rated measures has not been investigated. For example, the PDSS can be used to detect clients who are not responding to treatment for panic disorder, but a clinician may already be able to make this judgment without using this measure. Research needs to be conducted to demonstrate the incremental validity of self-rated and clinician-rated measures.

Although reliability and validity appear to be fair for many self-rated and clinician-rated measures, the evaluation of their validity has been limited. Rather than compare the results from one of these measures with the results of a structured interview or with another self-rated or clinician-rated measure, it would be helpful to use behavioral assessment methods to evaluate validity. This approach has rarely been used, but the results from one study are provocative. When behavioral assessment methods were used to evaluate the validity of clients' statements, clients were found to overestimate the frequency and intensity of their panic attacks on a structured interview and on a brief self-rated test (Margraf, Taylor, Ehlers, Roth, & Agras, 1987).

Behavioral Assessment Methods and Psychophysiological Assessment

Behavioral assessment methods and psychophysiological assessment can provide valuable information. For example, by using diary measures, one can ask a client to record and rate the frequency and intensity of panic attacks shortly after symptoms occur. Or one can monitor a client's eating or smoking habits. By making ratings shortly after symptoms or behaviors occur, the results are more likely to be accurate than when based on retrospective reports. The increased accessibility of palm-sized computers may eventually render it easier to collect and analyze self-monitoring data (data describing clients' ongoing behavior recorded by the clients themselves).

Behavioral assessment tests and other behavioral observation techniques can also provide valuable information. Behavioral assessment tests (also known as behavioral approach tests and behavioral avoidance tests) involve asking clients to enter situations that typically make them anxious, that they avoid, or both. For example, a client with a phobia can be instructed to approach a feared object (e.g., a spider) and a client with an obsessive-compulsive disorder can be instructed to switch off an electrical appliance and leave the room without checking it. During and after behavioral assessment tests, clients rate their level of anxiety. Other techniques include observing clients in role-play situations and in natural settings (without their being instructed to confront feared situations). For example, observations can be made of children in classrooms or of patients on psychiatric units.

Psychophysiological techniques can also provide valuable information. For example, a polysomnographic evaluation, which is conducted in a sleep lab, can provide valuable information about how well a client is sleeping (Savard & Morin, 2002). Similarly, measures of psychophysiological arousal can provide important information in the assessment of posttraumatic stress disorder, especially with respect to treatment process and outcome (Litz, Miller, Ruef, & McTeague, 2002). One team of investigators found that by playing a tape of combat sounds and measuring participants' heart rates, systolic blood pressure, and muscle tension with a forehead electromyogram, combat veterans with posttraumatic stress disorder could be discriminated from other veterans with 95.5% accuracy (Blanchard, Kolb, Pallmeyer, & Gerardi, 1982). Nevertheless, it will be important to cross-validate these findings in an independent sample. Because the psychophysiological assessment of other disorders has been confined largely to the laboratory, the extent to which these findings generalize to naturalistic settings remains unclear.

Global Measures of Personality and Psychopathology

Projective techniques and self-report personality inventories are designed to measure broad aspects of personality and psychopathology. Projective techniques include the Rorschach, Thematic Apperception Test (TAT), and human figure drawings. Self-report personality inventories include the Minnesota Multiphasic Personality Inventory–2 (MMPI–2; Butcher, Dahlstrom, Graham, Tellegen, & Kaemmer, 1989), the Personality Assessment Inventory (PAI; Morey, 1991), and the Millon Clinical Multiaxial Inventory–III (MCMI–III; Millon, 1994). Projective techniques are relatively unstructured: Stimuli are frequently ambiguous (e.g., inkblots, as in the case of the Rorschach) and response formats are typically open-ended (e.g., telling a story in response to a drawing of individuals interacting, as in the case of the TAT). In contrast, self-report personality inventories are relatively structured: Stimuli are fairly clear-cut (e.g., statements with which a client agrees or disagrees) and response formats are constrained (e.g., on the MMPI–2, one can make a response of "true" or "false"). In general, validity findings are more encouraging for self-report personality inventories than for projective techniques, although exceptions have been found (see Lilienfeld et al., 2000; Wood, Nezworski, Lilienfeld, & Garb, 2003).

Projective Techniques

A common argument for using projective techniques is that they can circumvent a client's purported defenses. According to this argument, they can be used to evaluate conscious and unconscious processes even when clients try to appear healthier or sicker than they really are. For example, some psychologists believe that when clients look at Rorschach inkblots and report what they see, they cannot invent faked responses because they do not know the true meaning of their Rorschach responses. However, research demonstrates that projective techniques are vulnerable to faking. For example, in one study (Albert, Fox, & Kahn, 1980), normal participants were instructed to fake paranoid schizophrenia. Presumed experts in the use of the Rorschach (Fellows of the Society for Personality Assessment) were unable to detect faking of psychosis. Diagnoses of malingering were made for 4% of the psychotic participants, 9% of the informed fakers (they were informed about the nature of disturbed thought processes and paranoid schizophrenia, but not about the Rorschach), 7% of uninformed fakers, and 2% of normal participants who were not instructed to fake. Diagnoses of psychosis were made for 48% of the psychotic participants, 72% of the informed fakers, 46% of the uninformed fakers, and 24% of the normal participants who were not instructed to fake.

A problem with many projective techniques is that they are difficult to score.[2] For example, the Comprehensive System (CS; Exner, 1993) is the most popular system for scoring the Rorschach. Exner (1993, p. 23), the developer of the CS, claimed that interrater reliability is better than .85 for all CS scores. However, results from recent studies indicate that this result is true for only about half of the CS scores (Acklin, McDowell, Verschell, & Chan, 2000; Nakata, 1999; Shaffer, Erdberg, & Haroian, 1999; but see Meyer et al., 2002). Furthermore, in one study (Guarnaccia, Dill, Sabatino, & Southwick, 2001), average scoring accuracy was only about 65%. In comparison, scoring is typically excellent for other types of tests (e.g., intelligence tests and personality inventories). For example, interrater reliability coefficients for the scoring of the Wechsler Adult Intelligence Scale, Third Edition (WAIS–III) have a median value of .95 and a minimum value of .90. Reliability for scoring the MMPI–2 is oftentimes even better: It is nearly perfect when responses are scored by a computer.

Another problem with projective techniques concerns the use of norms. Psychologists rarely use normative data when interpreting TAT protocols and human figure drawings, even though the availability of normative data can help to prevent the overperception of psychopathology. Furthermore, serious problems have surfaced regarding the normative data for the Rorschach. Exner (2001b) recently reported that his 1993 CS adult normative sample contained an error of enormous magnitude: The sample was described as being composed of 700 distinct protocols but it actually contained 479 distinct protocols with 221 protocols counted twice. Subsequently, the CS adult normative sample has been revised (Exner, 2001b), but even this sample has been reported to contain errors (Meyer & Richardson, 2001). Moreover, Exner (personal communication, December 8, 2000) has refused to make the current CS adult normative sample available for examination, even though J. M. Wood, a prominent critic of the CS, offered to pay for any expenses that this would incur (J. M. Wood, personal communication, August 5, 2000).[3] Finally, and most important, the use of the CS norms is likely to lead to the overperception of psychopathology (Hamel, Shaffer, & Erdberg, 2000; Shaffer et al., 1999; Wood, Nezworski, Garb, & Lilienfeld, 2001b; also see Aronow, 2001; Exner, 2001a; Hunsley & Di Giulio, 2001; Meyer, 2001; Widiger, 2001; Wood, Nezworski, Garb, & Lilienfeld, 2001a). For example, in one study (Hamel et al., 2000), the Rorschach was administered to a group of 100 relatively normal school children. Children were excluded from the study if they had a history of mental disorder. Even though an independent measure (the Conners Parent Rating Scale–92; Conners, 1989) revealed that the children were healthier than average, the results for the Rorschach indicated that the typical child in the sample suffered from "a distortion of reality and faulty reasoning approaching psychosis" and "an affective disorder that includes many of the markers found in clinical depression" (p. 291).

The evidence for the construct validity of most projective techniques is at best mixed. In several meta-analyses, effect sizes for the Rorschach have ranged from $r = .25$ to .35, indicating that some positive findings have been reported (e.g., Garb, Florio, & Grove, 1998; Hiller, Rosenthal, Bornstein, Berry, & Brunell-Neuleib, 1999; Meyer & Archer, 2001; Parker, Hanson, & Hunsley, 1988). However, positive validity findings for the Rorschach, TAT, and human figure drawings have rarely been independently replicated (Lilienfeld et al., 2000).

---

[2] In fact, the TAT is rarely scored in clinical practice (see Lilienfeld et al., 2000).

[3] There has also been a heated argument over the accessibility of studies that have been cited to support the CS. Unpublished studies sponsored by Rorschach Workshops are frequently cited as evidence supporting the CS, but attempts to obtain copies of papers describing the studies have frequently been unsuccessful (Nezworski & Wood, 1995; Wood, Nezworski, & Stejskal, 1996a, 1996b; but also see Exner, 1995, 1996). Copies of all correspondence will be provided on request.

The following criteria for evaluating construct validity were proposed by Wood, Nezworski, and Stejskal (1996b): (a) test scores should demonstrate a consistent relation to a particular symptom, trait, or disorder; (b) results must be obtained in methodologically rigorous studies; and (c) results must be replicated by independent investigators. Few scores for the Rorschach, TAT, and human figure drawings satisfy these criteria. For the Rorschach, the criteria have been satisfied for scores intended to detect thought disorder and psychotic conditions marked by thought disorder (e.g., schizophrenia), predict psychotherapy outcome, and assess behaviors related to dependency (e.g., Acklin, 1999; Bornstein, 1999; Jorgensen, Andersen, & Dam, 2000; Meyer & Handler, 1997). For the TAT, the criteria have been satisfied for the assessment of achievement motives, the identification of child sexual abuse history, and the detection of borderline personality disorder (Spangler, 1992; Westen, Lohr, Silk, Gold, & Kerber, 1990; Westen, Ludolph, Block, Wixom, & Wiss, 1990). For human figure drawings, the criteria have been satisfied only for distinguishing global psychopathology from normality (Naglieri & Pfeiffer, 1992). Ironically, over half of the indexes that have been empirically supported are rarely used by psychologists in clinical practice. Some of these indexes are difficult to score, while others were not incorporated into Exner's Comprehensive System—the Rorschach scoring system that most clinicians use.

Most projective indexes, including those used widely in clinical practice, have received relatively little empirical support. In commenting on the CS, Meyer and Archer (2001) offered a related observation:

> Yet many variables given fairly substantial interpretive emphasis have received little or no attention (Weiner, 2001). These include the Coping Deficit Index, Obsessive Style Index, Hypervigilance Index, active-to-passive movement ratio, D-score, food content, anatomy and X-ray content, Intellectualization Index, and Isolation Index. (p. 496)

Moreover, in a comprehensive review of research on the relation between Rorschach scores and psychiatric diagnoses (Wood, Lilienfeld, Garb, Nezworski, 2000), Rorschach scores did not show a well-demonstrated relationship to major depressive disorder, posttraumatic stress disorder (PTSD), anxiety disorders other than PTSD, dissociative identity disorder, conduct disorder, psychopathy, or personality disorders. Despite these negative findings, Rorschach results continue to be used by psychologists for the diagnosis of these disorders. Similarly, although Rorschach results and human figure drawings are sometimes used by mental health professionals to help decide whether a child has been sexually abused (Oberlander, 1995), none of these indexes has been consistently supported (e.g., Garb, Wood, & Nezworski, 2000; Trowbridge, 1995).

Personality Inventories

Like the self-rated brief tests described earlier (e.g., measures of the severity of panic symptoms), self-report personality inventories require clients to indicate whether a statement describes them. However, contrary to widespread claims, self-report personality inventories do not require clients to be able to accurately describe their symptoms and personality traits. The "dynamics" of self-report personality inventories were described by Meehl (1945):

> A self-rating constitutes an intrinsically interesting and significant bit of verbal behavior, the nontest correlates of which must be discovered by empirical means. [The approach is free] from the restriction that the subject must be able to describe his own behavior accurately, ...
>
>   The selection of items is done on a thoroughly empirical basis using carefully selected criterion groups. (p. 297)

Thus, whereas the validity of brief self-rated tests rests on the content of items, the validity of self-report personality inventories rests on empirical research that relates test items (and test scales) to client characteristics. This approach has met with some success. For example, results from a meta-analysis indicate that the MMPI can be useful for detecting overreporting and underreporting of psychopathology (Berry, Baer, & Harris, 1991).

Scientific support for personality inventories has been mixed. The primary scales of some tests (e.g., the MMPI–2, the Personality Assessment Inventory) have generally been supported, whereas the validity evidence for the scales of other widely used tests (e.g., the Millon Clinical Multiaxial Inventory–III or MCMI–III) is weaker and less consistent. For example, Rogers, Salekin, and Sewell (1999) reviewed the research on the MCMI–III and concluded that it should not be used in forensic settings (also see Dyer & McCann, 2000; Rogers, Salekin, & Sewell, 2000). Even for the MMPI–2, half of the supplementary scales have not been consistently supported (e.g., Greene, 2000, pp. 218–269). Despite these negative findings, positive results have been consistently replicated by independent investigators for a large number of MMPI–2 scores. For example, research has demonstrated that Scale 4 (psychopathic deviate) is correlated positively with criminal behaviors and recidivism risk (see Greene, 2000, p. 148), whereas Scale 9 (hypomania) is correlated with such characteristics as impulsiveness, extraversion, and superficiality in social relationships (e.g., Graham, Ben-Porath, & McNulty, 1997). In clinical judgment studies, judgments have been more valid when psychologists have been given results from personality inventories than when given results from projective techniques (e.g., Garb, 1989, 1998, 2003). In fact, in several studies, validity actually decreased, at least slightly, when Rorschach results were made available in addition to brief biographical and/or questionnaire results (e.g., Whitehead, 1985).

In contrast to psychologists who use projective techniques, psychologists using self-report personality inventories almost always use norms. There is no evidence that the norms of major self-report personality inventories, such as the MMPI–2, are unrepresentative of American adults or adolescents in the community. Nor is there evidence that these norms make relatively normal individuals appear pathological.

CLINICAL JUDGMENT AND DECISION-MAKING

Experience, Training, and Clinical Judgment

When confronted with negative evidence regarding the validity of specific assessment instruments, such as projective techniques, some clinicians retort that their extensive clinical experience permits them to extract useful inferences from these instruments. In other words, the argument goes, validation studies fail to capture the rich and subtle information that highly seasoned practitioners can obtain from certain assessment measures. For example, in response to review articles demonstrating that a mere handful of Rorschach variables are empirically supported (e.g., Lilienfeld et al., 2000, 2001), several practitioners on messages to the Rorschach Discussion and Information Group recently maintained that the negative research evidence was largely irrelevant because their numerous years of clinical experience with the Rorschach endowed them with special judgmental and predictive powers.

Nevertheless, these superficially plausible arguments do not withstand careful scrutiny, because the relation between clinical experience and judgmental accuracy has been weak in most studies of personality and psychopathology assessment (Dawes, 1994). For example, when given MMPI (e.g., Graham, 1967) or Rorschach (e.g., Turner, 1966) protocols, clinicians did not produce more valid ratings of psychopathology or personality than did psychology graduate students (see Garb, 1989, 1998, for reviews). Nor is there evidence that presumed experts on certain personality measures outperform other clinicians. In one striking example, Levenberg (1975) asked clinicians to identify children as either normal or abnormal on the basis of their protocols on the Kinetic Family Drawing test, a commonly used human figure drawing measure. Whereas a group of doctoral-level psychologists was correct for 72% of cases, the author of two books on the Kinetic Family Drawing test was correct for only 47% of cases (see also Turner, 1966, for similar findings on the Rorschach).

One potential exception to the literature on the negligible relation between experience and accuracy derives from a study by Brammer (2002), who compared psychologists and psychology students on a task involving an artificial intelligence program that simulated a psychiatric interview with a client. The number of years of clinician experience was significantly associated ($r = .33$) with the number of correct diagnoses made, as well as with the number of diagnostically specific questions asked ($r = .51$). Brammer's findings raise the intriguing possibility that experience is related to validity on tasks that require clinicians to structure complex tasks, such as formulating a psychiatric diagnosis by honing in on potential problem areas and then asking progressively more specific questions (see also Clavelle & Turner, 1980).

Some clinicians could contend that although the overall relation between experience and accuracy tends to be weak, many clinicians in real world settings know which of their judgments are likely to be accurate. Nevertheless, for the use of projective techniques and some other assessment instruments, the relation between the validity of clinicians' judgments and their confidence in these judgments is generally poor. For example, Albert et al. (1980) found no significant relation between validity and confidence when practitioners were asked to use Rorschach protocols to detect malingering. For the MMPI, there is some evidence that confidence is positively related to the validity of clinicians' judgments, but only when these judgments are reasonably valid (e.g., Goldberg, 1965). That is, when psychologists use the MMPI to assist in making diagnoses, they tend to be able to say which of their diagnostic judgments are most likely to be correct.

In contrast to the dispiriting findings concerning the value of clinical experience for personality assessment judgments, the research literature supports the value of training on certain assessment instruments. For example, in several studies psychologists using MMPI protocols made more valid personality judgments than did lay judges (e.g., Aronson & Akamatsu, 1981; see Garb, 1998, for a review). Nevertheless, research does not support the value of training in the interpretation of projective protocols. For example, in one study (Gadol, 1969), clinical psychologists and undergraduates were equally accurate when asked to make personality ratings of psychiatric patients on the basis of Rorschach protocols. Similar findings emerged when psychologists were compared with lay judges in their ability to distinguish psychopathology from normality on the basis of human figure drawings or sentence completion tests (see Garb, 1998, for a review).

Why Clinicians Often Do Not Benefit From Experience

Why are practitioners often unable to benefit from clinical experience? Although the reasons are manifold (see Arkes, 1981; Dawes, Faust, & Meehl, 1989; Garb, 1989), we focus on five here. The first three concern the nature of the feedback available to clinicians, and the second two concern cognitive processes that influence the selection and interpretation of this feedback.

Nature of Feedback. First, in contrast to physicians in most domains of organic medicine, psychologists rarely receive clear-cut feedback concerning their judgments and predictions (Meehl, 1973). Instead, the feedback clinicians receive is often vague, ambiguous, and open to multiple interpretations. For example, if a clinician concludes that an adult client was sexually abused in childhood on the basis of an unstructured interview and Rorschach protocol, this judgment is difficult to falsify. If the client were to deny a past abuse history or express uncertainty about it, the clinician could readily maintain that the abuse was repressed (although the scientific evidence for repression is controversial; see Holmes, 1990) or otherwise forgotten. Moreover, when clinicians receive feedback regarding their predictions (e.g., forecasts of violence), it is often substantially delayed, thereby introducing the potential distorting effects of memory.

Second, clinicians typically have access to only a subset of the data needed for accurate judgments, a quandary referred to by Gilovich (1991) as the "missing data" problem. For example, clinicians may perceive certain psychological conditions (e.g., nicotine dependence) to be more chronic and unremitting than they are (see Schacter, 1982) because they are selectively exposed to individuals who remain in treatment. Cohen and Cohen (1984) referred to this effect as the "clinician's illusion." Moreover, one likely reason why many clinicians have not recognized that the Rorschach overpathologizes clients is that clinicians rarely administer this measure to normal individuals (Wood et al., 2000).

Third, some feedback that clinicians receive from clients is misleading. For example, some of the personality interpretations made by purported experts in personality assessment sound suspiciously like those of astrologers and palm readers (see Wood, Nezworski, Lilienfeld, & Garb, 2003). Meehl (1956) referred to an individual's tendency to accept highly generalized but nonobvious personality descriptions as the *P. T. Barnum effect*, after the circus entrepreneur who quipped that "I like to give a little something to everybody" and "A sucker is born every minute." Numerous studies demonstrate that most individuals presented with Barnum descriptions (e.g., "You have a great deal of unused potential," "At times you have difficulty making up your mind") find such descriptions to be highly compelling, particularly when they believe that these descriptions were tailored for them (Logue, Sher, & Frensch, 1992; Snyder & Larson, 1972). The P. T. Barnum effect demonstrates that personal validation, the informal method of validating test feedback by relying on respondents' acceptance of this feedback, is a highly fallible barometer of actual validity. In addition, because clients are often impressed by Barnum feedback, such feedback can fool clinicians into believing that their interpretations are more valid than they really are.

Cognitive Processes. Fourth, a substantial body of literature documents that individuals are prone to *confirmatory bias*, the tendency to selectively seek out and recall information consistent with one's hypotheses and to neglect information inconsistent with these hypotheses. Several investigators have found that clinicians fall prey to confirmatory bias when asked to recall information regarding clients. For example, Strohmer, Shivy, and Chiodo (1990) asked counselors to read three versions of a case history of a client, one containing an equal number of descriptors indicating good self-control and poor self-control, one containing more descriptors indicating good control than poor self-control, and one containing more descriptors indicating poor than good self-control. One week after reading this case history, psychotherapists were asked to offer as many factors they could remember that "would be helpful in determining whether or not [the client] lacked self-control" (p. 467). Therapists offered more information that would be helpful for confirming than disconfirming the hypothesis that the client lacked self-control, even in the condition in which the client was described as characterized primarily by good self-control descriptors.

In a related vein, there is evidence that clinicians are sometimes prone to *premature closure* in diagnostic decision making: they may tend to reach conclusions too quickly (Garb, 1998). For example, Gauron and Dickinson (1969) reported that psychiatrists who observed a videotaped interview frequently formed diagnostic impressions within 30 to 60 seconds. Premature closure may both reflect and produce confirmatory bias. It may reflect confirmatory bias because clinicians may reach rapid conclusions by searching only for data that confirm preexisting hypotheses. It may produce confirmatory bias by effectively halting the search for data that could disconfirm such hypotheses.

Fifth, investigators have shown that clinicians, like all individuals, are prone to *illusory correlation*, which has generally been defined as the perception of (a) a statistical association that does not actually exist or (b) a stronger statistical association than is actually present. Illusory correlations are likely to arise when individuals hold powerful a priori expectations regarding the covariation between certain events or stimuli. For example, many individuals are convinced that a strong correlation exists between the full moon and psychiatric hospital admissions, even though studies have demonstrated repeatedly that no such association exists (Rotton & Kelly, 1985).

In a classic study of illusory correlation, Chapman and Chapman (1967) examined why psychologists perceive clinically meaningful associations between signs (e.g., large eyes) on the Draw-A-Person (DAP) test (a commonly used human figure drawing task) and psychiatric symptoms (e.g., suspiciousness) even though research has demonstrated that these associations do not exist (Kahill, 1984). They presented undergraduate participants with DAP protocols that were purportedly produced by psychiatric patients with certain psychiatric symptoms (e.g., suspiciousness). Each drawing was paired randomly with two of these symptoms, which were listed on the bottom of each drawing. Undergraduates were asked to inspect these drawings and estimate the extent to which certain DAP signs co-occurred with these symptoms. Chapman and Chapman found that participants "discovered" that certain DAP signs tended to consistently co-occur with certain psychiatric symptoms, even though the DAP signs and symptoms had been randomly paired. For example, participants perceived large eyes in drawings as co-occurring with suspiciousness and broad shoulders in drawings as co-occurring with doubts about manliness. Interestingly, these are the same associations that tend to be perceived by clinicians who use the DAP (Chapman & Chapman, 1967). Illusory correlation has been demonstrated with other assessment instruments, including the Rorschach (Chapman & Chapman, 1969) and sentence completion tests (Starr & Katkin, 1969). Scientifically minded practitioners need to be aware of the phenomenon of illusory correlation, which suggests that clinicians can be convinced of the validity of assessment indicators in the absence of validity.

Group Biases in Judgment. A large number of studies have examined race, sex, and socioeconomic status (SES) biases in clinical judgment (Garb, 1997). *Bias* occurs when the validity of a clinical judgment or test differs by client race, sex, or SES. The most frequent type of bias discussed by psychologists is slope bias, which involves differences in validity coefficients across groups. When a test or clinical judgment yields a significantly higher validity coefficient in one group than another (slope bias), the test or judgment exhibits "differential validity" (Anastasi & Urbina, 1997). Note that the mere presence of group differences on a test is not sufficient to infer bias; bias requires that the clinical judgment or test be less valid for one group than another.

Sex Bias. Sex role-stereotypes are a cause for concern in the diagnosis of psychopathology, especially personality disorders. Histrionic personality disorder is more likely to be diagnosed in women and antisocial personality disorder is more likely to be diagnosed in men, even when client symptoms (e.g., seductiveness, manipulativeness) are identical in both groups. When given case histories that differed only by client gender, both male and female clinicians exhibit this bias (e.g., Adler, Drake, & Teague, 1990; Ford & Widiger, 1989). Ford and Widiger found that an analysis of the individual criteria for these diagnoses did not exhibit clinician bias, but that the full diagnoses did. This finding suggests that the bias is linked to clinicians' perceptions of the diagnoses themselves, not with the DSM criteria for these disorders.

Race Bias. In a number of studies conducted in clinical settings, race bias has been shown to occur in psychiatric diagnosis, the prescription of psychiatric medications, violence prediction, and child abuse reporting (Garb, 1997, 1998). When the effect of social class was controlled, race still emerged as an important predictor. African American and Hispanic patients were less likely to be diagnosed with a psychotic mood disorder and more likely to be diagnosed with schizophrenia compared with White patients exhibiting similar symptoms (e.g., Mukherjee, Shukla, Woodle, Rosen, & Olarte, 1983; Simon, Fleiss, Gurland, Stiller, & Sharpe, 1973). This occurred even when a diagnosis of schizophrenia was inappropriate. Additionally, African American patients received a larger number of antipsychotic medications, injections of antipsychotic medications, and psychiatric medications overall. Moreover, clinicians have exhibited race bias when predicting the occurrence of violence in institutional settings, including psychiatric wards and prisons. In these studies, they have overestimated the risk of violence for Black inpatients and inmates. However, for clients residing in the community, race bias was not found for the prediction of violence. Race was a potent predictor of failure to report child abuse: Cases of child abuse were less likely to be reported if the child was White than Black (Hampton & Newberger, 1985).

Social Class Bias. Social class bias has been demonstrated only sparsely in psychiatric diagnosis and treatment (Garb, 1997, 1998). One finding that has emerged is the relation of social class to psychotherapy decisions. Clinicians were more likely to recommend middle-class individuals than lower-class individuals for psychotherapy and expected them to do better in therapy when both groups were recommended. Additionally, middle-class clients were more likely to be recommended for insight-focused therapy, whereas lower-class clients received more recommendations for supportive therapy (see Garb, 1997, for a review).

METHODOLOGICAL RECOMMENDATIONS

Several methodological steps can be taken to improve the quality of psychological assessment and the judgments derived from psychological tests. First, more sophisticated procedures can be used to evaluate validity. For example, to evaluate the validity of diagnoses, one can use the LEAD standard (Spitzer, 1983; also see Garb, 1998, pp. 45–53). Use of the LEAD standard, which was described earlier, allows researchers to ascertain the validity of structured interviews and other assessment instruments. Second, the criteria proposed by Wood et al. (1996b) should be used to determine if an assessment instrument is valid for its intended purpose. For example, if positive validity findings have been obtained in two studies but not in two others, one would conclude that the assessment instrument does not meet the Wood et al. (1996b) criteria because the results were not consistently replicated.

A third recommendation is that item response theory (IRT) be used to construct and evaluate tests. IRT is an alternative to traditional (classical) test theory. It can be used as a methodological and statistical tool for a number of purposes including test construction, evaluating a test, and using person-fit indexes to assess how well a trait (or construct) describes an individual. For example, using person-fit indexes, one may conclude that a trait is not relevant to a person if the person responds in an idiosyncratic manner (e.g., endorses severe but not moderate symptoms of depression). IRT also permits test constructors to determine which items are most discriminating at different levels of the trait in question. For example, IRT analyses could reveal that a measure of depression adequately distinguishes nondepressed from moderately depressed individuals, but not moderately from severely depressed individuals. Although well established in achievement and aptitude testing, IRT has been applied infrequently to personality assessment. This is partly because cognitive constructs are better understood than personality constructs. Put another way, construct validity issues have been more formidable for personality measurement. However, in recent years, IRT has been applied successfully to personality assessment. For example, historically, linear factor analyses have been used to describe the structure of the MMPI and MMPI–2. Because MMPI and MMPI–2 items are dichotomous (true–false), and because linear factor analysis assumes that ratings are normally distributed and not dichotomous, it is more appropriate to use nonlinear factor analysis or multidimensional IRT methods. Using IRT to uncover the factor structure of the MMPI–2, Waller (1998) found important differences between his results and those of previous factor analyses.

Fourth, the use of computers for making judgments and decisions is becoming increasingly important in the assessment of psychopathology. Findings from a recent meta-analysis (Grove, Zald, Lebow, Snitz, & Nelson, 2000) suggest that computer programs can be successfully developed for this purpose. The utility of these programs derives from well-established (although still largely neglected) findings that actuarial (statistical) formulas based on empirically established relations between predictors and criteria are almost always superior or at least equal to clinical judgment (Dawes et al., 1989; Grove & Meehl, 1996). However, relatively few well-validated computer programs are available for clinical tasks (Garb, 2000). As observed by Wood, Garb, Lilienfeld, and Nezworski (2002):

> *Substantial progress has been made in developing computerized algorithms to predict violence, child abuse and neglect, and recidivism among juvenile offenders.... However, there are still no well-validated algorithms for making diagnoses, predicting behavior, describing personality traits and psychopathology, or making treatment decisions. (p. 534)*

Similarly, Snyder (2000) concluded that popular computer programs that have been used for years to interpret test results (e.g., for the MMPI–2 and the Rorschach) are inadequately validated. Research is needed to develop and validate new computer programs that provide valid descriptions of a client's personality and psychopathology.

CONCLUSIONS

Judging and assessing psychopathology is an activity fraught with potential error and bias. However, by attending to research findings, psychologists can avoid using test scores that are invalid, and they can become familiar with the strengths and weaknesses of clinical judgment. In this way, errors that are potentially detrimental to clients can be avoided. For example, the use of the CS norms for interpreting Rorschach protocols can lead to false positives in the assessment of psychopathology. By not using the CS norms, or by using them with extreme caution, one can avoid making harmful judgments such as misdiagnosing normal clients as pathological.[4]

Some psychologists argue that although scientific research is important, we should also rely on clinical experience to determine if an assessment instrument is valuable. Indeed, some even argue that when research and clinical experience conflict, we should place a higher premium on the latter. Psychologists are frequently encouraged to use the Rorschach and other projective

---

[4]For a case history describing a client who was apparently harmed by interpretations of the Rorschach, see Garb, Wood, Lilienfeld, and Nezworski (2002).

techniques because they seem to provide rich clinical data (e.g., Karon, 2000). However, clinical experience can be fallible for a host of reasons including biased feedback, illusory correlation, and confirmatory bias (Dawes et al., 1989; Garb, 1998). The scientific method, not clinical experience, is the best method for minimizing error and resolving controversies. Scientific techniques, such as double-blind designs and control groups, are tools that researchers have developed to protect themselves from being misled (Lilienfeld, 2002). As McFall (1991) noted:

> *[There is a] commonly offered rationalization that science doesn't have all the answers yet, and until it does, we must do the best we can to muddle along, relying on our clinical experience, judgment, creativity, and intuition (cf., Matarazzo, 1990). Of course, this argument reflects the mistaken notion that science is a set of answers, rather than a set of processes or methods by which to arrive at answers. Where there are lots of unknowns—and clinical psychology certainly has more than its share—it is all the more imperative to adhere as strictly as possible to the scientific approach. Does anyone seriously believe that a reliance on intuition and other unscientific methods is going to hasten advances in knowledge? (pp. 76–77)*

Finally, as noted by McFall (cited in Trull & Phares, 2001, p. 62), one feature that should distinguish clinical and counseling psychologists from most other mental health professionals is their scientific training. To ignore research findings because they make us feel uncomfortable is to neglect our most distinctive and positive attribute: our training in, and our willingness to be guided by, science.

REFERENCES

Acklin, M. W. (1999). Behavioral science foundations of the Rorschach test: Research and clinical applications. *Assessment, 6,* 319–326.

Acklin, M. W., McDowell, C. J., Verschell, M. S., & Chan, D. (2000). Interobserver agreement, intraobserver reliability, and the Rorschach Comprehensive System. *Journal of Personality Assessment, 74,* 15–47.

Adler, D. A., Drake, R. E., & Teague, G. B. (1990). Clinicians' practices in personality assessment: Does gender influence the use of DSM-III Axis II? *Comprehensive Psychiatry, 31,* 125–131.

Albert, S., Fox, H. M., & Kahn, M. W. (1980). Faking psychosis on the Rorschach: Can expert judges detect malingering? *Journal of Personality Assessment, 44,* 115–119.

Alterman, A. I., Snider, E. C., Cacciola, J. S., Brown, L. S., Jr., Zaballero, A., & Siddiqui, N. (1996). Evidence of response set effects in structured research interviews. *Journal of Nervous and Mental Disease, 184,* 403–410.

American Educational Research Association, American Psychological Association, & National Council on Measurement in Education (1999). *Standards for educational and psychological testing.* Washington, DC: American Educational Research Association.

American Psychiatric Association (1980). *Diagnostic and statistical manual of mental disorders* (3rd ed.). Washington, DC: Author.

American Psychiatric Association (1994). *Diagnostic and statistical manual of mental disorders* (4th ed.). Washington, DC: Author.

Anastasi, A., & Urbina, S. (1997). *Psychological testing* (7th ed.). New York: Macmillan.

Antony, M. M., & Barlow, D. H. (Eds.) (2002). *Handbook of assessment and treatment planning for psychological disorders.* New York: Guilford.

Arkes, H. R. (1981). Impediments to accurate clinical judgment and possible ways to minimize their impact. *Journal of Consulting and Clinical Psychology, 49,* 323–330.

Aronow, E. (2001). CS norms, psychometrics, and possibilities for the Rorschach technique. *Clinical Psychology: Science and Practice, 8,* 383–385.

Aronson, D. E., & Akamatsu, T. J. (1981). Validation of a Q-sort task to assess MMPI skills. *Journal of Clinical Psychology, 37,* 831–836.

Baker, S. L., Patterson, M. D., & Barlow, D. H. (2002). Panic disorder and agoraphobia. In M. M. Antony & D. H. Barlow (Eds.), *Handbook of assessment and treatment planning for psychological disorders* (pp. 67–112). New York: Guilford.

Beck, A. T., & Steer, R. A. (1990). *Manual for the Beck Anxiety Inventory*. San Antonio, TX: Psychological Corporation.

Beck, A. T., Steer, R. A., & Brown, G. K. (1996). *Beck Depression Inventory Manual* (2nd ed.). San Antonio, TX: Psychological Corporation.

Berry, D. T. R., Baer, R. A., & Harris, M. J. (1991). Detection of malingering on the MMPI: A meta-analysis. *Clinical Psychology Review, 11*, 585–598.

Beutler, L. E., & M. L. Malik (Eds.) (2002). *Rethinking the DSM: A Psychological Perspective*. Washington, DC: American Psychological Association.

Blanchard, E. B., Kolb, L. C., Pallmeyer, T. P., & Gerardi, R. J. (1982). A psychophysiological study of posttraumatic stress disorder in Vietnam veterans. *Psychiatric Quarterly, 54*, 220–229.

Blashfield, R. K., & Herkov, M. J. (1996). Investigating clinician adherence to diagnosis by criteria: A replication of Morey and Ochoa (1989). *Journal of Personality Disorders, 10*, 219–228.

Bornstein, R. F. (1999). Criterion validity of objective and projective dependency tests: A meta-analytic assessment of behavioral prediction. *Psychological Assessment, 11*, 48–57.

Brammer, R. (2002). Effects of experience and training on diagnostic accuracy. *Psychological Assessment, 14*, 110–113.

Brockington, I. F., Kendell, R. E., & Leff, J. P. (1978). Definitions of schizophrenia: Concordance and prediction of outcome. *Psychological Medicine, 8*, 387–398.

Brown, T. A., Di Nardo, P., & Barlow, D. H. (1994). *Anxiety Disorders Interview Schedule for DSM-IV*. San Antonio, TX: Psychological Corporation.

Brown, T. A., Di Nardo, P. A., Lehman, C. L., & Campbell, L. A. (2001). Reliability of DSM-IV anxiety and mood disorders: Implications for the classification of emotional disorders. *Journal of Abnormal Psychology, 110*, 49–58.

Butcher, J. N., Dahlstrom, W. G., Graham, J. R., Tellegen, A., & Kaemmer, B. (1989). *Manual for the administration and scoring of the MMPI-2*. Minneapolis: University of Minnesota Press.

Chapman, L. J., & Chapman, J. P. (1967). Genesis of popular but erroneous psychodiagnostic observations. *Journal of Abnormal Psychology, 72*, 193–204.

Chapman, L. J., & Chapman, J. P. (1969). Illusory correlation as an obstacle to the use of valid psychodiagnostic signs. *Journal of Abnormal Psychology, 74*, 271–280.

Clavelle, P. R., & Turner, A. D. (1980). Clinical decision-making among professionals and paraprofessionals. *Journal of Clinical Psychology, 36*, 833–838.

Cohen, P., & Cohen, J. (1984). The clinician's illusion. *Archives of General Psychiatry, 41*, 1178–1182.

Conners, K. (1989). *Manual for Conners' rating scales*. North Tonawanda, NY: Multi-Health Systems.

Cronbach, L. J., & Meehl, P. E. (1955). Construct validity in psychological tests. *Psychological Bulletin, 52*, 281–302.

Dawes, R. M., Faust, D., & Meehl, P. E. (1989). Clinical versus actuarial judgment. *Science, 243*, 1668–1674.

Dawes, R. M. (1994). *House of cards: Psychology and psychotherapy built on myth*. New York: Free Press.

Dyer, F. J., & McCann, J. T. (2000). The Millon clinical inventories, research critical of their forensic application, and Daubert criteria. *Law and Human Behavior, 24*, 487–497.

Exner, J. E. (1993). *The Rorschach: A comprehensive system: Vol. 1: Basic Foundations* (3rd ed.). New York: Wiley.

Exner, J. E. (1995). Comment on "Narcissism in the Comprehensive System for the Rorschach." *Clinical Psychology: Science and Practice, 2*, 200–206.

Exner, J. E. (1996). Comment on "The Comprehensive System for the Rorschach: A Critical Examination." *Psychological Science, 7*, 11–13.

Exner, J. E. (2001a). A comment on "The Misperception of Psychopathology: Problems with the Norms of the Comprehensive System for the Rorschach." *Clinical Psychology: Science and Practice, 8*, 386–388.

Exner, J. E. (2001b). *A Rorschach workbook for the Comprehensive System* (5th ed.). Asheville, NC: Rorschach Workshops.

Faraone, S. V., & Tsuang, M. T. (1994). Measuring diagnostic accuracy in the absence of a "gold standard." *American Journal of Psychiatry, 151*, 650–657.

Finn, S. E., & Kamphuis, J. H. (1995). What a clinician needs to know about base rates. In J. Butcher (Ed.), *Clinical personality assessment: Practical approaches* (pp. 224–235). New York: Oxford University Press.

Fleiss, J. (1981). *Statistical methods for rates and proportions* (2nd ed.). New York: Wiley.

Ford, M., & Widiger, T. (1989). Sex bias in the diagnosis of histrionic and antisocial personality disorders. *Journal of Consulting and Clinical Psychology, 57*, 301–305.

Gadol, I. (1969). The incremental and predictive validity of the Rorschach test in personality assessments of normal, neurotic, and psychotic subjects. *Dissertation Abstracts, 29*, 3482B. (UMI No. 69-4469).

Garb, H. N. (1989). Clinical judgment, clinical training, and professional experience. *Psychological Bulletin, 105*, 387–396.

Garb, H. N. (1996). The representativeness and past-behavior heuristics in clinical judgment. *Professional Psychology: Research and Practice, 27*, 272–277.

Garb, H. N. (1997). Race bias, social class bias, and gender bias in clinical judgment. *Clinical Psychology: Science and Practice, 4*, 99–120.

Garb, H. N. (1998). *Studying the clinician: Judgment research and psychological assessment.* Washington, DC: American Psychological Association.

Garb, H. N. (2000). Computers will become increasingly important for psychological assessment: Not that there's anything wrong with that! *Psychological Assessment, 12*, 31–39.

Garb, H. N. (2003). Incremental validity and the assessment of psychopathology in adults. *Psychological Assessment, 15*, 508–520.

Garb, H. N., Florio, C. M., & Grove, W. M. (1998). The validity of the Rorschach and the Minnesota Multiphasic Personality Inventory: Results from meta-analyses. *Psychological Science, 9*, 402–404.

Garb, H. N., Wood, J. M., Lilienfeld, S. O., & Nezworski, M. T. (2002). Effective use of projective techniques in clinical practice: Let the data help with selection and interpretation. *Professional Psychology: Research and Practice, 33*, 454–463.

Garb, H. N., Wood, J. M., & Nezworski, M. T. (2000). Projective techniques and the detection of child sexual abuse. *Child Maltreatment, 5*, 161–168.

Gauron, E. F., & Dickinson, J. K. (1969). The influence of seeing the patient first on diagnostic decision-making in psychiatry. *American Journal of Psychiatry, 126*, 199–205.

Gawande, A. (2000). When doctors make mistakes. In J. Cohen (Series Ed.) & J. Gleick (Vol. Ed.), *Best American science writing 2000* (pp. 1–22). New York: Harper Collins. (Reprinted from *The New Yorker*, 1999).

Gilovich, T. (1991). *How we know what isn't so.* New York: Free Press.

Goldberg, L. R. (1965). Diagnosticians versus diagnostic signs: The diagnosis of psychosis versus neurosis from the MMPI. *Psychological Monographs, 79* (9, Whole No. 602).

Graham, J. R. (1967). A Q-sort study of the accuracy of clinical descriptions based on the MMPI. *Journal of Psychiatric Research, 5*, 297–305.

Graham, J. R., Ben-Porath, Y. S., & McNulty, J. L. (1997). Empirical correlates of low scores on the MMPI-2 scales in an outpatient mental health setting. *Psychological Assessment, 9*, 386–391.

Greene, R. L. (2000). *The MMPI-2: An interpretive manual.* Needham Heights, MA: Allyn & Bacon.

Grove, W. M., & Meehl, P. E. (1996). Comparative efficiency of informal (subjective, impressionistic) and formal (mechanical, algorithmic) prediction procedures: The clinical-statistical controversy. *Psychology: Public Policy and Law, 2*, 293–323.

Grove, W. M., Zald, D. H., Lebow, B. S., Snitz, B. E., & Nelson, C. (2000). Clinical versus mechanical prediction: A meta-analysis. *Psychological Assessment, 12*, 19–30.

Guarnaccia, V., Dill, C. A., Sabatino, S., & Southwick, S. (2001). Scoring accuracy using the Comprehensive System for the Rorschach. *Journal of Personality Assessment, 77*, 464–474.

Hamel, M., Shaffer, T. W., & Erdberg, P. (2000). A study of nonpatient preadolescent Rorschach protocols. *Journal of Personality Assessment, 75*, 280–294.

Hampton, R. L., & Newberger, E. H. (1985). Child abuse incidence and reporting by hospitals: Significance of severity, class and race. *American Journal of Public Health, 75*, 56–60.

Harkness, A. R., & Lilienfeld, S. O. (1997). Individual differences science for treatment planning: Personality traits. *Psychological Assessment, 9*, 349–360.

Henry, B., Moffitt, T. E., Caspi, A., Langley, J., & Silva, P. A. (1994). On the "Remembrance of Things Past": A longitudinal evaluation of the retrospective method. *Psychological Assessment, 6*, 92–101.

Holmes, D. S. (1990). The evidence for repression: An examination of sixty years of research. In J. L. Singer (Ed.), *Repression and dissociation: Implications for personality theory, psychopathology, and health* (pp. 85–102). Chicago: University of Chicago Press.

Hiller, J. B., Rosenthal, R., Bornstein, R. F., Berry, D. T. R., & Brunell-Neuleib, S. (1999). A comparative meta-analysis of Rorschach and MMPI validity. *Psychological Assessment, 11*, 278–296.

Hunsley, J., & Di Giulio, G. (2001). Norms, norming, and clinical assessment. *Clinical Psychology: Science and Practice, 8*, 378–382.

Jorgensen, K., Andersen, T. J., & Dam, H. (2000). The diagnostic efficiency of the Rorschach Depression Index and the Schizophrenia Index: A review. *Assessment, 7*, 259–280.

Kahill, S. (1984). Human figure drawing in adults: An update of the empirical evidence, 1967–1982. *Canadian Psychology, 25*, 269–292.

Karon, B. P. (2000). The clinical interpretation of the Thematic Apperception Test, Rorschach, and other clinical data: A reexamination of statistical versus clinical prediction. *Professional Psychology: Research and Practice, 31*, 230–233.

Levenberg, S. B. (1975). Professional training, psychodiagnostic skill, and Kinetic Family Drawings. *Journal of Personality Assessment, 39*, 389–393.

Lilienfeld, S. O. (2002). When worlds collide: Social science, politics, and the Rind et al. (1998) child sexual abuse meta-analysis. *American Psychologist, 57*, 176–188.

Lilienfeld, S. O., Wood, J. M., & Garb, H. N. (2000). The scientific status of projective techniques. *Psychological Science in the Public Interest, 1*, 27–66.

Lilienfeld, S. O., Wood, J. M., & Garb, H. N. (2001, May). What's wrong with this picture? *Scientific American, 284*, 80–87.

Litz, B. T., Miller, M. W., Ruef, A. M., & McTeague, L. M. (2002). Exposure to trauma in adults. In M. M. Antony & D. H. Barlow (Eds.), *Handbook of assessment and treatment planning for psychological disorders* (pp. 215–258). New York: Guilford.

Loevinger, J. (1957). Objective tests as instruments of psychological theory. *Psychological Reports, 3*, 635–694.

Logue, M. B., Sher, K. J., & Frensch, P. A. (1992). Purported characteristics of adult children of alcoholics: A possible "Barnum effect." *Professional Psychology: Research and Practice, 23*, 226–232.

Margraf, J., Taylor, C. B., Ehlers, A., Roth, W. T., & Agras, W. S. (1987). Panic attacks in the natural environment. *Journal of Nervous and Mental Disease, 175*, 558–565.

Matarazzo, J. D. (1990). Psychological assessment versus psychological testing: Validation from Binet to the school, clinic, and courtroom. *American Psychologist, 45*, 999–1017.

McFall, R. M. (1991). Manifesto for a science of clinical psychology. *Clinical Psychologist, 44*, 75–88.

McFall, R. M., & Treat, T. A. (1999). Quantifying the information value of clinical assessments with signal detection theory. *Annual Review of Psychology, 50*, 215–241.

Meehl, P. E. (1945). The dynamics of "structured" personality tests. *Journal of Clinical Psychology, 1*, 296–303.

Meehl, P. E. (1956). Wanted–A good cookbook. *American Psychologist, 11*, 263–272.

Meehl, P. E. (1973). Why I do not attend case conferences. In P. E. Meehl, *Psychodiagnosis: Selected papers* (pp. 225–302). Minneapolis: University of Minnesota Press.

Meehl, P. E. (1986). Diagnostic taxa as open concepts: Metatheoretical and statistical questions about reliability and construct validity in the grand strategy of nosological revision. In T. Millon & G. Klerman (Eds.), *Contemporary directions in psychopathology* (pp. 215–231). New York: Guilford.

Meehl, P. E., & Rosen, A. (1955). Antecedent probability and the efficiency of psychometric signs, patterns, or cutting scores. *Psychological Bulletin, 52*, 194–216.

Meyer, G. J. (2001). Evidence to correct misperceptions about Rorschach norms. *Clinical Psychology: Science and Practice, 8*, 389–396.

Meyer, G. J., & Archer, R. P. (2001). The hard science of Rorschach research: What do we know and where do we go? *Psychological Assessment, 13*, 486–502.

Meyer, G. J., & Handler, L. (1997). The ability of the Rorschach to predict subsequent outcome: A meta-analysis of the Rorschach Prognostic Rating Scale. *Journal of Personality Assessment, 69*, 1–38.

Meyer, G. J., Hilsenroth, M. J., Baxter, D., Exner, J. E., Fowler, J. C., Piers, C. C., & Resnick, J. (2002). An examination of interrater reliability for scoring the Rorschach Comprehensive System in eight data sets. *Journal of Personality Assessment, 78*, 219–274.

Meyer, G. J., & Richardson, C. (2001, March). *An examination of changes in Form Quality codes in the Rorschach Comprehensive System from 1974 to 1995*. Presented at the midwinter meeting of the Society for Personality Assessment, Philadelphia.

Millon, T. (1994). *The Millon Clinical Multiaxial Inventory-III manual*. Minneapolis, MN: National Computer Systems.

Molinari, V., Ames, A., & Essa, M. (1994). Prevalence of personality disorders in two geropsychiatric inpatient units. *Journal of Geriatric Psychiatry and Neurology, 7*, 209–215.

Morey, L. C. (1991). *Personality Assessment Inventory: Professional manual*. Tampa: Psychological Assessment Resources.

Morey, L. C., & Ochoa, E. S. (1989). An investigation of adherence to diagnostic criteria: Clinical diagnosis of the DSM-III personality disorders. *Journal of Personality Disorders, 3*, 180–192.

Mukherjee, S., Shukla, S., Woodle, J., Rosen, A. M., & Olarte, S. (1983). Misdiagnosis of schizophrenia in bipolar patients: A multiethnic comparison. *American Journal of Psychiatry, 140*, 1571–1574.

Naglieri, J. A., & Pfeiffer, S. I. (1992). Performance of disruptive behavior-disordered and normal samples on the Draw-A-Person: Screening Procedure for Emotional Disturbance. *Psychological Assessment, 4*, 156–159.

Nakata, L. M. (1999). Interrater reliability and the Comprehensive System for the Rorschach: Clinical and non-clinical protocols (Doctoral dissertation, Pacific Graduate School of Psychology, 1999). *Dissertation Abstracts International, 60*, 4296B.

Nezworski, M. T., & Wood, J. M. (1995). Narcissism in the Comprehensive System for the Rorschach. *Clinical Psychology: Science and Practice, 2*, 179–199.

Nunnally, J. (1978). *Psychometric theory* (2nd ed.). New York: McGraw-Hill.

Oberlander, L. B. (1995). Psycholegal issues in child sexual abuse evaluations: A survey of forensic mental health professionals. *Child Abuse & Neglect, 19,* 475–490.

Parker, K. C. H., Hanson, R., & Hunsley, J. (1988). MMPI, Rorschach, and WAIS: A meta-analytic comparison of reliability, stability, and validity. *Psychological Bulletin, 103,* 367–373.

Rogers, R. (1995). *Diagnostic and structured interviewing: A handbook for psychologists.* Odessa, FL: Psychological Assessment Resources.

Rogers, R., Salekin, R. T., & Sewell, K. W. (1999). Validation of the Millon Clinical Multiaxial Inventory for Axis II disorders: Does it meet the *Daubert* standard? *Law and Human Behavior, 23,* 425–443.

Rogers, R., Salekin, R. T., & Sewell, K. W. (2000). The MCMI-III and the *Daubert* standard: Separating rhetoric from reality. *Law and Human Behavior, 24,* 501–506.

Rotton, J., & Kelly, I. W. (1985). Much ado about the full moon: A meta-analysis of lunar-lunacy research. *Psychological Bulletin, 97,* 286–306.

Sartorius, N., Kaelber, C. T., Cooper, J. E., Roper, M. T., Rae, D. S., Gulbinat, W., Ustun, T. B., & Regier, D. A. (1993). Progress toward achieving a common language in psychiatry: Results from the field trial of the clinical guidelines accompanying the WHO classification of mental and behavioral disorders in *ICD-10. Archives of General Psychiatry, 50,* 115–124.

Savard, J., & Morin, C. M. (2002). Insomnia. In M. M. Antony & D. H. Barlow (Eds.), *Handbook of assessment and treatment planning for psychological disorders* (pp. 523–555). New York: Guilford.

Schacter, S. (1982). Recidivism and self-cure of smoking and obesity. *American Psychologist, 37,* 436–444.

Shaffer, T. W., Erdberg, P., & Haroian, J. (1999). Current nonpatient data for the Rorschach, WAIS-R, and MMPI-2. *Journal of Personality Assessment, 73,* 305–316.

Shear, M. K., Brown, T. A., Barlow, D. H., Money, R., Sholomskas, D. E., Woods, S. W., Gorman, J. M., & Papp, L. A. (1997). Multicenter collaborative Panic Disorder Severity Scale. *American Journal of Psychiatry, 154,* 1571–1575.

Simon, R. J., Fleiss, J. L., Gurland, B. J., Stiller, P. R., & Sharpe, L. (1973). Depression and schizophrenia in hospitalized black and white mental patients. *Archives of General Psychiatry, 28,* 509–512.

Snyder, C. R., & Larson, G. R. (1972). A further look at student acceptance of general personality interpretations. *Journal of Consulting and Clinical Psychology, 38,* 384–388.

Snyder, D. K. (2000). Computer-assisted judgment: Defining strengths and liabilities. *Psychological Assessment, 12,* 52–60.

Spangler, W. D. (1992). Validity of questionnaire and TAT measures of need for achievement: Two meta-analyses. *Psychological Bulletin, 112,* 140–154.

Spitzer, R. L. (1983). Psychiatric diagnosis: Are clinicians still necessary? *Comprehensive Psychiatry, 24,* 399–411.

Starr, B. J., & Katkin, E. S. (1969). The clinician as an aberrant actuary: Illusory correlation and the Incomplete Sentences Blank. *Journal of Abnormal Psychology, 74,* 670–675.

Steiner, J. L., Tebes, J. K., Sledge, W. H., & Walker, M. L. (1995). A comparison of the Structured Clinical Interview for DSM-III-R and clinical diagnoses. *Journal of Nervous and Mental Disease, 183,* 365–369.

Strohmer, D. C., Shivy, V. A., & Chiodo, A. L. (1990). Information processing strategies in counselor hypothesis testing: The role of selective memory and expectancy. *Journal of Counseling Psychology, 37,* 465–472.

Trowbridge, M. M. (1995). Graphic indicators of sexual abuse in children's drawings: A review of the literature. *The Arts in Psychotherapy, 22,* 485–493.

Trull, T. J., & Phares, E. J. (2001). *Clinical Psychology* (6th ed.). Belmont, CA: Wadsworth.

Turner, D. R. (1966). Predictive efficiency as a function of amount of information and level of professional experience. *Journal of Projective Techniques and Personality Assessment, 30,* 4–11.

Waller, N. G. (1998). Searching for structure in the MMPI. In S. E. Embretson & S. L. Hershberger (Eds.), *The new rules of measurement* (pp. 185–217). Mahwah, NJ: Lawrence Erlbaum Associates.

Weiner, I. B. (2000). Using the Rorschach properly in practice and research. *Journal of Clinical Psychology, 56,* 435–438.

Weiner, I. B. (2001). Advancing the science of psychological assessment: The Rorschach Inkblot Method as exemplar. *Psychological Assessment, 13,* 423–432.

Westen, D., Lohr, N., Silk, K. R., Gold, L., & Kerber, K. (1990). Object relations and social cognition in borderlines, major depressives, and normals: A Thematic Apperception Test analysis. *Psychological Assessment, 2,* 355–364.

Westen, D., Ludolph, P., Block, M. J., Wixom, J., & Wiss, F. C. (1990). Developmental history and object relations in psychiatrically disturbed adolescent girls. *American Journal of Psychiatry, 147,* 1061–1068.

Whitehead, W. C. (1985). Clinical decision making on the basis of Rorschach, MMPI, and automated MMPI report data (Doctoral dissertation, University of Texas Southwestern Medical Center at Dallas, 1985). *Dissertation Abstracts International, 46,* 2828.

Widiger, T. A. (2001). The best and the worst of us? *Clincial Psychology: Science and Practice, 8,* 374–377.

Widiger, T. A. (2002). Personality disorders. In M. M. Antony & D. H. Barlow (Eds.), *Handbook of assessment and treatment planning for psychological disorders* (pp. 453–480). New York: Guilford.

Wood, J. M., Garb, H. N., Lilienfeld, S. O., & Nezworski, M. T. (2002). Clinical assessment. *Annual Review of Psychology, 53,* 519–543.

Wood, J. M., Lilienfeld, S. O., Garb, H. N., & Nezworski, M. T. (2000). The Rorschach test in clinical diagnosis: A critical review, with a backward look at Garfield (1947). *Journal of Clinical Psychology, 56,* 395–430.

Wood, J. M., Nezworski, M. T., Garb, H. N., & Lilienfeld, S. O. (2001a). Problems with the norms of the Comprehensive System for the Rorschach: Methodological and conceptual considerations. *Clinical Psychology: Science and Practice, 8,* 397–402.

Wood, J. M., Nezworski, M. T., Garb, H. N., & Lilienfeld, S. O. (2001b). The misperception of psychopathology: Problems with the norms of the Comprehensive System for the Rorschach. *Clinical Psychology: Science and Practice, 8,* 350–373.

Wood, J. M., Nezworski, M. T., Lilienfeld, S. O., & Garb, H. N. (2003). *What's wrong with the Rorschach? Science confronts the controversial inkblot test.* San Francisco, CA: Jossey-Bass.

Wood, J. M., Nezworski, M. T., & Stejskal, W. J. (1996a). The Comprehensive System for the Rorschach: A critical examination. *Psychological Science, 7,* 3–10.

Wood, J. M., Nezworski, M. T., & Stejskal, W. J. (1996b). Thinking critically about the Comprehensive System for the Rorschach: A reply to Exner. *Psychological Science, 7,* 14–17.

6

Biological Bases of Psychopathology

Robert H. Howland
University of Pittsburgh School of Medicine

The biological basis of psychological disorders has been the subject of extensive study and passionate debate (Guze, 1989). All formulations of psychopathology must incorporate biological factors, because biology is the study of life processes. Psychopathology is the manifestation of disordered processes in various brain systems that mediate psychological functions. Thus, disturbances in such brain functions as perception, learning, thought, memory, emotions, communications, and language have biological underpinnings (Buck, 1999). Contemporary research has tended to focus on the study of particular disorders. However, there is a developing awareness that various psychopathological states are not limited to specific disorders (Cloninger, 1999). In this chapter, I will review some aspects of the neurobiology and genetics of depression, anxiety, mania, psychosis, and personality, which will support a general conceptual model of psychopathology as a complex interaction among genetically influenced neurobiological behavioral traits, dysregulation of various brain systems, and the central nervous system (CNS) response to environmental influences and stress (Cooper, 2001; Denenberg, 2000).

ABNORMALITIES OF NEUROBIOLOGICAL RESPONSE SYSTEMS

The earliest theories of the biological basis of various psychological disorders suggested dysfunction of CNS systems subserved by key neurotransmitters: norepinephrine (NE), serotonin (5-hydroxytryptamine or 5-HT), and dopamine (DA). These neurotransmitters were found to regulate vital bodily functions that often are disturbed in patients with psychological disorders (e.g., energy, sleep, appetite, libido, and psychomotor behavior). Dysregulation of NE, 5-HT, and DA systems, individually or in combination, also was believed to be more broadly associated with psychopathological states of depression, anxiety, mania, and psychosis (Kahn & Davis, 1995; Maes & Meltzer, 1995; Ninan & Cummins, 2003; Schatzberg & Schildkraut, 1995; Willner, 1995). Moreover, the first effective pharmacological treatments for depression and anxiety (tricyclic and monoamine oxidase inhibitor antidepressant drugs) were shown to have effects that enhanced NE and/or 5-HT neurotransmission, and the first effective pharmacological treatments for mania and psychosis (antipsychotic drugs such as chlorpromazine) were shown to block DA neurotransmission. Subsequent research has disconfirmed the most simplistic models of altered neurotransmitter levels in the pathophysiology of psychological disorders, but has yielded substantial evidence of disturbed neurotransmitter function in different brain regions of subgroups of people with depression, various forms of anxiety, mania, and psychosis. In addition, this research has revealed the staggering complexity of integrated CNS response systems. Examples of such complexity include the identification of dozens of additional peptide and amino acid neurotransmitters, recognition that neurons can express receptors for several different types of neurotransmitters (enabling direct "cross-talk" between various neuronal systems), and elucidation of intracellular mechanisms of gene transduction (Duman, Heninger, & Nestler, 1997; Nemeroff, 1998).

Noradrenergic Systems

Almost all of the NE cell bodies in the brain are located in the locus ceruleus (LC), located in the rostral pons of the brain stem. Noradrenergic neurons project widely from the LC to the thalamus, hypothalamus, limbic system, basal ganglia, and cerebral cortex (Kandel, Schwartz, & Jessell, 1991; Kingsley, 2000). Such diffuse distribution reflects the broad role of NE in initiating and maintaining limbic and cortical arousal, as well as modulation of other neural systems. For example, noradrenergic projections to the amygdala and hippocampus have been implicated in behavioral sensitization to stress (Ferry, Roozendaal, & McGaugh, 1999), which is relevant to understanding some aspects of the pathophysiology of depression and anxiety (Ninan & Cummins, 2003). Stimulation of the medial forebrain bundle, another major NE pathway in the brain, enhances attention and increases levels of goal-directed or reward-seeking behavior (Aston-Jones, Rajkowski, & Cohen, 1999), suggesting a role for NE in the pathophysiology of hypomanic and manic states (Depue & Iacono, 1989). In support of this relationship, longitudinal studies of bipolar disorder show increased urinary NE metabolite levels following shifts from depression into mania, and lithium treatment decreases NE turnover in manic patients (Schatzberg & Schildkraut, 1995). These findings support the hypothesis that NE modulates the switch process in bipolar disorder (Bunney, Goodwin, Murphy, House, & Gordon, 1972).

Perception of novel or threatening stimuli is relayed from the cerebral cortex to the LC via the thalamus and hypothalamus. This input can provoke an almost immediate increase in NE activity from the LC. In addition, pathways from the cerebral cortex also can stimulate release of the hypothalamic neuropeptide corticotrophin releasing hormone (CRH), which can "turn on" the LC and synergistically mediate the response to external stimuli or stress (Nestler, Alreja, & Aghajanian, 1999). Cognitive processes affecting perception thus can amplify or dampen NE cellular responses to internal or external stimuli, which is consistent with the possibility that dysregulation of these NE systems might contribute to pathological states of anxiety, such as panic attacks, social anxiety, and phobias (Mathew, Coplan, & Gorman, 2001). The peripheral nervous system response to stress is triggered by the LC, which stimulates the release of NE and the glucocorticoid hormone cortisol from the adrenal glands.

The activity of NE neurons is regulated in part by the autoinhibitory effects of noradrenergic autoreceptors. Thus, neuronal release of NE immediately begins to decrease the sensitivity of LC neurons to repeated firing. Noradrenergic receptors also are located on serotonergic cell bodies, and stimulation of these heteroceptors activates inhibitory 5-HT neurons. A sustained increase in LC firing (e.g., in response to persistent stress) also causes the number of noradrenergic receptors to decrease, a process known as down-regulation or desensitization. Together, noradrenergic autoinhibition, noradrenergic receptor down-regulation, and activation of colocalized inhibitory 5-HT tracts constitute the counterregulatory forces that promote homeostasis in the face of sustained stress (i.e., NE-mediated arousal). With chronic stress, however, NE stores will become depleted because demand or turnover eventually will exceed synthetic capacity. When this occurs, there will be diminished autoinhibitory noradrenergic and 5-HT input to the LC, resulting in dysregulated NE neurotransmission and increased firing of the LC. Over time, the net effect is that CNS NE neurotransmission will decrease, but peripheral nervous system output of NE and cortisol from the adrenal glands may remain high.

The behavioral consequences of acute stress on NE systems include heightened anxiety (including panic symptoms), fearfulness, and psychomotor agitation. For this reason, dysregulation of NE systems have been implicated in the pathophysiology of various anxiety disorders, which often are responsive to antidepressant drug treatment. There also is some evidence that increased NE activity may contribute to the genesis of psychotic symptoms. In addition to blocking the effects of DA, some antipsychotic drugs also block noradrenergic receptors, which might contribute to their clinical effects in the treatment of psychosis. By contrast, chronic stress on NE systems leads to decreased exploratory and consummatory behavior, a state described in animal models of depression as learned helplessness (Maier & Seligman, 1976). Although not synonymous with depression in humans, learned helplessness in animals can be viewed as an analogous state of CNS "exhaustion" associated with reductions of NE levels in the CNS and elevated cortisol activity (Weiss & Kilts, 1998). Not surprisingly, antidepressant drugs, which decrease the turnover of NE and decrease the firing rate of LC neurons (Ressler & Nemeroff, 1999), can normalize the behaviors associated with learned helplessness in animals.

Serotonergic Systems

Most of the 5-HT in the brain is synthesized in dorsal raphé nuclei of the brain stem. These 5-HT neurons project to the cerebral cortex, hypothalamus, thalamus, basal ganglia, septum, and hippocampus (Kandel et al., 1991; Kingsley, 2000). Serotonin pathways are largely colocalized with NE pathways and generally have tonic and inhibitory effects that counterbalance NE activity. Serotonergic input to the thalamus facilitates appetite and input to the anterior hypothalamus helps to regulate such circadian rhythms as sleep–wake cycles, body temperature, and hypothalamic-pituitary-adrenal axis function (Bunney & Bunney, 2000; Duncan, 1996). Tonic 5-HT neurotransmission is necessary for affiliative behavior (Insel & Winslow, 1998) and for the expression of goal-directed motor and consummatory behaviors that are primarily mediated by NE and DA. Animals with lower basal 5-HT levels generally have lower rankings on social dominance hierarchies than do animals with higher levels (Higley, Mehlman, & Higley et al., 1996; Higley, Mehlman, & Poland et al., 1996). Conversely, a rise in social dominance is accompanied by an increase in 5-HT levels (Mehlman et al., 1995).

The basal level of 5-HT neurotransmission in primates is partly under genetic control (Higley, Mehlman, & Higley et al., 1996). In humans, the heritability of 5-HT neurotransmission could be mediated by genes for the 5-HT transporter, the enzymes involved in 5-HT synthesis or degradation, or 5-HT receptor subtypes (Mann, Brent, & Arango, 2001). Studies investigating specific genes are underway throughout the world. For example, genetic polymorphisms of the 5-HT transporter gene, which is involved in the reuptake of 5-HT at brain synapses and is the site of action of serotonin reuptake inhibitor antidepressant drugs, have been associated with depression, anxiety, and some personality temperaments and traits (e.g., neuroticism and negative emotionality) (Murphy et al., 2001).

Chronic stress will down-regulate 5-HT-1A receptors, leading eventually to depletion of 5-HT stores (López, Liberzon, Vázquez, Young, & Watson, 1999; Weiss & Kilts, 1998). In animal models of depression, this state is associated with weight loss, decreased sleep, and decreased exploratory behavior. In humans, brain imaging studies have found dysfunction of 5-HT-1A receptors in depression (Drevets et al., 1999; Staley Malison, & Innis, 1998). Interestingly, the experimental elimination of tryptophan (a 5-HT precursor) from food in unaffected relatives of people with depression or mania can induce depression symptoms (Quintin et al., 2001). Decreased 5-HT neurotransmission is not specific to any particular psychological disorder, but has been consistently linked to an increased risk of completed suicide, potentially lethal suicide attempts, and other violent, life-threatening behaviors (Maes & Meltzer, 1995; Mann, Brent, & Arango, 2001). Animals with lower basal 5-HT levels are more impulsive and aggressive, mice lacking 5-HT-1B receptors are more aggressive, and treatment with serotonergic antidepressant drugs decreases impulsive aggression (Fairbanks, Melega, Jorgensen, Kaplan, & Mcguire, 2001). Hence, decreased 5-HT activity may be a more enduring, traitlike phenomenon that is associated with impulsivity and aggression.

Decreased inhibitory 5-HT activity can lead to increased release of NE, DA, CRH, and the excitatory amino acid neurotransmitter glutamate (Sasaki-Adams & Kelley, 2001; Weiss & Kilts, 1998). This effect may partly explain the association between low levels of 5-HT and the development of manic symptoms, psychosis, and anxiety states. For example, there is indirect evidence that low levels of 5-HT are associated with a vulnerability to develop manic episodes (Chouinard, Young, Bradwejn, & Annable, 1983), reflecting the failure of inhibitory control over the increases in NE and DA that are associated with switches into mania (Bunney et al., 1972; Schatzberg, Rothschild, Langlais, Bird, & Cole, 1985). Also, hallucinogenic drugs that affect 5-HT systems, such as lysergic acid diethylamide (LSD), cause psychotic symptoms, and antipsychotic drugs that block 5-HT in addition to DA are effective in treating psychotic symptoms. These observations have led to the view that interactions between 5-HT and DA may be involved in the pathophysiology of psychosis (Roth & Meltzer, 1995). Finally, in animal studies, mice lacking 5-HT-1A receptors show increased anxiety-like behavior (Fairbanks et al., 2001), and various serotonergic drugs are effective in the treatment of anxiety. Although dysregulation of 5-HT has been implicated in the etiology of obsessive-compulsive disorder in particular, based on the distinct therapeutic benefits of potent serotonergic antidepressant drugs, it is more likely that 5-HT modulates the activity of brain circuits involving the orbitofrontal cortex and basal ganglia in this disorder (Delgado & Moreno, 1998). Altogether, these findings are consistent with the broader role of 5-HT neurotransmission as a modulator of CNS stress response systems.

Dopaminergic Systems

There are four principal DA pathways in the brain (Kandel et al., 1991; Kingsley, 2000). The tuberoinfundibular system projects from the hypothalamus to the pituitary gland and inhibits secretion of the hormone prolactin. The nigrostriatral system, which helps to regulate psychomotor activity, originates from the substantia nigra and projects to the basal ganglia. The mesolimbic pathway begins in the ventral tegmentum and projects to the nucleus accumbens, amygdala, hippocampus, medial dorsal nucleus of the thalamus, and cingulate gyrus. The mesolimbic DA pathway modulates emotional expression and goal-directed or consummatory behavior. The mesocortical DA pathway, which projects from the ventral tegmentum orbitofrontal and prefrontal cerebral cortex, subserves motivation, initiation of goal-directed tasks, cognitive processes, and social behavior.

Chronic stress reduces DA levels and results in behavioral changes suggestive of depression (Willner, 1995). For example, decreased DA activity has been implicated in the development of psychomotor retardation, anhedonia, and impaired cognition seen in depression. Studies of antidepressant drugs have found that treatment can reverse or prevent the DA dysfunction caused by chronic stress (Cuadra, Zurita, Gioino, & Molina, 2001; Willner, 1997). Similarly, negative symptoms of psychosis (i.e., poverty of speech and thought, affective flattening, anhedonia, social withdrawal, inattention, anergia, and cognitive impairment) may result from decreased functioning of mesocortical DA neurons in the prefrontal cortex (Kahn and Davis, 1995). Negative symptoms may improve with drugs that selectively enhance prefrontal DA neurotransmission.

By contrast, increased mesolimbic DA activity may lead to positive symptoms of psychosis (i.e., hallucinations and delusions) in patients with severe depression, schizophrenia, and severe mania. Elevated cortisol levels can increase DA activity, which may contribute to the development of psychotic symptoms in these patients as well as in patients who take high doses of glucocorticoid drugs such as prednisone (Schatzberg & Rothschild, 1992). Also, increased mesocortical and mesolimbic DA activity may be related to such manic symptoms as euphoria, grandiosity, hyperactivity, hypersexuality, and disinhibited behaviors (Depue & Iacono, 1989; Schatzberg et al., 1985; Swerdlow & Koob, 1987). Brain imaging studies have found that DA-2 receptors are up-regulated in mania compared to depression and that DA-2 receptor up-regulation is greater in psychotic mania than in nonpsychotic mania (Pearlson et al., 1995). Chronic or high-dose treatment with stimulant drugs, which enhance DA function, can also cause a syndrome indistinguishable from mania (Willner, 1995). Patients with bipolar disorder are more susceptible than other depressed patients to the mood-elevating effects of drugs affecting DA (including antidepressants), which can often precipitate hypomanic or manic episodes (Bunney et al., 1972; Willner, 1995). Lithium and antipsychotic drugs can attenuate some of the DA stimulated behaviors in animals (Swerdlow & Koob, 1987) and are clinically effective in the treatment of mania and psychosis. Interestingly, DA blocking drugs may be effective in treating some patients with severe anxiety, suggesting a possible role for DA systems in the pathophysiology of some anxiety states.

Gamma amino butyric acid (GABA) has inhibitory effects on NE and DA pathways. GABA receptors are densely localized in the thalamus and ascending mesocortical and mesolimbic systems (Kingsley, 2000; Paul, 1995). Chronic stress can reduce or deplete GABA levels in these regions of the brain (Weiss & Kilts, 1998). Decreased GABA function could lead to increased DA activity, contributing to the development of psychomotor agitation, anxiety, mania, and psychosis. Benzodiazepine drugs attach to GABA receptors, which might dampen DA activity and explain their therapeutic benefits in the treatment of anxiety, mania, and psychosis (Paul, 1995).

STRESS AND THE HYPOTHALAMIC-PITUITARY-ADRENAL (HPA) AXIS

The perception of stress is linked to adrenal gland activity by pathways extending from the cerebral cortex and hypothalamus to the pituitary gland. The stress-responsive glucocorticoid hormone cortisol is released by the adrenal gland in response to a wide variety of physical and psychosocial stresses. The HPA axis is partly under the control of phasic NE (activating) and tonic 5-HT (inhibitory) neurotransmission. In the hypothalamus, the neuropeptide CRH is released in response to stimulation from NE and glutamate inputs, typically in response to the perception of stress or threat. CRH then triggers release of adrenocorticotrophic hormone (ACTH), which travels from the pituitary gland to the adrenal gland, where glucocorticoid hormones are synthesized and released. Cortisol binds to glucocorticoid receptors on various cells throughout the body, which regulate the immune system, glucose and lipid metabolism, and other cellular functions that facilitate short-term survival in response to overwhelming or life-threatening stress (Holsboer, 2000). Ordinarily, the HPA axis is tightly regulated by a redundant, multilevel system of negative feedback inhibitory control at the level of the hypothalamus, pituitary gland, adrenal gland, and hippocampus. As acute stresses pass or resolve, elevated plasma cortisol levels in healthy humans will normalize within minutes or hours.

Sustained hypercortisolism can result from increased CRH drive (from the hypothalamus or higher cerebral cortical areas of the brain), increased secretion of ACTH (e.g., from a pituitary tumor), diminished inhibitory feedback from dysfunctional hippocampal glucocorticoid receptors, unrestrained noradrenergic stimulation from the locus ceruleus, diminished serotonergic inhibition, or the failure of one or more mechanisms of feedback inhibition (Holsboer, 1995; Howland & Thase, 1999). Neurons containing CRH are diffusely located throughout the cerebral cortex, especially within the thalamus, amygdala, and other components of the limbic system. Studies measuring CRH synthesis demonstrate that these brain regions "light up" immediately following exposure to stress (Holsboer, 1995). Because CRH activates the LC, which in turn further stimulates the thalamus, hypothalamus, and amygdala, sustained stress can provoke a "reverberating circuit" or a positive feedback loop, resulting in destabilization of the HPA axis (Holsboer, 2000; Nemeroff, 1998).

Sustained hypercortisolism can impair HPA axis feedback inhibition (Bremner, 1999). For example, prolonged ACTH stimulation can cause adrenal hypertrophy, resulting in increased synthesis and release of cortisol. The cells expressing glucocorticoid receptors in the hippocampus are sensitive to very high concentrations of cortisol and will eventually die (Sapolsky, 2000). Hippocampal cell death due to sustained hypercortisolism is most likely to occur early in development and later in old age. For example, exposure to stress early in life can permanently impair normal regulation of HPA axis activity (Kaufman, Plotsky, Nemeroff, & Charney, 2000; McEwen, 2000). In animal models of early trauma, brief periods of maternal separation can result in long-standing changes in stress responses, which can be partly compensated for by competent maternal behavior (Coplan et al., 2001). Stress in later life accelerates the slow decline in the integrity of HPA axis regulation that occurs normally with aging. The age-dependent change in HPA axis regulation is due to the death of hippocampal glucocorticoid receptor cells.

Evidence of hypercortisolism and dysregulation of HPA axis activity is typically found in 40% to 60% of depressed people, but is more commonly associated with older age, psychotic symptoms, severe depression and anxiety, psychomotor agitation, weight loss, insomnia, and suicidality (Howland & Thase, 1999). The types of HPA axis abnormalities seen in depression are also found in mania, although usually to a less severe degree than in depression (Cookson, 1985; Linkowski et al., 1994; Schmider et al., 1995). Interestingly, the HPA axis may be relatively quiescent in depression characterized by low energy, such as bipolar depression (Geracioti, Loosen, & Orth, 1997), but may become overactive in psychotic mania (Cookson, 1985; Linkowski et al., 1994; Schmider et al., 1995), possibly related to decreased and increased activation, respectively, of the dopaminergic mesocorticolimbic system. In addition, a significant minority of people with acute schizophrenia, posttraumatic stress disorder, and other anxiety disorders have abnormal HPA axis activity. Hypercortisolism also is associated with memory and other cognitive impairments, which may reflect neuronal atrophy and cell death in the prefrontal cortex and hippocampus (Belanoff, Gross, Yager, & Schatzberg, 2001).

Because hypercortisolism tends to coaggregate with various measures of NE, 5-HT, and DA dysfunction, drugs with direct or indirect effects on these neurotransmitter systems tend to normalize dysregulation of the HPA axis (Holsboer, 1995; Maes & Meltzer, 1995; Schatzberg & Schildkraut, 1995). For example, antidepressant drugs initiate an effect at 5-HT or NE receptors, and these receptors activate membrane-bound G proteins and various enzymes (Duman et al., 1997; Shelton, 2000). These enzymes catalyze the formation of "second messengers," such as cyclic adenomonophosphate (cAMP) and diacylglycerol. The second messengers, in turn, activate intracellular enzymes that phosphorylate the gene transcription factor CREB (*cAMP response element binding* protein). CREB appears to be the first common step shared by antidepressants that selectively modulate NE or 5-HT neurotransmission (Shelton, 2000). Phosphorylated CREB regulates the activity of various gene products related to stress responses, including CRH, glucocorticoid receptors, brain derived neurotrophic factor (BDNF), and the BDNF receptor (Duman et al., 1997; Shelton, 2000). BDNF is particularly important because it has been shown to stimulate neurogenesis (the growth of neuronal cells). Lithium, antidepressants, and other psychotropic drugs have been shown to increase BDNF levels and reduce hypercortisolism, which reverse neuronal atrophy and cell death in the prefrontal cortex and hippocampus (Duman, Malberg, & Thome, 1999; Manji, Moore, & Chen, 2000).

The excitatory amino acid glutamate is one of the most widely distributed neurotransmitters in the CNS, modulating the effect of other neurotransmitters (Kingsley, 2000). Glutamate binds to the N-methyl-D-aspartate (NMDA) receptor and, in excess, can have neurotoxic effects similar to hypercortisolism. Glutamate can cause degeneration of cells in the hippocampus and amygdala, which have high concentrations of NMDA receptors (Mathew, Coplan, Smith et al., 2001), and this effect might contribute to the neurotoxic effects of increased cortisol, further decreasing negative feedback that activates the HPA axis (McEwen et al., 1992). Thus, glutamate likely contributes to the progressive, deleterious neurocognitive effects of chronic stress in patients with depression, anxiety, mania, and psychosis (Mathew, Coplan, Smith et al., 2001). There is developing evidence that various psychotropic drugs might work in part via direct or indirect effects on NMDA receptor systems (Anand et al., 2000).

BRAIN CIRCUITS AND PSYCHOPATHOLOGY

Computed axial tomography (CAT) and magnetic resonance imaging (MRI) scans provide sensitive and noninvasive methods to visualize different brain structures. Studies in patients with mood disorders have found ventricular enlargement, cortical atrophy, sulcal widening, and abnormal lesions (especially the periventricular area, basal ganglia, and thalamus) (Elkis, Friedman, Wise, & Meltzer, 1995; Sheline, 2000; Soares & Mann, 1997; Strakowski et al., 1993). These abnormalities are associated with advanced age, illness severity, symptom chronicity, and increased cortisol levels (Coffey, Wilkinson, Weiner, Ritchie, & Aque, 1993). Mood disorder patients also have brain changes in the hippocampus, amygdala, caudate nucleus, putamen, and prefrontal cortex, which are important structures in the mesocorticolimbic system (Coffey et al., 1993; Krishnan, Hays, & Blazer, 1997). These changes may reflect the neurodegenerative effects of recurrent episodes of depression and mania. Some of these abnormalities are surprisingly similar to the brain changes found in patients with schizophrenia, who typically have decreased gray matter, enlarged ventricles, and abnormalities in the hippocampus, prefrontal cortex, caudate nucleus, thalamus, and corpus callosum (Weinberger, 1995). Studies of patients with different anxiety disorders have found brain changes in the temporal lobes, amygdala, hippocampus, orbitofrontal cortex, caudate nucleus, and thalamus (Talbot, Mathew, & Laruelle, 2003).

In contrast to these studies, which visualize brain structures, other brain imaging technologies are used to visualize and measure brain function (i.e., cerebral blood flow and cerebral metabolism). These technologies include functional magnetic resonance imaging (fMRI), magnetic resonance spectroscopy (MRS), and positron emission tomography (PET) (Whalen et al., 1998). Experimentally provoked emotions (e.g., arousal and sadness) have been shown to increase cerebral blood flow to the thalamus, medial prefrontal cortex, and left amygdala in healthy persons (Lane, Reiman, Ahern, Schwartz, & Davidson, 1997; Liotti et al., 2000;

Mayberg et al., 1997; Mayberg et al., 1999). These studies of healthy persons suggest the potential involvement and relevance of these limbic-cortical regions in pathological states of depression. Indeed, in various studies of depressed patients, functional brain changes have been found in the orbital and medial prefrontal cortex, thalamus, amygdala, hippocampus, and striatum (caudate, putamen, and nucleus accumbens). This work has lead to the development of a model of depression comprised of a limbic-cortical-striatal-pallidal-thalamic neuroanatomic circuit, involving pathological increased activity in the amygdala, decreased hippocampal volume, and abnormal prefrontal cortical function (Drevets, 2000a; Sheline, 2000).

Abnormal and asymmetrical phosphorus metabolism has been found in the frontal lobes of patients with bipolar disorder compared to normal controls (Deicken, Fein, & Weiner, 1995; Kato et al., 1995) and in the left frontal lobe and basal ganglia of patients with unipolar depression (Moore, Christensen, Lafer, Fava, & Renshaw, 1997). Right versus left hemispheric differences in cerebral blood flow or metabolism may distinguish depressed and manic patients, with greater left hemisphere decreases in depression compared to greater right hemisphere changes in mania (Ketter et al., 1994; Mayberg, 1994). Interestingly, decreased cerebral blood flow and glucose metabolism in the prefrontal cortex of patients with unipolar and bipolar depressions is reversed following shifts from depression into mania (Baxter et al., 1985; Ketter et al.; Mayberg, 1994). These findings suggest that neuroanatomic circuits involving dysregulation of frontal lobe functioning are a specific abnormality in mood disorders (George, Ketter, & Post, 1994; Powell & Miklowitz, 1994; Sheline, 2003).

There is developing evidence that antidepressants, lithium, and anticonvulsant drugs may partially normalize some of the functional brain changes in mood disorders (Brody et al., 2001; Drevets, 2000b; Martin, Martin, Rai, Richardson, & Royall, 2001) and also might enhance compensatory neural circuits (Mayberg et al., 2000; Post, Speer, Hough, & Xing, 2003; Sheline et al., 2001). Limbic hypermetabolism is suppressed by effective antidepressant drug therapy, but reemerges when patients are taken off medication (Drevets, 2000b). Bremner et al. (1997) found that tryptophan depletion of recently remitted, antidepressant-treated subjects provoked increased activity in the amygdala. Hence, the amygdala could represent a key juncture in the limbic-cortical-striatal-pallidal-thalamic neuroanatomic emotional circuit that mediates the perception and transduction of stress into mood symptoms and episodes (Sheline, 2003).

The experimental induction of anxiety in normal persons leads to changes in the medial prefrontal cortex, anterior cingulate cortex, orbitofrontal cortex, anterior temporal cortex, parahippocampal gyrus, and amygdala, suggesting the potential relevance of these regions in pathological states of anxiety (Talbot, Mathew, & Laruelle, 2003). Brain imaging studies in pathological anxiety states have suggested some overlap with the brain circuits and neural pathways involved in depression (Talbot et al., 2003), which is consistent with the known clinical and genetic relationship between depression and anxiety (Ninan & Cummins, 2003). For example, in patients with panic disorder, reduced activity has been observed in hippocampal, parahippocampal, and inferior frontal regions of the brain (Gorman, Kent, Sullivan, & Coplan, 2000). In posttraumatic stress disorder, reductions in hippocampal volume are a consistent finding, along with decreased activity of the anterior cingulate gyrus and increased activity in the amygdala (Talbot et al., 2003). Finally, in obsessive-compulsive disorder, there is a highly consistent pattern of increased activity in cortico-striatal-thalamic-cortical cortical circuits involving the orbitofrontal cortex and anterior cortex, with especially important contributions from basal ganglia structures (i.e., caudate, putamen, and nucleus accumbens) (Micallef & Blin, 2001). To some extent, the brain structures and circuits implicated in the pathophysiology of anxiety disorders have also been identified as being an important part of the neurobiological systems involved in learning and conditioning. This finding is relevant to learning theory perspectives on the etiology of anxiety disorders as well as cognitive and behavioral treatment approaches for anxiety disorders (Bouton, Mineka, & Barlow, 2001; Chorpita & Barlow, 1998). For example, conditioning theories suggest that when stimuli (e.g., events or situations) are paired with anxiety (e.g., panic attacks), the learning that may occur can allow the stimuli to trigger anxiety when they are encountered again. Hence, cognitive psychotherapy (which focuses on thoughts and perceptions) and behavioral therapies (which focus on exposure and relaxation) may be effective in the treatment of anxiety disorders because they target these aspects of learning and conditioning. Similar to studies in mood disorders, drug and psychotherapy treatments may partially normalize some of the functional brain changes seen in anxiety disorders (Baxter et al., 2000).

In patients with schizophrenia, functional brain imaging studies have demonstrated profound reductions in prefrontal cortex function, which is correlated clinically with the presence of negative symptoms of psychosis and significant cognitive impairment (Gur, 1995). By contrast, functional changes in the hippocampus, parahippocampal gyrus, amygdala, and temporal cortex (with greater left than right hemispheric dysfunction) have been observed, and these appear to be correlated with the presence of thought disorder, auditory hallucinations, and language disturbances (Gur & Gur, 2000). Finally, some studies suggest dysfunction in the basal ganglia, which have been associated with such clinical symptoms as emotional withdrawal, blunted affect, and psychomotor retardation in schizophrenia (Gur & Gur, 2000).

GENETICS

Family, twin, and adoption studies have clearly shown that mood disorders aggregate within families, but there is some degree of genetic specificity that distinguishes major depression and bipolar disorder (Merikangas & Kupfer, 1995). Moreover, these studies also suggest that bipolar disorder may have a greater genetic liability than major depression, but that nongenetic environmental factors are substantially important in the etiology of mood disorders. Similar family, twin, and adoption studies also have found that anxiety disorders are strongly familial and under genetic control (Hettema, Neale, & Kendler, 2001), but that there is some degree of genetic overlap among some of the anxiety disorders and between depression and anxiety, and that there is a significant nongenetic environmental component as well (Maier, 2003). Family, twin, and adoption studies strongly indicate that schizophrenia aggregates in families and that a substantial proportion of that aggregation results from genetic factors (Bailer et al., 2002; Harrison & Owen, 2003). However, there is some evidence that schizophrenia and major mood disorders may be genetically related, perhaps reflecting a common genetic liability for the development of psychosis, which can occur in schizophrenia, severe depression, and mania (Bailer et al., 2002).

Many twin and adoption studies confirm that hereditary factors influence the development of various personality traits and temperaments, such as those proposed by Eysenck (i.e., neuroticism, psychoticism, and extroversion) or by Cloninger (i.e., novelty seeking, harm avoidance, reward dependence, and persistence) (Aschauer & Schlogelhofer, 2003). The heritability of personality traits is consistent with the idea that biological factors underlie various dimensions of personality (Cloninger, Svrakic, & Przybeck, 1993; Plomin & Caspi, 1998). For example, different personality traits may correspond to the behavioral expression of specific neurotransmitter systems in the brain (e.g., NE, 5-HT, and DA). This theory provides some rationale for the use of psychotropic drugs (e.g., antidepressants and antipsychotics) in the treatment of some personality disorders (Bond, 2001; Aschauer & Schlogelhofer, 2003). For example, serotonergic antidepressant drugs, which are effective in the treatment of various anxiety disorders, are used clinically to treat patients who have anxiety-related personality disorders (e.g., avoidant or obsessive-compulsive personalities) or traits (e.g., neuroticism). Similarly, antipsychotic drugs, which block the effects of dopamine and are used to treat psychotic disorders, are used clinically to treat psychotic-like personality disorders (e.g., paranoid personality). Hereditary and biological factors may help explain the relationship between personality and various psychological disorders. For example, schizotypal personality and schizophrenia may represent two aspects of a psychotic-like spectrum (Berenbaum, Taylor, & Cloninger, 1994). In adoption studies, biological relatives of persons with schizophrenia tend to have a higher prevalence of schizophrenia and schizotypal personality disorder. Therefore, what is genetically transmitted may not be a specific liability for schizophrenia alone, but rather some type of general liability for oddness, poor psychosocial functioning, and/or psychosis. Hereditary and biological factors underlying personality traits also might be a way to understand the concept of vulnerability in the development of psychopathology, such as a genetic phenotype expressing illness or a genetic susceptibility to environmental stress contributing to illness (McGue & Bouchard, 1998). For example, some work has suggested that anxiety and depression are variable expressions of a heritable trait of neuroticism (Eley & Plomin, 1997). Hence, both conditions share the same genetic vulnerability, but the differential alternative expression as anxiety or as depression must be due to distinct nongenetic environmental factors.

The use of various molecular genetics techniques is a very active area of research in psychopathology. For example, a vulnerability to develop early-onset recurrent major depression has been linked to a genetic region containing the CREB gene, which regulates the activity of various gene products related to stress responses (Zubenko et al., 2003). Extensive work also has focused on other plausible candidate genes in mood disorders, such as those related to NE, 5-HT, and DA receptors, transporters, and metabolic enzymes as well as G proteins and other components of second messenger cellular signaling neuronal pathways. Many recent studies have examined genetic polymorphisms of the 5-HT transporter gene, which is involved in the reuptake of 5-HT at brain synapses and is the site of action of serotonin reuptake inhibitor antidepressant drugs (Murphy et al., 2001). These studies have found that certain polymorphisms of the 5-HT transporter gene are associated with neuroticism and negative emotionality (personality traits associated with depression and anxiety). Of particular interest, a recent study found that people with short copies of the 5-HT transporter gene exhibited more depressive symptoms, diagnosable depression, and suicidality in relation to stressful life events than people who had long copies of the gene (Caspi et al., 2003). In other words, a functional polymorphism of the 5-HT transporter gene was found to moderate the influence of environmental stress on depression rather than causing depression. This finding is one example of how genes and environment interact to cause psychopathology. Other studies also have provided evidence of genetic–environmental interactions in depression and anxiety (Cadoret et al., 1996; Silberg, Rutter, Neale, & Eaves, 2001). Developing work has found substantial evidence that genetic–environmental interactions influence the expression of personality traits (Lesch, Greenberg, Higley, Bennett, & Murphy, 2002; Ozkaragoz & Noble, 2000) and that the heritability of many behavioral traits may be greater in permissive than in restrictive environments (Kendler, 2001). Finally, in schizophrenia, recent studies have found an association with the gene for catechol-O-methyltransferase (COMT), which metabolizes neurotransmitters, influences frontal lobe function, and regulates cortical DA activity (Harrison & Owen, 2003), but genetic–environmental interactions are also clearly important in the development of psychosis (Cannon, Kendell, Susser, & Jones, 2003; Van Os, Hanssen, Bak, Bijl, & Vollebergh, 2003).

Various psychopathological states are clearly associated with a wide range of neurobiological disturbances, some overlapping and others more distinct or specific. In addition to obvious vegetative requirements for survival, the biological aspects of CNS function must be rooted in evolutionary processes that resulted in the development of perception, learning, thought, memory, emotions, communication, and language (Gilbert, 1998; Smith, 1993). These functions are critical for interacting with and adapting to the social and physical environment and would necessitate the development of a well-regulated set of CNS responses to environmental stresses. The genetic and biological correlates of what are conceptualized as personality traits and temperaments also must be rooted in evolutionary processes (Bouchard & Loehlin, 2001), perhaps relevant to the development of a behavioral repertoire and an information processing system that mediates interaction with and adaptation to the social and physical environment, analogous to the role of behavioral traits in animals (Gosling, 2001; Weiss, King, & Figuerdo, 2000). Why certain forms of psychopathology persist evolutionarily may partly reflect the adaptive function of underlying traits and temperaments that become maladaptive in response to social, cultural, or environmental stress (Brody, 2001; Haensly & Reynolds, 1993; Leckman & Mayes, 1998; Wilson, 1998). More florid psychopathology may also occur as a result of neurodevelopmental aberrations or the dysregulation of neurobiological systems (Crow, 1995; Stein & Bouwer, 1997). Various forms of psychopathology may then be viewed as the result of unique interactions among genetically determined biological functions and/or behavioral traits, sporadic and/or spontaneous neurobiological anomalies, and environmental stressors or insults, each of which may operate on a particular region of the CNS and/or affect the CNS at a particular time of neurodevelopment. From this perspective, then, the nature–nurture approach to psychopathology is a false dichotomy that should be replaced by a deeper appreciation of the profound and complex dynamical interactions among genes, biology, and the environment (Kendler, 2001; Rose, 2001).

REFERENCES

Anand, A., Charney, D. S., Oren, D. A., Berman, R. M., Hu, X. S., Cappiello, A., & Krystal, J. H. (2000). Attenuation of the neuropsychiatric effects of ketamine with lamotrigine. Support for hyperglutamatergic effects of N-methyl-D-aspartate receptor antagonists. *Archives of General Psychiatry, 57*, 270–276.

Aschauer, H. N., & Schlogelhofer, M. (2003). Anxiety, depression, and personality. In S. Kasper, J. A. den Boer, & J. M. Ad Sitsen (Eds.), *Handbook of Depression and Anxiety* (2nd ed., pp. 91–110). New York: Marcel Dekker.

Aston-Jones, G., Rajkowski, J., & Cohen, J. (1999). Role of locus coeruleus in attention and behavioral flexibility. *Biological Psychiatry, 46*(9), 1309–1320.

Bailer, U., Leisch, F., Meszaros, K., Lenzinger, E., Willinger, U., Strobl, R., Heiden, A., Gebhardt, C., Doge, E., Fuchs, K., Sieghart, W., Kasper, S., Hornik, K., & Aschauer, H. N. (2002). Genome scan for susceptibility loci for schizophrenia and bipolar disorder. *Biological Psychiatry, 52*, 40–52.

Baxter, L. R., Ackermann, R. F., Swendlow, N. R., Brody, A., Saxena, S., Schwartz, J. M., Gregortich, J. M., Stoessel, P., & Phelps, M. E. (2000). Specific brain system mediation of obsessive-compulsive disorder responsive to either medication or behavior therapy. In W. K. Goodman, & M. V. Rudorfer (Eds.), *Obsessive-Compulsive Disorder: Contemporary Issues In Treatment* (pp. 573–609). Mahwah, NJ: Erlbaum Associates.

Baxter, L. R., Phelps, M. E., Mazziotta, J. C., Schwartz, J. M., Gerner, R. H., Selin, C. E., & Sumida, R. M. (1985). Cerebral metabolic rates for glucose in mood disorders: Studies with positron emission tomography and fluorodeoxygulcose F18. *Archives of General Psychiatry, 42*, 441–447.

Belanoff, J. K., Gross, K., Yager, A., & Schatzberg, A. F. (2001). Corticosteroids and cognition. *Journal of Psychiatric Research, 35*, 127–145.

Berenbaum, S. A., Taylor, M. A., & Cloninger, C. R. (1994). Family study of schizophrenia and personality. *Journal of Abnormal Psychiatry, 103*(3), 475–484.

Bond, A. J. (2001). Neurotransmitters, temperament and social functioning. *European Neuropsychopharmacology, 11*, 261–274.

Bouchard, T. J., & Loehlin, J. C. (2001). Genes, evolution, and personality. *Behavior Genetics, 31*(3), 243–273.

Bouton, M. E., Mineka, S., & Barlow, D. H. (2001). A modern learning theory perspective on the etiology of panic disorder. *Psychological Review, 108*(1), 4–32.

Bremner, J. D. (1999). Does stress damage the brain? *Biological Psychiatry, 45*(7), 797–805.

Bremner, J. D., Innis, R. B., Salomon, R. M., Staib, L. H., Ng, C. K., Miller, H. L., Bronen, R. A., Krystal, J. H., Duncan, J., Rich, D., Price, L. H., Malison, R., Dey, H., Soufer, R., & Charney, D. S. (1997). Positron emission tomography measurement of cerebral metabolic correlates of tryptophan depletion-induced depressive relapse. *Archives of General Psychiatry, 54,* 364–374.

Brody, J. F. (2001). Evolutionary recasting: ADHD, mania and its variants. *Journal of Affective Disorders, 65,* 197–215.

Brody, A. L., Saxena, S., Stoessel, P., Gillies, L. A., Fairbanks, L. A., Alborzian, S., Phelps, M. E., Huang, S. C., Wu, H. M., Ho, M. L., Ho, M. K., Au, S. C., Maidment, K., & Baxter, J. R., Jr. (2001). Regional brain metabolic changes in patients with major depression treated with either paroxetine or interpersonal therapy: Preliminary findings. *Archives of General Psychiatry, 58,* 631–640.

Buck, R. (1999). The biological affects: A typology. *Psychological Review, 106*(2), 301–336.

Bunney, W. E., & Bunney, B. G. (2000). Molecular clock genes in man and lower animals: Possible implications for circadian abnormalities in depression. *Neurospychopharmacology, 22*(4), 335–345.

Bunney, W. E. J., Goodwin, F. K., Murphy, D. L., House, K. M., & Gordon, E. K. (1972). The "switch process" in manic-depressive illness: II: Relationship to catecholamines, REM sleep, and drugs. *Archives of General Psychiatry, 27,* 304–309.

Cadoret, R. J., Winokur, G., Langbehn, D., Troughton, E., Yates, W. R., & Stewart, M. A. (1996). Depression spectrum disease, I: The role of gene-environment interaction. *American Journal of Psychiatry, 153*(7), 892–899.

Cannon, M., Kendell, R., Susser, E., & Jones, P. (2003). Prenatal and perinatal risk factors for schizophrenia. In R. M. Murray & P. B. Jones (Eds.), *The Epidemiology of Schizophrenia* (pp. 74–99). New York: Cambridge University Press.

Caspi, A., Sugden, K., Moffitt, T. E., Taylor, A., Craig, I. W., Harrington, H., McClay, J., Mill, J., Martin, J., Braithwaite, A., & Poulton, R. (2003). Influence of life stress on depression: Moderation by a polymorphism in the 5–HTT gene. *Science, 301,* 386–389.

Chorpita, B. F., Barlow, D. H. (1998). The development of anxiety: The role of control in the early environment. *Psychological Bulletin, 124*(1), 3–21.

Chouinard, G., Young, S. N., Bradwejn, J., & Annable, L. (1983). Tryptophan in the treatment of depression and mania. *Advanced Biological Psychiatry, 10,* 47–66.

Cloninger, C. R. (1999). A new conceptual paradigm from genetics and psychobiology for the science of mental health. *Australian New Zealand Journal of Psychiatry, 33*(2), 174–186.

Cloninger, C. R., Svrakic, D. M., & Przybeck, T. R. (1993). A psychobiological model of temperament and character. *Archives of General Psychiatry, 50*(12), 975–990.

Coffey, C. E., Wilkinson, W. E., Weiner, R. D., Ritchie, J. C., & Aque, M. (1993). The dexamethasone suppression test and quantitative cerebral anatomy in depression. *Biological Psychiatry, 33,* 442–449.

Cookson, J. C. (1985). The neuroendocrinology of mania. *Journal of Affective Disorders, 8,* 233–241.

Cooper, B. (2001). Nature, nurture and mental disorder: Old concepts in the new millennium. *British Journal of Psychiatry, 178*(Suppl. 40), s91–s102.

Coplan, J. D., Smith, E. L. P., Altemus, M., Scharf, B. A., Owens, M. J., Nemeroff, C. B., Gorman, J. M., & Rosenblum, L. A. (2001). Variable foraging demand rearing: Sustained elevations in cisternal cerebrospinal fluid corticotropin-releasing factor concentrations in adult primates. *Biological Psychiatry, 50*(3), 200–204.

Crow, T. J. (1995). A Darwinian approach to the origins of psychosis. *British Journal of Psychiatry, 167*(1), 12–25.

Cuadra, G., Zurita, A., Gioino, G., & Molina, V. (2001). Influence of different antidepressant drugs on the effect of chronic variable stress on restraint-induced dopamine release in frontal cortex. *Neuropsychopharmacology, 25*(3), 384–394.

Deicken, R. F., Fein, G., & Weiner, M. W. (1995). Abnormal frontal lobe phosphorous metabolism in bipolar disorder. *American Journal of Psychiatry, 152*(6), 915–918.

Delgado, P. L., & Moreno, F. A. (1998). Different roles for serotonin in anti-obsessional drug action and pathophysiology of obsessive-compulsive disorder. *British Journal of Psychiatry, 173*(Suppl. 35S), 21–25.

Denenberg, V. H. (2000). Evolution proposes and ontogeny disposes. *Brain & Language, 73*(2), 274–296.

Depue, R. A., & Iacono, W. G. (1989). Neurobehavioral aspects of affective disorders. *Annual Review of Psychology, 40,* 457–492.

Drevets, W. C. (2000a). Neuroimaging studies of mood disorders. *Biological Psychiatry, 48,* 813–829.

Drevets, W. C. (2000b). Functional anatomical abnormalities in limbic and prefrontal cortical structures in major depression. *Progress in Brain Research, 126,* 413–431.

Drevets, W. C., Frank, E., Price, J. C., Kupfer, D. J., Holt, D., Greer, P. J., Huang, Y., Gautier, C., & Mathis, C. (1999). PET imaging of serotonin 1A receptor binding in depression. *Biological Psychiatry, 46*(10), 1375–1387.

Duman, R. S., Malberg, J., & Thome, J. (1999). Neural plasticity to stress and antidepressant treatment. *Biological Psychiatry, 46,* 1181–1191.

Duman, S., Heninger, G. R., & Nestler, E. J. (1997). A molecular and cellular theory of depression. *Archives of General Psychiatry, 54,* 597–606.

Duncan, W. C., Jr. (1996). Circadian rhythms and the pharmacology of affective illness. *Pharmacology Therapy*, *71*(3), 253–312.

Eley, T. C., & Plomin, R. (1997). Genetic analyses of emotionality. *Current Opinion In Neurobiology*, *7*, 279–284.

Elkis, H., Friedman, L., Wise, A., & Meltzer, H. Y. (1995). Meta-analyses of studies of ventricular enlargement and cortical sulcal prominence in mood disorders. Comparisons with controls or patients with schizophrenia. *Archives of General Psychiatry*, *52*, 735–746.

Fairbanks, L. A., Melega, W. P., Jorgensen, M. J., Kaplan, J. R., & Mcguire, M. T. (2001). Social impulsivity inversely associated with CSF 5-HIAA and fluoxetine exposure in vervet monkeys. *Neuropsychopharmacology*, *24*(4), 370–378.

Ferry, B., Roozendaal, B., & McGaugh, J. L. (1999). Role of norepinephrine in mediating stress hormone regulation of long-term memory storage: A critical involvement of the amygdala. *Biological Psychiatry*, *46*(9), 1140–1152.

George, M. S., Ketter, T. A., & Post, R. M. (1994). Prefrontal cortex dysfunction in clinical depression. *Depression*, *2*, 59–72.

Geracioti, T. D., Loosen, P. T., & Orth, D. N. (1997). Low cerebrospinal fluid corticotropin-releasing hormone concentrations in eucortisolemic depression. *Biological Psychiatry*, *42*, 166–174.

Gilbert, P. (1998). Evolutionary psychopathology: Why isn't the mind designed better than it is? *British Journal of Medical Psychology*, *71*(4), 353–373.

Gorman, J. M., Kent, J. M., Sullivan, G. M., & Coplan, J. D. (2000). Neuroanatomical hypothesis of panic disorder, revised. *American Journal of Psychiatry*, *157*(4), 493–505.

Gosling, S. D. (2001). From mice to men: What can we learn about personality from animal research? *Psychological Bulletin*, *127*(1), 45–86.

Gur, R. (1995). Functional brain-imaging studies in schizophrenia. In F. E. Bloom & D. J. Kupfer (Eds.), *Psychopharmacology: The fourth generation of progress* (pp. 1185–1192). New York: Raven.

Gur, R. E., & Gur, R. C. (2000). Schizophrenia: Brain structure and function. In B. J. Sadock and V. A. Sadock (Eds.), *Comprehensive Textbook of Psychiatry* (7th ed., pp. 1117–1129). Philadelphia, PA: Lippincott Williams and Wilkins.

Guze, S. B. (1989). Biological psychiatry: Is there any other kind? *Psychological Medicine*, *19*(2), 315–323.

Haensly, P. A., & Reynolds, C. R. (1993). Whither goes DNA—an intelligent creative process? Or, creativity emanating from psychotic traits? *Psychological Inquiry*, *4*(3), 200–204.

Harrison, P. J., & Owen, M. J. (2003). Genes for schizophrenia? Recent findings and their pathophysiological implications. *Lancet*, *361*, 417–419.

Hettema, J. M., Neale, M. C., & Kendler, K. S. (2001). A review and meta-analysis of the genetic epidemiology of anxiety disorders. *American Journal of Psychiatry*, *158*(10), 1568–1578.

Higley, J. D., Mehlman, P. T., Higley, S. B., Fernald, B., Vickers, J., Lindell, S. G., Taub, D. M., Suomi, S. J., & Linnoila, M. (1996). Excessive mortality in young free-ranging male nonhuman primates with low cerebrospinal fluid 5-hydroxyindoleacetic acid concentrations. *Archives of General Psychiatry*, *53*, 537–543.

Higley, J. D., Mehlman, P. T., Poland, R. E., Taub, D. M., Vickers, J., Suomi, S. J., & Linnoila, M. (1996). CSF testosterone and 5-HIAA correlate with different types of aggressive behaviors. *Biological Psychiatry*, *40*(11), 1067–1082.

Holsboer, F. (1995). Neuroendocrinology of mood disorders. In F. E. Bloom & D. J. Kupfer (Eds.), *Psychopharmacology: The fourth generation of progress* (pp. 957–969). New York: Raven.

Holsboer, F. (2000). The corticosteroid receptor hypothesis of depression. *Neuropsychopharmacology*, *23*(5), 477–501.

Howland, R. H., & Thase, M. E. (1999). Affective disorders. Biological aspects. In T. Millon, P. Blaney, & R. Davis (Eds.), *Oxford textbook of psychopathology* (pp. 166–202). Oxford: Oxford University Press.

Insel, T. R., & Winslow, J. T. (1998). Serotonin and neuropeptides in affiliative behaviors. *Biological Psychiatry*, *44*(3), 207–219.

Kahn, R. S., & Davis, K. L. (1995). New developments in dopamine and schizophrenia. In F. E. Bloom & D. J. Kupfer (Eds.), *Psychopharmacology: The fourth generation of progress* (pp. 1193–1203). New York: Raven.

Kandel, E. R., Schwartz, J. H., & Jessell, T. M. (1991). *Principles of neural science* (3rd ed.). New York: Elsevier.

Kato, T., Shioiri, T., Murashita, J., Hamakawa, H., Takahashi, Y., Inubushi, T., & Takahashi, S. (1995). Lateralized abnormality of high energy phosphate metabolism in the frontal lobes of patients with bipolar disorder detected by phase-encoded ^{31}P-MRS. *Psychological Medicine*, *25*, 557–566.

Kaufman, J., Plotsky, P. M., Nemeroff, C. B., & Charney, D. S. (2000). Effects of early adverse experiences on brain structure and function: Clinical implications. *Biological Psychiatry*, *48*, 778–790.

Kendler, K. S. (2001). Twin studies of psychiatric illness: An update. *Archives of General Psychiatry*, *58*, 1005–1014.

Ketter, T. A., George, M. S., Ring, H. A., Pazzaglia, P., Marangell, L., Kimbrell, T. A., & Post, R. M. (1994). Primary mood disorders: Structural and resting functional studies. *Psychiatric Annals*, *24*(12), 637–642.

Kingsley, R. E. (2000). *Concise text of neuroscience* (2nd ed.). Philadelphia: Lippincott Williams & Wilkins.

Krishnan, K. R. R., Hays, J. C., & Blazer, D. G. (1997). MRI-Defined vascular depression. *American Journal of Psychiatry*, *154*(4), 497–501.

Lane, R. D., Reiman, E. M., Ahern, G. L., Schwartz, G. E., & Davidson, R. J. (1997). Neuroanatomical correlates of happiness, sadness, and disgust. *American Journal of Psychiatry*, *154*(7), 926–933.

Leckman, J. F., & Mayes, L. C. (1998). Understanding developmental psychopathology: How useful are evolutionary accounts? *Journal of the American Academy of Child Adolescent Psychiatry*, *37*(10), 1011–1021.

Lesch, K. P., Greenberg, B. D., Higley, J. D., Bennett, A., & Murphy, D. L. (2002). Serotonin transporter, personality, and behavior: Toward a dissection of gene-gene and gene-environment interaction. In J. Benjamin & R. P. Ebstein (Eds.), *Molecular Genetics and the Human Personality* (pp. 109–135). Washington, DC: American Psychiatric Publishing.

Linkowski, P., Kerhofs, M., Van Onderbergen, A., Hubain, P., Copinschi, G., L'Hermite-Baleriaux. M., Leclercq, R., Brasseur, M., Mendlewicz, J., & Van cauter, E. (1994). The 24-hour profiles of Cortisol, prolactin, and growth hormone secretion in mania. *Archives of General Psychiatry*, *51*, 616–624.

Liotti, M., Mayberg, H. S., Brannan, S. K., McGinnis, S., Jerabek, P., & Fox, P. T. (2000). Differential limbic-cortical correlates of sadness and anxiety in healthy subjects: Implications for affective disorders. *Biological Psychiatry*, *48*, 30–42.

López, J. F., Liberzon, I., Vázquez, D. M., Young, E. A., & Watson, S. J. (1999). Serotonin 1A receptor messenger RNA regulation in the hippocampus after acute stress. *Biological Psychiatry*, *45*(7), 934–937.

Maes, M., & Meltzer, H. Y. (1995). The serotonin hypothesis of major depression. In F. E. Bloom & D. J. Kupfer (Eds.), *Psychopharmacology: The fourth generation of progress* (pp. 933–944). New York: Raven.

Maier, S. F., & Seligman, M. E. P. (1976). Learned helplessness: Theory and evidence. *Journal of Experimental Psychology*, *105*, 3–46.

Maier, W. (2003). Genetics of anxiety. In S. Kasper, J. A. den Boer, J. M. Ad Sitsen (Eds.), *Handbook of Depression and Anxiety* (2nd ed., pp. 189–205). New York: Marcel Dekker.

Manji, H. K., Moore, G. J., & Chen, G. (2000). Clinical and preclinical evidence for the neurotrophic effects of mood stabilizers: Implications for the pathophysiology and treatment of manic-depressive illness. *Biological Psychiatry*, *48*, 740–754.

Mann, J. J., Brent, D. A., & Arango, V. (2001). The neurobiology and genetics of suicide and attempted suicide: A focus on the serotonergic system. *Neuropsychopharmacology*, *24*(5), 467–477.

Martin, S. D., Martin, E., Rai, S. S., Richardson, M. A., & Royall, R. (2001). Brain blood flow changes in depressed patients treated with interpersonal psychotherapy or venlafaxine hydrochloride. Preliminary findings. *Archives of General Psychiatry*, *58*, 641–648.

Mathew, S. J., Coplan, J. D., Gorman, J. M. (2001). Neurobiological mechanisms of social anxiety disorder. *American Journal of Psychiatry*, *158*(10), 1558–1567.

Mathew, S. J., Coplan, J. D., Smith, E. L. P., Schloepp, D. D., Rosenblum, L. A., & Gorman, J. M. (2001). Glutamate-hypothalamic-pituitary-adrenal axis interactions: Implications for mood and anxiety disorders. *CNS Spectrums*, *6*(7), 555–564.

Mayberg, H. S. (1994). Functional imaging studies in secondary depression. *Psychiatric Annals*, *24*, 643–647.

Mayberg, H. S., Brannan, S. K., Mahurin, R. K., Jerabek, P. A., Brickman, J. S., Tekell, J. L., Silva, J. A., McGinnis, S., Glass, T. G., Martin, C. C., & Fox, P. T. (1997). Cingulate function in depression: A potential predictor of treatment response. *Clinical Neuroscience and Neuropathology*, *8*(4), 1057–1061.

Mayberg, H. S., Brannan, S. K., Tekell, J. L., Silva, J. A., Mahurin, R. K., McGinnis, S., & Jerabek, P. A. (2000). Regional metabolic effects of fluoxetine in major depression: Serial changes and relationship to clinical response. *Biological Psychiatry*, *48*(8), 830–843.

Mayberg, H. S., Liotti, M., Brannan, S. K., McGinnis, S., Mahurin, R. K., Jerabek, P. A., Silva, J. A., Tekell, J. L., Martin, C. C., Lancaster, J. L., & Fox, P. T. (1999). Reciprocal limbic-cortical function and negative mood: Converging PET findings in depression and normal sadness. *American Journal of Psychiatry*, *156*(5), 675–682.

McEwen, B. S. (2000). Effects of adverse experiences for brain structure and function. *Biological Psychiatry*, *48*, 721–731.

McEwen, B. S., Angulo, J., Cameron, H., Chao, H. M., Daniels, D., Gannon, M. N., Gould, E., Mendelson, S., Sakai, R., Spencer, R., & Woolley, C. (1992). Paradoxical effects of adrenal steroids on the brain: Protection versus degeneration. *Biological Psychiatry*, *31*, 177–199.

McGue, M., & Bouchard, T. J. (1998). Genetic and environmental influences on human behavioral differences. *Annual Review of Neuroscience*, *21*, 1–24.

Mehlman, P. T., Higley, J. D., Faucher, I., Lilly, A. A., Taub, D. M., Vickers, J., Suomi, S. J., & Linnoila, M. (1995). Correlation of CSF 5-HIAA concentration with sociality and the timing of emigration in free-ranging primates. *American Journal of Psychiatry*, *152*(6), 907–913.

Merikangas, K. R., & Kupfer, D. J. (1995). Mood disorders: genetic aspects. In H. I. Kaplan & B. J. Sadock (Eds.), *Comprehensive Textbook of Psychiatry* (6th ed., pp. 1102–1116). Baltimore: Walkins.

Micallef, J., & Blin, O. (2001). Neurobiology and clinical pharmacology of obsessive-compulsive disorder. *Clinical Neuropharmacology, 24*(4), 191–207.

Moore, C. M., Christensen, J. D., Lafer, B., Fava, M., & Renshaw, P. F. (1997). Lower levels of nucleoside triphosphate in the basal ganglia of depressed subjects: A phosphorous-31 magnetic resonance spectroscopy study. *American Journal of Psychiatry, 154*, 116–118.

Murphy, D. L., Li, Q., Engel, S., Wichems, C., Andrews, A., Lesch, K. P., & Uhl, G. (2001). Genetic perspectives on the serotonin transporter. *Brain Research Bulletin, 56*(5), 487–494.

Nemeroff, C. B. (1998). Psychopharmacology of affective disorders in the 21st century. *Biological Psychiatry, 44*(7), 517–525.

Nestler, E. J., Alreja, M., & Aghajanian, G. K. (1999). Molecular control of locus coeruleus neurotransmission. *Biological Psychiatry, 46*(9), 1131–1139.

Ninan, P. T., & Cummins, T. K. (2003). Neurobiology of anxiety and depression. In S. Kasper, J. A. den Boer, & J. M. Ad Sitsen (Eds.), *Handbook of Depression and Anxiety* (2nd ed., pp. 331–347), New York: Marcel Dekker.

Ozkaragoz, T., & Noble, E. P. (2000). Extraversion: Interaction between D2 dopamine receptor polymorphisms and parental alcoholism. *Alcohol, 22*(3), 139–146.

Paul, S. M. (1995). GABA and glycine. In F. E. Bloom & D. J. Kupfer (Eds.), *Psychopharmacology: The fourth generation of progress* (pp. 87–94). New York: Raven.

Pearlson, G. D., Wong, D. F., Tune, L. E., Ross, C. A., Chase, G. A., Links, J. M., Dannals, R. F., Wilson, A. A., Ravert, H. T., & Wagher, H. N., & DePaulo, R. (1995). In Vivo D2 dopamine receptor density in psychotic and nonpsychotic patients with bipolar disorder. *Archives of General Psychiatry, 52*, 471–477.

Plomin, R., & Caspi, A. (1998). DNA and personality. *European Journal of Personality, 12*, 387–407.

Post, R. M., Speer, A. M., Hough, C. J., & Xing, G. (2003). Neurobiology of bipolar illness: Implications for future study and therapeutics. *Annals of Clinical Psychiatry, 15*(2), 85–94.

Powell, K. B., & Miklowitz, D. J. (1994). Frontal lobe dysfunction in the affective disorders. *Clinical Psychology Review, 14*, 525–546.

Quintin, P., Benkelfat, C., Launay, J. M., Arnulf, I., Pointereau-Bellenger, A., Barbault, S., Alvarez, J. C., Varoquaux, O., Perez-Diaz, F., Jouvent, R., & Leboyer, M. (2001). Clinical and neurochemical effect of acute tryptophan depletion in unaffected relatives of patients with bipolar affective disorder. *Biological Psychiatry, 50*(3), 184–190.

Ressler, K. J., & Nemeroff, C. B. (1999). Role of norepinephrine in the pathophysiology and treatment of mood disorders. *Biological Psychiatry, 46*(9), 1219–1233.

Rose, S. (2001). Moving on from old dichotomies: Beyond nature-nurture towards a lifeline perspective. *British Journal of Psychiatry, 178*(Suppl. 40), s3–s7.

Roth, B. L., & Meltzer, H. Y. (1995). The role of serotonin in schizophrenia. In F. E. Bloom & D. J. Kupfer (Eds.), *Psychopharmacology: The fourth generation of progress* (pp. 1215–1227). New York: Raven.

Sapolsky, R. M. (2000). The possibility of neurotoxicity in the hippocampus in major depression: A primer on neuron death. *Biological Psychiatry, 48*, 755–765.

Sasaki-Adams, D. M., & Kelley, A. E. (2001). Serotonin-dopamine interactions in the control of conditioned reinforcement and motor behavior. *Neuropsychopharmacology, 25*(3), 440–452.

Schatzberg, A. F., & Rothschild, A. J. (1992). Psychotic (delusional) major depression: Should it be included as a distinct syndrome in DSM-IV? *American Journal of Psychiatry, 149*(6), 733–745.

Schatzberg, A. F., Rothschild, A. J., Langlais, P. J., Bird, E. D., & Cole, J. O. (1985). A corticosteroid/dopamine hypothesis for psychotic depression and related states. *Journal of Psychiatry Research, 19*, 57–64.

Schatzberg, A. F., & Schildkraut, J. J. (1995). Recent studies on norepinephrine systems in mood disorders. In F. E. Bloom & D. J. Kupfer (Eds.), *Psychopharmacology: The fourth generation of progress* (pp. 911–920). New York: Raven.

Schmider, J., Lammers, C. H., Gotthardt, U., Dettling, M., Holsboer, F., & Heuser, J. E., (1995). Combined dexamethasone/corticotropin-releasing hormone test in acute and remitted manic patients, in acute depression, and in normal controls: 1. *Biological Psychiatry, 38*, 797–802.

Sheline, Y. I. (2000). 3D MRI studies of neuroanatomic changes in unipolar major depression: The role of stress and medical comorbidity. *Biological Psychiatry, 48*(8), 793–800.

Sheline, Y. I. (2003). Neuroimaging studies of mood disorder effects on the brain. *Biological Psychiatry, 54*, 338–352.

Sheline, Y. I., Barch, D. M., Donnelly, J. M., Ollinger, J. M., Snyder, A. Z., & Mintun, M. A. (2001). Increased amygdala response to masked emotional faces in depressed subjects resolves with antidepressant treatment: An fMRI study. *Biological Psychiatry, 50*(9), 651–658.

Shelton, R. C. (2000). Cellular mechanisms in the vulnerability to depression and response to antidepressants. *Psychiatric Clinics of North America, 23*, 713–729.

Silberg, J., Rutter, M., Neale, M., & Eaves, L. (2001). Genetic moderation of environmental risk for depression and anxiety in adolescent girls. *British Journal of Psychiatry, 179*, 116–121.

Smith, C. U. (1993). Evolutionary biology and psychiatry. *British Journal of Psychiatry, 162*, 149–153.

Soares, J. C., & Mann, J. J. (1997). The anatomy of mood disorders-review of structural neuroimaging studies. *Biological Psychiatry, 41*(1), 86–106.

Staley, J. K., Malison, R. T., & Innis, R. B. (1998). Imaging of the serotonergic system: Interactions of neuroanatomical and functional abnormalities of depression. *Biological Psychiatry, 44*(7), 534–549.

Stein D. J., & Bouwer, C. (1997). A neuro-evolutionary approach to the anxiety disorders. *Journal of Anxiety Disorders, 11*(4), 409–429.

Strakowski, S. M., Wilson, D. R., Tohen, M, Woods, B. T., Douglass, A. W., & Stoll, A. L. (1993). Structural brain abnormalities in first-episode mania. *Biological Psychiatry, 33*, 602–609.

Swerdlow, N. R., & Koob, G. F. (1987). Dopamine, schizophrenia, mania, and depression: Toward a unified hypothesis of cortico-straito-pallido-thalamic function. *Behavioral and Brain Sciences, 10*, 197–245.

Talbot, P. S., Mathew, S. J., & Laruelle, M. (2003). Brain imaging in depression and anxiety. In S. Kasper, J. A. den Boer, & J. M. Ad Sitsen (Eds.), *Handbook of Depression and Anxiety* (2nd ed., pp. 289–329), New York, Marcel Dekker.

Van Os, J., Hanssen, M., Bak, M., Bijl, R. V., & Vollebergh, W. (2003). Do urbanicity and familial liability coparticipate in causing psychosis? *American Journal of Psychiatry, 160*, 477–482.

Weinberger, D. R. (1995). Neurodevelopmental perspectives on schizophrenia. In F. E. Bloom & D. J. Kupfer (Eds.), *Psychopharmacology: The fourth generation of progress* (pp. 1171–1183). New York: Raven.

Weiss, A., King, J. E., & Figuerdo, A. J. (2000). The heritability of personality factors in chimpanzees (Pan troglodytes) (2000). *Behavior Genetics, 30*(3), 213–221.

Weiss, J. M., & Kilts, C. D. (1998). Animal models of depression and schizophrenia. In A. F. Schatzberg & C. B. Nemeroff (Eds.), *Textbook of Psychopharmacology* (2nd ed., pp. 89–131). Washington, DC: American Psychiatric Press.

Whalen, P. J., Rauch, S. L., Etcoff, N. L., McInerney, S. C., Lee, M. B., & Jenike, M. A. (1998). Masked presentations of emotional facial expressions modulate amygdala activity without explicit knowledge. *Journal of Neuroscience, 18*(1), 411–418.

Willner, P. (1997). The mesolimbic dopamine system as a target for rapid antidepressant action. *International Clinical Psychopharmacology, 12*(Suppl. 3), S7–S14.

Willner, P. (1995). Dopaminergic mechanisms in depression and mania. In F. E. Bloom & D. J. Kupfer (Eds.), *Psychopharmacology: The fourth generation of progress* (pp. 921–931). New York: Raven.

Wilson, D. R. (1998). Evolutionary epidemiology and manic depression. *British Journal of Medical Psychology, 71*(4), 375–395.

Zubenko, G. S., Maher, B., Hughes, H. B., Zubenko, W. N., Stiffler, J. S., Kaplan, B. B., & Marazita, M. L. (2003). Genome-wide linkage survey for genetic loci that influence the development of depressive disorders in families with recurrent, early-onset, major depression. *American of Journal of Medical Genetics Part B (Neuropsychiatric Genetics), 123B*, 1–18.

II

COMMON ADULT, ADOLESCENT, AND CHILD DISORDERS

Anxiety Disorders

S. Lloyd Williams
Stuttgart, Germany

People are anxious about many different things, and to many different degrees, but nearly everyone knows about anxiety from firsthand experience. We speak about ourselves and others using a vocabulary rich with words about feeling anxious, tense, nervous, afraid, worried, scared, and the like. We use such terms not only to describe feelings, but to explain behaviors. We say that someone did (or did not do) something because she was afraid or because he was nervous. Scientists too have held that fear and anxiety (terms this paper will treat as synonyms) cause many behaviors, normal and abnormal, adaptive and maladaptive. This anxiety theory of behavior is widely accepted by those who help people with psychological problems. But the meaning of anxiety, and its power to strongly influence behavior, are far from clear.

THE CONCEPT OF ANXIETY DISORDER

Anxiety also denotes sets of proposed mental illnesses called *anxiety disorders*, as in the title of this chapter. The theory that some psychological problems are anxiety disorders, or are caused by anxiety disorders, derives from the medical model that views people's psychological problems as psychopathology, symptoms, psychiatric syndromes, mental illnesses, mental disorders, and related disease-like conditions. Anxiety disorder theory is embodied in detail in leading psychiatric organizations' official manuals of mental disorders (American Psychiatric Association, 1994, DSM–IV; 1980, DSM–III; 1987, DSM–III–R; World Health Organization, 1992, ICD–10). From the author's social cognitive perspective (Williams & Cervone, 1998; cf. Bandura, 1969, 1978, 1986), mental disorders, including anxiety disorders, do not exist. Rather, psychological problems exist. Psychological problems differ from mental disorders in fundamental ways that greatly affect how we study problems and help people solve them.

This chapter will focus on a number of problem dimensions, including maladaptive avoidance behavior and compulsive rituals, subjective feelings of fear and panic, disturbing thoughts, and autonomic hyperarousal. These are compelling psychological realities, problems in their own right, whereas anxiety disorders are abstractions devised by committees. The elusive relationship between mental disorders and psychological response dimensions is evident in the way DSM-IV and ICD-10 call problem responses *symptoms* of disorder, but do not explain how a response can define a disorder yet be a symptom of the disorder at the same time. Abstract disorders concretely influence research on avoidance and fear, including the selection of participants, the measurement of their problems, and the choice of experimental and correlational (i.e., independent) variables and treatment interventions. These practices have many negative implications because anxiety disorders do not correspond closely to psychological reality.

Disorders Distort Psychological Reality

Mental illness/disorder as a scientific concept distorts our view of psychological responses in many ways, a few of which I will convey here so readers will know why the chapter does not run through the usual proposed anxiety disorders, but presents instead a psychological view of problems that rejects the concept of mental disorder altogether (see Williams, in preparation, for a fuller exposition).

No Cohesive Distinctive Anxiety Disorder Grouping Exists

The term anxiety disorders implies falsely that the diverse problems so labeled actually belong together in a special distinctive way. In reality, no such cohesive distinctive grouping exists, as we will see in considering the related issue of construct validity of anxiety disorder. The burden of proof lies heavily on advocates of anxiety disorder theory. Avoidant and compulsive behaviors, frightened feelings, disturbing thoughts, physiological hyperarousal, and all the other responses employed to define anxiety disorders occur widely in psychological life, far beyond the narrow confines of proposed anxiety disorders. The concept of anxiety disorder thus captures remarkably little of the psychological phenomena with which it concerns itself. And far from showing orderly clustering of their problems, people said to have a given anxiety disorder tend to show idiosyncratic combinations of problems and as a group are highly heterogeneous with respect to the actual individual problems they display. Indeed, having almost any problem greatly increases the likelihood of having almost any other problem (Boyd et al., 1987), which directly challenges the medical model's ideal of distinct neat clusterings of particular responses in disorders, and of these disorders into groupings such as anxiety disorders.

"Anxiety Disorder" Is Formally Invalid

The anxiety disorder concept formally lacks construct validity, as it lacks both convergent validity and discriminant validity (Campbell & Fiske, 1959) because the diverse alleged anxiety disorder problem dimensions/responses tend to be only modestly correlated with one another (Lang, 1985; Rachman, 1976), and yet can be highly correlated with allegedly distinct phenomena such as depressed mood and other problems (Clark, Watson, & Reynolds, 1995). This chapter will return to the problem of construct validity again after it discusses in more detail the meaning of anxiety in later sections. Note that unidimensional, unitary constructs, such as current anxiety as rated on a simple intensity scale (Walk, 1956), are not burdened with construct validation requirements. But multidimensional constructs that lack construct validity suffer from a fatal flaw that we ignore at our scientific and therapeutic peril.

Human Problems Are Dimensional, Not Dichotomous

Psychological problems such as avoidance, fear, and intrusive thinking are plainly dimensional and graduated, not dichotomous. Each varies in intensity and frequency in degrees, from being little or no problem to being a severely distressing and/or incapacitating problem, with many importantly different levels of problem intensity in between. In contrast, an anxiety disorder is all or none: a person either has it or does not have it. Diagnosing anxiety disorder thus means gathering dimensional information (e.g., number of panicky sensations, amount of time spent in avoidance rituals, extent of phobic disability, etc.), then giving up that information in exchange for a dichotomous illness judgment: disordered or not disordered. This is a very bad trade. Transforming a graduated dimensional variable into a dichotomous category is "willful discarding of information. It has been shown that when you so mutilate a variable, you typically reduce its squared correlation with behavior about 36% (Cohen, 1983). Don't do it" (Cohen, 1990, p. 1307). The social cognitive view sees psychological continuity between problem and nonproblem responses (Bandura, 1978, 1986; Williams & Cervone, 1998), holding that the same kinds of psychobiological factors influence both. This fundamental continuity leaves no role for mental disorders in the explanation of behavior.

"Disorder" Excludes Real Problems

Many problems of avoidance, rituals, fear, and bothersome scary thoughts, both mild and severe, are systematically excluded from the scope of mental disorders either outright or by placement in a nonspecific disorder category (e.g., Bienvenu, Nestadt, & Eaton, 1998; Marshall, Olfson, Hellman, Blanco, Guardino, & Struening, 2001), either way denying people the alleged benefits of the disorder-based explanatory scheme. Some call the problems excluded from disorderhood "subthreshold disorders," a delightfully nonsensical term that seems to mean disorders that are not disorders. Subthreshold whatever-they-ares result in part from arbitrarily high and otherwise psychologically questionable cutoff scores that define disorder. For example, to count an anxiety attack as a panic attack for diagnosing panic disorder, DSM–IV requires that some attacks be accompanied by at least four responses from a longer list, although an attack with only one or two such responses (for example, a smothering sensation and a feeling of imminent death) can be intense and have serious psychological sequelae (Katerndahl & Realini, 1993; Margraf, Taylor, Ehlers, Roth, & Agras, 1987). The psychological dimensional approach measures problems across their full intensity range, from none to extreme, without any cutoffs or exclusion rules arbitrarily fixed in advance.

Disorders Are Disconnected From Responses

At the heart of the distorting effects of mental disorder is that a disorder is disconnected from the underlying psychological responses it consists of. The difficulty is less when a mental disorder is based on a single underlying psychological dimension, but an anxiety disorder usually is constructed of multiple dissimilar problem dimensions simultaneously, and these dimensions can be little correlated with one another. Because only some of the problems need be present for a positive diagnosis, saying someone has a certain anxiety disorder can convey little definite information about his or her actual problems. Consider the discrepancies between panic *attack* (the psychological phenomenon/dimension/response) and panic *disorder* (the proposed mental illness), and between agoraphobic *avoidance* (the response) and agoraphobic *disorder* (the proposed illness). Briefly, a panic attack is a sudden surge of intense fear, and agoraphobic avoidance is avoidance of certain activities/settings in the community (Marks, 1987; Mathews, Gelder, & Johnston, 1981; Williams, 1985; we will consider both panic and agoraphobia in more detail in later sections).

Brown and Barlow (2002) observed, "a DSM–IV diagnosis of panic disorder with agoraphobia conveys no information about frequency and intensity of panic attacks and the severity of agoraphobic avoidance" (p. 325). A person alleged to have this mental disorder can suffer from any level of panic attacks including none, and any level of agoraphobic avoidance including none, and indeed can have none of either. In DSM–IV, people who either avoid or fear agoraphobic activities have panic disorder whether they have panic attacks or not, as long as they were at least briefly bothered by panic at any past time, however remote. Moreover, DSM–IV agoraphobic disorders (i.e., panic disorder with agoraphobia and agoraphobia without history of panic disorder) require only that the person need a companion or feel anxious in agoraphobic settings, not that he or she avoid them (ICD–10 requires avoidance behavior). So a person can suffer from DSM–IV panic disorder with agoraphobia despite having neither panic attacks nor agoraphobic avoidance. Such a diagnosis conveys little about someone's problems.

Another source of discordance between panic as response and panic as disorder arises because panic disorder causes (or consists of) some kinds of panic attacks but not others. For example, panic attacks are not DSM–IV panic disorder (or its symptoms) if they occur in relation to various phobias, obsessions, compulsions, and stress, as panic attacks very often do (Barlow, 1987). Even more restrictively, ICD–10 panic attacks are not panic disorder if the people who suffer from them are depressed, phobic of almost anything (including agoraphobic), or experience high anxiety between panic attacks, all of which panicky people very often do (Barlow, 2002). The complex and clashing diagnostic exclusion rules point plainly to great arbitrariness in the concepts of panic disorder and agoraphobic disorder, as well as to the failure of disorders to characterize their own underlying psychological dimensions. Panic attacks and agoraphobic avoidance can co-occur, but they are largely uncorrelated (Craske & Barlow, 1987), and they are remedied by somewhat different approaches (Craske, 1999). Each dimension is separate and important in its own right, and is better viewed that way.

Bodily Causes of Behavior Are Not Mental Illnesses

Bodily processes have a bearing on avoidance, fear, and scary thoughts (Barlow, 2002), as they do on nearly every facet of human functioning. The relationship between bodily causes and mental illnesses is a point of widespread confusion. A bodily process and a mental illness are quite different things. For example, bodily processes are physical (i.e., they consist of internal biochemical events, anatomical structures, and the like, measured only physically and objectively) whereas mental illnesses are mental (i.e., they are defined largely by subjective thoughts and feelings, social behaviors, etc.). In just about any psychological theory bodily processes play a role in nearly every human response, so bodily influence says nothing about disease. A bodily organ being affected by a bodily process does not mean the organ is diseased, and likewise a mental state being affected by a bodily process does not mean the mental state is diseased. Nor does it mean that mental states or behavior can be reduced to bodily processes. Mental states in their own right can explain behavior, and they must be understood on their own terms (Bandura, 1986, 1997; Salkovskis, 1996b; Williams & Cervone, 1998). This chapter later reviews findings that people's consciousness can predict their future anxious feelings and avoidant behaviors accurately, indeed far more accurately than can any measure of biophysiology. But even if physiological measures strongly predicted avoidance, avoidant behavior still would be neither a mental illness nor mental disorder.

PROBLEMS DESCRIBED

Avoidance Behavior: Phobic Avoidance

The social cognitive perspective on the importance of behavioral functioning is that although it is not the only important dimension of psychosocial adaptation, for many purposes it is the most important one (Williams & Cervone, 1998). People's paths through life, and their inward fulfillments and sufferings along the way, have a lot to do with what they do, and do not do, outwardly. Outward behavior is fundamental to meeting one's responsibilities, to maintaining social relationships, and to achieving most valued personal goals. To suffer anxiety in shops and social gatherings is bad indeed, but to be unable to go into them is worse, undermining people's very ability to physically sustain themselves and foreclosing any chance of a near-normal life.

Needless avoidance in at least mild and transitory forms is widespread in psychological life, but when avoidance is limiting and persistent one speaks of phobia. Phobias illustrate prototypically the "neurotic paradox" of self-defeating behavior in which a person is unable to do a very ordinary action although she (or he) is otherwise quite competent, wishes to function normally, possesses the necessary cognitive-motoric skills, and is well aware that her disability is senseless. Behavioral disability is fundamentally important in its own right as limiting a person's ability to live a normal life, but also because what people do outwardly (and cannot do) powerfully affects for better or worse how they think and feel inwardly (Bandura, 1997; Williams, 1995, 1996a). Phobic avoidance and compulsive rituals torture people by robbing them of social and recreational possibilities and even of their livelihoods, by humiliating and depressing them, and by lowering their self-esteem and quality of life (Bandura, 1978; Steketee & Barlow, 2002; Marks, 1987).

Avoidance of activities/stimuli must be distinguished from fearful feelings toward activities/ stimuli, as the two are not highly correlated (Carr, 1979; Lang, 1985; Mineka, 1979; Rachman, 1976). The term *phobia* can apply to either pattern—for example, diagnosing phobic disorder requires avoidance behavior in ICD–10, but DSM–IV accepts anxiety about particular things without avoidance of them as phobic disorder. This section emphasizes phobic avoidance behavior, whereas later sections address subjective anxiety and scary thoughts.

Phobias vary widely in object, severity, and generality. Some phobias are of highly specific objects or activities (e.g., riding elevators or encountering cats or loud people), whereas generalized phobic patterns can encompass a wide range of seemingly dissimilar activities. Any specific phobia can be a generalized problem when it is severe enough or when the feared object/activity is found in diverse places (e.g., spiders or strangers; Bandura, 1978; Marks, 1987). Specific phobias tend to occur with other specific phobias, so the distinction between specific and generalized phobias can be difficult to make in any case (Hoffman, Lehman, & Barlow, 1997; Lipsitz, Barlow, Mannuzza, Hoffman, & Fyer, 2002). A specific phobia can be heterogeneous; for example, a dental-phobic person might dread the confinement, the needle, the drilling, the scents, allergic reactions, panic attacks, or various scary social possibilities (e.g., Moore, Brodsgaard, & Birn, 1991), so "dental phobia" conveys only a limited amount about an individual's problems.

Multiphobic conditions can occur in constellations such as *agoraphobia*, in which a person is simultaneously phobic of at least a few and possibly many or all of about 15 or so distinct community activities such as leaving home alone, using public transportation, shopping, tolerating heights, crossing bridges, riding elevators or escalators, driving a car, and being in an audience (Marks, 1987; Williams, 1985). Phobias of social scrutiny or of being embarassed or of causing embarassment to others can accompany agoraphobia or occur separately from it. Social phobias are common. Great heterogeneity exists between individuals and across different cultural contexts in the number, kinds, and patterning of multiphobic and agoraphobic individuals' fears and in their concomitant problems such as panic attacks, mood problems, worry, and many other psychological difficulties (Brown & Barlow, 2002; Hoffman & Barlow, 2002; Williams, 1985).

As mentioned earlier, excessive avoidance and/or fearful feelings about particular things are common far beyond the problems that diagnostic manuals deem official phobic disorders.

All of the DSM–IV and ICD–10 proposed anxiety disorders, including obsessive-compulsive disorder, generalized anxiety disorder, and various stress disorders, are defined in significant part by maladaptive behavioral avoidance of, and/or fearful feelings about, specifiable activities or objects, in other words, by phobias. Some sexual phobias are called sexual dysfunctions; some phobias of having a bodily deformity, body dysmorphic disorder; some disease phobias, hypochondriasis; some phobias of gaining weight, anorexia nervosa; and so on. Avoidance behaviors and frightened feelings toward particular activities/objects certainly can have individual distinctive psychological features and thematic concerns not shared among all phobias. But they are phobias nonetheless.

Avoidance Behavior: Compulsive Rituals

An important variant of dysfunctional avoidance behavior is compulsive behavioral rituals, such as excessive cleaning, repeating, checking, counting, arranging, hoarding, or other action that the person feels compelled to do. It is difficult to exaggerate the heartbreaking extent of functional impairment and strangeness of behavior that can be found in people with severe compulsions (Rachman & Hodgson, 1980; Steketee & Barlow, 2002). Less extreme but nonetheless troubling compulsions appear to be quite common (Muris, Merckelbach, & Clavan, 1997). And diverse problem behaviors other than those defined by DSM or ICD as obsessive-compulsive disorder, such as tics, hair pulling, rituals connected with self-starvation, dysmorphophobia, and other problems can be compulsive in nature (Yaryura-Tobias & McKay, 2002). Compulsions are usually accompanied by obsessive intrusive thoughts, by a sense that they prevent harm or danger, by a subjective feeling of fear or discomfort that declines with the compulsive act, and by rational recognition that the behavior is excessive, but none of these four is invariably present even in severe cases (Rachman & Hodgson, 1980; Steketee & Barlow, 2002).

Phobia and compulsion can be viewed as different points along a passive-avoidance versus active-avoidance continuum. At one end, a person passively refrains from activities, as a restaurant-phobic person simply stays away from restaurants. In the continuum's middle are active maneuvers to avoid or manage phobic threats, such as a bridge-phobic man driving far out his way to work every day to avoid a large bridge. At the most active end are effortful rituals performed at length to avoid a dreaded possibility. Phobic and compulsive behaviors often co-occur and overlap (Rachman & Hodgson, 1980). For example, a woman who dreaded being burglarized remained fully dressed in bed every night atop the bedcovers (phobia), and spent much time before bed checking and rechecking her window and door locks (compulsion). Although most people with phobias do not have marked compulsions, they often engage in subtle self-protective rituals in coping with phobia-related activities (Salkovskis, 1991; Williams, 1985), and most people with marked compulsions are phobic about compulsion-provoking circumstances, such as compulsive handwashers who phobically avoid contact with contaminating objects like door handles.

Cognitive compulsions also exist, in which people perform thought rituals, such as mentally checking, counting, reciting, or arranging. Compulsions may occur in response to external stimuli or in response to obsessions, intrusive unwanted thoughts, images, or impulses often experienced as alien, aversive, or frightening. At times the provoking activities/stimuli and obsessive thoughts operate in concert. For example, when one man stepped off a curb he had not to think "Damn God!" else he would be eternally damned; usually unsure if he had done it right, he had to step back and repeat it over and over. Obsessive thoughts and compulsive behaviors are partly independent dimensions. Some individuals have obsessions but not compulsions, others have compulsions but not obsessions, and others (perhaps 80%) have some kind of mixture of both. Either can predominate, and theories and treatments concerning each are importantly different (Rachman, 1998; Salkovskis, 1996a; Steketee & Barlow, 2002). Therefore, the general severity of a person's compulsions and obsessions would be characterized far better by two separate dimensional scores than by a diagnosis (or not) as obsessive-compulsive disorder. We will discuss obsessions in more detail later when we consider bothersome thoughts.

Anxiety

Unimodal, Multimodal, and Polymodal Anxiety

Scientists have long conceived anxiety in diverse ways. Anxiety can be defined unimodally by a single kind of response such as the subjective intensity of fear (Walk, 1956) or objective physiological arousal (Mowrer, 1960). More commonly anxiety is defined multimodally by both subjective anxiety and physiological responses, and sometimes by certain thought patterns as well. The extreme of multimodal definitions I call polymodal anxiety includes expansive contents (Lang, 1985) to be discussed later. The social cognitive view is that for most purposes the dissimilar responses are better kept separate, conceptually and terminologically, rather than lumped into an all-purpose but not very meaningful anxiety category, so social cognitive theory calls the various responses by their individual names.

Subjective Anxiety

Being afraid means above all feeling afraid, consciously, without which anxiety has no meaning. Fear in consciousness is to some extent ineffable, indescribable in words, but people can meaningfully indicate how intensely afraid they feel by rating a scale, for example, from 0 (not anxious or afraid) to 10 (extremely anxious and afraid). Fear intensity scales from 0 to 100, or 0 to 8, with variant instruction sets and anchor values, are widely used. This sort of definition has the large advantage of not imposing meanings on anxiety other that what people themselves mean by simple anchoring terms such as anxious, afraid, and the like. Subjective anxiety has meaning in relation to the psychological context in which people experience it, and anxiety intensity ratings indicate straightforwardly how much particular activities, objects, or images frighten people (Hersen, 1973; Walk, 1956; Wolpe, 1958).

Physiological Anxiety

Anxiety is widely considered to be in part physiological response, mainly autonomic arousal and its associated neurochemical mechanisms. People commonly report scary experiences and feelings in part by describing how their heart raced, they broke out in a sweat, and so on. Because autonomic arousal per se can be measured physically, without reference to people's conscious-ness, it is a favored index of fear among investigators who judge subjective feelings to be private events inaccessable to science. Defining anxiety as physiological arousal gets peo-ple's unscientific inner feelings out of the way, but at a high scientific price. Although people are more physically aroused when feeling strong emotions generally, autonomic arousal pat-terns do not correspond to particular subjective feeling states (Hoehn-Saric, 1998; Lacey, 1967; Zajonc & McIntosh, 1992), and frightened and panicky people show many patterns of phys-iological arousal, including none (Carr, 1979; Ehlers, 1993; Margraf et al., 1987; Morrow & Labrum, 1978; Taylor et al., 1986). Physiological arousal without subjective fear is common, as when people exercise, feel sexual interest, or merely hear a familiar voice (Lang, 1985). Calling autonomic arousal anxiety creates confusion about how anxious someone is because different autonomic responses correlate little with one another and can even change in different directions in an individual during treatment (Bandura, 1969; Rachman & Hodgson, 1974). The large gap between physiology and subjective feeling means that bodily responses per se cannot be anxiety, but must be considered on their own terms (Williams, 1987).

Perception of Physiological Arousal

In social cognitive theory, physiological arousal per se has less impact on behavior than does the person's perception and interpretation of physiological arousal (Cioffi, 1991; Clark, 1986; Salkovskis & Warwick, 1986). Bodily perceptions can become a focus of obsessive worrying and can give rise to defensive actions, such as seeking medical help for a racing heart or ritually carrying a bottle of water against a possible dry mouth. Bodily perceptions are implicated too in panic attacks and illness phobias (Clark, 1986; Salkovskis & Warwick, 1986). Yet people, including those with avoidance and fear-related problems, are remarkably inaccurate at perceiving how much they are sweating or their heart is beating (Ehlers, 1993; Mandler, 1962; Pennebaker, 1982). The inaccuracy of bodily perceptions is curiously ignored by DSM–IV and ICD–10, which allow diagnosticians to measure accelerated heart rate either by a biometric apparatus or by the diagnosed person's subjective impressions, two little-related indicants.

Trait Anxiety

Theorists have conceived anxiety not only as a transitory feeling state, but an enduring personality trait, a disposition to generally see circumstances as threatening and to react with fear (e.g., Cattell & Scheier, 1961; Spielberger, 1983). Trait anxiety is usually measured by asking people to rate the self-descriptiveness of various brief general statements. Variant trait conceptions and traitlike inventories abound that measure anxiety in general, without respect to context. People certainly do differ from one another in how much they are generally distressed (or disabled, or bedeviled by bothersome thoughts), but in every case they are troubled by certain definite things and not by others (e.g., Chambless, Beck, Gracely, & Grisham, 2000). Social cognitive theory predicts marked shifts in behavior, thought, and feeling depending on context (Bandura, 1969; Beck, 1976; Williams, 1985). Variation in an individual's trait-relevant behavior across situations is simply ignored by generalized traits, as is the idiosyncratic configuration of particular problem responses from one person to another. Such variation cannot in principle be explained by differences in generalized tendencies to be anxious or neurotic, or to think catastrophic thoughts, feel negative affect, or be frightened by perceived bodily arousal.

Trait scores have some predictive ability, but rarely can they reliably explain even 15% of the variance in behavior, often far less (Bandura, 1986; Mischel, 1990; Williams & Cervone, 1998). Because psychological treatments involve the person having direct mental and physical commerce with the specific things he or she fears, avoids, ritualizes over, or intrusively thinks about (Barlow, 2002; Craske, 1999), knowing someone's average tendency to be anxious gives therapists little useful information for helping people change. Diverging from the trait approach, the social cognitive approach measures particular problem responses in direct relation to particular problem circumstances, in the natural environment if possible, and otherwise in a particularly defined psychological context (Williams, 1985). Context-sensitive social cognitions accurately predict and explain problem behaviors, as we will see later.

Psychiatric Anxiety

Manuals of mental disorders rely on anxiety as a description, a cause, and an effect of diverse mental illnesses, but are unclear and internally inconsistent in how they define and talk about anxiety. Psychiatric anxiety is multimodal anxiety and comes in three rather different forms:

the phenomenon of anxiety, the proposed symptoms of anxiety disorder, and panic attacks, each of which differs between ICD–10 and DSM–IV.

Psychiatric Anxiety as a Proposed Multimodal Phenomenon. In DSM–IV's glossary, anxiety is "the apprehensive anticipation of future danger or misfortune accompanied by a feeling of dysphoria or somatic symptoms of tension" (p. 764). ICD–10's definition of anxiety is looser (note the term "usually" in what follows) yet more elaborate: "Primary symptoms of anxiety . . . usually involve elements of (a) apprehension (worries about future misfortunes, feeling 'on edge', difficulty in concentrating, etc.); (b) motor tension (restless fidgeting, tension headaches, trembling, inability to relax); and (c) autonomic overactivity (lightheadedness, sweating, tachycardia . . . dizziness, dry mouth, etc.)" (p. 140). Note that neither definition incorporates avoidance behavior. (Curiously, DSM–IV panic does not necessarily involve apprehension of danger or harm, but then it does not necessarily involve feeling afraid either). The requirement for danger thoughts in DSM–IV anxiety, and their optional inclusion in ICD–10 anxiety, transform danger thoughts from anxiety's cause into its very definition, thereby rendering Beck's (1976) danger theory of anxiety null and void because a cause cannot directly cause itself. For conceptual and research clarity, it seems better to keep danger thoughts out of the definition of feeling afraid to enable exploring the role of danger thoughts in making people feel afraid.

Psychiatric Anxiety as a Symptom of Anxiety Disorder. DSM–IV and ICD–10 each propose that varied cognitive, emotional, behavioral, physiological, and perceptual responses (somewhat different between the two manuals) are anxiety disorder symptoms. Some proposed anxiety symptoms are anxiety (e.g., fearful subjective feelings, physiological hyperarousal), whereas other anxiety symptoms are not anxiety (e.g., obsessive thoughts, phobic behaviors), according to each manual's definition of anxiety (see the preceding paragraph). Because the terms anxiety, anxiety symptoms, and anxiety disorder symptoms are widely used as interchangeable, it seems that the diagnostic manuals' efforts to set things straight have if anything further beclouded anxiety's already foggy meaning.

Psychiatric Anxiety as Panic Attack. Psychiatric manuals also emphasize panic attacks, a variant form of anxiety. Panic attacks are sudden rushes of intense fear (or in DSM–IV, discomfort) that can be disturbing and can leave a lasting residue of dread and disability (Barlow, 2002; Craske, 1999; Rachman & Maser, 1988). Yet people have panic attacks who do not have or develop serious problems in connection with them (Norton, Cox, & Malan, 1992; Wilson, Sandler, Asmundson, Ediger, Larsen, & Walker, 1992). Panic attacks can vary widely in intensity, duration, frequency, number and kind of accompanying sensations/reactions, and other graduated dimensions (Craske, 1999). The DSM–IV definition of panic attack, widely used in research, is a discrete period of rapidly mounting intense fear or discomfort accompanied by at least a small subset of about twenty-five listed thoughts, feelings, perceptions, and physiological or other sensations. The twenty-five responses are sorted into thirteen categories, with responses in at least four of the thirteen categories needed for the attack to be an official DSM–IV panic attack, as mentioned earlier. Notably, avoidance behavior is not part of this definition. DSM–IV calls the twenty-five responses symptoms of panic, but of course they are panic per se rather than its symptoms. Terms such as panic responses or panic features serve better because the term panic symptoms absurdly implies that panic attacks cause or produce their own defining characteristics.

Controversy exists as to whether panic differs from simply rapidly mounting anxiety (Barlow, 2002). The similarities seem much larger than the differences (Craske, 1999). Virtually

every one of the twenty-five panic responses listed in DSM–IV is commonly included in definitions of plain old anxiety. For example, of the twenty-one items in the Beck Anxiety Inventory
(Beck, Epstein, Brown, & Steer, 1988), fifteen are DSM–IV panic responses. Although panic,
like anxiety, is conventionally defined and conceived in part as bodily arousal, the actual relationship between bodily arousal and panic, like that between bodily arousal and subjective
anxiety, is not very strong, with many reported panic attacks having no evident accompanying
autonomic arousal, and with high rapid autonomic arousal often not being experienced as scary
or panicky by an individual (Craske, 1999; Ehlers, 1993; Taylor et al., 1986). As the essence
and sine qua non of anxiety is the subjective feeling of anxiety, the essence and sine qua non
of panic is the subjective feeling of panic.

The concept of spontaneous (or uncued or unexpected) panic was proposed by Klein (1980)
as being importantly different from ordinary phobic anxiety because it was unlinked to particular stimuli, and early theories considered panic to be a biologically triggered event (Barlow,
2002; Klein, 1980). Panic attacks vary dimensionally in their apparent relation to specific
environmental circumstances, with some seeming to come unexpectedly and others being perceived as more likely or less likely in given circumstances. Apart from people's perception of
a cue, cued and uncued panic attacks are similar (Craske, 1991, 1999). The social cognitive
view is that even unexpected anxiety and panic often occur in relation to discrete psychological events, but these can be cognitive events such as catastrophic interpretations of perceived
bodily states (e.g., Clark, 1986; Clark et al., 1997; Craske, 1991) and loss of self-efficacy for
maintaining cognitive control (Williams & LaBerge, 1994). Panic can be highly responsive to
environmental and psychological manipulations and interventions (Clark, 1993; Craske, 1999;
Rapee, 1993, 1995; Williams & Falbo, 1996).

Multimodal Anxiety Plus: The Three-Systems Analysis

Most kinds of anxiety are defined by nonbehavioral responses. The three-systems analysis
(Lang, 1985) goes further and throws in maladaptive behavior itself, the very phenomenon
anxiety was supposed to explain. Lang (1985) states, "the data of anxiety . . . are measurable
responses which fall into three general categories of behavior" consisting of "verbal reports of
distress, fear related behavioral acts," and "patterns of visceral and somatic activation" (Lang,
1985, p. 133–134). The verbal report category has come to include nearly everything people
can say about their multimodal fear responses (Craske, 1999). People no doubt think, feel, act,
and respond physiologically, all at once, in nearly every facet of their lives. But as a theory of
avoidant behavior the three systems analysis is stillborn. The emotion of anxiety was to be the
cause of problem behavior. Asserting that the emotion and the behavior are one and the same,
namely anxiety, robs both of meaning.

The three-systems analysis does not specify psychological causes except to reject conscious
thought and feeling as causes of anything. The verbal report category is sometimes called the
cognitive system, yet it consists not of conscious cognitions or conscious emotions but of
"verbal reports of distress, i.e., reports of anxiety, fear, dread, panic, and associated complaints
of worry, obsessions, inability to concentrate, insecurity, and the like" (Lang, 1985, p. 133).
Lang (1985) states plainly that these reports have little real meaning: "Feeling states are
completely private and represent a poor data resource for the clinician preparing to undertake
treatment," and "their unavailability to . . . observers appears to deny any possibility of scientific
investigation" (p. 131). Fortunately, "peculiarities of behavior" and "a variety of [physiological]
symptoms . . . are more yielding to objective analysis" (Lang, 1985, p. 131). This rejection of
private experience is profoundly anticognitive. Surprisingly, this "language behavior" concept,
despite its similarity to B. F. Skinner's (1957) "verbal behavior" concept, has been credited

with having laid the foundation for acceptance of cognition in clinical psychology (Hawton, Salkovskis, Kirk, & Clark, 1989, p. 10). It is not clear how cognitive approaches benefited from a theory that private experience is a poor data source for therapists, is unavailable to observers, and lies beyond any possibility of scientific investigation. Nobody ever doubted that people report having thoughts and feelings. The cognitive revolution in psychology was about finally accepting that these reports of thoughts and feelings have direct psychological meaning and need to be taken seriously on their own terms (see, e.g., Bandura, 1969).

Polymodal Anxiety: Bioinformational Theory

The three-systems view was not a causal theory so much as a proposed list of anxiety responses. Bioinformational theory (Cook, Melamed, Cuthbert, McNeil & Lang, 1988; Lang, 1985; Lang, Cuthbert, & Bradley, 1998) tries to unify the discordant proposed anxiety systems by means of a fear structure (also called a fear program or emotion prototype), a largely unconscious associative network of memory nodes containing diverse interacting elements, including propositions about stimuli, responses, and their verbal/semantic meanings, as well as efferent codes, motor programs, concrete action imagery, cognitive schemas, action subprograms, and dozens of other descriptive contents linked to diverse neurophysiological substrates. The fear structure thus expands anxiety to encompass nearly everything. Its meaning network seems to touch the entire human mental faculty and its biophysiological mechanisms the entire human body. Indeed, bioinformational theory leaves the reader wondering where anxiety ends and the rest of the human being, if any, begins.

In this theory "emotions . . . are fundamentally to be understood as behavioral acts" (Lang, 1985, p. 140), insofar as the deep emotional prototype initially produces a fear reaction unified across response modes, but inhibitory neural pathways selectively abort some fear responses before they are realized in expression (Lang, 1985; Lang et al., 1998). Transmuting fearful emotion into avoidant behavior is quite a feat of psychic alchemy given their well-known empirical disassociation (Barlow, 2002; Carr, 1979; Lang, 1985; Mineka, 1979; Rachman, 1976; Schwartz, 1989; Seligman & Johnston, 1973). Why the prototype would abort its own efferent signals and why evolution would construct special neural pathways to achieve this self-cancelling objective are not clear. The theory's testable claims, for example, that fear arousal is necessary or sizably advantageous for treatment benefit (Foa & McNally, 1996), clash with long-settled findings (Mathews et al., 1981; Rachman & Hodgson, 1974, 1980; White & Barlow, 2002; Williams, 1987). Otherwise, the theory is hard to evaluate because it provides no clear measures of its many distinctive elements (Williams, 1996b). Bioinformational research (e.g., Cook et al., 1988; Lang et al., 1998; Lang, Levin, Miller, & Kozak, 1983) has failed to measure bioinformational processes per se, and has focused on predictions that do not seem relevant to the prototype-matching hypothesis, for example, that snake–phobic people differ from public speaking–phobic people in their multimodal anxiety reactions toward snakes and public speaking (Lang et al., 1983). Barlow (2002) wrote well that accepting bioinformational theory's deep psychic unity of fear and avoidance "demands a leap of faith" (p. 57).

Bioinformational theory incorporates the latest terminology from neuroscience, cognitive science, and cyberscience, but it is a big step backward. Progress in solving human problems requires theories that stake claims that are meaningful (reasonably operationalized) and believable (not already disconfirmed). Mowrer's (1960) two-factor autonomic arousal theory, Beck's (1976) danger cognitions theory, and Bandura's (1997) self-efficacy theory each state plainly in operational terms what causes avoidant behavior, let the evidence show what it will. Bioinformational theory's polyform phenomena governed by myriad interacting unconscious and neurobiological mechanisms can tell us little about people's problems. Perhaps worse, the theory makes people into walking avoidance machines, emotion prototypes unconsciously bio-computing propositional data and outputting fear expressions that reprogram with prototype-mismatching input. Social cognitive people, in contrast, feel emotions and think thoughts in consciousness, they act in accordance with their appraisal of their circumstances and themselves, and they exercise conscious personal agency as they actively master their problems in thought and deed (Bandura, 1997; Williams & Cervone, 1998).

Construct Invalidity of Multimodal Anxiety and Anxiety Disorders

The construct validity of complex personality entities such as multimodal anxiety or anxiety disorders requires at a minimum that the parts of the proposed entity must display internal coherence or convergent validity by correlating highly with one another, and external distinctiveness or discriminant validity by the parts correlating little with ostensibly dissimilar entities (Campbell & Fiske, 1959), as mentioned earlier. In other words, subjective fear and elevated heart rate should correlate well with one another because both are anxiety (or anxiety disorder), whereas anxious feelings and depressed feelings should be little correlated because they are allegedly distinct entities. Of course, just the opposite is empirically true. The chapter has reviewed the low correlations among the proposed indices of multimodal anxiety, and of anxiety disorder, a pattern sometimes called desynchrony but perhaps better called convergent invalidity. The multimodal anxiety constructs also lack discriminant validity, as mentioned earlier, in that anxiety and depression inventories tend to correlate over .70 with one another (Clark et al., 1995) and anxiety disorder diagnoses correlate with many other diagnoses (Boyd et al., 1987; Brown & Barlow, 2002). The lack of construct validity refutes the very existence, as meaningful psychological entities, of multimodal anxiety and of anxiety disorders.

Note that construct validity is not at issue for unitary social cognitive response constructs such as perceptions of danger (Beck, 1976), perceptions of self-efficacy (Bandura, 1997), or subjective feelings of anxiety intensity (Walk, 1956; Williams, 1985), because these constructs do not try to incorporate dissimilar psychological responses into a single multimodal psychic entity. Particular human problem dimensions certainly do exist, and subjective feelings of anxiety certainly do exist, but multimodal anxiety entities do not.

Bothersome Thoughts

People with marked fear and/or dysfunctional avoidance show distinctive problem-related changes in their conscious thinking. Some characteristic thoughts are also proposed cognitive mechanisms of fear and avoidance (e.g., Bandura, 1997; Beck, 1976), which we will consider in the later section on causal theories. This section considers cognitions that are problems in their own right. Troublesome intrusive thoughts, difficult to control or dismiss, can come as obsessive preoccupations, excessive worries, scary images, mad impulses, catastrophic expectations, or horrifying recollections (e.g., Borkovec, Shadick, & Hopkins, 1991; Frost & Steketee, 2002; Rapee & Barlow, 1991). Some bothersome thoughts are neither fear-provoking nor resisted but simply consume too much time and thereby interfere with the person's life, whereas others can be alien frightening ideas that the person avoids by phobic maneuvers or by neutralizing rituals or thoughts (Steketee & Barlow, 2002). All of the various problematic cognitions tend to occur especially often in people with any pattern of notable avoidance or fear. People with phobias, for example, often perceive danger, worry, obsess, and have intrusive disturbing recollections, anticipations, and nightmares about what they avoid (Bandura, 1978; Marks, 1987).

Indeed, bothersome thoughts of many kinds, including obsessions, worries, intrusions, and even hallucinations and delusions, are common in psychological life generally (Johns & Van

Os, 2001; Norton et al., 1992; Steketee & Barlow, 2002). People who seek help for obsessions or worries or identify themselves as worriers appear to have somewhat more frequent and frightening thoughts on the average than those who do not, but the two groups' problem thoughts greatly overlap and are sometimes not clearly distinguishable in content, duration, how much the person resists them, of even in the anxiety, avoidance, or compulsive rituals they occasion (Borkovec et al., 1991; Craske, Rapee, Jackel, & Barlow, 1989; Rachman & de Silva, 1978; Salkovskis & Harrison, 1984). A dimension of major importance distinguishing whether intrusive thoughts are problematic appears to be their perceived controllability (Borkovec et al., 1991; Craske et al., 1989) and whether people beset by intrusions conclude that they cannot effectively manage the worrisome future possibilities (Aikins & Craske, 2001).

One can examine many different dimensions of thought for different purposes, but the boundaries between the intrusive, the worrisome, the persistent, and the obsessive are not hard and fast. Worries and obsessions are similar in being repetitive and time-consuming, having recurrent themes, and often being experienced as uncontrollable. Differentiating worry from obsession is perhaps possible in principle (Turner, Beidel, & Stanley, 1992), but the two are substantially correlated and in practice can be hard to tell apart (Freeston, Ladouceur, Rheaume, Letarte, Gagnon, & Thibodeau, 1994; Wells & Papageorgiou, 1998). Maladaptive worry is also not always clearly distinct from constructive preparatory problem solving, as both involve considering possible dangers and how to deal with them (Craske, 1999).

Nor are the boundaries between the excessive, the unreasonable, and the delusional entirely sharp. People with avoidance, panic, or scary thoughts often recognize that these are out of proportion to objective facts, but such "insight" is highly variable across situations and between individuals, and is thus eminently dimensional in character (e.g., Williams & Watson, 1985; Williams, Turner, & Peer, 1985). Why DSM–IV requires insight into the unreasonableness of fear in specific and social phobic disorders, but not in agoraphobic or other proposed anxiety disorders, is not clear. People with obsessions and compulsions, as well as thoughts of danger and dysfunctional avoidance, may or may not accept that their thoughts and actions are senseless, and some obsessions are plainly delusional (O'Dwyer & Marks, 2000; Steketee & Barlow, 2002; Yaryura-Tobias & McKay, 2002). People with psychotic problems frequently display obsessions, compulsions, phobias, and traumatic stress reactions (Cassano, Pini, Saettoni, & Dell'Osso, 1999; Cosoff & Hafner, 1998; Neria, Bromet, Sievers, Lavelle, & Fochtmann, 2002), and worry and anxiety appear to contribute to delusional distress (Freeman & Garety, 1999; Krabbendam, Janssen, Bak, Bijl, de Graaf, & van Os, 2002).

In various ways DSM–IV distorts the study of intrusions, worry, obsessions, danger perceptions, and delusions (cf. Persons, 1986) as psychological dimensions by declaring arbitararily, for example, that excessive worries about everyday things cannot be obsessions, and that the worries in generalized anxiety disorder cannot concern being away from family, gaining weight, being very ill, public embarassment, and other things people worry about a lot, and that the danger beliefs in some phobias cannot be delusional. The social cognitive approach studies worry, obsessions, danger beliefs, and delusions as graduated psychological dimensions, unconcerned about trespassing on diagnostic turf, and indeed expecting each problem response to covary with other problems. This is neither to deny that for particular purposes one can make meaningful distinctions between kinds of intrusive upsetting thoughts, nor to deny that certain patterns of co-occurring problem thoughts and behaviors might be of distinctive interest, but that there is little sacred about any particular way of defining problem thinking, and arbitrary rules about what contents worries (for example) shall have (and may not have) make for a self-hindered start of a research program to understand the nature of excessive worrying.

CAUSES OF AVOIDANCE, ANXIETY, AND BOTHERSOME THOUGHTS

Causes of Avoidance Behavior

This review focuses on current psychological causes of problems, although historical factors, including developmental, genetic, biological, and social learning influences, have been studied extensively (Barlow, 2002; Craske, 1999, Rachman, 1977). Sometimes phobias develop straightforwardly, for example, instated by brief social modeling experiences alone in monkeys (Mineka, Davidson, Cook, & Keir, 1984) or emerging full-blown in people from a single brief traumatic experience. Most phobias have unclear or ambiguous developmental histories, in which multiple biological, social, psychological, and environmental factors appear to interact (Rachman, 1977). In the social cognitive approach, historical influences operate in the present primarily via conscious cognitive process that sustain avoidance and that can be easily measured here and now in conjunction with avoidance.

Avoidance and rituals are correlated to some extent with countless specific inner states, including feelings, cognitions, sensations, and perceptions (Barlow, 2002; Steketee & Frost, 2002), any of which could in principle play a role in causing the avoidant behavior. Isolating inner psychological causes of avoidance requires at a minimum identifying the inner states that correlate most strongly with avoidance behavior. Only the relatively strong inner predictors of behavior are likely to emerge as distinctive independent causes of behavior. Finding strong psychological predictors of avoidance behavior took a very long time because for decades anxious feelings, not problematic thoughts, dominated the research agenda.

Anxiety Theory of Avoidance Behavior

Maladaptive avoidance behavior was a principal psychological phenomenon that the concept of anxiety was originally intended to explain. Anxiety was the hypothetical cause and avoidant behavior was the explained effect. The psychoanalytic conception that an anxiety drive arising from unconscious threats found symbolic expression in particular neurotic self-defeating behaviors was reformulated in learning terms by two-factor theory (Mowrer, 1960), which held that anxiety comes to control avoidant behavior in a two-part (classical plus operant conditioning) process. First the person learns to be afraid of a previously neutral stimulus after experiencing it paired with an aversive stimulus. Then the anxiety provoked by the now-conditioned stimulus motivates the person to avoid that conditioned stimulus, and the decline in anxiety resulting from avoidance rewards the avoidance (Mowrer, 1960; Wolpe, 1958). Two-factor theory dominated the study of avoidance for decades and continues to have loyal adherents, although a series of reviews in the late 1960s and 1970s (Bandura, 1969; Bolles, 1975; Carr, 1979; Mineka, 1979; Rachman, 1976; Rachman & Hodgson, 1974; Schwartz, 1978, 1989; Seligman & Johnston, 1973) revealed fundamental problems that two-factor theory has never solved (Williams, 1987). Attempts have been made to resurrect anxiety conditioning theories by importing social cognitive concepts and reframing them in anxiety conditioning terms (e.g., Foa & McNally, 1996; Davey, 1992). I have questioned elsewhere the wisdom of putting new cognitive wine in old conditioning bottles (Williams, 1996b). Why cling to the awkward old conditioning terminology and concepts when the more straightforward and parsimonious (cognitively simple) language of social cognition is available? Directly fatal to anxiety theories of behavior in general, including two-factor conditioning theory, is the consistent lack of strong association between anxiety and avoidance behavior, which no amount of reframing can change.

Although Mowrer (1960) was concerned with subjective feelings of anxiety, he operationally defined anxiety as autonomic arousal. But peripheral physiology is as little related to phobic or compulsive behaviors as it is to feelings of subjective fear (Bandura, 1969; Lang, 1985; Mineka, 1979; Schwartz, 1989; Seligman & Johnston, 1973; Williams, 1987). Indeed, autonomic reactions are highly unstable in response to a given stimulus (Holden & Barlow, 1986) and thus lack the statistical reliability needed to strongly cause much of anything, especially highly stable responses like compulsions and phobias.

Subjective feelings of anxiety are somewhat better correlated with avoidant behavior (e.g., Williams, Dooseman, & Kleifield, 1984; Williams et al., 1985), but often account for less than 10% of the variance in avoidance (Lang, 1985). Feeling very afraid without avoiding is common, as in many panic victims who do not have marked phobias, and in terrified but frequent fliers. Severe phobic avoidance or compulsion with little or no fear is also well documented (Carr, 1979; Spitzer & Williams, 1985) and is noted by both DSM–IV and ICD–10. Bridge-phobic commuters fearlessly leave home hours early each day and calmly drive far around large bridges (Williams, 1985). Indeed, most human avoidance behavior is fearless: people usually fill fuel tanks and lock doors in emotional tranquility (Carr, 1979). Easily executed apparently effective avoidance maneuvers, even quite maladaptive ones, leave nothing to be afraid of. The main driver of phobic and compulsive behavior clearly is not subjective fear.

Panic Theory of Avoidance

A variation on anxiety theory, embodied in DSM–IV but not in ICD–10, holds that agoraphobic behavior is caused by panic or panic-like reactions. As panic is highly similar to anxiety, so panic theory founders on the same rock that sank two-factor anxiety theory: Panic does not correlate much with agoraphobic behavior (Craske & Barlow, 1988). Panic can be accompanied by extensive phobias, but often it is not, and agoraphobia is common without current panic and without history of panic attacks (e.g, Magee, Eaton, Wittchen, McGonagne, & Kessler, 1996). Panic is also common with many problems other than agoraphobia (Barlow, 1987; Cosoff & Hafner, 1998) and occurs in people who have no particular problems at all (Norton et al., 1992). Therefore, panic does not have even a distinctive relationship to agoraphobia, never mind a strong causal relationship to it.

Social Cognitive Theory of Avoidance

Social cognitive theory and a family of related cognitive theories explain avoidant behavior, anxiety, and disturbing thoughts in terms of predominantly conscious cognitive processes (e.g., Bandura, 1997; Beck, 1976; Beck, Emery, & Greenberg, 1985; Clark, 2001; Leary & Kowalski, 1995; Maddux, 1995a; Rachman, 1998; Salkovskis, 1996a, 1998; Williams, 1995, 1996a; Williams & Cervone, 1998). I call these collectively social cognitive theories (although they do not all identify themselves that way) because they explain problems by people's particular beliefs, expectations, and judgments about particular things, as representable vividly to themselves in awareness, and about which they can communicate directly and meaningfully. The social cognitive view is that nonconscious factors exert their effects on action largely through the final common pathways of conscious thought (Bandura, 1997; Beck, 1976; Beck et al., 1985; Salkovskis, 1996b). Social cognitions are not generalized traitlike cognitive or information-processing styles, but specific thoughts about self and circumstances. Such specificity enables, in principle and in practice as we will see, predicting the idiosyncratic patterning of individuals' responding across situations and time.

Social cognitive theories emphasize various kinds of conscious thought, of which outcome expectations and self-efficacy judgments are especially important (Bandura, 1986; Beck, 1976;

Williams & Cervone, 1998). Outcome expectations refer to people's beliefs about the possible outcomes of their own actions, such as encountering possible dangers or facing high likelihood of being harmed (e.g., "if I try to pet the dog, it will surely bite me"), anticipated anxiety (e.g., "if I walk by it, I will get very scared"), and anticipated panic ("probably I would panic"). Danger thoughts are central elements in a family of cognitive theories derived from the pioneering work of Beck (1976) and addressing phenomena such as phobia, panic, anxiety, obsession, compulsion, and traumatic stress (e.g., Beck et al., 1985; Clark, 1986, 1999, 2001; Salkovskis, 1998) in terms of various danger-related thought patterns. Another family of cognitive theories emphasizes anticipated anxiety or anticipated panic, holding that avoidance can be motivated by a fear of fear, or aversion to becoming afraid, panicky, or physiologically aroused (e.g., Chambless & Gracely, 1989; Kirsch, 1990).

Self-efficacy judgments constitute another class of cognitions, people's judgments about their ability to execute courses of action irrespective of anticipated outcomes (e.g., "I don't think I could touch the dog if I tried"). Self-efficacy theory (Bandura, 1988, 1997) holds that avoidance, fear, and scary thoughts arise largely because people have lost their belief that they can act effectively and exercise control in the circumstances (Leary & Kowalski, 1995; Maddux, 1995a; Maddux, Norton, & Leary, 1988; Schwarzer, 1992; Williams, 1995, 1996a). Perceived control is intimately related to self-efficacy because feeling in control requires feeling able to enact controlling responses. Personal control has major implications for lowering anxiety (Barlow, 2002; Borkovec et al., 1991; Craske et al., 1991; Mineka & Kelly, 1989).

Williams (1995, 1996a) reviewed a number of studies by different investigators that examined the power of people's self-efficacy judgments to predict their approach behavior toward real phobic threats, and compared it to the power of perceived danger, anticipated anxiety, and/or anticipated panic to predict approach behavior (see also Öst, Ferebee, & Furmark, 1997). Self-efficacy was consistently the most accurate single predictor of approach behavior, usually accounting for more than half the variance, with rs usually in the range of .70 to .80, followed by anticipated anxiety and anticipated panic, which were also strongly predictive of behavior. Perceived danger was generally a weak predictor of behavior. Importantly, self-efficacy consistently remained a strong predictor of behavior when the alternative cognitive factors such as anticipated anxiety were held constant, whereas the alternative factors consistently lost power to significantly predict behavior with self-efficacy held constant (Öst et al., 1997; Williams, 1995, 1996a; Williams et al., 1984, 1985; Williams, Kinney, & Falbo, 1989). Self efficacy also remains an accurate predictor of future approach behavior when indices of previous behavior are controlled statistically or are unavailable and when other noncausal interpretations are implausible (Bandura, 1997; Williams, 1995, 1996a). For example, Williams et al. (1989) found that when agoraphobics were given performance exposure treatment for only some of their phobic areas (e.g., shopping, heights), the generalized behavioral improvements in their untreated phobias (e.g., driving) were best predicted by changes in self-efficacy toward the generalized threats. These data make clear that people's beliefs about their abilities have a strong causal bearing on their phobic avoidance and disability.

Causes of Anxiety

Causes of Subjective Anxiety

The preceding section compared possible cognitive causes of behavior. One can also compare possible cognitive causes of subjective fear. In the studies summarized by Williams (1995, 1996a), anticipated anxiety and anticipated panic correlated about $r = .75$ with later anxiety rated during the behavioral test, whereas self-efficacy correlated only about $r = .50$ with later subjective anxiety ratings. Anticipated anxiety and anticipated panic each continued to strongly predict performance anxiety when either self-efficacy or perceived danger was held constant, whereas the latter two factors lost all significant predictiveness of anxiety with anticipated panic held constant. The superiority of anticipated anxiety/panic over self-efficacy in predicting later subjective anxiety corresponds to an oft-observed phenomenon: a phobic person expressing simultaneously high self-efficacy and high anticipated anxiety/panic for a task and then doing the task without difficulty but experiencing high anxiety (Williams, 1985, 1986, 1996a). Bandura (1988) proposed that self-efficacy for controlling scary thoughts (cf. Kent & Gibbons, 1984; Salkovskis & Harrison, 1984) also plays a role in anxiety, and this thought control self-efficacy factor does have predictive power beyond that of conventional self-efficacy measures, but anticipated anxiety and anticipated panic remain the overriding social cognitive predictors of anxiety arousal (Zane & Williams, 1993). The data suggest strongly that seeing oneself as being vulnerable to anxiety or panic is in some way causally connected to actually experiencing anxiety (Kirsch, 1990; Williams, 1986), although why and how this connection comes about is unclear (Bandura, 1995; Maddux, 1995b).

Danger perceptions are weak predictors of subjective anxiety (Williams et al., 1985, 1989; Williams & Watson, 1985). And strikingly, danger ideas are absent from agoraphobic people's thoughts when they are trying to do the things they most dread (Williams, Kinney, Harap, & Liebmann, 1997).

Information Processing in Trait Anxiety and Anxiety Disorders

Most research on the role of cognition in anxiety has been guided by one of two broad theoretical approaches: the *social cognition model* and the *information-processing model*. Social cognitive approaches emphasize people's conscious conclusions, such as their beliefs, expectations, judgments, and similar kinds of thoughts, in relation to themselves and their circumstances, which can potentially be expressed openly in an interview or on a self-report questionnaire. Social cognitivists then relate those thoughts directly to people's psychological functioning in actual community environments. In contrast, the information-processing approach seeks biases, both conscious and unconscious, in anxious individuals' attention to, perception of, interpretation of, and memory for anxiety-promoting information (Mathews & McLeod, 1994, 2002; McNally, 1999). Information-processing research has related processing biases mostly to general psychological states such as trait anxiety level or diagnostic status rather than to coping behavior in the community per se.

Information-processing experiments often infer cognitive operations indirectly rather than asking people about them. In typical attention experiments, for example, people selected for having (or not having) a certain problem respond to brief verbal stimuli related to various anxiety/danger themes or to benign themes, and their responses (often reaction times on subtasks ostensibly unrelated to the words' meanings) are examined for average intergroup differences in how the words are processed as a function of their meanings. This research has found that individuals suffering from a given problem differ from nonproblem individuals in how they process some information, for example being generally more attentive to negative information related to their problem (Mathews & McLeod, 1994, 2002; McNally, 1999). Less clear is whether such biases tell us much distinctive about trait anxiety and diagnostic status, or simply that people are biased to attend to personally-relevant information of any kind, positive or negative. Not all kinds of cognitive operations are equivalently biased in anxious individuals. For example, on explicit memory tasks, anxious individuals tend not to show evidence of information-processing biases (Mathews & McLeod, 1994, 2002; McLeod, 1999; McNally, 1999).

Social cognitive theories concur that how people process problem-related information contributes to problem responses. For example, people's interpretations of why they succeeded in doing scary tasks during phobia treatment affect how much beneficial information they gain from those successes (Williams & Kinney, 1997). The more they attribute success to the therapist rather than to themselves, the less they gain in self-efficacy and behavioral ability. Attributions explain significant variation in benefit beyond that explained by the level of past behavioral successes (Williams & Kinney, 1997).

Laboratory information-processing research often uses attenuated problem-relevant stimuli consisting of verbal material presented to participants in a safe context, and it measures experimental responses, such as latency to detect a probe or to name a color appearing on a computer screen, rather than problem responses per se. Much information-processing research addresses psychological constructs with unclear behavioral referents, such as trait anxiety level or diagnostic status. The artificiality of the experimental stimuli and responses, and the indefiniteness of the psychological conditions being explained, leave inherently unclear how any observed biases relate to people's actual fears, thoughts, and avoidance behaviors in the natural environment.

Processing biases, like other proposed inner causes, need to establish that they are not simply more of countless psychological measures that modestly but significantly predict trait anxiety scores or mental disorder diagnoses. Trait-like general biases for seeing broad classes of information as threatening, like personality traits of all kinds, have little ability to explain the idiosyncratic patterning of people's problems across situations, whereas specific social cognitions encounter no such explanatory limit. Processing of complex meaning information with awareness is powerful, but processing information without any awareness is hard to convincingly demonstrate (e.g., Kouider & Depoux, 2004). Many laboratory information-processing bias effects are less than robust, being eliminated or even reversed in direction by theoretically minor variations in experimental stimuli, subjects, or responses (Mathews & McLeod, 1994, 2002; McNally, 1999). And little evidence exists that any proposed unconscious processing bias strongly predicts actual avoidance behavior and subjective fear remotely as accurately as do the conscious social cognitions that this chapter has already reviewed (Williams, 1996a).

Intriguing recent work has shown effects of induced information-processing biases on experienced anxious feelings (Mathews & McLeod, 2002), suggesting a direct link to human discomfort. The social cognitive view is that anxious people are biased in their processing of not only threat information per se, but of evidence of inability, of personal responsibility, of vulnerability to anxious feelings, and other self-undermining cognitions, which function not as generalized traits, but in attunement with specific psychological and physical contexts.

Panic

Much work has been done on social cognitive factors in panic attacks (e.g., Clark, 1986; Rapee, 1993). Most early work on panic focused on physiological causes (reviewed in detail by Barlow, 2002), and indeed a variety of physical influences, including sodium lactate, carbon dioxide, caffeine, vigorous exercise, rapid breathing, and others can induce panic in vulnerable individuals. The sheer variety of bodily influences on panic suggests the possibility of a common psychological mechanism (Clark, 1986). Psychological models of panic generally conceive it as resulting from perception of threat (Beck et al., 1985), in particular, a vicious cycle of perceiving bodily sensations, interpreting them catastrophically, therefore feeling afraid and apprehensive, which provokes more bodily sensations to be interpreted catastrophically, and so on (Clark, 1986; Rachman & Maser, 1988; Rapee, 1993). A self-efficacy analysis places emphasis also on the belief that one can prevent, limit, or control panic or the thoughts that give rise to it, or function effectively despite panic (Williams & LaBerge, 1994). Evidence supports a role for cognition in panic, including a mediating influence of psychological and environmental manipulations on biological panic induction (Clark, 1993; Rapee, 1993), as well as for cognitive interventions in treatment (discussed later).

Causes of Bothersome Thoughts

Social cognitive theories hold that bothersome thoughts occur in the normal stream of consciousness (Rachman & de Silva, 1978) but become problematic as people appraise, interpret, and respond to them maladaptively. It is less the occurrence of danger thoughts than the belief that one cannot manage potential dangers that gives danger thoughts power to scare (Bandura, 1988). Recent theorizing on obsessions has emphasized an excessive sense of responsibility for potential harmful effects and a corresponding impulse to take preventative actions. When people try to avoid or suppress bothersome intrusions by neutralizing rituals, these can serve merely to increase the thought's frequency and to undermine the sense of control, producing both anxiety and greater efforts to exert control, and so on in a vicious cycle (Rachman, 1998; Salkovskis, 1996a; Steketee & Barlow, 2002). General cognitive deficit theories of obsession fail because, like traits, they are unable to account for the pronounced situational specificity of obsessions (Salkovskis, 1996a). Theories of worry view it as reinforced by anxiety reduction, by a sense of control, or by perceived risk reduction (Borkovec, et al., 1991; Craske, 1999). A sense of control over scary thoughts and self-efficacy for exercising such control appear important (Bandura, 1988; Kent & Gibbons, 1987) and lack of self-efficacy for solving problems is implicated in generalized anxiety and worry (Aikins & Craske, 2001).

TREATMENT

Psychological approaches to helping people overcome avoidance and rituals, subjective fear and panic attacks, and worries, obsessions, and intrusive bothersome thoughts have achieved notable successes in recent decades, although much room for improvement remains (Barlow, 2002; Chambless & Peterman, 2004; Craske, 1999). Nevertheless, the findings make amply clear that behavioral, social, and cognitive methods can greatly improve these problems in many cases.

Treatment of Avoidance and Rituals

Helping people overcome behavioral disabilities is important in its own right, of course, but also because reducing avoidance behaviors robustly reduces the subjective fear, panic, obsessions, intrusive thoughts, and depressed mood that tend to go with them.

Performance-Based Exposure Treatments

Historically pivotal to phobia treatment was the development of systematic desensitization (Wolpe, 1958) and related methods that guide people to imagine doing avoided activities, and vicarious methods (e.g., Bandura, Blanchard, & Ritter, 1969) in which people watch others doing the activities. The next major advance was performance-based treatments, in which people directly perform their avoided activities (e.g., Agras, Leitenberg, & Barlow, 1968; Bandura et al., 1969). In performance-based treatment of rituals the person engages in ritual-provoking activities (e.g., touches the door handle, or thinks "Damn God") but then refrains from the rituals (Rachman & Hodgson, 1980), a method known widely as exposure plus response prevention. Performance-based methods are reliably more effective than methods based on the person only imagining or viewing the activities (Bandura et al., 1969; Emmelkamp & Wessels, 1975; Steketee & Barlow, 2002).

Guided mastery treatment focused entirely on reducing avoidance behavior without explicitly addressing, thinking and feeling can completely eliminate specific phobias and their cognitive and emotional accompaniments within a few hours in the majority of cases (Bandura, 1997; Öst, 1996). The benefits of performance-focused exposure treatment for complex phobias and compulsions are many (Craske, 1999; Rachman & Hodgson, 1980; White & Barlow, 2002). Indeed, phobia treatment is a major ingredient in the treatment of anxiety, panic, stress reactions, and bothersome intrusive thoughts, all of which may be sustained in large part by subtle or gross avoidance behaviors that insulate people from corrective learning experiences (Clark, 1999; Keane & Barlow, 2002; Salkovskis, 1991; Williams, 1985).

Guided Mastery

Imagery-based, vicarious, and performance-based treatments are sometimes called collectively exposure treatments, following the conception that treatment is like a classical extinction procedure in which unreinforced exposure to the conditioned stimulus deconditions fear and avoidance (e.g., Foa & McNally, 1996; Marks, 1978). Commerce with relevant stimuli is required for learning just about anything, but identical durations of exposure to phobic stimuli routinely result in highly disparate degrees of change in phobic behavior, between individuals and between groups (e.g., Bandura et al., 1969; Bandura, Jeffrey, & Wright, 1974; Williams et al., 1984, 1985). The exposure conception points to outer stimuli instead of inner psychological processes, and portrays treatment and behavior change in passive mechanistic deconditioning terms. The social cognitive approach holds that people overcome phobias and compulsions actively in thought and deed (Williams, 1990). By this interpretation, an agoraphobic woman is not exposed to stores, she shops in them; and store stimuli do not extinguish her phobia, she masters it.

In treatment based on self-efficacy theory or guided mastery treatment (Williams, 1990) the therapist seeks to build a strong sense of self-efficacy by fostering people's performance accomplishments. Although the proposed self-efficacy mechanism is cognitive, the recommended procedure is performance, because firsthand behavioral success conveys the most dependable information that one really can do something. The therapist assists people to succeed at tasks that otherwise would be too difficult, and guides them to do tasks proficiently, free of embedded rituals and restrictions that limit their feeling of success. Assisting people to tackle phobic and compulsive problems usually produces better results than does simply encouraging them to expose themselves to scary stimuli and refrain from ritualizing without much help (Abramowitz, 1996; Bandura et al., 1974; Feske & Chambless, 1995; Öst, Salkovskis, & Hellstrom, 1991; Williams et al., 1984; 1985; Williams & Zane, 1989). Cognitive therapies designed to help people lower their overestimates of danger and to adopt more helpful ways of thinking are widely used to treat behavioral avoidance and rituals, but these do not seem to have a reliable impact beyond that achieved by performance methods alone (Feske & Chambless, 1995; Hope, Heimberg, & Bruch, 1995; McLean, Whittal, Thordarson, Taylor, Söchting, Koch, Paterson, & Anderson, 2001; Steketee & Barlow, 2002; Williams & Rappoport, 1983).

Treatment of Anxiety

Subjective Anxiety

People usually feel anxious about something in particular, and often avoid it as well. As mentioned earlier, mastering the avoidance behavior alone often eliminates any accompanying subjective anxiety as a by-product (e.g., Bandura et al., 1969; Öst et al., 1991; Williams et al., 1984). When people can do an activity but feel anxious doing it, social cognitive analyses suggest counteracting subtle avoidance maneuvers, defensive activities, and self-protective rituals that circumscribe their sense of mastery and therefore promote continued anxious feelings (Williams, 1985; Williams & Zane, 1989; Zane & Williams, 1993). This phenomenon is sometimes interpreted in light of safety signals (Clark, 2001; Salkovskis, 1991). When people stop the defensive activities and perform in a proficient varied manner, the anxiety usually goes away quickly (Salkovskis, 1991; Williams & Zane, 1989). Of course subjective anxiety can be treated by guiding people to imagine themselves encountering stressors and coping effectively with them, and by a variety of relaxation and cognitive reappraisal methods (Beck, 1976; Rapee & Barlow, 1991; Wolpe, 1958).

Panic Attacks

Most people with panic attacks display some avoidance behavior, gross or subtle (Salkovskis, 1991), and performance-based therapies for agoraphobic avoidance can have a notable impact on panic attacks (Barlow, 2002; Williams & Falbo, 1996; Michelson, Mavissakalian, & Marchione, 1988). Several treatment methods specifically focused on panic include social cognitive therapies designed to increase rational appraisal and to decatastrophize thinking, somatic interventions to induce autonomic arousal or other bodily responses associated with panic (sometimes called interoceptive exposure), and breathing and relaxation techniques designed to normalize and calm physiological arousal (Craske, 1999; Rachman & Maser, 1988; White & Barlow, 2002).

Early studies of the panic-focused methods applied in combination found them to have strikingly positive effects, enduringly eliminating panic attacks in 85% or more of panicky individuals (Craske, 1999; Rachman & Maser, 1988). In apparent contrast, performance-based therapies initially appeared to reduce panic attacks only moderately. It now appears that the advantage of panic-focused therapies was largely an artifact of subject selection differences. Most studies of panic-focused treatments for panic excluded panicky people who had significant phobias, whereas studies of performance exposure treatments for panic included or even selected for severe agoraphobic disability (Williams & Falbo, 1996). When panicky people who varied widely in agoraphobic disability were given psychological treatments, irrespective of treatment condition significantly more of those with few phobias (96%) became panic-free than did those with many phobias (52%; Williams and Falbo, 1996). A meta-analysis of 13 recent studies of panic treatment by cognitive-behavioral therapies, with diverse selection criteria, found rates of panic-free participants after treatment ranging from 53% to 85%, with a mean of 71% (Chambless & Peterson, in press). Even so, panic-focused methods still have been formally tested mostly on the easier panickers to help and will need to be evaluated further for relieving panic in people who are highly phobic, compulsive, and otherwise disabled. The strongly positive effects of several different psychological interventions, including performance exposure, with many disabled panicky individuals establishes psychological methods as potent treatments for panic.

Treatment of Bothersome Thoughts

Helping people with bothersome thoughts often involves a combination of elements administered together. Perhaps the most widely used technique, regardless of whether the thoughts are worries, obsessions, flashbacks, or visualized future calamities, is with phobia exposure techniques (i.e., enactive or imaginal performance). Worries and obsessions are often accompanied by mental or behavioral avoidance reactions or neutralizing rituals, reassurance-seeking, and other responses that paradoxically maintain and increase intrusions (Craske, 1999; Keane & Barlow, 2002; Rachman, 1998; Salkovskis, 1996a). In a mental equivalent of compulsion treatment, the person deliberately thinks the intrusive thought then practices not mentally reacting to it. Sometimes this kind of thought practice is cast as a behavioral experiment to test and disconfirm problematic beliefs. Cognitive treatments (Clark, 1999; Craske, 1999) involve dialogue aimed at conveying that obsessions are normal, challenging excessive responsibility beliefs and catastrophic meanings, increasing tolerance of uncertainty, and altering problem imagery, but without trying to decrease the number of intrusive thoughts directly (Clark, 1999; Salkovskis, 1996a).

Pharmacological Treatments

This chapter has focused on non-biological causes and treatments, but drugs appear also to have a role to play, so a few general comments on drug treatment are in order. Psychological treatments are more effective than any known drug for some problems such as specific phobias, and appear superior to drugs for panic attacks as well (Barlow, 2002). Generalized phobias, panic, obsessions, and compulsions improve from certain drugs more than from placebo pills (Barlow, 2002), and it appears that some individuals benefit from drugs more than from the psychological treatments they have had. But drug treatments are beset by distinct therapeutic difficulties, including the tendency for problems to return when the drug is withdrawn, whereas psychological treatment benefits tend to be more enduring. People often cannot physically tolerate a drug, may not be allowed to take it (e.g., pregnant women), or may reject the idea of drugs of their own accord. Chemical dependency and drug tolerance/withdrawal reactions including strong rebound and exacerbating effects are common. There is a relative paucity of research comparing pharmacological treatment with psychological treatment and combined treatment although many individuals receive both in practice (Craske, 1999), and of drug research for some kinds of problems such as traumatic stress reactions. Drug treatment research encounters distinctive methodological problems such as high positive response rates among placebo control subjects, difficulty maintaining blindness in drug dispensers and outcome assessors because of visible common side effects, subject attrition due to drug intolerance, and other thorny research problems that limit understanding of drug benefits. Because psychological treatments for most of the problems we have discussed are substantially beneficial to the average individual, and drugs while sometimes beneficial have serious potential shortcomings, it seems generally advisable for therapists to use psychological methods first but be prepared to use pharmacological agents when psychological treatments alone are insufficient.

PREVALENCE OF DISORDER OR DISTRIBUTION OF DIMENSIONAL SCORES?

The rates at which psychological problems occur in the community have been measured for the most part indirectly as prevalence rates of categorical mental disorders rather than directly as frequency distributions of dimensional scores. Probably just about everybody has experienced needless avoidance, fears, and unpleasant thoughts now and again, so their prevalence as mental disorders is largely in the eye of the beholder, dependent on which responses and cutoff criteria one chooses to define disorder and on how assessors actually operationalize the definitions (Williams, in preparation). For example, in one analysis the prevalence of DSM–III generalized anxiety disorder dropped from 45% to 9% of the population when the required duration of anxiety increased from one month to six months and the minimum number of anxiety-defining responses increased from three to six (Breslau & Davis, 1985).

Prevalence of social phobic disorder ranges from about 2% to 19% of the population, depending on cutoff scores and on how diagnostic interviewers pose their questions (Stein,

Walker, & Forde, 1994). Markedly varying prevalence rates are found for posttraumatic stress disorder mainly because of DSM's imprecise nonoperational definitions (e.g., Kessler, Sonnega, Bromet, Hughes, & Nelson, 1995). The impact of ambiguous decision rules is evident in a recent reanalysis of epidemiological findings applying the DSM–IV clinical significance criterion, which changed the United States national prevalence of mental illnesses by 19.2 million people at a single stroke (Narrow, Rae, Robins, & Regier, 2002). It is clear that the prevalence of problems in the population would be far better characterized by distributions of problem dimension scores than by frequency counts of the presence or absence of proposed mental disorders. Nevertheless, estimated prevalences of mental illnesses (e.g., Kendler, 1994) show beyond any doubt that serious psychological problems of the kinds we have been considering are widespread.

I have approached anxiety disorders by encouraging readers to question both anxiety and disorders. Calling psychological phenomena by their own proper names without a pseudo-unifying anxiety label removes a comforting illusion of understanding, but helps us see problem phenomena more clearly on their own terms. Perhaps more important is to deeply question disorder theory. Most critics of psychiatric diagnosis oddly conclude with a wish to use psychological dimensions to develop a better system of categorizing mental disorders. I disagree fundamentally. Here and now dimensions do everything good that disorders do, only much better, and without all the distortions. Far from subordinating psychological science to the medical model, which would be like the victorious General Grant surrendering his army to the defeated General Lee in Mark Twain's tall tale, psychological scientists can celebrate the demise of the medical model and never look back. Needed is not a better understanding of psychopathology and mental illness, but of people's psychological problems. Social cognitive theories achieve notable successes in explaining and ameliorating difficult problems without the need of embracing disjointed multimodal psychic states, including anxiety disorders. We act not because of multimodal anxiety or anxiety disorders, but above all because of our conscious thoughts about our circumstances and ourselves.

Author Note: I thank Dianne Chambless for her helpful comments on a draft of this paper.

REFERENCES

Abramowitz, J. S. (1996). Variants of exposure and response prevention in the treatment of obsessive-compulsive disorder: A meta-analysis. *Behavior Therapy*, *27*, 583–600.

Agras, W. S., Leitenberg, H., & Barlow, D. H. (1968). Social reinforcement in the modification of agoraphobia. *Archives of General Psychiatry*, *19*, 423–427.

Aikins, D. E., & Craske, M. G. (2001). Cognitive theories of generalized anxiety disorder. *Psychiatric Clinics of North America*, *24*, 57–74.

American Psychiatric Association (1994). *Diagnostic and statistical manual of mental disorders* (4th ed., DSM–IV; 3rd ed., DSM–III, 1980; 3rd rev. ed., DSM–III–R, 1987). Washington, DC: Author.

Bandura, A. (1969). *Principles of behavior modification*. New York: Holt, Rinehart, & Winston.

Bandura, A. (1978). On paradigms and recycled ideologies. *Cognitive Therapy and Research*, *2*, 79–103.

Bandura, A. (1986). *Social foundations of thought and action: A social cognitive theory*. Englewood Cliffs, NJ: Prentice-Hall.

Bandura, A. (1988). Self-efficacy conception of anxiety. *Anxiety Research*, *1*, 77–98.

Bandura, A. (1995). On rectifying conceptual ecumenism. In J. E. Maddux (Ed.), *Self-efficacy, adaptation, and adjustment* (pp. 347–375). New York: Plenum.

Bandura, A. (1997). *Self-efficacy: The exercise of control*. New York: Freeman.

Bandura, A., Blanchard, E. B., & Ritter, B. (1969). Relative efficacy of desensitization and modeling approaches for inducing behavioral, affective, and attitudinal changes. *Journal of Personality and Social Psychology*, *13*, 173–199.

Bandura, A., Jeffrey, R. W., & Wright, C. L. (1974). Efficacy of participant modeling as a function of response induction aids. *Journal of Abnormal Psychology, 83*, 35–64.

Barlow, D. H. (1987). The classification of anxiety disorders. In G. L. Tischler (Ed.), *Diagnosis and classification in psychiatry* (pp. 223–242). Cambridge: Cambridge University Press.

Barlow, D. H. (2002). *Anxiety and its disorders*. New York: Guilford.

Beck, A. T. (1976). *Cognitive therapy and the emotional disorders*. New York: International Universities Press.

Beck, A. T., Emery, G., & Greenberg, R. L. (1985). *Anxiety disorders and phobias: A cognitive perspective*. New York: Basic Books.

Beck, A. T., Epstein, N., Brown, G., & Steer, R. A. (1988). An inventory for measuring clinical anxiety: Psychometric properties. *Journal of Consulting and Clinical Psychology, 56*, 893–897.

Bienvenu, O. J., Nestadt, M. B., & Eaton, W. W. (1998). Characterizing generalized anxiety: Temporal and symptomatic thresholds. *Journal of Nervous and Mental Disease,* 186:51–56.

Bolles, R. C. (1975). *Learning theory*. New York: Holt, Rinehart, & Winston.

Borkovec, T. D., Shadick, R. N., & Hopkins, M. (1991). The nature of normal and pathological worry. In R. M. Rapee & D. H. Barlow (Eds.), *Chronic anxiety: Generalized anxiety disorder and mixed anxiety-depression* (pp. 29–51). New York: Guilford.

Boyd, J. H., Burke, J. D., Gruenberg, E., Holzer, C. E., Rae, D. S., George, L. K., Karno, M., Stoltzman, R., McEvoy, L., & Nestadt, G. (1987). The exclusion criteria of DSM–III. In G. L. Tischler (Ed.), *Diagnosis and classification in psychiatry* (pp. 403–424). Cambridge: Cambridge University Press.

Breslau, N., & Davis, G. C. (1985). Further evidence on the doubtful validity of generalized anxiety disorder. *Psychiatry Research, 16*, 177–179.

Brown, T. A., & Barlow, D. H. (2002). Classification of anxiety and mood disorders. In D. Barlow (Ed./author), *Anxiety and its disorders* (pp. 292–327). New York: Guilford.

Campbell, D. T., & Fiske, D. (1959). Convergent and discriminant validation by the multitrait-multimethod matrix. *Psychological Bulletin, 56*, 81–105.

Carr, A. T. (1979). The psychopathology of fear. In W. Sluckin (Ed.), *Fear in animals and man* (pp. 199–235). New York: Van Nostrand Reinhold.

Cassano, G. B., Pini, S., Saettoni, M., & Dell'Osso, L. (1999). Multiple anxiety disorder comorbidity in patients with mood spectrum disorders with psychotic features. *American Journal of Psychiatry, 156*, 474–476.

Cattell, R. B., & Scheier, I. H. (1961). *The meaning and measurement of neuroticism and anxiety*. New York: Ronald Press.

Chambless, D. L., Beck, A. T., Gracely, E. J., & Grisham, J. R. (2000). Relationships of cognitions to fear of somatic symptoms: A test of the cognitive theory of panic. *Depression and Anxiety, 11*, 1–9.

Chambless, D. L., & Gracely, E. J. (1989). Fear of fear and the anxiety disorders. *Cognitive Therapy and Research, 13*, 9–20.

Chambless, D. L., & Peterman, M. (in press-2004). Cognitive behavior therapy for generalized anxiety disorder and panic disorder: The second decade. In R. L. Leahy (Ed.). *New frontiers of cognitive therapy*. New York: Guilford.

Cioffi, D. (1991). Beyond attentional strategies: A cognitive-perceptual model of somatic interpretation. *Psychological Bulletin, 109*, 25–41.

Clark, D. M. (1986). A cognitive approach to panic. *Behaviour Research and Therapy, 24*, 461–470.

Clark, D. M. (1993). Cognitive mediation of panic attacks induced by biological challenge tests. *Advances in Behaviour Research and Therapy, 15*, 75–84.

Clark, D. M. (1999). Anxiety disorders: Why they persist and how to treat them. *Behaviour Research and Therapy, 37*(Suppl.), S5–S27.

Clark, D. M. (2001). A cognitive perspective on social phobia. In W. R. Crozier & L. E. Alden (Eds.), *International handbook of social anxiety: Concepts, research, and interventions relating to the self and shyness* (pp. 405–430). Chichester: Wiley.

Clark, D. M., Salkovskis, P. M., & Chalkley, A. J. (1985). Respiratory control as a treatment for panic attacks. *Journal of Behavior Therapy and Experimental Psychiatry, 16*, 23–30.

Clark, D. M., Salkovskis, P. M., Öst, L.-G., Breitholtz, E., Koehler, K. A., Westling, B. E., Jeavons, A., & Gelder, M. (1997). Misinterpretation of body sensations in panic disorder. *Journal of Consulting and Clinical Psychology, 65*, 203–213.

Clark, L. A., Watson, D., & Reynolds, S. (1995). Diagnosis and classification of psychopathology: Challenges to the current system and future directions. *Annual Review of Psychology, 46,* 121–153.

Cohen, J. (1983). The cost of dichotomization. *Applied Psychological Measurement, 7*, 249–253.

Cohen, J. (1990). Things I have learned (so far). *American Psychologist, 45*, 1304–1312.

Cook, E. W., Melamed, B. G., Cuthbert, B. N., McNeil, D. W., & Lang, P. J. (1988). Emotional imagery and the differential diagnosis of anxiety. *Journal of Consulting and Clinical Psychology, 56*, 734–740.

Cosoff, S. J., & Hafner, R. J. (1998). The prevalence of comorbid anxiety in schizophrenia, schizoaffective disorder and bipolar disorder. *Australian and New Zealand Journal of Psychiatry, 32,* 67–72.

Craske, M. G. (1991). Phobic fear and panic attacks: The same emotional states triggered by different cues? *Clinical Psychology Review, 11,* 599–620.

Craske, M. G. (1999). *Anxiety disorders: Psychological approaches to theory and treatment.* Boulder, CO: Westview.

Craske, M. G., & Barlow, D. H. (1988). A review of the relationship between panic and avoidance. *Clinical Psychology Review, 8,* 667–685.

Craske, M. G., Bunt, R., Rapee, R. M., & Barlow, D. H. (1991). Perceived control and controllability during in vivo exposure: Spider phobics. *Journal of Anxiety Disorders, 5,* 285–292.

Craske, M. G., Rapee, R. M., Jackel, L., & Barlow, D. H. (1989). Qualitative dimensions of worry in DSM-III-R generalized anxiety disorder subjects and nonanxious controls. *Behaviour Research and Therapy, 27,* 397–402.

Davey, G. C. L. (1992). Classical conditioning and the acquisition of human fears and phobias: A review and synthesis of the literature. *Advances in Behaviour Research and Therapy, 14,* 29–66.

Ehlers, A. (1993). Interoception and panic disorder. *Advances in Behaviour Research and Therapy, 15,* 3–21.

Emmelkamp, P. M. G., & Wessels, H. (1975). Flooding in imagination vs. flooding in vivo: A comparison with agoraphobics. *Behaviour Research and Therapy, 13,* 7–15.

Feske, U., & Chambless, D. L. (1995). Cognitive behavioral versus exposure only treatment for social phobia: A meta-analysis. *Behavior Therapy, 26,* 695–720.

Foa, E. B., & McNally, R. J. (1996). Mechanisms of change in exposure therapy. In R. Rapee (Ed.), *Current controversies in the anxiety disorders* (pp. 329–343). New York: Guilford.

Freeman, D., & Garety, P. A. (1999). Worry, worry processes, and the dimensions of delusions: An exploratory investigation of a role for anxiety processes in the maintenance of delusional distress. *Behavioural and Cognitive Psychotherapy, 27,* 47–62.

Freeston, M. H., Ladouceur, R., Rheaume, J, Letarte, H., Gagnon, F., & Thibodeau, N. (1994). Self-report of obsessions and worry. *Behaviour Research and Therapy, 32,* 29–36.

Frost, R. O., & Steketee, G. (2002). *Cognitive approaches to obsessions and compulsions: Theory, assessment, and treatment.* Elsevier: Oxford.

Hawton, K., Salkovskis, P. M., Kirk, J., & Clark, D. M. (1989). *Cognitive behaviour therapy for psychiatric problems.* Oxford: Oxford University Press.

Hersen, M. (1973). Self-assessment of fear. *Behavior Therapy, 4,* 241–257.

Hoehn-Saric, R. (1998). Psychic and somatic anxiety: Worries, somatic symptoms, and physiological changes. *Acta Psychiatrica Scandinavica, 98*(Suppl. 393), 32–38.

Hoffman, S. G., & Barlow, D. H. (2002). Social phobia (social anxiety disorder). In D. H. Barlow, *Anxiety and its disorders* (pp. 454–476). New York: Guilford.

Hoffman, S. G., Lehman, C. L., & Barlow, D. H. (1997). How specific are specific phobias? *Journal of Behavior Therapy and Experimental Psychiatry, 28,* 233–240.

Holden, A. E., & Barlow, D. H. (1986). Heart rate and heart rate variability recorded in vivo in agoraphobcs and nonphobics. *Behavior Therapy, 17,* 25–42.

Hope, D. A., Heimberg, R. G., & Bruch, M. A. (1995). Dismantling cognitive-behavioral group therapy for social phobia. *Behaviour Research and Therapy, 33,* 637–650.

Johns, L. C., & Van Os, J. (2001). The continuity of psychotic experiences in the general population. *Clinical Psychology Review, 21,* 1125–1141.

Katerndahl, D. A., & Realini, J. P. (1993). Lifetime prevalence of panic states. *American Journal of Psychiatry, 150,* 246–249.

Keane, T. M., & Barlow, D. H. (2002). Posttraumatic stress disorder. In D. H. Barlow (Ed./author), *Anxiety and its disorders* (pp. 418–453). New York: Guilford.

Kendler, K. S. (1994). Lifetime and 12-month prevalence of DSM–III–R psychiatric disorders in the United States: Results from the National Comorbidity Survey. *Archives of General Psychiatry, 51,* 8–19.

Kent, G., & Gibbons, R. (1987). Self-efficacy and the control of anxious cognitions. *Journal of Behavior Therapy and Experimental Psychiatry, 18,* 33–40.

Kessler, R. C., Sonnega, A., Bromet, E., Hughes, M., & Nelson, C. B. (1995). Posttraumatic stress disorder in the National Comorbidity Survey. *Archives of General Psychiatry, 52,* 1048–1060.

Kirsch, I. (1990). *Changing expectations.* Belmont, CA: Brooks-Cole.

Klein, D. F. (1980). Anxiety reconceptualized. *Comprehensive Psychiatry, 21,* 411–427.

Kouider, S., & Dupoux, E. (2004). Partial awareness creates the "illusion" of subliminal semantic priming. *Psychological Science, 15,* 75–81.

Krabbendam, L., Janssen, I., Bak, M., Bilj, R. V., de Graaf, R., & Van Os, J. (2002). Neuroticism and low self-esteem as risk factors for psychosis. *Social Psychiatry and Psychiatric Epidemiology, 37,* 1–6.

Lacey, J. I. (1967). Somatic response patterning and stress: Some revisions of activation theory. In M. H. Appley & R. Trumbull (Eds.), *Psychological stress: Issues in research* (pp. 14–42). New York: Appleton Century Crofts.

Lang, P. J. (1985). The cognitive psychophysiology of emotion: Fear and anxiety. In A. H. Tuma & J. D. Maser (Eds.), *Anxiety and the anxiety disorders* (pp. 131–170). Hillsdale, NJ: Lawrence Erlbaum Associates.

Lang, P. J., Cuthbert, B. N., & Bradley, M. M. (1998). Measuring emotion in therapy: Imagery, activation, and feeling. *Behavior Therapy, 29*, 655–674.

Lang, P. J., Levin, D. N., Miller, G. A., & Kozak, M. J. (1983). Fear behavior, fear imagery, and the psychophysiology of emotion: The problem of affective response intregration. *Journal of Abnormal Psychology, 92*, 275–306.

Leary, M. R., & Kowalski, R. M. (1995). The self-presentational model of social phobia. In R. G. Heimberg, M. R. Liebowitz, D. A. Hope, & F. R. Schneier (Eds.), *Social phobia: diagnosis, assessment, treatment* (pp. 94–112). New York: Guilford.

Lipsitz, J. D., Barlow, D. H., Mannuzza, S., Hoffman, S. G., & Fyer, A. J. (2002). Clinical features of four DSM-IV-specific phobia subtypes. *Journal of Nervous and Mental Disease, 190*, 471–478.

Maddux, J. E. (Ed.) (1995a). *Self-efficacy, adaptation, and adjustment: theory, research, application.* New York: Plenum.

Maddux, J. E. (1995b). Looking for common ground: A comment on Kirsch and Bandura. In J. Maddux (Ed.), *Self-efficacy, adaptation, and adjustment: Theory, research, application* (pp. 377–385). New York: Plenum.

Maddux, J. E., Norton, L. W., & Leary, M. R. (1988). Cognitive components of social anxiety: An investigation of the integration of self-presentational theory and self-efficacy theory. *Journal of Social and Clinical Psychology, 6*, 180–190.

Magee, W. J., Eaton, W. W., Wittchen, H.-U., McGonagne, K. A., & Kessler, R. C. (1996). Agoraphobia, simple phobia, and social phobia in the National Comorbidity Survey. *Archives of General Psychiatry, 53*, 159–168.

Mandler, G. (1962). Emotion. In R. Brown, E. Galanter, E. Hess, & G. Mandler (Eds.), *New directions in psychology: Vol. 1.* (pp. 269–343). New York: Holt, Rinehart, & Winston.

Margraf, J., Taylor, C. B., Ehlers, A., Roth, W. T., & Agras, W. S. (1987). Panic attacks in the natural environment. *Journal of Nervous and Mental Disease, 175*, 558–565.

Marks, I. M. (1978). Behavioral psychotherapy of adult neurosis. In S. L. Garfield & A. E. Bergin (Eds.), *Handbook of psychotherapy and behavior change* (pp. 493–547). New York: Wiley.

Marks, I. M. (1987). *Fears, phobias, and rituals.* New York: Oxford.

Marshall, R. D., Olfson, M., Hellman, F., Blanco, C., Guardino, M., & Struening, E. L. (2001). Comorbidity, impairment, and suicidality in subthreshold PTSD. *American Journal of Psychiatry, 158*, 1467–1473.

Mathews, A. M., Gelder, M. G., & Johnston, D. W. (1981). *Agoraphobia: Nature and treatment.* New York: Guilford.

Mathews, A. M., & MacLeod, C. (1994). Cognitive approaches to emotion and emotion disorders. *Annual Review of Psychology, 45*, 25–50.

Mathews, A., & MacLeod, C. (2002). Induced processing biases have causal effects on anxiety. *Cognition and Emotion, 16*, 331–354.

McLean, P. D., Whittal, M. L., Thordarson, D. S. Taylor, S., Söchting, I., Koch, W. J., Paterson, R., & Anderson, K. W. (2001). Cognitive versus behavioral therapy in the group treatment of obsessive compulsive disorder. *Journal of Consulting and Clinical Psychology, 69*, 205–214.

Michelson, L., Mavissakalian, M., & Marchione, M. (1988). Cognitive, behavioral, and psychophysiological treatments of agoraphobia: A comparative outcome investigation. *Behavior Therapy, 19*, 97–120.

Mineka, S. (1979). The role of fear in theories of avoidance learning, flooding, and extinction. *Psychological Bulletin, 86*, 985–1010.

Mineka, S., Davidson, M., Cook, M., & Keir, R. (1984). Observational conditioning of snake fear in rhesus monkeys. *Journal of Abnormal Psychology, 93*, 344–372.

Mineka, S., & Kelly, K. A. (1989). The relationship between anxiety, lack of control and loss of control. In A. Steptoe and A. Appels (Eds.), *Stress, personal control and health* (pp. 163–191). New York: Wiley.

Mischel, W. (1990). Personality dispositions revisited and revised: A view after three decades. In L. A. Pervin (Ed.), *Handbook of personality: Theory and research* (pp. 111–164). New York: Guilford.

Moore, R., Brodsgaard, I., & Birn, H. (1991). Manifestations, acquisition and diagnostic categories of dental fear in a self-referred population. *Behaviour Research and Therapy, 29*, 51–60.

Morrow, G. R., & Labrum, A. H. (1978). The relationship between psychological and physiological measures of anxiety. *Psychological Medicine, 8*, 95–101.

Mowrer, O. H. (1960). *Learning theory and behavior.* New York: Wiley.

Muris, P., Merckelbach, H., & Clavan, M. (1997). Abnormal and normal compulsions. *Behaviour Research and Therapy, 35*, 249–252.

Narrow, W. E., Rae, D. S., Robins, L. N., Regier, D. A. (2002). Revised prevalence estimates of mental disorders in the United States. *Archives of General Psychiatry, 59*, 115–123.

Neria, Y., Bromet, E. J., Sievers, S., LaVelle, J., & Fochtmann, L. J. (2002). Trauma exposure and post-traumatic stress disorder in psychosis: Findings from a first-admission cohort. *Journal of Consulting and Clinical Psychology, 70,* 246–251.

Norton, G. R., Cox, B. J., & Malan, J. (1992). Nonclinical panickers: A critical review. *Clinical Psychology Review, 12,* 121–139.

O'Dwyer, A., & Marks, I. M. (2000). Obsessive-compulsive disorder and delusions revisited. *British Journal of Psychiatry, 176,* 281–284.

Öst, L.-G. (1996). Long term effects of behavior therapy for specific phobias. In M. R. Mavissakalian & R. F. Prien (Eds.), *Long term treatments of the anxiety disorders.* Washington, DC: American Psychiatric Press.

Öst, L.-G., Ferebee, I., & Furmark T. (1997). One-session group therapy of spider phobia: Direct versus indirect treatments. *Behaviour Research and Therapy, 35,* 721–732.

Öst, L.-G, Salkovskis, P., & Hellstrom, K. (1991). One-session therapist-directed exposure vs. self-exposure in the treatment of spider phobia. *Behavior Therapy, 22,* 407–422.

Pennebaker, J. W. (1982). *The psychology of physical symptoms.* New York: Springer-Verlag.

Persons, J. (1986). The advantages of studying psychological phenomena rather than psychiatric diagnoses. *American Psychologist, 11,* 1252–1260.

Rachman, S. (1976). The passing of the two-stage theory of fear and avoidance: Fresh possibilities. *Behaviour Research and Therapy, 14,* 125–131.

Rachman, S. (1977). The conditioning theory of fear acquisition: A critical examination: *Behaviour Research and Therapy, 15,* 375–387.

Rachman, S. (1998). A cognitive theory of obsessions: Elaborations. *Behaviour Research and Therapy, 36,* 385–401.

Rachman, S., & de Silva, P. (1978). Abnormal and normal obsessions. *Behavior Research and Therapy, 16,* 233–248.

Rachman, S., & Hodgson, R. (1974). I. Synchrony and desynchrony in fear and avoidance. *Behaviour Research and Therapy, 12,* 311–318.

Rachman, S., & Hodgson, R. (1980). *Obsessions and compulsions.* Englewood Cliffs, NJ: Prentice-Hall.

Rachman, S., & Maser, J. D. (Eds.) (1988). *Panic: psychological perspectives.* Hillsdale, NJ: Lawrence Erlbaum.

Rapee, R. M. (1993). Psychological factors in panic disorder. *Advances in Behavior Research and Therapy, 15,* 85–102.

Rapee, R. M. (1995). Psychological factors influencing the affective response to biological challenge procedures in panic disorder. *Journal of Anxiety Disorders, 9,* 59–74.

Rapee, R. M., & Barlow, D. H. (Eds.) (1991). *Chronic anxiety.* New York: Guilford.

Salkovskis, P. M. (1991). The importance of behavior in the maintenance of anxiety and panic: A cognitive account. *Behavioural Psychotherapy, 19,* 6–19.

Salkovskis, P. M. (1996a). Cognitive-behavioral approaches to the understanding of obsessional problems. In R. M. Rapee (Ed.), *Current controversies in the anxiety disorders* (pp. 103–133). New York: Guilford.

Salkovskis, P. M. (1996b). Understanding of obsessive-compulsive disorder is not improved by redefining it as something else. In R. M. Rapee (Ed.), *Current controversies in the anxiety disorders* (pp. 191–200). New York: Guilford.

Salkovskis, P. M. (1998). Psychological approaches to the understanding of obsessional problems. In R. P. Swinson, M. M. Anthony, S. Rachman, & M. A. Richter (Eds.), *Obsessive-compulsive disorder: Theory, research,and treatment* (pp. 33–50). New York: Guilford.

Salkovskis, P. M., & Harrison, J. (1984). Abnormal and normal obsessions: A replication. *Behaviour Research and Therapy, 22,* 549–552.

Salkovskis, P. M., & Warwick, H. M. C. (1986). Morbid preoccupations, health anxiety and reassurance: A cognitive-behavioural approach to hypochondriasis. *Behaviour Research and Therapy, 24,* 597–602.

Schwartz, B. (1978). *Psychology of learning and behavior.* New York: Norton.

Schwartz, B. (1989). *Psychology of learning and behavior* (3rd ed.). New York: Norton.

Schwarzer, R. (Ed.)(1992). *Self-efficacy: Thought control of action.* Washington DC: Hemisphere.

Seligman, M. E. P., & Johnston, J. C. (1973). A cognitive theory of avoidance learning. In F. J. McGuigan & D. B. Lumsden (Eds.), *Contemporary approaches to conditioning and learning* (pp. 69–110). Washington, DC: Winston & Sons.

Skinner, B. F. (1957). *Verbal behavior.* New York: Appleton-Century-Crofts.

Spielberger, C. D. (1983). *Manual for the State-Trait Anxiety Inventory.* Palo Alto, CA: Consulting Psychologists.

Spitzer, R. L., & Williams, J. B. W. (1985). Proposed revisions in the DSM-III classification of anxiety disorders based on research and clinical experience. In A. H. Tuma & J. D. Maser (Eds.), *Anxiety and the anxiety disorders* (pp. 759–773). Hillsdale, NJ: Lawrence Erlbaum Associates.

Stein, M. B., Walker, J. R., & Forde, D. R., (1994). Setting diagnostic thresholds for social phobia: Considerations from a community study of social anxiety. *American Journal of Psychiatry, 152,* 408–412.

Steketee, G., & Barlow, D. H. (2002). Obsessive-compulsive disorder. In D. H. Barlow, *Anxiety and its disorders* (pp. 516–550). New York: Guilford.

Taylor, C. B., Sheikh, J., Agras, W. S., Roth, W. T., Margraf, J., Ehlers, A., Maddock, R. J., & Gossard, D. (1986). Ambulatory heart rate changes in patients with panic attacks. *American Journal of Psychiatry, 143,* 478–482.

Turner, S. M., Beidel, D., & Stanley, M. A. (1992). Are obsessional thoughts and worry different cognitive phenomena? *Clinical Psychology Review, 12*, 257–270.

Walk, R. D., (1956). Self ratings of fear in a fear-invoking situation. *Journal of Abnormal and Social Psychology, 52*, 171–178.

Wells, A., & Papageorgiou, C. (1998). Relationships between worry, obsessive-compulsive symptoms and meta-cognitive beliefs. *Behaviour Research and Therapy, 36*, 899–913.

White, K. S., & Barlow, D. H. (2002). Panic disorder and agoraphobia. In D. H. Barlow, *Anxiety and its disorders* (pp. 328–379). New York: Guilford.

Williams, S. L. (in preparation). *The case against anxiety disorders.*

Williams, S. L. (1985). On the nature and measurement of agoraphobia. *Progress in Behavior Modification, 19*, 109–144.

Williams, S. L. (1986, August). Self-appraisal determinants of defensive behavior and emotional arousal. In R. Ganellen (Chair), *Agoraphobia: Cognitive contributions*. Symposium conducted at the meeting of the American Psychological Association, Washington, DC.

Williams, S. L. (1987). On anxiety and phobia. *Journal of Anxiety Disorders, 1*, 161–180.

Williams, S. L. (1990). Guided mastery treatment of agoraphobia: Beyond stimulus exposure. *Progress in Behavior Modification, 26*, 89–121.

Williams, S. L. (1995). Self-efficacy, anxiety, and phobic disorders. In J. Maddux (Ed.), *Self-efficacy, adaptation, and adjustment: Theory, research, and application* (pp. 69–107). New York: Plenum.

Williams, S. L. (1996a). Therapeutic changes in phobic behavior are mediated by changes in perceived self-efficacy. In R. Rapee (Ed.), *Current controversies in the anxiety disorders* (pp. 344–368). New York: Guilford.

Williams, S. L. (1996b). Overcoming phobia: Unconscious bioinformational deconditioning or conscious cognitive reappraisal? In R. Rapee (Ed.), *Current controversies in the anxiety disorders* (pp. 373–376). New York: Guilford.

Williams, S. L., & Cervone, D. (1998). Social cognitive theories of personality. In D. F. Barone, M. Hersen, & V. B. Van Hasselt (Eds.), *Advanced personality* (pp. 173–207). New York: Plenum.

Williams, S. L., Dooseman, G., & Kleifield, E. (1984). Comparative effectiveness of guided mastery and exposure treatments for intractable phobias. *Journal of Consulting and Clinical Psychology, 52*, 505–518.

Williams, S. L., & Falbo, J. (1996). Cognitive and performance-based treatments for panic attacks in people with varying degrees of agoraphobic disability. *Behaviour Research and Therapy, 34*, 253–264.

Williams, S. L., & Kinney, P. J. (1997, November). Variation in response to agoraphobia treatment as a function of causal attributions for performance success. In S. Bouchard (Chair), *Factors associated with failure in the treatment of panic disorder with agoraphobia*. Symposium at the meeting of the Association for Advancement of Behavior Therapy, Miami, FL.

Williams, S. L., Kinney, P. J., & Falbo, J. (1989). Generalization of therapeutic changes in agoraphobia: The role of perceived self-efficacy. *Journal of Consulting and Clinical Psychology, 57*, 436–442.

Williams, S. L., Kinney, P. J., Harap, S., & Liebmann, M. (1997). Thoughts of agoraphobic people during scary tasks. *Journal of Abnormal Psychology, 106*, 511–520.

Williams, S. L., & LaBerge, B. (1994). Panic disorder with agoraphobia. In C. G. Last & M. Hersen (Eds.), *Adult behavior therapy casebook* (pp. 107–123). New York: Plenum.

Williams, S. L., & Rappoport, A. (1983). Cognitive treatment in the natural environment for agoraphobics. *Behavior Therapy, 14*, 299–313.

Williams, S. L., Turner, S. M., & Peer, D. F. (1985). Guided mastery and performance desensitization treatments for severe acrophobia. *Journal of Consulting and Clinical Psychology, 53*, 237–247.

Williams, S. L., & Watson, N. (1985). Perceived danger and perceived self-efficacy as cognitive determinants of acrophobic behavior. *Behavior Therapy, 16*, 237–247.

Williams, S. L., & Zane, G. (1989). Guided mastery and stimulus exposure treatments for severe performance anxiety in agoraphobics. *Behaviour Research and Therapy, 27*, 237–247.

Wilson, K. G., Sandler, L. S., Asmundson, G. J. G., Ediger, J. M., Larsen, D. K., & Walker, J. R. (1992). Panic attacks in the nonclinical population: an empirical approach to case identification. *Journal of Abnormal Psychology, 101*, 460–468.

Wolpe, J. (1958). *Psychotherapy by reciprocal inhibition*. Stanford, CA: Stanford University Press.

World Health Organization (1992). *The ICD-10 classification of mental and behavioural disorders: Clinical description and diagnostic guidelines*. Geneva: Author.

Yarura-Tobias, J. A., & McKay, D. (2002). Obsessive compulsive disorder and schizophrenia: a cognitive perspective of shared pathology. In R. O. Frost & G. Steketee (Eds.), *Cognitive approaches to obsessions and compulsions: Theory, assessment, and treatment* (pp. 251–267). Oxford: Pergamon.

Zajonc, R. B., & McIntosh, D. N. (1992). Emotions research: some promising questions and some questionable promises. *Psychological Science, 3*, 70–74.

Zane, G., & Williams, S. L. (1993). Performance-related anxiety in agoraphobia: Treatment procedures and cognitive mechanisms of change. *Behavior Therapy, 24*, 625–643.

8

Mood Disorders

Rick Ingram
University of Kansas

Lucy Trenary
University of Colorado

Depression is not a recent phenomenon. Although descriptions of conditions resembling depression can be found in the Old Testament of the Bible, it was Hippocrates in the fourth century B.C. who hypothesized that melancholia stemmed from an imbalance of black bile. Even more modern conceptions of depression were suggested by Aretaeus of Cappadocia around 120 A.D., who described melancholia as being characterized by sadness, a tendency toward suicide, feelings of indifference, and psychomotor agitation. It was not until the early 20th century that theorists such as Abraham (1911–1960) and Freud (1856–1939) began to recognize the importance of psychological and emotional factors in the development of depression.

Today depression is not only widely recognized as a significant public health concern, but its prevalence rates are increasing so much that some researchers have argued that the public faces a depression epidemic (Seligman, 1990). Depression is associated with a wide variety of problems including social withdrawal, occupational disability, and interpersonal turmoil. Furthermore, depression is frequently a chronic condition; relapse and recurrence rates are quite high (Hammen, 1991a; Ingram, Miranda, & Segal, 1998), and individuals who experience recurrent depression are also at considerable risk for developing dysthymia as well as other psychiatric conditions. Apart from the emotional misery that is linked to depression, suicide and suicide attempts are not uncommon during depressive episodes. Even over and above suicide rates, data also show that depression is related to earlier mortality (Saz & Dewey, 2001).

In this chapter we examine a number of facets of mood disorders. Although mood disorders include both unipolar depression and bipolar disorder, the majority of our focus is on unipolar depression. We start by briefly describing the various mood disorders presented in the fourth edition of the *Diagnostic and Statistical Manual of Mental Disorders* (American Psychiatric Association, 2000), noting the approach taken by the DSM as well as discussing some limitations. We next move to a discussion of the epidemiology of depression and then provide some perspectives on gender differences and cultural issues in depression. Following this, we examine theory and research on depression. In particular, we discuss the role of stress in depression with specific reference to diathesis–stress hypotheses, and then examine biologically based models of depression and psychologically based models. We conclude with an examination of data on the prevention of depression and data on biological and psychological approaches to treatment.

DEFINITIONS AND DESCRIPTIONS OF MOOD DISORDERS

Issues in Defining Mood Disorders

Psychopathological constructs such as depression can be viewed in a variety of ways. For instance, Nurcombe (1992) has argued that the term *depression* can be used to indicate a mood state, a symptom or sign, a syndrome consisting of a constellation of symptoms, a disorder that allows for the identification of a group of individuals, or a disease that is associated with biochemical or genetic abnormalities. Similarly, Kendall, Hollon, Beck, Hammen, and Ingram (1987) note that depression can be a symptom (e.g., being sad), a syndrome (e.g., a constellation of signs and symptoms that cluster together), or a mental disorder. Although each use of these definitions is a legitimate descriptor of a state or condition, they can be the source of confusion when used interchangeably. Adding to possible confusion, a number of specific subtypes of depression have been proposed. For instance, a relatively early distinction differentiated between reactive depressions, which were thought specifically to be associated with stressful events, and endogenous depression, which was less related to stress and more associated with internal dysregulation. With few exceptions there has been little agreement on the nature of specific subtypes. This is not to suggest, however, that subtypes do not exist, but rather that these subtypes are difficult to pin down conceptually and empirically. Indeed, there is wide consensus that there may be a number of types of depression, and that depression itself is a label for a heterogeneous group of conditions that result in a similar symptom constellation, but that may have very different causes and courses. Despite this uncertainty over the nature of the various types of depression, the most widely used set of definitions of depression is incorporated in the *Diagnostic Statistical Manual*, fourth edition (DSM–IV–TR), of the American Psychiatric Association.

The DSM is a taxonomic system of behavior categorization. Specifically, diagnostic categories in the DSM reflect an attempt to develop a taxonomy that differentiates and then classifies dysfunctional behavior. It is important to note, however, that such taxonomic systems are not fixed, but rather, evolve as concepts and paradigms shift and, correspondingly, become more complex with a deeper appreciation of natural phenomena. Indeed, psychiatric taxonomy illustrates just such an evolutionary process; since its introduction in 1952, the DSM has undergone four extensive revisions with depression being defined in somewhat different ways in each edition.

DSM-Defined Diagnoses

Mood disorders can be conceptualized as falling into two main categories: unipolar and bipolar disorders. The following represents the categorizations of mood disorders as described by the *Diagnostic Statistical Manual*, fourth edition (DSM–IV–TR). In brief, DSM–IV includes diagnoses for unipolar depression, dysthymic disorder, bipolar disorder, and cyclothymic disorder, as well as more minor categories, which include depressive disorder not otherwise specified, bipolar disorder not otherwise specified, mood disorder due to a general medical condition, substance-induced mood disorder, and mood disorder not otherwise specified. We focus here on a brief description of the major categories of mood disorders.

Unipolar Depression. In unipolar depression, an individual suffers from one or more major depressive episodes. A major depressive episode is defined as persisting for a period of at least two weeks, with the experience of at least one of two cardinal features. These two cardinal features are depressed mood and anhedonia, which is defined as a loss of pleasure in activities that are usually enjoyable. In total, individuals must endorse five of the following nine symptoms: depressed mood, anhedonia, appetite or weight changes, insomnia or hypersomnia, psychomotor agitation or retardation, loss of energy, feelings of worthlessness or guilt, diminished ability to concentrate or indecision, or suicide ideation. It is important to note that the depressed mood exemplifies a change from the person's normal functioning. In addition, symptoms and altered functioning must be associated with significant distress or impairment.

Dysthymic Disorder. Dysthymic disorder can best be thought of as a chronic, low-grade depression that lasts for at least two years. The same symptoms as in a major depressive episode are present, but in this case fewer and less severe symptoms are needed for a diagnosis. Because of the chronicity of dysthymic disorder, the depressed mood and associated symptoms often become integrated into a person's normal functioning (American Psychiatric Association, 2000). According to DSM–IV–TR, after the first two years of depressed mood, if a major depressive episode also occurs, the combination is referred to as double depression.

Bipolar Disorder. Bipolar I and Bipolar II are two main types of bipolar disorders. The presence of a manic or mixed episode defines Bipolar I. A depressive episode does not have to occur to fall into this category. A manic episode is defined as a period of at least one week where mood is abnormally expansive, elevated, or irritable. Three (or four if mood is irritable only) out of seven symptoms must also be endorsed: inflated self-esteem or grandiosity, decreased need for sleep, more talkative than usual, flight of ideas, distractibility, increase in goal-directed activity, and excessive involvement in pleasurable activities that are likely to have adverse consequences. Individuals with Bipolar I disorder may engage in a number of risky activities and often exhibit poor judgment. Besides a manic episode, one may also have a mixed episode to qualify for Bipolar I disorder. A mixed episode lasts at least a week, during which the criteria are met for both a major depressive episode and a manic episode on a daily basis with the individual's mood state alternating between these extremes.

Bipolar II disorder is characterized by one or more major depressive episodes accompanied by at least one hypomanic episode. Though similar to a manic episode, hypomanic symptoms last for a minimum of four days, as opposed to the seven required for mania. Individuals endorse the same number and types of symptoms as with mania. Functioning is not as greatly impaired, and psychotic features are not present.

Cyclothymic Disorder. Like dysthymia, cyclothymia is a chronic disorder (lasting at least two years) during which an individual fluctuates between depressive and hypomanic symptoms. Both classes of symptoms are of insufficient number, severity, and duration to warrant a diagnosis of a major depressive episode or hypomania. No major depressive, manic, or mixed episode can occur during the first two years, though they may co-occur with the cyclothymia once this initial period has passed.

Potential Problems With the DSM Classification System

The DSM represents one important way of conceptualizing depression. Indeed, it has become the "gold standard" in psychopathology research and practice—researchers design their studies based on DSM criteria, and clinicians give their patients a diagnosis aligned with the criteria in this manual. But it is important to understand that the classification system of the DSM is only one of many potential ways to conceptualize the construct of depression.

The two major ways to view depression are categorically and dimensionally. The DSM uses a categorical perspective, delineating distinct classes of mood disorders with definitive boundaries among them. Categorical views can be viewed as either-or constructs—either an individual is depressed or is not, with little in between. Moreover, clinical depression is seen as qualitatively distinct from the mildly depressed mood states that many people experience. Conversely, the dimensional approach views these disorders as existing on a continuum, ranging from less to more severe, without any clear and definitive boundaries or categories.

Like any classification system, the categorical method has both advantages and disadvantages. In the way of advantages, distinct categories facilitate clear communication about a particular disorder. For example, the severity and general clinical picture are fairly clear based on the language that the DSM provides, which provides a common language between and among clinicians and researchers. Hence, the categorical perspective simplifies the conceptualization of psychopathology and expedites clinical and research decision making (Trull, Widiger, & Guthrie, 1990).

On the other hand, problems inherent in such a system deal with the fact that categories force a vague and unclear phenomenon into specific and fixed compartments. Mood states are seen as qualitatively different from one another, when in fact they, or at least varying components of them, might exist on a continuum. Similarly, DSM uses somewhat arbitrary cutoffs and diagnostic symptoms. For example, why must someone have at least five out of nine possible symptoms (why not four or six?), and why are other features of the disorder (e.g., social withdrawal) not among the possible symptoms? A related point hinges on the apparent simplicity of a basic diagnosis. Although a categorical system makes communication easier, it may also disguise important differences. Two diagnoses of major depressive episode could manifest in very different manners, having completely distinct etiologies, symptom patterns, clinical courses, and treatment outcomes.

Course of Mood Disorders

Major depressive episode symptoms often develop over days to weeks, often beginning with a mild form that later escalates into a full-blown episode. The length of each individual episode can vary greatly from person to person, but untreated depressive disorders can last as long as six months to a year, and in some cases individuals may experience significant symptoms for up to two years (see Goodwin & Jamison, 1990). Many individuals completely recover from their symptoms, entering a period of full remission. Approximately 20% to 30% of individuals experiencing a major depressive disorder remit only partially from the episode and remain in a low-grade depressive state.

Unipolar Depression.   Unipolar depression has an average age of onset in the early- to mid-20s. Typically, the number of previous episodes is a good predictor of the probability of future episodes. Similarly, periods of remission tend to shorten with each passing episode. More than 80% of individuals who experience a major depressive episode will experience recurrent episodes (Kessler, 2002). Individuals with only partial remission are more likely to develop another episode, as well as being more likely to remit only partially in between future episodes. The DSM–IV–TR notes that naturalistic studies have shown that one year after being diagnosed with a major depressive episode, 40% of individuals still met criteria for the major depressive episode, 20% of individuals were in partial remission, and the remaining 40% evidenced no symptoms of depression (American Psychiatric Association, 2000).

Bipolar Disorder. Among individuals diagnosed with Bipolar I disorder, approximately 90% have more than one manic episode. Even though Bipolar I does not necessarily include a major depressive episode, 60% to 70% of manic (or hypomanic in Bipolar II) episodes occur immediately before or after a major depressive episode. Typically, individuals with bipolar disorders have more total episodes (including both depressive and manic or hypomanic) in their lives than those with unipolar depression. The time between episodes tends to decrease with increasing age. In addition, the presence of psychotic features indicates a greater likelihood of incomplete recovery between episodes, as well as indicating a greater propensity toward psychotic features in subsequent manic episodes.

Epidemiology, Gender, and Culture

Epidemiology. Point prevalence rates of current major depression are found to be 2% to 4% for adults (Kessler, 2002) (point prevalence rates estimate the number of people at a particular point in time who are experiencing the disorder). From another perspective, lifetime prevalence rates for major depression have been found to range anywhere from 6% to 25% (Kessler, 2002). Researchers speculate three reasons for this wide variation in lifetime prevalence estimates. The first is a true increase in the incidence of depression in more recent cohorts. Second, these more recent cohorts are also more willing to admit their depressive symptoms, thereby leading to an increase in prevalence findings. Last, methodological differences between diagnostic interviews may account for the discrepancy: More recent studies use more refined diagnostic interviews that are better able to detect mood disorders (Kessler, 2002).

Epidemiological studies have also found substantial comorbidity between depression and other disorders. The Epidemiologic Catchment Area Study (ECS) and the National Comorbidity Survey (NCS) are two large epidemiological studies that describe depression. Both use diagnostic interviews in assessing the population, and both show comorbidity rates of approximately 75% (Kessler, 2002). The most frequent Axis I comorbid (or co-occurring) conditions with depression are anxiety disorders, particularly generalized anxiety disorder, panic disorder, and posttraumatic stress disorder.

Gender Differences. Mood disorders, particularly unipolar depression, are characterized by substantial gender differences. About twice as many women as men suffer from major depression or dysthymia. Moreover, this gender difference persists across demographic and cultural groups as well as in different countries (Nolen-Hoeksema, 2002). Gender differences seem to arise around the age of 12 or 13 years (possibly coinciding with the onset of puberty); before this time depression is uncommon, but boys and girls are equally affected. Additionally, data from epidemiological studies show that adult gender differences are due to a greater number of initial onsets of depression in women, as opposed to a difference in length or frequency of depressive episodes (Nolen-Hoeksema, 2002).

Interestingly, few gender differences in incidence of bipolar disorders are found. Some differences, however, have been found in the type of bipolar disorder experienced. For example, women are typically diagnosed first with a major depressive episode and men with a manic episode. Correspondingly, women typically have more major depressive episodes whereas men typically have more manic episodes (American Psychiatric Association, 2000).

Cultural Factors. Culture can affect both the conceptualization and manifestation of depression. There are two main approaches that researchers take to understand these culturally based manifestations: ethnographic and biomedical. The ethnographic approach, typically taken by anthropologists, argues that persons in non-Western cultures may indeed experience the same symptoms that are defined as depressive in Western cultures, but that these symptoms may have different meanings. In contrast, the biomedical approach assumes that if the particular symptoms are present, then the disorder exists. For example, numerous studies of depressive symptomatology in non-Western cultures have documented high rates of depressive disorders as they are defined by the constellation of depressive symptoms articulated in the DSM. Although the biomedical approach does not entirely discount the role of culture, cultural meanings of symptoms are de-emphasized. Psychologists and psychiatrists typically use the biomedical approach.

There are significantly varied meanings of depression across cultures. Western culture has influenced the definition of depression in three ways (Tsai & Chentsova-Dutton, 2002). First, Western culture values positive emotions and feeling good about oneself, and definitions and diagnoses of depression hinge on the absence of such positive feelings. Second, Western cultures tend to view a healthy individual as independent and autonomous, thereby explaining depression as an internal disturbance. In non-Western cultures, where connectedness among people is apt to be more highly valued than individuation, depressive symptoms are more likely to be seen as the result of interpersonal difficulties. This is not to say that depression in Western societies does not involve interpersonal difficulties, but rather that compared to the non-Western world, autonomy is likely to be valued more than interconnectedness. Lastly, Western culture views depression as the result of disturbance in either the mind or the body; in contrast, non-Western cultures have a more holistic perspective in which mind and body are inextricably connected. These differences could lead to different symptom presentations. For example, individuals in non-Western cultures typically present more somatization than do individuals in Western cultures. Thus, while cross-cultural research has identified a core expression of depressive disorders that exist in varying degrees across cultures, it appears that symptomatology is more "psychological" in Western societies and more "somatized" in non-Western societies.

Numerous factors can be responsible for variations in prevalence rates and frequency of symptoms across cultures, ethnic groups, and even geographic locations (e.g., actual differences in depression rates; varying degrees of poverty; different ways of thinking about depression; depressive symptoms included in and defined as another illness; methodological differences in the assessment of depression, etc.) (Tsai & Chentsova-Dutton, 2002). It is thus important to keep in mind that depression goes beyond DSM's definition and its manner of operationalizing the construct and may have very different meanings in different cultural groups.

THEORY AND RESEARCH IN DEPRESSION

Genes, biochemistry, social skills, negative life events, interpersonal interactions, and cognitive and affective processes are all involved in varying ways and degrees in the development and course of depression. However, distinctions among these varying approaches to depression have become increasingly blurred. For example, life events are recognized as the cornerstone in many episodes of depression, but various life event models now attempt explicitly to integrate notions of vulnerability, cognitive mediation, interpersonal behavior, and brain function. However, although some progress has been made toward an integration of the various aspects of depression, few integrative models of depression exist. Thus, in this chapter we will examine contemporary approaches according to their single-variable points of origin, but it is important to bear in mind that even though we individually describe these various origins, they in fact interact to varying degrees in different cases of depression.

The Role of Stress in Depression

The link between an adverse social environment and depression has been recognized for centuries. Although there are a number of different aspects of social adversity (e.g., poverty), stressful life events are typically considered to be a core correlate of depression. The majority of research consistently finds a strong relationship between the experience of stressful life events and the onset of depression (Monroe & Hadjiyannakis, 2002). Even though the link between stress and depression is well documented, the nature of this link is complex and far from completely understood. Stress is anything but a simple concept, and it defies comprehensive exposition in a single chapter. Yet, we will discuss several important themes and questions that are important to recognize in understanding the relationship between stress and depression. Although most models emphasize the role of stress in the etiology of depression, we also need to ask about the role stress plays in different subtypes of depression and in the course of depression (e.g., degree and duration of symptoms, remission and recovery, relapse or recurrence). (Monroe & Hadjiyannakis, 2002). Even this discussion, however, barely touches on the complexities of stress. For example, can depression only be triggered by major life events, or is a series of chronic minor life events sufficient? Stress may consist of events that independently happen to people, but depressed individuals also may play a role in generating stress that prolongs depression (Hammen, 1991b).

Data have suggested that approximately 50% of depressed individuals experienced severe stress before onset (Mazure, 1998). Such data show that stress plays a role in depression, but they also show that other factors are important. For example, not all individuals who experience significant stress develop depression, nor do all individuals who develop depression experience significant stress. To account for this difference, most modern theories of depression rely on diathesis–stress perspectives. Diathesis refers to a predisposition, or vulnerability, to an illness, and although not all models of depression emphasize a diathesis, most contemporary theories do make use of the idea to some degree. There is also general agreement that events perceived as stressful trigger vulnerability processes that bring about depression (Ingram et al., 1998).

The nature of the diathesis–stress relationship is complex. Some models, for example, suggest an inverse relationship between stress and diatheses, such that as the degree or severity of the diathesis increases, less stress is necessary to initiate a depressive episode (Ingram et al., 1998). Alternatively, some perspectives argue that both severe stress and a strong diathesis are necessary to elicit depression (Monroe & Hadjiyannakis, 2002). Whatever its nature, the diathesis–stress idea is one that we will come back to frequently as we discuss theory and research in depression.

Depression Models and Approaches

Theory and research on depression is both remarkably abundant and remarkably diverse. Numerous theories of depression have been proposed and literally thousands of empirical reports examining various aspects of depression have been published in psychological and psychiatric journals. These theories and research span a variety of different models of depression ranging from biological to psychological to social/environmental. We review here the major models, theories, and important findings that may be informative about such causal factors.

Biomedical Models

Biomedical models encompass several different areas of assumption and inquiry. Three related approaches are genetic, biological, and neuroscience perspectives.

Genetic Approaches.   Genetic models argue that at least some of the variance in the development of depression is linked to genetic factors (Wallace, Schneider & McGuffin, 2002). Data that inform genetic models come from one of three different sources: family studies, twin studies, and adoption studies. Family study methods are based on the observation that depression runs in families (Hammen, 1991a) and that to the extent that depression vulnerability is inherited, mood-disorders should cluster within a family. The most direct approach to evaluating this clustering is to interview family members using a standardized diagnostic interview to determine the number and type of mood-related disorders that occur among relatives (Faraone, Tsuang, & Tsuang, 1999). The more familial history there is of mood disorders, the more evidence there is that the disorder, or the propensity to the disorder, is inherited. However, because families share not only genes but also share environments, family studies have difficulty disentangling genetic factors from environmental factors.

Twin studies are in some respects an extension of family studies, but compare concordance rates for monozygotic (identical) twins, who are genetically identical (100% shared genes), to dizygotic (fraternal) twins whose genes are similar (about 50% on average) but not identical. Concordance rates refer to the likelihood that both twins will be diagnosed with the disorder; to the extent that genetically identical monozygotic twins have higher concordance rates than genetically similar dizygotic twins, genetic factors are thought to play a significant role in the disorder. For example, McGuffin, Katz, and Rutherford (1991) found concordance rates of 58% in monozygotic twins as compared to 28% in dizygotic twins. Likewise, Kendler Neale, Kessler, Heath, and Eaves (1992) found rates of 44% in monozygotic twins and 19% in dizygotic twins. In both cases the degree of concordance was about twice as high for monozygotic twins and thus strongly suggests a genetic component to depression.

Although superior to family studies, twin studies are not without limitations. For example, twin studies rely on the assumption that environments are identical for twins, but this may not always be the case if twins who are identical in appearance are treated more similarly than twins who look like same-aged siblings. Hence, environment cannot be completely ruled out as a contributing factor in concordance rates, although environmental influences are in most cases probably reasonably similar (Kendler & Gardner, 1998). Other methodological issues (e.g., small samples in many studies, questions about generalizibility to nontwins) may also limit the validity of twin studies (Wallace et al., 2002).

The most powerful genetic method is the adoption study. Adopted children are genetically similar to their biological parents but have nothing genetically in common with their adoptive parents. They share, however, a psychosocial environment with the adopted families. Evidence for a genetic role in depression is thus found when adopted children with a biological family history of depression are also more likely than adopted children without a biological family history of depression to experience a mood disorder. This finding is particularly true if children are adopted at a young age and have had less opportunity to be exposed to the psychosocial environment of the biological family, which may be confounded with purely genetic influences. The major disadvantage of these studies is pragmatic in that they are costly and difficult to conduct. As a result, relatively few adoption studies on genetic factors in depression have been published, and those that have been published suffer from the types of problems that often result from logistically difficult-to-conduct studies (e.g., small sample sizes).

Although each of these methods has limitations, when taken together, these data have provided some estimates of the degree to which depression is influenced by genes. Kendler et al. (1992) have suggested that the heritably of milder forms of depression ranges anywhere from 20% to 45%, with estimates for more severe cases of depression (e.g., those requiring hospitalization) ranging as high as 70% (Malhi, Moore, & McGuffin, 2000). Genetic contributions for recurrent or chronic cases of depression may also be higher than those for single episodes.

Thus, depending on type and severity of the disorder, data suggest that the heritability of depression is anywhere from moderate to high. Even this range, however, is mitigated by other factors, such as gender differences; for example, heritability appears to be stronger in women than in men.

Given the complexity of depression and its recognized subtypes, it is unlikely that a single gene will ever be found that is linked to depression. Moreover, it is important to consider what is being inherited. As we have noted, there is a reasonably broad consensus that depression is not inherited, but that a predisposition or vulnerability to depression is. As we also noted, other factors such as stress determine whether this susceptibility ever becomes realized in a diagnosable depressive disorder. Thus, even though heritability does play a potentially large role in at least some types of depression, environmental features also clearly have a considerable part in the etiology of depression. Genes may set the stage more or less for depression and its various forms, but consistent with diathesis–stress concepts, a variety of other factors are likely to determine whether depression occurs.

Biological Bases of Depression. Biological functioning in depression is every bit as complex as the genetic variables that influence the disorder. This is partly because genes and biology are closely intertwined but also because biological systems themselves are connected in multifaceted and interactive ways. Moreover, both biological function and genetics are intricately tied to brain structure and functioning, which we will examine in the next section.

The earliest biological views were relatively straightforward and suggested that deficits in catecholamine norepinephrine (NE) and indoleamine serotonin (5-HT) were causally related to depression (Schildkraut, 1965). These neurotransmitters were first suspected to play a role in depression because they had been found to control several areas of physical functioning (e.g., sleep and appetite) that are sometimes disrupted in depression. Deficits in dopamine were suggested somewhat later also to contribute to depressive disorders (Korf & van Praag, 1971). However, although dysfunction in these systems does appear to play a role in at least in some forms of depression (Thase, Jindal, & Howland, 2002), the relationship between these monoamines and other biological disturbances now appears to be much more complicated than the early theories suggested.

Even though research on biological aspects of depression is rapidly evolving, current thinking centers on several possible areas of pathophysiological processes (Thase et al., 2002). For example, a subgroup of depressed individuals appears to excrete low levels of a metabolite for NE (3-methoxy-4hydroxyphenylglycol, or MHPG), thus suggesting that a reduction in NE may be involved in some depressions (Ressler & Nemeroff, 1999). Other studies have shown that low levels of a metabolite for 5-HT are found in some subgroups of depressed individuals (Maes & Meltzer, 1995). Interestingly, diminished 5-HT function may be related to behaviors that are characteristic of some cases of depression (e.g., suicidality), although these behaviors may characterize other disorders as well. For this reason, 5-HT disruption may be a more general deficit in psychopathology rather than one specifically linked to depression.

Third, high levels of cortisol (a hormone) have been found in some groups of depressed individuals. Cortisol is regulated by the adrenal cortex and is excreted in times of stress. However, cortisol also returns to normal levels when the individual is no longer depressed. Interestingly, when a synthetic cortisol known as dexamethasone is administered, nondepressed people show a suppression of naturally occurring cortisol, a procedure known as a dexamethasone suppression test (DST). However, this suppression is not observed in a subset of depressed people. For these particular depressed individuals, hypercortisol secretion may reflect an exaggerated stress response that is not seen in individuals who experience stress without becoming depressed. Although the DST was originally thought to have great potential as a diagnostic indicator of depression, the fact that only some, but not all, depressed people fail to suppress cortisol has diminished this enthusiasm. Nevertheless, these data do suggest that sustained or excessive cortisol secretion may reflect an important biological process in some forms of depression.

Some evidence suggests that sleep neurophysiology and circadian rhythms may be disturbed in depression. Other evidence suggests that decreased slow wave sleep and the intensification of rapid eye movement (REM) sleep occur among depressed individuals. REM sleep occurs several times throughout the night at approximately 90-minute intervals. Some research suggests that the first REM sleep interval for some depressed people occurs earlier than the normal 90 minutes. Moreover, some depressed people show evidence of all three sleep abnormalities. Such sleep disturbances, along with other factors such as hypercortisol excretion, may reflect a disruption in circadian rhythms, although it is unclear if this disruption plays an etiological role in depression or if it is the result of a more primary dysregulation in biological functioning.

Such data clearly show evidence of biological dysregulation in depression. However, several qualifications are in order. Although data have shown a variety of biological processes that appear to be disturbed in depression, these processes do not characterize all cases of depression, nor are they necessarily specific to depression. Some biological processes appear to be stable in some depressions, such as decreased 5-HT and some sleep disturbances such as decreased slow wave sleep. Other processes, however, appear to be more characteristic of the depressed state (e.g., hypercortisol), and tend to normalize as individuals recover. In many cases, individuals who show evidence of these diffuse biological disturbances typically are older, more severely depressed, have more vegetative symptoms, and experience recurrent episodes of depression. Moreover, many of these processes may reflect the effect of stress that is severe and/or sustained. These studies do not suggest that some forms of depression have purely biological causes and that others have purely psychosocial causes. They do suggest, however (along with results showing that many of these abnormalities run in families and thus appear to have a genetic component), that some forms of depression (particularly very severe forms) may have a much stronger biological component that others.

Affective Neuroscience. Affective neuroscience focuses on the neural processes that are linked to emotion. Research in affective neuroscience uses a variety of methods such as examining the link between brain damage and impaired functioning. However, the use of imaging techniques such as functional magnetic resonance imaging (fMRI) has become increasingly common in recent years. fMRI creates images of the oxygen in the blood flow to brain areas that are active and can thus be used to assess the role and function of brain structures and regions during various tasks. Mapping this activation provides a window into how the brain functions in depressed (and nondepressed) states and can thus help to chart the brain circuitry that may be involved in depression. Knowledge of this circuitry may have implications for understanding various patterns of cognitive and behavioral deficits in depression and ideally might also provide insight into the onset, maintenance, and remission of depression.

Affective neuroscience approaches to depression usually have focused most attention on the prefrontal cortex, anterior cingulate cortex, hippocampus, and amygdala (Davidson, Pizzagalli, & Nitschke, 2002). Although these structures serve numerous functions, in general, the prefrontal cortex is that part of the cortex that is most evolved in primates and that plays a substantial role in goal-directed activities such as planning and formulating strategies. To accomplish desired goals, the prefrontal cortex sends signals to other parts of the brain, inhibiting some areas and disinhibiting others. The anterior cingulate cortex is typically involved in selective attention and emotion and thus appears to be involved in the perception of emotionally relevant information. The hippocampus is a part of the limbic system and is involved in the consolidation of memory; it is linked to the representation of emotion-evoking events, which may be particularly important in understanding the neural circuitry underlying an emotional state such as depression. The amygdala is also part of the limbic system. This structure is also involved in the memory for emotionally significant events and is also connected to other brain regions and serves to signal to these areas when stimuli important to the person require additional processing (Davidson, Pizzagalli, & Nitschke, 2002).

Although knowledge of the brain circuitry of depression is far from complete, several promising findings have emerged. For example, some depressed individuals exhibit decreased activation in the prefrontal cortex (Drevets, 1998), particularly on the left side (Davidson, 1993). This decreased activation may be responsible for the disruption of goal-directed activities that frequently characterize depression (DSM–IV). Interestingly, some studies have found that the young children of depressed mothers exhibit a similar pattern of left-side hypoactivation (Hammen, 2001), suggesting a genetic link to this brain abnormality. Drevets et al. (1997) reported that the prefrontal cortices of depressed individuals with a family history of depression were significantly smaller than the prefrontal cortexes of nondepressed controls. No such differences were found in comparisons between depressed individuals without a family history and normal controls. These findings offer more evidence for a genetic link in at least in some forms of depression.

Decreases in the activation of the anterior cingulate cortex have also been found in depressed individuals and may be linked to the social withdrawal, poor coping, and anhedonia that is sometimes seen in depression (Davidson et al., 2002). Some data have also shown reduced hippocampal volume in depressed patients. One hypothesis concerning this reduced volume is that the hippocampus may atrophy because it contains high levels of cortisol (a glucocorticoid) receptors; glucocorticoids, which are known to be neurotoxic, lead to cell loss. Because the hippocampus is involved in encoding environmental context, one result of this atrophy may be deficits in the ability to process social information, leading to the preservation of depressed mood in situations that should provoke positive or neutral affect (Davidson et al., 2002).

The hippocampus is strongly connected to the amygdala, another brain region closely linked to depression (Drevets, 2001). In particular, the amygdala has been shown to be hyperactivated in depressed individuals and may be responsible for the maintenance of the sad mood that is a hallmark of depression (Dougherty & Rauch, 1997). Not only is the amygdala linked to the perseveration of a sad mood, amygdala hyperactivation may result from the failure of the prefrontal cortex to inhibit this region. (Siegle, Steinhauer, Thase, Stenger, & Carter, 2002). Recall that one function of the PFC, which may become hypoactive in depression, is to regulate other areas of the brain to initiate the attainment of goals. Thus failure of the prefrontal cortex to inhibit the amygdala may precipitate the maintenance of emotional information processing in depression that not only perpetuates a sad mood, but also interferes with adaptive functioning. Moreover, Siegle et al. (2002) have shown evidence of sustained activity of the amygdala in depressed people in a manner that is consistent with observations of the rumination of negative information. Rumination has long been theorized to be an important process in depression (Beck, 1967; Ingram, 1984).

The prefrontal cortex, anterior cingulate cortex, hippocampus, and amygdala form a circuit that is extensively interconnected. Certainly other areas of the brain are involved in depression, but this circuit appears to play a key role in at least some forms of depression and may have a genetic link. Much remains to be learned, however, about the neural circuitry of depression. For example, although some data have suggested that neural deficits continue after depression has remitted, it is still unclear if these deficits are linked to the cause of depression, might co-occur with depression, or might arise as a result of depression. Moreover, because these brain regions are densely connected, it is difficult to determine whether one region is primarily linked to depression (whereas other connected regions are of a more secondary nature) and this primary region in turn affects the other connected areas of the brain. Likewise, the abnormalities linked to depression may reside in the connections between structures rather than in the structures themselves. Despite numerous questions and the complexity of the issues that are inherent in affective neuroscience, significant strides have been made in gaining some insight into how the brain functions in depression.

Psychosocial Approaches to Depression: Cognitive Models

Cognitive approaches to the conceptualization, assessment, and treatment of depression have expanded rapidly over the past several decades and are probably the predominant psychosocial approach to depression today. Even though there are several specific cognitive models of depression, the primary assumption that underlies all cognitive models is that certain cognitive negative processes are related in some fashion to vulnerability, onset, course, and/or alleviation of the disorder.

Irrational Belief Models.   Early theories emphasized a relatively simple linear association between thinking errors and the onset of emotionally troublesome states. These theories can be traced to the development of the pioneering cognitive-behavioral interventions that focused on the treatment of psychological dysfunction through procedures designed to correct errors in thinking. Albert Ellis' approach is probably the first of these models. In the most recent revision of Ellis' theory (Ellis, 1996), he argues that depression-prone people tend to hold overly rigid standards that are applied to one's own performance, the performance of others, and life events. Because these standards are too rigid, they are considered to be irrational. Consequently, the person who (irrationally) expects too much of himself or herself, other people, or life in general, is likely to be disappointed and, ultimately, become depressed.

Learned Helplessness and Hopelessness Theory.   The helplessness theory of depression evolved from an earlier emphasis on learned helplessness in depression. This work began with Seligman, who observed that animals who were unable to control negative events often developed behavior that "looked like" depressive symptoms. Based on these observations, Seligman developed a theory of human depression that focused on depressed individuals' expectations that they were helpless to control aversive outcomes (see Seligman, 1975). Perhaps because of its intuitive appeal and apparent simplicity, learned helplessness theory generated an enormous amount of research (Abramson, Seligman, & Teasdale, 1978).

Even though much of the research on learned helplessness was supportive of the basic tenants of the theory (e.g., that depressed people tended to display more features of helplessness than nondepressed people), other research highlighted some substantial shortcomings. In response to these shortcomings, the theory was reformulated in 1978 as an attributional theory that focused on how attributions about the causes of events were linked to depression (Abramson et al., 1978). In particular, the theory proposed that making global, stable, and internal attributions for negative events and making specific, unstable, external attributions for positive events leads to depression. In 1989, Abramson, Metalsky, and Alloy (1989) refined this theory into the hopelessness theory of depression and suggested that hopelessness depression represented a specific subtype of depression that is caused by the expectation that highly desired outcomes will not occur, or that highly aversive outcomes will occur and that no response available to the individual will change the likelihood of these outcomes.

Dysfunctional Cognitive Schema Theories. The most widely known cognitive model that focuses on dysfunctional structures was proposed by Beck (1967). The model has been elaborated and refined several times (e.g., Beck, 2002), but the basic elements have remained the same. In particular, the model argues that dysfunctional cognitive self-structures, or schemas, are the central elements in the onset and maintenance of depression.

A schema is a stored body of knowledge that interacts with incoming information to influence selective attention and memory search. Self-schemas organize the personal meaning that individuals assign to information. In the case of depression, these schemas incorporate a significant amount of negative self-relevant information and guide how information is abstracted from social settings and processed. That is, the information to which attention is drawn becomes increasingly congruent with the schematic knowledge structures directing the search (Segal, 1988). As a result, these dysfunctional schemas become self-perpetuating and increasingly biased over time because input that may disconfirm or contradict the information encoded in a schema receives insufficient processing. Schemas are also closely linked with affective structures, and in the case of depression, are hypothesized to form the genesis of the disorder because they cause and perpetuate negative cognitive tendencies (Ingram et al., 1998).

Even though the focus of Beck's theory is on schemas and negative thinking in general, he also hypothesized two specific types of concepts represented within cognitive structures that reflect different subtypes of depression. In particular, sociotropic individuals value positive interchange with others and focus on acceptance, support, and guidance from others. Moreover, these individuals also tend to be highly self-critical (Blatt & Homann, 1992). Autonomous individuals, on the other hand, value independence, mobility, and achievement. Blatt (1974) has suggested somewhat similar ideas and has argued that depressed individuals can be either anaclitic or introjective. Anaclitic depression is characterized by feelings of helplessness, weakness, depletion, and being unloved whereas introjective depression is characterized by feelings of being unworthy, unlovable, guilty, and having failed to live up to expectations and standards. In all cases, when stressors congruent with these themes are experienced (e.g., the dissolution of a relationship for anaclitic or sociotropic individuals or a perceived failure at work or school for autonomous/introjective individuals), dysfunctional cognitive structures become active and depression results.

Research has tended to support a link between these dimensions and depression, although there is a consensus that the sociotropic/anaclitic dimensions are more strongly related to depression than the autonomous/introjective dimensions (Enns & Cox, 1997). However, some methodological problems have been shown to exist within this literature, which were underscored in a recent review by Coyne and Whiffen (1995). They noted, for example, that many individuals score high on both subtypes, something counter to the prediction of the theory. Clearly this area is promising but in need of sounder methodology.

Network Theories. Some conceptualizations of depression have focused on theoretical assumptions derived specifically from cognitive psychology. Although quite similar to conceptualizations that focus on cognitive schemas, cognitive network approaches emphasize somewhat different structural assumptions about the nature of schemas and accentuate information processing as the key factor in depression. For example, network theories suggest that the initial experience of depression results from the activation of affective structures that are responsible for a sad or depressed mood and that when these structures are activated, negative cognitions become similarly activated (Ingram, 1984). Moreover, once activated these structures provide access to more extensive and elaborate processing of depressive information. This spreading activation feeds back to affective structures that have previously become associated with sadness and depression and thus results in the spiraling from the normative depressive mood experienced by most people into more significant and debilitating depression. After becoming fully activated, these networks serve to perpetuate depression until the affective/cognitive activity level eventually decays or is altered (e.g., by treatment).

Interacting Cognitive Subsystems.   Teasdale and colleagues (Teasdale & Barnard, 1993; Teasdale, 1999) have proposed a comprehensive information processing model of depression called the interacting cognitive subsystems (ICS) framework. This framework attempts to account for virtually all aspects of information processing (Siegle & Ingram, 1996) and suggests that different aspects of experience are represented by patterns of different kinds of information, or mental codes. For example, at a superficial level, experience is coded in visual, auditory, and proprioceptive inputs, but at deeper levels, patterns of sensory codes are represented by intermediate codes (e.g., sensory data that form letters are represented by combinations of letters into words and sentences). At deeper levels of encoding, mental codes are formed that create meaning (e.g., a sentence conveys both information and meaning) that can be linked to emotions. In the ICS framework, emotional reactions are produced when patterns of low-level meanings and patterns of sensory-derived input produce emotion-laden representations of the self. Production of a depressed state occurs when these depressogenic schematic models are created and is maintained because these models are continually reproduced in day-to-day experience. When the production of these models stops, the depression abates.

Evaluation of Cognitive Models.   An enormous body of empirical research has investigated the various claims of various cognitive models. Support for certain aspects of these models is quite strong. For example, there is little doubt that when depressed, individuals do in fact experience the types of negative cognition that are hypothesized to result from depressive schemas or to emanate from dysfunctional attributional styles (Ingram et al., 1998). Moreover, studies have found these results regardless of whether these cognitive constructs are assessed using self-report methods or performance-based information-processing tasks. Related lines of research have also suggested that adverse early experiences may create some of the cognitive conditions that seem to be related to the experience of depression (Ingram, 2001; Ingram et al., 1998).

Despite this body of research, several significant aspects of cognitive models have yet to be consistently verified empirically. Recall that cognitive models are typically causal models and not simply models of the cognitive correlates of depressed states. Yet, a number of studies have shown that many of the negative cognitive features of depressed states seem to disappear when depression remits. The inability to detect such cognitive functioning in remitted states provides some suggestion that these cognitions were merely correlates of or consequences of the depressed state, not causes of it. At first, these findings seemed to undermine the most critical assumptions of these cognitive ideas—that negative thoughts cause depression. However, because cognitive models of depression are invariably diathesis–stress models, studies that failed to incorporate this relationship did not provide critical tests of the model (Segal & Ingram, 1994). More appropriate tests have generally been supportive of the diathesis–stress idea. In particular, studies that attempt to model stress in the laboratory typically find that depressive cognition returns under these stressful conditions (Ingram et al., 1998).

One of the more comprehensive studies designed to assess the role of cognition in depression is the Temple-Wisconsin Cognitive Vulnerability to Depression project (Alloy & Abramson, 1999). This longitudinal study examined the proposals of both the hopelessness model and cognitive schema theory as represented by Beck's model (1967). Specifically, a group of individuals were assessed who, on entry into college, were identified as possessing negative inferential styles or negative self-schemas. Among the researchers' findings, those identified as being at high cognitive risk were in fact more likely to experience depression at some point in the future (Alloy & Abramson et al., 1999). Hence, data from this project suggest that cognitive factors do in fact predict the eventual onset of depression.

Psychosocial Approaches to Depression: Interpersonal Approaches

Although the cognitive approach focuses on the internal processes involved in depression, other approaches suggest that people get depressed because of problematic interactions with others. In particular, interpersonal approaches focus on the behaviors, especially the social behaviors, of the depressed individual and suggest that these behaviors contribute to the cause and maintenance of depression. Before discussing this approach, however, it is important to clarify that perspectives on the social origins and nature of depression do not necessarily represent a specific model of depression. As Hammen (1999) has aptly noted, this approach is not sufficiently articulated theoretically to be considered a psychosocial model.

There is little doubt that the interpersonal functioning of depressed individuals can be significantly disrupted. A large body of research shows that depressed individuals are prone to marital and relationship difficulties (Whisman, 2001), occupational problems (Tennant, 2001), impaired parenting (Garber & Flynn, 2001), and difficulties in daily interpersonal functioning (Dill & Anderson, 1999). It is easy to see how the features of the depressed state may be linked to some of these interpersonal problems. For example, not only is social withdrawal considered a pervasive feature of depression, some specific symptoms of depression, such as concentration difficulties, may pave the way for problems in relating to others.

A large and growing body of research has sought to examine the interpersonal context in which depression occurs. The first ideas on the interpersonal nature of depression were proposed by Coyne, who assigned a central role to the manner in which the social environment responds to the interpersonal behavior of the depressed individual. According to Coyne's proposals (1999), the occurrence of stressful life events leads to a display of depressive symptoms by the depressed individual. These symptoms include withdrawal from interactions, expressions of helplessness and hopelessness, and irritability and agitation. The goal of the depressed person is to gain reassurance regarding his or her self-worth and acceptance by others. Initially, individuals respond with genuine concern and support for the person. The effects of this reassurance, however, are short-lived, and the depressed person continues to seek reassurance of his or her self-worth. The persistence of a depressive display, however, eventually becomes aversive to others, and some people in the depressed person's social network may express anger and irritation at the depressed person whereas others start to find suitable excuses to avoid further interactions. The depressed person accurately interprets these behaviors as rejection, leading to intensified efforts by the depressed person to seek reassurance. Thus, a cycle based on the perceived or actual rejection by others is generated that is unpleasant to both the depressed person and to others who continue to remain in the depressed person's social environment.

Interpersonal perspectives thus argue that depression is fundamentally interpersonal in nature (see Joiner & Coyne, 1999). Interpersonal approaches have also been refined and extended since Coyne's original work. For example, investigators have focused on interpersonal topics in depression ranging from life stress and coping, to the role of self-esteem, and to the relationships between cognitive models and interpersonal approaches (Gotlib & Hammen, 1992).

Causal Factors in the Interpersonal Approach. Joiner (2002) has proposed three possible ways that interpersonal factors may create risk for depression. First, impaired social skills may cause the interactional disruptions that lead to depression. Although many individuals who are depressed do display limited social skills, and although the idea that social skill deficits characterize depression-prone people has been around for a while (e.g., Lewinsohn, 1985), few studies show that these deficits precede depression. Such temporal antecedence is a necessary condition for demonstrating that a factor plays a causal role in depression (Garber & Hollon, 1991).

A related but second possibility is that depression-prone individuals display general interpersonal inhibition, which creates risk for depression. Such inhibition suggests that depressed individuals tend to be socially avoidant or shy and that these inhibitions lead to disrupted social functioning and depression. Although data reliably show that these inhibitions occur in the depressed state (Joiner, 2002), little research has addressed the possibility that these processes lead to depression.

A third possibility, and one that is associated with cognitive models, is that an excessive amount of interpersonal dependency creates risk for depression. A number of studies have shown a link between depressive symptoms and dependency (Zuroff & Fitzpatrick, 1995), making it a reasonable candidate for creating risk. Some research has supported this proposition. For instance, Stader and Hokanson (1998) demonstrated that feelings of dependency preceded elevations in depressive symptoms, although these feelings remained even after the depressive symptoms diminished. Although data such as these are suggestive, more extensive longitudinal research will be necessary to determine how much of a role dependency plays in the onset of depressive episodes.

The onset of depression is only one element of the causal cycle in depression (Ingram et al., 1998). Depression can last for months or years, sometimes even with treatment, and interpersonal processes may play a critical role in maintaining the depressed state. The excessive reassurance seeking that is the cornerstone of interpersonal models suggests pathways whereby depression may be maintained. The interference with social bonds that this process may lead to indicates that social support will be diminished and interpersonal rejection will be increased. A number of studies have revealed this process in depressed individuals (Joiner, 2002). Moreover, these behaviors may also be related to increases in stress (Hammen, 1991b), thus making depression more difficult to escape. Regardless of whether these problematic interactions are involved in the onset of depression or in the maintenance of depression, the interpersonal approach is an important perspective in understanding depression.

TREATMENT AND PREVENTION

Prevention

Treating cases of depression will always be an important focus of therapists. However, some researchers have argued that a better approach to treatment is prevention of the disorder before it has occurred (Albee, 2000). There is little argument that preventing depression would provide considerably greater benefits to society and to individuals than does the treatment of one depressed individual at a time. Though promising, however, research on the prevention of depression is a young field. For instance, there are few reports of prevention efforts that occurred before the 1990s. Prevention researchers typically adapt and apply treatments that have been shown to be effective for treating depression to individuals who are not yet depressed but who are at risk for depression.

For the most part, prevention trials to date have proven somewhat successful in reducing the incidence of depression (Munoz, Le, Clarke, & Jaycox, 2002). Moreover, the data tend to show that those who are most helped by prevention programs are children and adolescents (Ingram, Odom, & Mitchusson, 2004). The majority of prevention research has focused on psychosocial treatment methods, frequently with an emphasis on modifying cognitive factors. Research shows the promise of these methods and offers individuals the possibility of new learning and of modifying cognitive and behavioral functioning that may have lasting effects.

Biological Approaches to Treatment

Pharmacotherapy for depression has become increasingly common. Indeed, because of their demonstrated effectiveness, the use of antidepressants as the front-line treatment against depression has soared. Antidepressant medications fall into the categories of monoamine oxidize (MAO) inhibitors, tricyclic antidepressants, and selective serotonin reuptake inhibitors (SSRIs). All of these drugs work by increasing the levels of norepinephrine and/or serotonin. Researchers, however, are still unsure as to the exact mechanisms by which these medications achieve their effects.

Monoamine Oxidize Inhibitors. Monoamine oxidize (MAO) inhibitors were the first antidepressant medications, accidentally discovered in the 1950s when one such drug (iproniazid) failed to cure tuberculosis but inadvertently ameliorated the patient's depressive symptoms (Pinel, 2000). This class of drugs increases the level of monoamines (e.g., serotonin and norepinephrine) by inhibiting the enzymes that would otherwise break down these neurotransmitters. Currently, MAO inhibitors have been relegated to third- or fourth-line antidepressants, mostly because of dietary restrictions that are required with their use (Gitlin, 2002). Such dietary restrictions have been termed the "cheese effect" because certain foods that contain an amine called tyramine cannot be eaten because they can raise blood pressure dangerously high (wine and cheese are two such restricted foods). In addition, MAO inhibitors have potentially perilous drug-to-drug interactions that can lead to hypertension or death (these other medications include over-the-counter cold remedies, as well as SSRIs). Other less serious side effects include anxiety, nausea, dizziness, insomnia, weight gain, and sexual dysfunction.

Tricylcic Antidepressants. So named because of their three-ringed structure, tricyclic antidepressants were also developed in the 1950s. Similar to the MAO inhibitors, these drugs were discovered when imipramine proved unsuccessful in treating schizophrenia (Pinel, 2000). Tricyclics function by blocking the reuptake of serotonin and norepinephrine, thereby causing an increase in these neurotransmitters. These antidepressants consistently show good efficacy and are therefore frequently used as the reference drugs in evaluating new treatments (Gitlin, 2002). Disadvantages of tricyclics include the need to increase the dosage slowly to full effect as well as several deleterious side effects such as heart arrhythmias, tachycardia, constipation, urinary problems, sedation, weight gain, blurry vision, and dry mouth (Gitlin, 2002).

Selective Serotonin Reuptake Inhibitors. Developed in the 1990s, selective serotonin reuptake inhibitors (SSRIs) are currently the most commonly prescribed antidepressants and include brand names such as Prozac, Paxil, and Zoloft. As the name implies, SSRIs inhibit the reuptake of serotonin, thereby increasing the level of serotonin in the brain. Their widespread use is due to the fact that they require only one dose daily, as well as to their limited side effects, such as nausea, insomnia, nervousness, sedation, and sexual side effects (Gitlin, 2002). Quite often, the nausea, insomnia, and nervousness diminish after the first few weeks of treatment. SSRIs are roughly equal in effectiveness to tricyclics, although some data have recently emerged that suggest that SSRIs are not much superior to placebo effects (Kirsch & Sapirstein, 1998). Exactly what roles variables such as beliefs have in the effectiveness of SSRIs must await further research.

Psychosocial Treatment Approaches

Dating from Freud's area, depression has been treated with a variety of psychosocial methods. Currently the dominant psychosocial approaches for the treatment of depression are cognitive-behavioral therapy and interpersonal therapy. Both have demonstrated considerable efficacy in the treatment of the disorder, but other more specialized methods have also been used with some success. For instance, marital therapy has been used in cases where marital functioning and depression appear to be entangled. Some other approaches, for example, brief dynamic therapy and behavioral therapy, have also shown some evidence of efficacy (Depression Guideline Panel, 1993). However, because of space limitations, we focus on cognitive therapy and interpersonal therapy.

Cognitive Therapy.   Before discussing cognitive therapy, several caveats are in order. First, there are a number of different approaches to modifying dysfunction that fall within the domain of cognitive therapy. Our focus is on cognitive therapy as developed by Beck (e.g., Beck, Rush, Shaw & Emery, 1979), largely because this particular version of cognitive therapy has been empirically evaluated the most extensively and because it was the first psychotherapy approach to focus explicitly on the modification of cognitive factors. Second, while at initial glance it might appear that the development of cognitive treatment methods would follow from theory and research on the cognitive factors in depression, it was in fact the early success of cognitive therapy that stimulated much of the theory and research on cognitive processes. Last, even though the goal of these approaches is the modification of cognitive factors that are presumed to play an important role in both the onset and maintenance of depressed states, most cognitive approaches also make considerable use of behavioral methods to help achieve these ends. Hence, cognitive and cognitive-behavioral are terms that can be used interchangeably.

The goal of cognitive therapy in the treatment of depression (and in other disordered states) is to teach individuals to recognize and modify dysfunctional beliefs and cognitions (Beck et al., 1979). To do so, cognitive therapists make use of collaborative empiricism, which entails working together with the patient to test the validity of negative thinking processes that are embedded in the patient's meaning system and, where possible, modify them. Thus, the goal is first to help patients recognize the thoughts that may be maintaining depression, and then to test the validity of these thoughts. Cognitive therapists use a variety of methods, but tend to rely heavily on Socratic questioning and behavioral experiments to achieve these goals. Socratic questioning takes the form of asking questions such as "What is the evidence for this belief?" and "Are there other ways to view the situation?"; and if the belief is accurate, "What is the meaning of this?" Initially these methods should help the patient minimize distress in a particular situation, but can also be used in other situations and after therapy has ended to deal with future stressful situations. Behavioral experiments are exercises designed to help the patient test the validity of the belief.

What is the empirical evidence for the efficacy of cognitive therapy? Cognitive therapy is among the most extensively tested treatments for depression and is widely recognized as one of the most effective psychosocial treatments available (Hollon, Haman, & Brown, 2002). Well-controlled studies have suggested that cognitive therapy produces outcomes that are roughly equivalent to psychopharmacological interventions (Hollon et al., 2002). In addition, cognitive therapy may substantially reduce the rate of relapse (the return of the treated episode) (e.g., Evans et al., 1992) and recurrence (the appearance of a new episode) (e.g., Fava, Rafanelli, Grandi, Conti, & Belluardo, 1998).

Combining cognitive therapy with medication may modestly enhance positive response rates (Conti, Plutchik, Wild, & Karasu, 1986), but such conclusions are not without quali-fication. For example, superior efficacy for combined approaches may be obtained only for cases of depression that are more severe or complex or that have a high degree of comorbidity. Alternatively, combined therapy and medication may enhance responsiveness for those indi-viduals who are not responsive to either treatment alone. Practice guidelines typically call for the addition of a different approach if symptoms are not reduced within six to eight weeks (American Psychiatric Association, 2000). Thus, it appears that in some cases medication may enhance the effects of cognitive therapy.

Interpersonal Psychotherapy. Interpersonal approaches can trace their origin to the more psychoanalytic approaches of Adolph Meyer and Harry Stack Sullivan and explicitly rely on the interpersonal theories of personality proposed by these early theories. These approaches view interpersonal difficulties concerning grief, role disputes, role transitions, or interpersonal deficits as the core problems in depression. Interpersonal therapy also assigns a "sick role" to the patient to remove guilt about the diagnosis of depression. Whereas cognitive therapy provides a fairly structured set of therapeutic methods, interpersonal therapy is typically unstructured.

After an assessment of depressive symptoms, patients are asked to describe in detail the nature of their interpersonal relationships and difficulties, which provides a basis for the ther-apist to focus on one or two of the major areas of interpersonal functioning (e.g., grief, role disputes, role transitions, or interpersonal deficits). If grief is the focus, the therapist attempts to help the patient mourn in a healthy way and, when appropriate, to develop new relationships. Role transitions (e.g., the loss of a job) are dealt with by helping the patient to acquire new skills that will facilitate a positive transition. When a role dispute is the focus of treatment (e.g., difficulties in a close relationship such as marriage), the therapist works with the patient to try to resolve the dispute. Such resolutions can take the form of renegotiating the nature of the relationship or might take the form of dissolution of the relationship. In this latter case, grief at the loss of the relationship may also become a focus of therapy. Finally, if interpersonal deficits are the focal point of treatment, the therapist helps the patient develop more effective social skills through role playing and related methods.

Considerable research supports the efficacy of interpersonal therapy for depression. An initial study reported by Weissman et al. (1979) found that interpersonal therapy was equivalent in efficacy to medication (amitriptyline). Studies have also suggested that the combination of psychopharmacological approaches and interpersonal therapy is effective, with some evidence to suggest that the combination is better than either treatment alone (DiMasico et al., 1979).

SUMMARY

This chapter began with a basic overview of the major classes of mood disorders, with a primary focus on unipolar depression. The discussion of the DSM–IV–TR noted required symptoms for mood disorders, the general course of mood disorders, and issues in defining the idea of depression. Epidemiological data, gender differences, and cultural issues were explored. Some epidemiological studies estimate lifetime prevalence rates of depression to be as high as 25%, although these figures may depend on the way depression is defined and in what culture depression is assessed. About twice as many women suffer from unipolar depression as men, though there are few gender differences in bipolar disorders. Cultural issues explore how depression can be manifested and conceptualized differently in various cultures, and although DSM-inspired notions of depression rely heavily on Western society, depression may be thought of very differently in other cultures.

There are a number of models of depression, as well as corresponding research findings. Diathesis–stress conceptualizations focus on the interaction between internal and external sources in the development of depression, and although not universally the case, most theories of depression reflect such perspectives to some degree. Biomedical models focus on genetics, biological evidence, and affective neuroscience perspectives. Genetic perspectives look to family studies, twin studies, and adoption studies, which show familial clusters of mood disorders as evidence for genetic contributions to depression. In the area of biological approaches to depression, several pathophysiological processes have been noted, such as serotonin and norepinephrine dysregulation, high levels of cortisol, and sleep disturbances. Affective neuroscience, which focuses on neural processes linked to emotion, has suggested abnormalities of the prefrontal cortex, the anterior cingulate cortex, the hippocampus, and the amygdala. Each of these perspectives has provided important insights into the nature of depression, but our understanding of biomedical processes is still far from complete.

The other major approaches to depression are psychosocial approaches. The common theme among cognitive models is that negative cognitive processes play an important role in the cause and course of depression. Empirical studies affirm a number of aspects of these cognitive models. Although some research points to the causal validity of these models, key causal contributions have not yet been demonstrated. Interpersonal approaches also represent a psychosocial view of depression, but focus on interactional patterns as key features in depression. As with cognitive models, interpersonal approaches vary, but tend to converge on the idea that troubled interaction patterns may both cause and maintain depression. Also, as with cognitive models, while some research has been supportive, the major variables in this approach have yet to be definitively shown to play a key role in the cause and course of depression.

Lastly we examined various forms of treatment and prevention for mood disorders. Paralleling the two major areas of depression theory and research, the two main approaches to treatment are biological and psychosocial. Biological treatment entails the use of pharmacotherapy, with the three main types of antidepressant medications consisting of MAO inhibitors, tricyclics, and SSRIs. All of these can be effective for certain groups of people, although SSRIs are prescribed most often because their efficacy is at least equal to other drugs and because of their limited side effects. Major psychosocial interventions include cognitive therapy and interpersonal psychotherapy. Cognitive therapy aims to help individuals recognize and modify their dysfunctional beliefs. Socratic questioning and behavioral experiments are two techniques that cognitive therapists use. Data have repeatedly shown the efficacy of such approaches. Interpersonal psychotherapy focuses on the areas of grief, role disputes, role transitions, or interpersonal deficits as the core issues that are addressed in therapy. As with cognitive therapy, a considerable body of research supports the efficacy of this psychosocial intervention.

Significant strides have been made in understanding the core factors involved in depression, as well as mechanisms that may be involved in its onset and course. As significant as these strides have been, however, much is still unknown about the essential features of depression. Most depression theorists believe that there are different subtypes of depression, and although these all result in similar symptom constellations, they may have different causes, courses, and correlates. This heterogeneity has implications not only for theory and research on depression, but also for prevention and treatment efforts; prevention programs and treatment specifically tailored to the causal factors in different kinds of depressive disorders may dramatically improve positive outcomes. From a more general perspective, this heterogeneity illustrates a concept that is important to keep in mind in any exploration of depression. Mood disorders are dynamic constructs whose understanding hinges on definitions and cultural contexts. The key to unlocking the secrets of depression may therefore lie in cataloging the different subtypes of the disorders that we call depression, and then examining the biological and psychological factors that contribute to their various causes and courses. This goal is unlikely to be attainable in the foreseeable future, but it is a worthy aspiration for clinicians, theorists, and researchers who wish to understand the nature of depression.

REFERENCES

Abramson, L. Y., Metalsky, G. I., & Alloy, L. B. (1989). Hopelessness depression: A theory-based subtype of depression. *Psychological Review, 96*, 358–372.

Abramson, L. Y., Seligman, M. E. P., & Teasdale, J. (1978). Learned helplessness in humans: Critique and reformulation. *Journal of Abnormal Psychology, 87*, 49–74.

Albee, G. W. (2000). Critique of psychotherapy in American Society. In C. R. Snyder & R. E. Ingram (Eds.), *Handbook of psychological change: Psychotherapy processes and practices for the 21st century*. New York: Wiley.

Alloy, L. B., & Abramson, L. Y. (1999). The Temple-Wisconsin Cognitive Vulnerability to Depression project: Conceptual background, design, and methods. *Journal of Cognitive Psychotherapy, 13*, 227–262.

American Psychiatric Association. (2000). *Diagnostic and statistical manual of mental disorders* (4th ed. text revision). Washington D.C.: Author.

Beck, A. T. (1967). *Depression: Causes and treatment*. Philadelphia: University of Pennsylvania Press.

Beck, A. T. (2002). Cognitive models of depression. In R. L. Leahy & T. E. Dowd (Eds.), *Clinical advances in cognitive psychotherapy: Theory and application* (pp. 29–61). New York: Springer.

Beck, A. T., Rush, A. J., Shaw, B. F., & Emery, G. (1979). *Cognitive therapy of depression*. New York: Guilford.

Blatt, S. J. (1974). Level of object representation in anaclitic and introjective depression. *Psychoanalytic Study of the Child, 29*, 107–157.

Blatt, S. J., & Homann, E. (1992). Parent-child interaction in the etiology of dependent and self-critical depression. *Clinical Psychology Review, 12*, 47–91.

Conti, H. R., Plutchik, R., Wild, K. V., & Karasu, T. B. (1986). Combined psychotherapy and pharmacotherapy for depression. *Archives of General Psychiatry, 43*, 471–479.

Coyne, J. C. (1999). Thinking interactionally about depression: A radical restatement. In T. E. Joiner & J. C. Coyne (Eds.), *The interactional nature of depression* (pp. 365–392). Washington, DC: American Psychological Association.

Coyne, J. C., & Whiffen, V. E. (1995). Issues in personality as diathesis for depression: The case of sociotropy dependency and autonomy self criticism. *Psychological Bulletin, 118*, 358–378.

Davidson, R. J. (1993). Cerebral asymmetry and emotion: Conceptual and methodological conundrums. *Cognition and Emotion, 7*, 115–138.

Davidson, R. J., Pizzagalli, D., & Nitschke, J. B. (2002). The representation and regulation of emotion in depression: Perspectives from affective neuroscience. In I. H. Gotlib & C. L. Hammen (Eds.), *Handbook of depression* (3rd ed.) (pp. 219–244). New York: Guilford.

Depression Guideline Panel. (1993). *Depression in primary care: Vol. 2. Treatment of major depression* (Clinical Practice Guideline No. 5, AHCPR Publication No. 9300551). Rockville, MD: Department of Health and Human Services, Public Health Service, Agency for Health Care Policy and Research.

Dill, J. C., & Anderson, C. A. (1999). Loneliness, shyness and depression: The etiology and interrelationships of everyday problems in living. In T. E. Joiner & J. C. Coyne (Eds.), *The interactional nature of depression* (pp. 93–126). Washington, DC: American Psychological Association.

DiMascio, A., Weissman, M. M., Prusoff, B. A., Neu, C., Zwilling, M., & Klerman, G. L. (1979). Differential symptom reduction by drugs and psychotherapy in acute depression. *Archives of General Psychiatry, 36*, 1450–1456.

Dougherty, D., & Rauch, S. L. (1997). Neuroimaging and neurobiological models of depression. *Harvard Review of Psychiatry, 5*, 138–159.

Drevets, W. C. (1998). Functional neuroimagining studies of depression: The anatomy of melancholia. *Annual Review of Medicine, 49*, 341–361.

Drevets, W. C. (2001). Neuroimagining and neuropathological studies of depression: Implications for the cognitive-emotional features of mood disorders. *Current Opinion in Neurobiology, 11*, 240–249.

Drevets, W. C., Price, J. L., Simpson, J. R. J., Todd, R. D., Reich, T., Vannier, M., & Raichle, M. E. (1997). Subgenial prefrontal cortex abnormalities in mood disorders. *Nature, 386*, 824–827.

Ellis, A. (1996). *Better, deeper and more enduring brief therapy: The rational emotive behavior therapy approach*. New York: Brunner/Mazel.

Enns, M., & Cox, B. (1997). Personality dimensions and depression: Review and commentary. *Canadian Journal of Psychiatry, 42*, 274–284.

Evans, M. D., Hollon, S. D., & DeRubies, R. J. (1992). Differential relapse following cognitive therapy and pharmacotherapy for depression. *Archives of General Psychiatry, 49*, 802–808.

Faraone, S. V., Tsuang, T., & Tsuang, D. (1999). *Genetic of mental disorders: A guide for students, clinicians, and researchers.* New York: Guilford.

Fava, G. A., Rafanelli, C., Grandi, S., Conti, S., & Belluardo, P. (1998). Prevention of recurrent depression with cognitive-behavioral therapy. *Archives of General Psychiatry, 55*, 816–820.

Garber, J., & Flynn, C. (2001). Predictors of depressive cognitions in young adolescents. *Cognitive Therapy and Research, 4*, 353–376.

Garber, J., & Hollon, S. (1991). What can specificity designs say about causality in psychopathology research? *Psychological Bulletin, 110*, 129–136.

Gitlin, M. J. (2002). Pharmacological treatment of depression. In I. H. Gotlib & C. L. Hammen (Eds.), *Handbook of depression* (3rd ed.) (pp. 360–382). New York: Guilford.

Goodwin, F. K., & Jamison, K. R. (1990). *Manic-depressive illness.* New York: Oxford University Press.

Gotlib, I. H., & Hammen, C. L. (1992). *Psychological aspects of depression: Toward a cognitive-interpersonal integration.* Chichester, England: Wiley.

Hammen, C. (1991a). *Depression runs in families: The social context of risk and resilience in children of depressed mothers.* New York: Springer-Verlag.

Hammen, C. (1991b). The generation of stress in the course of unipolar depression. *Journal of Abnormal Psychology, 100*, 555–561.

Hammen, C. (1999). The emergence of an interpersonal approach to depression. In T. E. Joiner & J. C. Coyne (Eds.), *The interactional nature of depression* (pp. 21–36). Washington, DC: American Psychological Association.

Hammen, C. L. (2001). Vulnerability to depression in adulthood. In R. E. Ingram & J. M. Price (Eds.), *Vulnerability to psychopathology: Risk across the lifespan* (pp. 226–257). New York: Guilford.

Hollon, S. D., Haman, K. L., & Brown, L. L. (2002). Cognitive-behavioral treatment of depression. In I. H. Gotlib & C. L. Hammen (Eds.), *Handbook of depression* (3rd ed.) (pp. 383–403). New York: Guilford.

Ingram, R. E. (1984). Toward an information processing analysis of depression. *Cognitive Therapy and Research, 8*, 443–478.

Ingram, R. E. (2001). Developing perspectives on the cognitive-developmental origins of Depression: Back is the future. *Cognitive Therapy and Research, 25*, 497–504.

Ingram, R. E., Miranda, J., & Segal, Z. (1998). *Cognitive vulnerability to depression.* New York: Guilford.

Ingram, R. E., & Odom, M., & Mitchusson, L. (2004). Secondary prevention of depression: Risk, vulnerability and intervention. In D. J. A. Dozois & K. S. Dobson (Eds.), *The prevention of anxiety and depression: Theory, research, and practice.* (pp. 205–231). Washington, DC: American Psychological Association.

Joiner, T. E. (2002). Depression in its interpersonal context. In I. H. Gotlib & C. L. Hammen (Eds.), *Handbook of depression* (3rd ed.) (pp. 295–313). New York: Guilford.

Joiner, T. E., & Coyne, J. C. (1999) (Eds.). *The interactional nature of depression.* Washington, DC: American Psychological Association.

Kendall, P. C., Hollon, S. D., Beck, A. T., Hammen, C. L., & Ingram, R. E. (1987). Issues and recommendations regarding use of the Beck Depression Inventory. *Cognitive Therapy and Research, 11*, 289–299.

Kendler K., & Gardner, C. O. (1998). Twins studies of adult psychiatric and substance dependence disorders. *Psychological Medicine, 28*, 625–633.

Kendler, K., Neale, M., Kessler, R., Heath, A., & Eaves, L. (1992). Major depression and generalized anxiety disorder. *Archives of General Psychiatry, 49*, 716–722.

Kessler, R. C. (2002). Epidemiology of depression. In I. H. Gotlib & C. L. Hammen (Eds.), *Handbook of depression* (3rd ed.) (pp. 23–42). New York: Guilford.

Kirsch, I., & Sapirstein, G. (1998). Listening to Prozac but hearing placebo: A meta analysis of antidepressant medication. *Prevention & Treatment, 1*, Article 0002a.

Korf, J., & van Praag, H. H. (1971). Retarded depressions and the dopamine hypothesis. *Psychopharmacologia, 19*, 199–203.

Lewinsohn, P. (1985). A behavioral approach to depression. In J. C. Coyne (Ed.), *Essential papers in depression.* New York: NYU Press.

Maes, M., & Meltzer, H. Y. (1995). The serotonin hypothesis of major depression. In F. E. Bloom & D. J. Kupfer (Eds.), *Psychopharmacology: The fourth generation of progress* (pp. 933–944). New York: Raven.

Malhi, G. S., Moore, J., & McGuffin, P. (2000). The genetics of major depression. *Current Psychiatry Reports, 2*, 165–169.

Mazure, C. M. (1998). Life stressors as risk factors in depression. *Clinical Psychology: Science and Practice*, *5*, 291–313.

McGuffin, P., Katz, R., & Rutherford, J. (1991). Nature, nurture, and depression: A twin study. *Psychological Medicine*, *21*, 329–335.

Monroe, S. M., & Hadjiyannakis, K. (2002). The social environment and depression: Focusing on severe life stress. In I. H. Gotlib & C. L. Hammen (Eds.), *Handbook of depression* (3rd ed.) (pp. 314–341). New York: Guilford.

Munoz, R., Le, H., Clarke, G., & Jaycox, L. (2002). Preventing the onset of major depression. In I. H. Gotlib & C. L. Hammen (Eds.), *Handbook of depression* (3rd ed.) (pp. 343–359). New York: Guilford.

Nolen-Hoeksema, S. (2002). Gender differences in depression. In I. H. Gotlib & C. L. Hammen (Eds.), *Handbook of depression* (3rd ed.) (pp. 492–509). New York: Guilford.

Nurcombe, B. (1992). The evolution and validity of the diagnosis of major depression in childhood and adolescence. In D. Cicchetti & S. L. Toth (Eds.), *Developmental perspectives on depression*. Rochester, NY: University of Rochester Press.

Pinel, J. P. J. (2000). *Biopsychology*. Needman Heights, MA: Pearson Education.

Ressler, K. J., & Nemeroff, C. B. (1999). Role of norepinephrine in the pathophysiology and treatment of mood disorders. *Biological Psychiatry*, *46*, 1219–1233.

Saz, P., & Dewey, M. (2001). Depression, depressive symptoms and mortality in persons aged 65 and over living in the community: A systematic review of the literature. *International Journal of Geriatric Psychiatry*, *16*, 622–630.

Schildkraut, J. J. (1965). The catecholamine hypothesis of affective disorders: A review of supporting evidence. *American Journal of Psychiatry*, *122*, 509–522.

Segal, Z. V., (1988). Appraisal of the self-schema construct in cognitive models of depression. *Psychological Bulletin*, *103*, 147–162.

Segal, Z. V. & Ingram, R. E. (1994). Mood priming and construct activation in tests of cognitive vulnerability to unipolar depression. *Clinical Psychology Review*, *14*, 663–695.

Seligman, M. E. P. (1975). *Helplessness: On depression, development, and death*. San Francisco: Freeman.

Siegle, G. J., & Ingram, R. E. (1996). The big picture. *Contemporary Psychology*, *41*, 163–164.

Siegle, G. J., Steinhauer, S. R., Thase, M. E., Stenger, A., & Carter, C. S. (2002). Can't shake that feeling: Event–related fMRI assessment of sustained amygdala activity in response to emotional information in depressed individuals. *Biological Psychiatry*, *51*, 693–707.

Seligman, M. E. P. (1990). Why is there so much depression today: The waxing of the individual and the waning of the commons. In R. E. Ingram, (Ed.), *Contemporary psychological approches to depression: Theory, research, and treatment* (1–9). New York, Plenum Press.

Stader, S. R., & Hokanson, J. E. (1998). Psychosocial antecedents of depressive symptoms: An evaluation using daily experiences methodology. *Journal of Abnormal Psychology*, *107*, 17–26.

Teasdale, J. D. (1999). Multi-level theories of cognition-emotion relations. In T. Dalgleish & M. Power (Eds.), *Handbook of cognition and emotion* (pp. 665–681). Chichester, England: Wiley.

Teasdale, J. D., & Barnard, P. J. (1993). *Affect, cognition, and change*. Hillsdale, NJ: Lawrence Erlbaum Associates.

Tennant, C. (2001). Work-related stress and depressive disorders. *Journal of Psychosomatic Research*, *51*, 697–704.

Thase, M E., Jindal, R., & Howland, R. H. (2002). Biological aspects of depression. In I. H. Gotlib & C. L. Hammen (Eds.), *Handbook of depression* (3rd ed.) (pp. 192–218). New York: Guilford.

Trull, T. J., Widiger, T. A., & Guthrie, P. (1990). Categorical versus dimensional status of borderline personality disorder. *Journal of Abnormal Psychology*, *99*, 40–48.

Tsai, J. L., & Chentsova-Dutton, Y. (2002). Understanding depression across cultures. In I. H. Gotlib & C. L. Hammen (Eds.), *Handbook of Depression* (3rd ed.) (pp. 467–491). New York: Guilford.

Wallace, J., Schneider, T., & McGuffin, P. (2002). In I. H. Gotlib & C. L. Hammen (Eds.), *Handbook of depression* (3rd ed.) (pp. 169–191). New York: Guilford.

Weissman, M., Prusoff, B. A., DiMascio, A., Neu, C., Goklaney, M., & Klerman, G. (1979). The efficacy of drugs and psychotherapy in the treatment of acute depressive episodes. *American Journal of Psychiatry*, *136*, 555–558.

Whisman, M. A. (2001). The association between depression and marital dissatisfaction. In S. R. H. Beach (Ed), *Marital and family processes in depression: A scientific foundation for clinical practice* (pp. 3–24). Washington, DC: American Psychological Association.

Zuroff, D. C., & Fitzpatrick, D. K. (1995). Depressive personality styles: Implications for adult attachment. *Personality and Individual Differences*, *18*, 253–365.

9

Schizophrenia

Elaine Walker
Annie Bollini
Karen Hochman
Lisa Kestler
Emory University

Schizophrenia is among the most debilitating of mental illnesses. It is typically diagnosed between 20 and 25 years of age, a stage of life when most people gain independence from parents, develop intimate romantic relationships, plan educational pursuits, and begin work or career endeavors (DeLisi, 1992). Because the clinical onset usually occurs during this pivotal time, the illness can have a profound negative impact on the individual's opportunities for attaining social and occupational success, and the consequences can be devastating for the adult life course. Furthermore, although treatment approaches and the prognosis for schizophrenia may differ among nations and ethnic groups, the illness knows no national boundaries. Across cultures, estimates of the lifetime prevalence of schizophrenia range around 1%, or one out of 100 (Keith, Regier, & Rae, 1991; Kulhara, & Chakrabarti, 2001; Torrey, 1987), although the prognosis may differ among countries (Kulhara & Chakrabarti, 2001).

The origins of this devastating mental disorder have continued to elude researchers, despite many decades of scientific research. To date, no single factor has been found to characterize all patients with the illness. This holds for potential etiological factors, as well as clinical phenomena. Schizophrenia patients vary in symptom profiles, developmental histories, family backgrounds, cognitive functions, and even brain morphology and neurochemistry. Although this variation has led some to express dismay at our chances of ever finding the cause of schizophrenia, there is reason to be optimistic. Research efforts have succeeded in revealing numerous pieces of what is now recognized as a complex puzzle of etiological processes.

The consensus in the field, based on findings from various lines of research, is that (a) schizophrenia is a brain disease, (b) its etiology involves the interplay between genetic and environmental factors, (c) multiple developmental pathways eventually lead to disease onset, and (d) brain maturational processes play a role in the etiological process. In this chapter, we provide an overview of the current state of our knowledge about schizophrenia. We will begin with a discussion of history and phenomenology, then proceed to a description of some of the key findings that have shed light on the illness.

HISTORY AND PHENOMENOLOGY

Written descriptions of patients experiencing psychotic symptoms have been recorded since antiquity. However, because psychotic symptoms can be a manifestation of a variety of disorders, it is unclear whether schizophrenia, as such, is an ancient or relatively new phenomenon. In the mid-to-late nineteenth century, European psychiatrists were investigating the etiology, classification, and prognoses of the various types of psychosis. At that time, the most common cause of psychosis was *tertiary syphilis*, although researchers were unaware that there was any link between psychosis and syphilis. The psychological symptoms of tertiary syphilis frequently overlap with symptoms of what we now call schizophrenia. The cause of syphilis was eventually traced to an infection with the spirochete, *Treponema pallidum*, and antibiotics were found to be effective for prevention and treatment of the disorder. This important discovery served to illustrate how a psychological syndrome can be produced by an infectious agent. It also sensitized researchers to the fact that similar syndromes might be the result of different causes.

Emil Kraepelin (1856–1926) was the medical director of the famous Heidelberg Clinic. He was the first to differentiate schizophrenia, which he referred to as '*dementia praecox*' (or dementia of the young) from manic-depressive psychosis (Kraepelin, 1913). He also lumped together hebephrenia, paranoia, and catatonia (previously thought to be distinct disorders), and classified all of them as variants of dementia praecox. He based this classification on similarities in age of onset and the tendency for all to involve poor prognosis. Kraepelin did not believe that any one symptom was diagnostic of dementia praecox, but instead based the diagnosis on the total clinical picture and observation of the evolution of symptoms. If a psychotic patient deteriorated over an extended period of time (months/years), the condition was assumed to be dementia praecox.

The expectation of negative outcome with the diagnosis of schizophrenia has continued to pervade the thinking of psychiatry. Although it is true that the majority of patients manifest a chronic course that entails lifelong disability, this is not always the case (Carpenter & Buchanan, 1994). The story of Dr. John Nash, professor and mathematician at Princeton, as told in the movie, *A Beautiful Mind*, illustrates this quite well. Yet, even today, the expectation of negative outcome infuses the mental health profession with an unfortunate sense of therapeutic nihilism.

The term *schizophrenia* was introduced at the beginning of the 20th century by Eugen Bleuler (1857–1939), a Swiss psychiatrist and the medical director of a mental hospital in Zurich (Howells, 1991, pp. xii, 95). The word is derived from two Greek words: *schizo*, which means to tear or to split, and *phren*, which has several meanings: In ancient times, the word *phren* meant the intellect or the mind. *Phren* also referred to the lungs and the diaphragm, which were believed to be the seat of emotions. Thus, the word schizophrenia literally means the splitting or tearing of the mind and emotional stability of the patient.

Bleuler classified the symptoms of schizophrenia into fundamental and accessory symptoms. The fundamental symptoms of schizophrenia are often reported in textbooks as the four As, although, in fact, there are six As and one D (Bleuler, 1911/1950). The fundamental symptoms are listed in Table 9.1. According to Bleuler, these symptoms are present in all patients, at all stages of the illness, and are *diagnostic* of schizophrenia.

Bleuler's accessory symptoms of schizophrenia included delusions, hallucinations, movement disturbances, somatic symptoms, and manic and melancholic states. He believed that these symptoms were not present in all schizophrenia patients and often occurred in other illnesses. For these reasons, the accessory symptoms were not assumed to be diagnostic of schizophrenia.

Further refinements in the diagnostic criteria for schizophrenia were proposed by Kurt Schneider in the mid 1900s. Like Bleuler, Kurt Schneider thought that certain key symptoms

TABLE 9.1

Bleuler's Fundamental Symptoms of Schizophrenia

Disturbances of association (loose, illogical thought processes)
Disturbances of affect (indifference, apathy, or inappropriateness)
Disturbances of attention
Ambivalence (conflicting thoughts, emotions, or impulses that are present simultaneously or in rapid succession)
Autism (detachment from social life with inner preoccupation)
Abulia (lack of drive or motivation)
Dementia (irreversible change in personality)

TABLE 9.2

The Schneiderian First Rank Symptoms

Thought echoing or audible thoughts (patients hear their thoughts out loud)
Thought broadcasting (patients believe that others can hear their thoughts out loud)
Thought intrusion (patients feel that some of their thoughts are from outside; that is, not originating in their own minds)
Thought withdrawal (patients believe that the cause of having lost track of a thought is that someone is taking their thoughts away)
Somatic hallucinations (unusual, unexplained sensations in one's body)
Passivity feelings (patients believe that their thoughts, feelings, or actions are controlled by another or others)
Delusional perception (a sudden, fixed, false belief about a particular everyday occurrence or perception

were diagnostic of schizophrenia (Schneider, 1959). In his classification, he referred to these diagnostic symptoms as first rank symptoms (see Table 9.2). He believed that, after certain medical causes of psychosis were ruled out, one could make the diagnosis of schizophrenia if one or more first rank symptom was present. Schneider's descriptions of the symptoms were more detailed and specific than were Bleuler's fundamental symptoms. Subsequent diagnostic criteria for schizophrenia have been heavily influenced by Schneider's approach.

In subsequent years, investigators began to make a distinction between positive and negative symptoms of schizophrenia (Harvey & Walker, 1987). The positive symptoms are those that involve an excess of ideas, sensory experiences, or behavior. Hallucinations, delusions, and bizarre behaviors fall in this category. Most of the first rank symptoms described by Schneider are also considered to be positive symptoms. Negative symptoms, in contrast, involve a decrease in behavior, such as blunted or flat affect, anhedonia (lack of enjoyment in pleasurable activities, and lack of motivation). These symptoms were emphasized by Bleuler.

During the middle of the twentieth century, different diagnostic criteria for schizophrenia became popular in different parts of the world. The Kraepelinian tradition, with its longitudinal requirements for diagnosis, identified patients with poorer long-term prognosis. In contrast, the Bleulerian and Schneiderian diagnostic systems allowed for a wider range of psychotic patients to be diagnosed with schizophrenia. Thus the patients diagnosed with these two systems tended to have a better prognosis than those diagnosed in the more stringent Kraepelinian tradition. The use of multiple diagnostic systems had a detrimental effect on research progress. Research findings from countries using different diagnostic criteria were not comparable, thus limiting the generalizability of the results.

The next generation of diagnostic systems evolved with the intent of achieving uniformity in diagnostic criteria and improving diagnostic reliability. Among these were the Feighner or St. Louis diagnostic criteria (Feighner, Robins, & Guze, 1972), and the Research Diagnostic Criteria developed by Robert Spitzer and his colleagues (Spitzer, Endicott, & Robins, 1978). These two approaches to the diagnosis of schizophrenia had a major impact on the criteria for schizophrenia contained in contemporary diagnostic systems, most notably, the *Diagnostic and Statistical Manual of Mental Disorders* (DSM).

The DSM is now the most widely used system for diagnosing schizophrenia and other mental disorders. The most recent version of the DSM is the DSM–IV–TR (APA, 2000). Using DSM–IV–TR criteria, schizophrenia can be diagnosed when signs and symptoms of the disorder have been present for 6 months or more (including prodromal and residual phases). The characteristic symptom criteria for schizophrenia include the following; (a) hallucinations, (b) delusions, (c) disorganized speech (e.g., frequent derailment or incoherence), (d) grossly disorganized or catatonic behavior, and (e) negative symptoms, that is, affective flattening, alogia or avolition.

At least two or more of these psychotic symptoms must be present for at least 1 month (or less if successfully treated). Only one of these symptoms is necessary if the delusions are bizarre or the hallucinated voices consist of a running commentary or of two voices conversing (both of these are derived from Schneider's first rank symptoms in Table 9-2). In addition to the clinical symptoms, there must be social/occupational dysfunction. Furthermore, significant mood disorder, such as depression or manic symptoms, must not be present. (This requirement would exclude individuals who meet criteria for major depressive disorder with psychotic symptoms and bipolar disorder with psychotic symptoms). Finally, general medical conditions or substance abuse that might lead to psychotic symptoms must be ruled out.

The four subtypes of schizophrenia described in DSM–IV are *paranoid, disorganized, catatonic, and undifferentiated*. The *paranoid* type is characterized by a preoccupation with delusions or hallucinations, but there is no disorganized speech, disorganized or catatonic behavior, or flat or inappropriate affect. This is the subtype with the best prognosis. In the *disorganized* type, all of the following are prominent: disorganized speech, disorganized behavior, and flat or inappropriate affect, but the criteria for the catatonic subtype are not met. This is the subtype with the worst prognosis. The *catatonic* type involves a clinical syndrome that is dominated by at least two of the following: motoric immobility, excessive purposeless motor activity (catatonic excitement), extreme negativism (purposeless resistance to movement and/or all instructions), mutism (absence of speech), peculiar voluntary movements (voluntary assumption of bizarre or unusual postures), stereotyped movements (repetitive, nonfunctional, yet voluntary), prominent mannerisms (repetitive gestures or expressions) or prominent facial grimacing, or echolalia (repetition of another person's words or phrases) or echopraxia (repetition of another person's actions). Finally, the *undifferentiated* subtype is diagnosed when the patient does not meet criteria for the previous subtypes, yet does meet the general criteria for schizophrenia. The inclusion of this subtype in the DSM–IV should remind us that these are artificially constructed categories, not distinct diagnostic entities with unique causes.

Two other diagnostic categories in the schizophrenia spectrum are worth noting. One is a category for individuals who have met criteria for schizophrenia in the past, but no longer do. This category is referred to as the *residual type*. This diagnosis is applied when there is a prominence of negative symptoms, or two or more attenuated characteristic symptoms, but no prominent delusions, hallucinations, catatonic symptoms, or disorganized behavior or speech. The other category, *schizophreniform disorder*, is for individuals whose symptoms do not meet the six-month criterion. This diagnosis is frequently made as a prelude to the diagnosis of schizophrenia, when the patient presents for treatment early in the course of the disorder.

Some individuals with this disorder, however, will recover completely and not suffer further episodes of psychosis.

It is important to emphasize that, despite advances in diagnosis, we still do not know the diagnostic boundaries of schizophrenia. Moreover, the boundaries between schizophrenia and mood disorders are obscure. Many individuals who meet criteria for schizophrenia show marked signs of depression or manic tendencies. These symptoms are sometimes present before the onset of schizophrenia, and frequently occur in combination with marked psychotic symptoms. As a result, the DSM–IV includes a diagnostic category called *schizoaffective disorder*. This disorder can be thought of as a hybrid between the mood disorders (bipolar disorder or major depression with psychotic features) and schizophrenia. The two subtypes are the *depressive* subtype (if the mood disturbance includes only depressive episodes) and the *bipolar* subtype (where the symptoms of the disorder have included either a manic or a mixed episode). Interestingly, the prognosis for patients with schizoaffective disorder is, on average, somewhere between that of schizophrenia and the mood disorders.

COGNITIVE AND EMOTIONAL ASPECTS OF SCHIZOPHRENIA

Among the most well-established aspects of schizophrenia are the cognitive deficits that accompany the illness. Schizophrenia patients manifest performance deficits on a broad range of cognitive tasks, from simple to complex (Green, Kern, Braff, & Mintz, 2000). One of the most basic is the deficit in the very earliest stages of visual information processing. Using a laboratory procedure called backward masking, researchers have shown that schizophrenia patients are slower in the initial processing of stimuli (Green, Nuechterlein, Breitmeyer, & Mintz, 1999). Among the higher-level cognitive functions, schizophrenia patients show deficits in verbal and spatial memory, abstract reasoning, psychomotor speed, and planning (Kuperberg & Heckers, 2000).

There are also deficits in thinking about social phenomena. Studies of social cognitive abilities in schizophrenia patients have consistently shown that patients are impaired in their ability to comprehend and solve social problems (Penn, Corrigan, Bentall, Racenstein, & Newman, 1997). Deficits in social cognition may be partially due to limitations in more basic cognitive processes, such as memory and reasoning. However, basic cognitive impairments do not account completely for the more pervasive and persistent social cognitive deficits observed in schizophrenia.

One of the diagnostic criteria for schizophrenia is blunted or inappropriate affect. It is, therefore, not surprising that patients show abnormalities in the expression of emotion in both their faces and verbal communications; specifically, less positive and more negative emotion (Brozgold et al., 1998). Further, they are less accurate than normal comparison subjects in their ability to label facial expressions of emotion (Penn, Combs, Ritchie, Francis, Cassisi, Morris, & Townsend, 2000; Walker et al., 1981). Patients with more severe impairments in their abilities to recognize and express emotion also have more problems in social adjustment.

THE ORIGINS OF SCHIZOPHRENIA

Psychological Theories

In the early part of the 20th century, psychosocial theories of schizophrenia dominated the literature. For example, Sigmund Freud, the father of psychoanalysis, believed that psychological processes resulted in the development of psychotic symptoms (Howells, 1991). In 1948, Frieda

Fromm-Reichmann proposed a psychological theory of schizophrenia that postulated that the disorder arose in response to rearing by a schizophrenogenic mother (Fromm-Reichmann, 1948). Although this hypothesis has fallen in disfavor because of lack of support from empirical research, it caused considerable suffering for families. The theory added to the stigma and burden of family members seeking treatment for their ill family members. Subsequently, family interaction models of the etiology of schizophrenia were offered by various theorists (Howells, 1991). Again, these contributed relatively little to our understanding of the etiology of schizophrenia, although they did eventually serve to highlight the importance of considering the role of the family in providing support for the recovering patient.

Biological Theories

Kraepelin, Bleuler, and other early writers on schizophrenia did not offer specific theories about the origins of schizophrenia. They did, however, suggest that there might be a biological basis for at least some cases of the illness. Likewise, contemporary ideas about the origins of schizophrenia focus on biological vulnerabilities that are assumed to be present at birth. Researchers have identified two sources of constitutional vulnerability: genetic factors and prenatal or obstetric factors. Both appear to have implications for fetal brain development.

The Genetics of Schizophrenia.   One of the most well established findings in schizophrenia research is that a vulnerability to the illness can be inherited (Gottesman, 1991). Behavior genetic studies utilizing twin, adoption, and family history methods have all yielded evidence that the risk for schizophrenia is elevated in individuals who have a biological relative with the disorder; the closer the level of genetic relatedness, the greater the likelihood the relative will also suffer from schizophrenia.

In a review of family, twin, and adoption studies conducted from 1916 to 1989, Irving Gottesman (1991) outlined the compelling evidence for the role of genetic factors in schizophrenia. Monozygotic (MZ) twins, who share nearly 100% of their genes, have the highest concordance rate for schizophrenia. Among MZ cotwins of patients with schizophrenia, 25% to 50% will develop the illness. Dizygotic (DZ) twins and other siblings share, on average, only about half of their genes. About 10% to 15% of the DZ cotwins of patients are also diagnosed with the illness. Furthermore, as genetic relatedness of the relative to the patient becomes more distant, such as from first degree (parents, siblings) to second degree relatives (grandparents, half-siblings, aunts, and uncles), the relative's lifetime risk for schizophrenia is reduced.

Adoption studies have provided evidence that the tendency for schizophrenia to run in families is primarily due to genetic factors rather than the environmental influence of being exposed to a mentally ill family member. In a seminal adoption study, Heston (1966) examined the rates of schizophrenia in adoptees with and without a biological parent who was diagnosed with the illness. He found higher rates of schizophrenia, and other mental illnesses, in the biological offspring of parents with schizophrenia, when compared to adoptees with no mental illness in biological parents. Similarly, in a Danish sample, Kety (1988) examined the rates of mental illness in the relatives of adoptees with and without schizophrenia. He found that the biological relatives of adoptees who suffered from schizophrenia had a significantly higher rate of schizophrenia than the adoptive relatives who reared them. Also, the rate of schizophrenia in the biological relatives of adoptees with schizophrenia was higher than in the relatives (biological or adoptive) of healthy adoptees. These adoption studies provide ample evidence for a significant genetic component in the etiology of schizophrenia.

Of course, adoption studies assume a genetic influence when adopted individuals are more similar to their biological parents than their adoptive parents. However, an environmental confound that cannot be ruled out is the intrauterine environment. As described later, there is an elevated rate of substance abuse among schizophrenia patients, so it is possible that the offspring of women with schizophrenia are exposed to more prenatal risk factors. To determine whether adoption findings are partially attributable to intrauterine factors, Kety (1988) examined paternal half-siblings (children with the same father and different mothers) who were adopted away and either developed schizophrenia or had healthy adult outcomes. If the intrauterine environment is increasing risk for schizophrenia in the biological offspring of women with the disorder, then paternal half-siblings should have lower concordance for schizophrenia. Kety found that the rate of schizophrenia in paternal half-siblings of schizophrenic adoptees (13%) was much greater than the rate of schizophrenia in half-siblings of normal adoptees (1.6%), suggesting that the elevated risk is attributable to genetic factors.

But more recent findings from an adoption study indicate that the genetic influences often act in concert with environmental factors. Tienari, Wynne, Moring, and Lahti (1994) conducted an adoption study in Finland, and found that the rate of psychoses and other severe disorders was significantly higher than in the matched control adoptees. However, the difference between the groups was detected only in adoptive families that were rated as dysfunctional. The genetic vulnerability was mainly expressed in association with a disruptive adoptive environment and was not detected in adoptees reared in a healthy, possibly protective, family environment. These findings are consistent with the prevailing diathesis–stress models of etiology.

Taken together, the findings from behavioral genetic studies of schizophrenia lead to the conclusion that the disorder involves multiple genes rather than a single gene (Gottesman, 1991). This conclusion is based on several observations, most notably the fact that the pattern of familial transmission does not conform to what would be expected form a single genetic locus or even a small number of genes. Consistent with this assumption, attempts to identify a genetic locus that accounts for a significant proportion of cases of schizophrenia have not met with success. Instead, researchers using molecular genetic techniques have identified several genes that may account for a very small proportion of cases. Candidate gene analyses and linkage studies have provided some evidence for the involvement of several specific genes, such as the serotonin type 2a receptor (5-HT2a) gene, the dopamine D3 receptor gene, and several chromosomal regions (i.e., regions on chromosomes 6, 8, 13, and 22) (Mowry & Nancarrow, 2001).

One of the most noteworthy genetic discoveries to date is the association between schizophrenia and chromosomal microdeletions in the q11 band of chromosome 22, usually referred to as the 22q11 deletion. The 22q11 deletion occurs in about .025% of the general population and is often accompanied by a physical syndrome that includes structural anomalies of the face, head, and heart. About 25% of individuals with the 22q11 deletion syndrome (DS) meet diagnostic criteria for schizophrenia, and approximately 2% of schizophrenia patients have the 22q11 deletion genotype, although the rate of 22q11 deletion may be higher in patients with an earlier onset (Bassett et al., 1998; Karayiorgou, Morris, & Morrow, 1995).

But beyond the well-established findings described here, there are some ongoing controversies surrounding the genetics of schizophrenia. One of these controversies concerns the specificity of the genetic liability for schizophrenia. Early behavioral genetic studies led to the conclusion that there were separable genetic liabilities for schizophrenia and the major affective disorders, namely, bipolar disorder and psychotic depression. But more recent evidence indicates that this is not the case. Using quantitative genetic techniques with large twin samples, researchers have shown that there is significant overlap in the genes that contribute to schizophrenia, schizoaffective disorder, and manic syndromes (Cardno, Rijsdijk, Sham, Murray, & McGuffin, 2002). Other studies have yielded similar results, leading many in the field to conclude that the genetic vulnerability does not conform to the diagnostic boundaries listed in DSM and other taxonomies (e.g., Potash et al., 2001). Rather, it appears that there is a genetic vulnerability to psychosis in general, and that the expression of this vulnerability can take the form of schizophrenia *or* an affective psychosis, depending on other genetic and acquired risk factors.

The second major controversy in the field concerns the magnitude and extent of the genetic vulnerability for schizophrenia. In other words, what is the relative importance of inherited vulnerability *versus* external factors that impinge on the developing individual. As mentioned earlier, we now know that the environment begins to have an impact before birth; prenatal events are linked with risk for schizophrenia, and some of these prenatal factors are discussed later. Thus, in order to index environmental events that contribute to acquired constitutional vulnerability, we must include both the prenatal and postnatal periods. At this point, however, researchers are not in a position to estimate the relative magnitude of the inherited and environmental contributors to the etiology of schizophrenia. Moreover, we do not yet know whether genetic vulnerability is present in all cases of schizophrenia. It is possible that some cases of the illness are solely attributable to environmental risk factors.

Furthermore, we do not know whether the genetic predisposition to schizophrenia is always expressed, although there is substantive evidence to indicate that it is not. We know that the concordance rate for schizophrenia in MZ twins is nowhere near 100%, which suggests that some genetically vulnerable individuals do not develop the illness. It is possible, however, that the genetic liability for schizophrenia sometimes results from a mutation that occurs in only the affected member of discordant MZ pairs. But findings from studies of discordant MZ twins indicate that the rate of schizophrenia is similar, and elevated, in the offspring of both the affected *and* nonaffected cotwins (Gottesman & Bertelsen, 1989; Kringlen & Cramer, 1989). In other words, the offspring of the normal MZ twin have a rate of schizophrenia similar to the offspring of the ill cotwin, even though they were not raised by a schizophrenic parent. This finding provides support for the notion that some individuals possess a genetic vulnerability for schizophrenia that they pass on to their offspring, despite the fact that they are never diagnosed with the illness. Thus, unexpressed genetic vulnerabilities for schizophrenia may be common in the general population. The presence of individuals who have an unexpressed genetic vulnerability to schizophrenia makes the work of genetic researchers much more difficult. At the same time, the evidence of unexpressed genotypes for schizophrenia leads us to inquire about factors that trigger the expression of illness in vulnerable individuals and to hope that this knowledge may, some day, lead to effective preventative interventions.

Prenatal and Perinatal Factors.   In addition to the support it provides for hereditary influences on schizophrenia, the behavior genetic literature clearly illustrates the relevance of environmental factors. Identifying these factors is a primary focus of many investigators, and the prenatal period has received greater attention in recent years. There is extensive evidence that obstetrical complications (OCs) have an adverse impact on the developing fetal brain and may contribute to vulnerability for schizophrenia. Birth cohort studies have shown that schizophrenia patients are more likely to have a history of OCs (Buka, Tsuang, & Lipsitt, 1993; McNeil, 1988; Dalman, Allebeck, Cullberg, Grunewald, & Koester, 1999). Included among these are pregnancy problems, such as toxemia and preeclampsia, and labor and delivery complications. A review of the OC literature by Cannon (1997) concluded that, among the different types of OCs, labor and delivery complications, which are often associated with hypoxia (fetal oxygen deprivation), were the most strongly linked with later schizophrenia. In the National Collaborative Perinatal Project, which involved over 9,000 children followed from birth through adulthood, the odds of adulthood schizophrenia increased linearly with an increasing number of hypoxia-related OCs (Cannon, Hollister, Bearden, & Hadley, 1997; Cannon, 1998).

Another prenatal event that has been linked with increased risk for schizophrenia is maternal viral infection. Researchers have found that the risk rate for schizophrenia is elevated for individuals born shortly after a flu epidemic (Barr, Mednick, & Munk-Jorgensen, 1990; Murray, Jones, O'Callaghan, & Takei, 1992) or after being prenatally exposed to rubella (Brown, Cohen, Harkavy-Friedman, & Babulas, 2001). The critical period appears to be between the fourth and sixth months of pregnancy. The findings from research on viral infection are consistent with reports on the season-of-birth effect in schizophrenia. Several studies have found that a disproportionate number of schizophrenic patients are born during the late winter months (Bradbury & Miller, 1985; Torrey, Miller, Rawlings, & Yolken, 1997). This timing may reflect seasonal exposure to viral infections, which are most common in late fall and early winter. Thus the fetus could have been exposed to the infection during the second trimester. The second trimester is an important time for brain development, and disruptions during this stage may lead to developmental abnormalities.

Studies of rodents and nonhuman primates have shown that prenatal maternal stress can interfere with fetal brain development and is associated with elevated glucocorticoid release and hippocampal abnormalities in the offspring (Smythe, McCormick, Rochford, & Meaney, 1994; Weinstock, 1996). Along the same lines, in humans, there is evidence that stressful events during pregnancy are associated with greater risk for schizophrenia and other psychiatric disorders in adult offspring. Researchers have found higher rates of schizophrenia in the offspring of women whose spouses had died during their pregnancies (Huttunen, 1989) and in women who were exposed to a military invasion during their pregnancies (van Os & Selten, 1998). It is likely that prenatal stress triggers the release of maternal stress hormones, which have been found to disturb fetal neurodevelopment and subsequent functioning of the hypothalamic-pituitary-adrenal axis, which, in turn influences behavior and cognition (Welberg & Seckl, 2001).

One of the chief questions confronting researchers is whether OCs act independently to increase risk for schizophrenia or, rather, have their effect in conjunction with a genetic vulnerability. One possibility is that the genetic vulnerability for schizophrenia involves an increased sensitivity to prenatal factors that interfere with fetal neurodevelopment (Cannon, 1997; 1998). It is also plausible that obstetrical events act independently of genetic vulnerabilities, although such effects would likely entail complex interactions among factors (Susser & Brown, 1999). For example, in order to produce the neurodevelopmental abnormalities that confer risk for schizophrenia, it may be necessary for a specific OC to occur during a critical period of cellular migration and/or in conjunction with other factors such as maternal fever or immune response. These possibilities are currently the focus of research.

BIOLOGICAL INDICATORS OF VULNERABILITY

Having identified two likely sources of vulnerability for schizophrenia, genetic and obstetrical factors, we now turn to the *nature* of vulnerability. Where does the weakness lie? Since the turn of the century, writers in the field of psychopathology had suspected that schizophrenia involved some biological abnormality in the brain (Bleuler, 1965). This assumption was based, in part, on the severity of the symptoms and the deteriorating clinical course. However, it was not until the advent of neuroimaging techniques that solid, empirical data were gathered to support this assumption.

Abnormalities in Brain Structure

The first reports on brain abnormalities in schizophrenia patients were based on computerized axial tomography (CAT) scans, and showed that they had enlarged brain ventricles, especially increased volume of the lateral ventricles (Dennert & Andreasen, 1983). As new techniques for brain scanning were developed, these findings were replicated and additional abnormalities were detected (Henn & Braus, 1999). Magnetic resonance imaging (MRI) revealed decreased frontal, temporal, and whole brain volume among people with schizophrenia (Lawrie & Abukmeil, 1998). More fine-grained analyses demonstrated reductions in the size of structures such as the thalamus and hippocampus. In fact, of all the regions studied, the hippocampus is one that has most consistently been identified as distinguishing people with schizophrenia from healthy controls (Schmajuk, 2001).

A landmark study of MZ twins discordant for schizophrenia was the first to demonstrate that these brain abnormalities were not solely attributable to genetic factors (Suddath, Christison, Torrey, Casanova, & Weinberger, 1990). When compared to their healthy identical cotwins, twins with schizophrenia were found to have smaller temporal lobe volumes, with the hippocampal region showing the most dramatic difference between the affected and nonaffected cotwins. Subsequent studies have confirmed smaller brain volumes among affected twins than among their healthy identical cotwins (Baare, van Oel, Pol, Schnack, Durston, Sitskoorn, & Kahn, 2001). These studies lend support to the hypothesis that the brain abnormalities observed in schizophrenia are at least partially due to factors that interfere with prenatal brain development.

Despite the plethora of research findings indicating the presence of abnormalities in the brains of patients with schizophrenia, however, no specific abnormality has yet been shown to be pathognomonic. In other words, there is no evidence that a specific morphological abnormality is unique to schizophrenia or characterizes all schizophrenia patients. The structural brain abnormalities observed in schizophrenia are, therefore, gross manifestations of the occurrence of a deviation in neurodevelopment that has implications for neurocircuitry function.

Neurotransmitters

The idea that schizophrenia involves an abnormality in neurotransmission has a long history. Initial neurotransmitter theories focused on epinephrine and norepinephrine. Subsequent approaches have hypothesized that serotonin, glutamate and/or gamma-amino butyric acid (GABA) abnormalities are involved in schizophrenia. But, compared to other neurotransmitters, dopamine has played a more enduring role in theorizing about the biochemical basis of schizophrenia. In this section we will review the major neurotransmitter theories of schizophrenia, with an emphasis on dopamine.

In the early 1950s, investigators began to suspect that dopamine might be playing a central role in schizophrenia. Dopamine is widely distributed in the brain and is one of the neurotransmitters that enables communication in the circuits that link subcortical with cortical brain regions (Jentsch, Roth, & Taylor, 2000). Since the 1950s, support for this idea has waxed and waned. In the past decade, however, there has been a resurgence of interest in dopamine, largely because research findings have offered a new perspective.

The initial support for the role of dopamine in schizophrenia was based on two indirect pieces of evidence (Carlsson, 1988); (a) drugs that reduce dopamine activity also serve to diminish psychotic symptoms, and (b) drugs that heighten dopamine activity exacerbate or trigger psychotic episodes. It was eventually discovered that antipsychotic drugs had their effect by blocking dopamine receptors, especially the D2 subtype that is prevalent in subcortical regions of the brain. The newer antipsychotic drugs, or atypical antipsychotics, have the advantage of causing fewer motor side effects. Nonetheless, they also act on the dopamine system by blocking various subtypes of dopamine receptors (Jentsch, Roth, & Taylor, 2000).

Early studies of dopamine in schizophrenia sought to determine whether there was evidence of excess neurotransmitter in schizophrenia patients. But concentrations of dopamine and its metabolites were generally not found to be elevated in fluids from schizophrenia patients (Carlsson, Hansson, Waters, & Carlsson, 1999). When investigators examined dopamine receptors, however, there was some evidence of increased densities. Both postmortem and functional MRI studies of patients' brains yielded evidence that the number of dopamine D2 receptors tends to be greater in patients than normal controls (Kestler, Walker, & Vega, 2001). Controversy has surrounded this literature, because antipsychotic drugs can change dopamine receptor density. Nonetheless, even studies of never-medicated patients with schizophrenia have shown elevations in dopamine receptors (Kestler et al., 2001).

Other abnormalities in dopamine transmission have also been found. It appears, for example, that dopamine synthesis and release may be more pronounced in the brains of people with schizophrenia than among normals (Lindstrom et al., 1999). When schizophrenia patients and normal controls are given amphetamine, a drug that enhances dopamine release, the patients show more augmented dopamine release (Abi-Dargham et al., 1998; Soares & Innis, 1999).

Glutamate is an excitatory neurotransmitter. Glutamatergic neurons are part of the pathways that connect the hippocampus, prefrontal cortex, and thalamus, all regions that have been implicated in schizophrenia. There is evidence of diminished activity at glutamatergic receptors among schizophrenia patients in these brain regions (Carlsson, Hansson, Waters, & Carlsson, 1999; Goff & Coyle, 2001; Tsai & Coyle, 2002). One of the chief receptors for glutamate in the brain is the N-methyl-D-aspartic acid (NMDA) subtype of receptor. It has been suggested that these receptors may be abnormal in schizophrenia. Blockade of NMDA receptors produces the symptomatic manifestations of schizophrenia in normal subjects, including negative symptoms and cognitive impairments. For example, administration of NMDA receptor antagonists, such as phencyclidine (PCP) and ketamine, induces a broad range of schizophrenic-like symptomatology in humans, and these findings have contributed to a hypoglutamatergic hypothesis of schizophrenia. Conversely, drugs that indirectly enhance NMDA receptor function can reduce negative symptoms and improve cognitive functioning in schizophrenia patients. It is important to note that the idea of dysfunction of glutamatergic transmission is not inconsistent with the dopamine hypothesis of schizophrenia, because there are reciprocal connections between forebrain dopamine projections and systems that use glutamate. Thus dysregulation of one system would be expected to alter neurotransmission in the other.

GABA is an inhibitory neurotransmitter. Some have suggested that its inhibitory effects may be increased in psychotic disorders (Squires & Saederup, 1991). On the other hand, the uptake and the release of GABA has been shown to be reduced in some studies of postmortem brain tissue from schizophrenia patients (Lewis, Pierri, Volk, Melchitzky, & Woo, 1999), and there are abnormalities in the interconnections among GABA neurons (Benes & Berretta, 2001). More specifically, there is evidence of a loss of cortical GABA interneurons. Current theories about the role of GABA in schizophrenia assume that it is important because cortical processes require an optimal balance between GABA inhibition and glutamatergic excitation.

The true picture of the neurochemical abnormalities in schizophrenia may be more complex than we would like to assume. All neurotransmitter systems interact in intricate ways at multiple levels in the brain's circuitry (Carlsson et al., 2001). Consequently, an alteration in the synthesis, reuptake, or receptor density affinity for any one of the neurotransmitter systems would be expected to have implications for one or more of the other neurotransmitter systems. Further, because neural circuits involve multiple segments that rely on different transmitters, it is easy to imagine how an abnormality in even one specific subgroup of receptors could result in the dysfunction of all the brain regions linked by a particular brain circuit.

COURSE AND PROGNOSIS

Assuming that genetic and obstetrical factors confer the vulnerability for schizophrenia, the diathesis must be present at birth. Yet, schizophrenia is typically diagnosed in late adolescence or early adulthood, with the average age of diagnosis in males about four years earlier than for females (Riecher-Rossler & Hafner, 2000). This fact raises intriguing questions about the developmental course before the clinical onset.

Premorbid Development

There is compelling evidence that there are signs of schizophrenia long before the illness is diagnosed. Most of these signs are subtle and do not reach the severity of clinical disorder. Nonetheless, when compared to children with healthy adult outcomes, children who later develop schizophrenia manifest deficits in multiple domains. In some of these domains, the deficits are apparent as early as infancy.

In the area of cognitive functioning, children who later develop schizophrenia tend to perform below their healthy siblings and classmates. This is reflected in lower scores on measures of intelligence and achievement and poorer grades in school (Aylward, Walker, & Bettes, 1984; Jones, Rodgers, Murray, & Marmot, 1994). Preschizophrenic children also show abnormalities in social behavior. They are less responsive in social situations, show less positive emotion (Walker & Lewine, 1990; Walker, Grimes, Davis, & Smith, 1993), and have poorer social adjustment than children with healthy adult outcomes (Done, Crow, Johnstone, & Sacker, 1994; Neumann, Walker, Lewine, & Baum, 1996). In our studies of the childhood home movies of schizophrenia patients, we found that the preschizophrenic children showed more negative facial expression of emotion than did their siblings as early as the first year of life, indicating that the vulnerability for schizophrenia is subtly manifested in the earliest interpersonal interactions (Walker et al., 1993).

Vulnerability to schizophrenia is also apparent in motor functions. When compared to their siblings with healthy adult outcomes, preschizophrenic children show more delays and abnormalities in motor development, including deficits in the acquisition of early motor milestones such as bimanual manipulation and walking (Walker, Savoi, & Davis, 1994). Deficits in motor function extend throughout the premorbid period and persist after the onset of the clinical illness (McNeil, Cantor-Graae, & Weinberger 2000). It is important to note that neuromotor abnormalities are not pathognomonic for schizophrenia, in that they are observed in children at risk for a variety of disorders, including learning disabilities and conduct and mood disorders. But they are one of several important clues pointing to the involvement of brain dysfunction in schizophrenia.

Despite the subtle signs of abnormality that have been identified in children at risk for schizophrenia, most do not manifest diagnosable mental disorders in childhood. Thus, while their parents may recall some irregularities in their development, most preschizophrenic children were not viewed as clinically disturbed. But the picture often changes in adolescence. Many adolescents who go on to develop schizophrenia show a pattern of escalating adjustment problems (Walker & Baum, 1998). They show a gradual increase in adjustment problems, including feelings of depression, social withdrawal, irritability, and noncompliance. But this developmental pattern is not unique to schizophrenia; adolescence is also the critical period for the expression of the first signs of mood disorders, substance abuse, and some other behavioral disorders. As a result, researchers view adolescence as a critical period for the emergence of various kinds of behavioral dysfunction (Walker, 2002).

Among the behavioral risk indicators sometimes observed in preschizophrenic adolescents are subclinical signs of psychotic symptoms. These signs are also the defining features of a DSM Axis II disorder, namely, *schizotypal personality disorder* (SPD). The diagnostic criteria for SPD include social anxiety or withdrawal, affective abnormalities, eccentric behavior, unusual ideas (e.g., persistent belief in extrasensory perception [ESP], aliens, extrasensory phenomena, etc.), and unusual sensory experiences (e. g., repeated experiences with confusing noises with peoples' voices, seeing objects move, etc.). Although the individual's unusual ideas and perceptions are not severe or persistent enough to meet criteria for delusions or hallucinations, they are recurring and atypical of the person's cultural context. An extensive body of research demonstrates genetic and developmental links between schizophrenia and SPD. The genetic link between SPD and schizophrenia has been documented in twin and family history studies (Kendler, McGuire, Gruenberg, & Walsh, 1995; Kendler, Neale, & Walsh, 1995; Raine & Mednick, 1995). The developmental transition from schizotypal signs to schizophrenia in young adulthood has been followed in several recent longitudinal studies, with researchers reporting that 20% to 40% of schizotypal youth eventually show an Axis I schizophrenia spectrum disorder (Miller et al., 2002; Yung et al., 1998). The remainder either show other adjustment problems or a complete remission of symptoms in young adulthood. Given the high rate of progression to schizophrenia, researchers are now attempting to determine whether schizotypal youth who will eventually manifest schizophrenia can be identified before the onset of the illness. This step is considered to be pivotal in efforts to develop secondary prevention programs.

Recent investigations have revealed that adolescents with SPD manifest some of the same functional abnormalities observed in patients with schizophrenia. For example, SPD youth show motor abnormalities (Walker, Lewis, Loewy, & Paylo, 1999), cognitive deficits (Diforio, Kestler, & Walker, 2000), and an increase in cortisol, a stress hormone that is elevated in several psychiatric disorders (Weinstein, Diforio, Schiffman, Walker, & Bonsall, 1999). These new findings may eventually aid in the identification of SPD adolescents who are at greatest risk for developing schizophrenia.

The Illness Onset

The onset of the first episode of schizophrenia may be sudden or gradual. As mentioned earlier, it is usually preceded by escalating adjustment problems, a period referred to as the *prodromal* phase (Lieberman et al., 2001). There is some evidence that longer untreated psychotic episodes may be harmful for schizophrenia patients and may result in a worse course of illness (Davidson & McGlashan, 1997). However, this conclusion is controversial, and some researchers suggest that the relation between longer duration of untreated psychosis and worse prognosis may be a product of poorer premorbid functioning and an insidious onset (Larsen et al., 2001).

People with schizophrenia vary in their course of illness and prognosis. Being male, gradual onset, early age of onset, poor premorbid functioning, and family history of schizophrenia are all associated with poorer prognosis (Gottesman, 1991). In addition, some environmental factors have been found to contribute to a worse outcome. For example, schizophrenia patients who live in homes where family members express greater negative emotion are more likely than those from warm, supportive families to have relapses (Butzlaff & Hooley, 1998). Also, exposure to stress has been found to exacerbate schizophrenia symptoms. Researchers have found an increase in the number of stressful events in the months immediately preceding a schizophrenia relapse (Ventura, Neuchterlein, Hardesty, & Gitlin, 1992).

As outlined, the prognosis for many schizophrenia patients is poor. Only 20% to 30% are able to lead somewhat normal lives, meaning they can live independently and/or maintain a job (Grebb & Cancro, 1989). The majority experience a more debilitating course, with 20% to 30% manifesting continued moderate symptoms and over half experiencing significant impairment the rest of their lives. Furthermore, patients with schizophrenia often suffer from other comorbid (i. e., co-occurring) conditions. For example, the rate of substance abuse among schizophrenia patients is very high, with as many as 47% in the community and 90% in prison settings meeting lifetime DSM–IV criteria for substance abuse or dependence (Regier et al., 1990).

Suicide is the leading cause of death among people with schizophrenia. It has been estimated that 25% to 50% of schizophrenia patients attempt suicide and 4% to 13% successfully commit suicide (Meltzer, 2001). Risk factors associated with suicide in this population include more severe accompanying depressive symptoms, being male, earlier onset, and recent traumatic events (Schwartz & Cohen, 2001).

THE TREATMENT OF SCHIZOPHRENIA

Researchers have not yet identified any psychological or biological cures for schizophrenia. However, significant progress has been made in the development of treatments that greatly improve the prognosis for the illness. Thus the quality of life for patients is now much better than it was at the turn of the century.

The first issue to be addressed in the evaluation and treatment of schizophrenia is safety. The risk of self-harm and potential for violence must be assessed. This is of particular importance because of the risk of suicide in patients with schizophrenia (Siris, 2001). Furthermore, a medical examination is typically administered in order to rule out other illnesses that can cause psychotic symptoms. This examination includes a review of the medical history, a physical examination, and laboratory tests. Many patients with schizophrenia have untreated medical conditions, such as nutritional deficiencies and infections, that are a result of their psychological and/or socioeconomic limitations (Goff, Heckers, & Freudenreich, 2001).

If a patient is not at acute risk to self or others, the next consideration becomes the type of treatment that would be most beneficial. There are several factors to consider. These include the person's living situation (many patients with schizophrenia are homeless), financial resources including health insurance, family and other available social support, the person's level of insight and willingness to accept treatment, past treatment history, and the person's preference.

The treatment of schizophrenia can be divided into three phases: the acute, stabilization, and maintenance phases (Kaplan & Sadock, 1998). In the acute phase, the goal of treatment is to reduce the severity of symptoms. This phase is usually of 4 to 8 weeks in duration. In the stabilization phase, the goal is to consolidate treatment gains. This usually takes about 6 months. Finally, during the maintenance phase, the symptoms are in remission (partial or complete). At this point, the goal of treatment is to prevent relapse and improve functioning.

Antipsychotic Medication

The mainstay of the biological treatment of schizophrenia is antipsychotic medication. The first effective biological treatment for schizophrenia, chlorpromazine (Thorazine), was developed in the 1950s. It was the first in a line of medications now referred to as the typical antipsychotics or neuroleptics. All of these medications act by blocking activity in the dopamine systems. The typical antipsychotic medications are classified as high, medium, and low potency and differ from each other in side-effect profiles (see Table 9.3). *High potency* neuroleptics tend to carry a higher risk of motor side effects, and are prescribed in low dosages. Some examples of high potency agents are Prolixin (fluphenazine), Stelazine (trifluoperazine), and Haldol (haloperidol). *Low potency* neuroleptics are prescribed in higher doses and have lower risk of motor side effects, but a higher risk of inducing seizures, antihistaminic effects (including sedation and weight gain), anticholinergic effects (including cognitive dulling, dry mouth, blurry vision, urinary hesitancy, and constipation), and antiadrenergic effects (including postural hypotension and sexual dysfunction). Examples of low potency neuroleptics include Thorazine (chlorpromazine), and Mellaril (thioridazine). *Medium potency* agents tend to have side effects

TABLE 9.3

Selected Antipsychotic Drugs

Drug	Route of Administration	Usual Daily Oral Dose	Sedation	Autonomic	Extrapyramidal Adverse Effects
Chlorpromazine	Oral, IM	200–600	+++	+++	++
Fluphenazine	Oral, IM, depot	2–20	+	+	+++
Trifluoperazine	Oral, IM	5–30	++	+	+++
Perphenazine	Oral, IM	8–64	++	+	+++
Haloperidol	Oral, IM, depot	5–20	+	+	+++
Loxapine	Oral, IM	20–100	++	+	++
Olanzapine	Oral	7.5–25	+	++	0?
Quetiapine	Oral	150–750	++	++	0?
Risperidone	Oral	2–16	+	++	+
Clozapine	Oral	150–900	+++	+++	0?

From Sadock & Sadock, 2000.

intermediate between the low and high potency drugs. Examples of these are Trilafon (perphenazine) and Loxapac (loxapine).

In the 1990s a new generation of antipsychotic medications became available for therapeutic use in Europe and North America. The new class of medication is referred to as the atypicals. Medications in this class share with each other a lower risk of both the early occurring and the late emerging (or tardive) movement disorders. The atypical antipsychotics include the following: Risperdal (risperidone), Zyprexa (olanzapine), Seroquel (quetiapine), Geodon (ziprazadone), and Clozaril (clozapine). They differ significantly from one another in terms of the neurotransmitter receptors that they occupy. Although all block dopamine neurotransmission to some extent, they vary in the extent to which they affect serotonin, glutamate, and other neurotransmitters. These atypical antipsychotics have become first line in the treatment of schizophrenia. The efficacy of the atypical antipsychotics for the treatment of positive symptoms is at least equivalent to that of the typical antipsychotics, and some studies suggest that they are more effective for negative symptoms and the cognitive impairment associated with the disorder. (Forster, Buckley, & Phelps, 1999).

Antipsychotic medications are usually administered orally. For patients who are not compliant with oral medication, injectible, long-lasting antipsychotic medication (referred to as depot medication) may be administered every few weeks. Two depot neuroleptics are commercially available in the United States: Prolixin (fluphenazine decanoate), and Haldol (haloperidol decanoate). Benefits of depot neuroleptics include the ease of use for the patient and the fact that compliance is easily monitored by the clinician. The risks are similar to the risks of all of the typical antipsychotics. The only additional risk is that of localized pain or swelling at the injection site.

Drug-induced movement disorders can be divided into early and late emerging syndromes (from Sadock & Sadock, 2000, table 12.8-3 p. 1207). Early emerging motor syndromes include pseudoparkinsonism, bradykinesia (decreased movement), rigidity, and dystonic reactions (sudden onset of sustained intense, uncontrollable muscle contraction commonly occurring in the facial and neck muscles). Tardive dyskinesia is a late emerging syndrome that includes irregular choreiform (twisting or wormlike) movements that usually involve the facial muscles, but can involve any voluntary muscle group. It is fortunate that the rate of tardive dyskinesia has declined since the introduction of atypical neuroleptics.

Mention should also be made of the neuroleptic malignant syndrome (NMS). This is a rare, idiopathic, life-threatening complication of neuroleptic medication. It is characterized by mental status changes (delirium), immobility, rigidity, tremulousness, staring, fever, sweating, and autonomic instability (labile blood pressure and tachycardia). Laboratory investigations often reveal an elevated white blood cell count (in the absence of infection), as well as other abnormalities. Treatment involves discontinuation of neuroleptic medication, supportive medical treatment, a peripheral muscle relaxant, and bromocriptine (a D2 receptor agonist) (Rosebush, & Mazurek, 2001).

Psychosocial Treatments of Schizophrenia

Although antipsychotic medication is the crucial first step in the treatment of schizophrenia, there is substantial evidence that psychosocial interventions can also be beneficial for both the patient and the family (Penn & Mueser, 1996). It is unfortunate that such treatments are not always available because of limited mental health resources. Nonetheless, it is generally agreed that the optimal treatment approach is one that integrates pharmacologic and psychosocial interventions.

A large body of research supports the use of family therapy, which includes psychoeducational and behavioral components, in treatment programs for schizophrenia (Bustillo, Lauriello, Horan, & Keith, 2001). Family therapy has been shown to reduce the risk of relapse, reduce family burden, and improve family members' understanding of and coping with schizophrenia.

Comprehensive programs for supporting the patient's transition back into the community have been effective in enhancing recovery and reducing relapse. One such program, called Assertive Community Treatment (ACT), was originally developed in the 1970s by researchers in Madison, Wisconsin (Bustillo et al., 2001; Sadock & Sadock, 2000). ACT is a comprehensive treatment approach for the seriously mentally ill living in the community. Patients are assigned to a multidisciplinary team (nurse, case manager, general physician, psychiatrist) that has a fixed caseload and a high staff/patient ratio (1:12). The team delivers all services to the patient when and where he or she needs them and is available to the patient at all times. Services include home delivery of medication, monitoring of physical and mental health status, *in vivo* social skills training, and frequent contact with family members. Studies suggest that ACT can reduce time spent in hospital, improve housing stability, and increase patient and family satisfaction.

Social skills training seeks to improve the overall functioning of patients by teaching the skills necessary to improve performance of activities of daily living, employment-related skills, and interaction with others (Bustillo et al., 2001; Penn & Mueser, 1996). Some social skills programs emphasize learning new skills through modeling. Others focus more on teaching patients better strategies for solving interpersonal problems or training them to read nonverbal cues of emotion in other people. Research indicates that all of these approaches to social skills training can improve social competence in the laboratory and in the clinic (Bustillo, 2001). However, it remains unclear to what extent this improvement in social competence translates into better functioning in the community.

The rate of competitive employment for the severely mentally ill has been estimated at less than 20% (Lehman, 1995); thus vocational rehabilitation has been a major focus of many treatment programs. Vocational rehabilitation programs have a positive influence on work-related activities, although they have not yet been shown to have a substantial impact on patients' abilities to obtain employment in the community (Lehman, 1995). Some evidence suggests that supported employment programs that provide assistance in maintaining good work habits produce better results than traditional vocational rehabilitation programs. Nonetheless, job retention remains a significant problem (Lehman et al., 2002), and little evidence supports

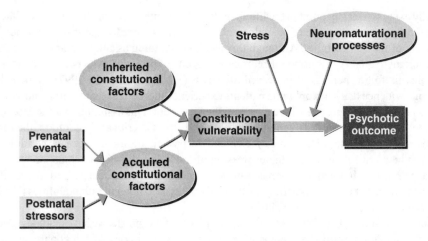

FIG. 9.1. A diathesis–stress model of the etiology of schizophrenia.

the contention that employment improves self-esteem or quality of life (Bustillo et al., 2001). Of course, employment has financial benefits for patients and may offer access to health care that would otherwise not be available.

Finally, cognitive behavior therapy for schizophrenia draws on the tenets of cognitive therapy that were originally developed by Beck and Ellis (Beck, 1976; Ellis, 1986). The theory is that normal psychological processes can play a role in specific psychotic symptoms. Cognitive behavior therapy (CBT) for psychosis challenges the notion of a discontinuity between psychotic and normal thinking. The normal cognitive mechanisms that are already being used in the nonpsychotic aspects of the patient's thinking can be used to help the psychotic individuals deal directly with their symptoms. Individual CBT emphasizes a collaborative relationship between patient and therapist. The therapist and patient jointly examine the patient's specific symptoms. The choice of target symptoms is based on the patient's preference and/or severity of the problems created by the psychotic symptom in question. Psychotic beliefs are never directly confronted, although specific psychotic symptoms such as hallucinations, delusions, and related problems are targeted for intervention (Dickerson, 2000). The few published randomized controlled trials available for review suggest that CBT is at least somewhat effective in reducing hallucinations and delusions in medication-resistant patients and as a complement to pharmacotherapy in acute psychosis (Bustillo et al., 2001).

This chapter has reviewed a broad range of scientific research on the nature and origins of schizophrenia. Spanning over a century, the efforts of investigators have yielded, piece by piece, a clearer view of the illness. The puzzle is not solved, but we can certainly claim progress toward a solution. The picture that has emerged is best described in the framework of the *diathesis–stress* model that has dominated the field for several decades.

Figure 9.1 illustrates a contemporary version of the diathesis–stress model. This particular model postulates that constitutional vulnerability (i.e., the *diathesis*) emanates from both inherited and acquired constitutional factors. The inherited factors are genetically determined characteristics of the brain that influence its structure and function. Acquired vulnerabilities arise mainly from prenatal events that compromise fetal neurodevelopment.

Whether the constitutional vulnerability is a consequence of genetic factors, environmental factors, or a combination of both, the model assumes that vulnerability is, in most cases, congenital. But the assumption that vulnerability is present at birth does not imply that it will be clinically expressed at any point in the life span. Rather, the model posits that two sets of factors determine the postnatal course of the vulnerable individual. First, external stress influences the expression of the vulnerability. Although this is a long-standing assumption among theorists, it is important to qualify this notion. Empirical research has provided evidence that episodes of schizophrenia follow periods of increased life stress (Walker & Diforio, 1997). Nonetheless, there is no evidence that schizophrenia patients experience more stress than healthy individuals, but rather that they are more sensitive to stress when it occurs. This assumption is the essence of the model—the interaction between vulnerability and stress is critical. In addition, the model assumes that neuromaturation is a key element. In particular, adolescence/early adulthood appears to be a critical period for the expression of the vulnerability for schizophrenia. Thus some aspects(s) of brain maturational processes during the postpubertal period are likely playing an important role in triggering the clinical expression of latent vulnerabilities (Walker, 1994; Walker, Walder, & Reynolds, 2001).

In summary, although we have not found all the pieces of the puzzle, we have made significant progress in moving toward a comprehensive account of the etiology of schizophrenia. In the coming years, we can expect research to yield important information about the precise nature of the brain vulnerabilities associated with schizophrenia and the mechanisms involved in the interaction of congenital vulnerability with subsequent life stress and neuromaturation.

REFERENCES

Abi-Dargham, A., Gil, R., Krystal, J., Baldwin, R. M., Seibyl, J. P., Bowers, M., van Dyck, C. H., Charney, D. S., Innis, R. B., & Laruelle, M. (1998). Increased striatal dopamine transmission in schizophrenia: Confirmation in a second cohort. *American Journal of Psychiatry, 155*, 761–767.

American Psychiatric Association. (2000). *Diagnostic and statistical manual of mental disorders* (4th ed., text rev.). Washington, DC: Author.

Aylward, E., Walker, E., & Bettes, B. (1984). Intelligence in schizophrenia: Meta-analysis of the research. *Schizophrenia Bulletin, 10*, 430–459.

Baare, W. F., van Oel, C. J., Pol H. E., Schnack, H. G., Durston, S., Sitskoorn, M. M., & Kahn, R. S. (2001). Volumes of brain structures in twins discordant for schizophrenia. *Archives of General Psychiatry, 58*(1), 33–40.

Barr, C. E., Mednick, S. A., & Munk-Jorgensen, P. (1990). Exposure to influenza epidemics during gestation and adult schizophrenia: A 40-year study. *Archives of General Psychiatry, 47*, 869–874.

Bassett, A. S., Hodgkinson, K., Chow, E. W., Correia, S., Scutt, L. E., Weksberg, R. (1998). 22q11 deletion syndrome in adults with schizophrenia. *American Journal of Medical Genetics, 81*, 328–337.

Beck, A. T. (1976). Cognitive therapy and the emotional disorders. 356pp.

Benes, F. M., & Berretta, S. (2001). GABA ergic interneurons: Implications for understanding schizophrenia and bipolar disorder. *Neuropsychopharmacology, 25*(1), 1–27.

Bleuler, E. (1950). *Group of schizophrenias* (J. Zinkin, Trans.). (1950), New York: International Universities Press. (Original work published 1911)

Bleuler, M. (1965). Conception of schizophrenia within the last fifty years and today. *International Journal of Psychiatry, 1*(4), 501–523.

Bradbury, T. N., & Miller, G. A. (1985). Season of birth in schizophrenia: A review of evidence, methodology, and etiology. *Psychological Bulletin, 98*, 569–594.

Brown, A. S., Cohen, P., Harkavy-Friedman, J., & Babulas, V. (2001). Prenatal rubella, premorbid abnormalities, and adult schizophrenia. *Biological Psychiatry, 49*, 473–486.

Brozgold, A. Z., Borod, J. C., Martin, C. C., Pick, L. H., Alpert, M., & Welkowitz, J. (1998). Social functioning and facial emotional expression in neurological and psychiatric disorders. *Applied Neuropsychology, 5*(1), 15–23.

Buka, S. L., Tsuang, M. T., & Lipsitt, L. P. (1993). Pregnancy/delivery complications and psychiatric diagnosis: A prospective study. *Archives of General Psychiatry, 50*, 151–156.

Bustillo, J. R., Lauriello, J., Horan, W. P., & Keith, S. J. (2001). The psychosocial treatment of schizophrenia: An update. *The American Journal of Psychiatry, 158*, 163–175.

Butzlaff, R. L., & Hooley, J. M. (1998). Expressed emotion and psychiatric relapse. *Archives of General Psychiatry, 55*, 547–552.

Cannon, T. D. (1997). On the nature and mechanisms of obstetric influences in schizophrenia: A review and synthesis of epidemiologic studies. *International Review of Psychiatry*, *9*, 387–397.

Cannon, T. D. (1998). Genetic and perinatal influences in the etiology of schizophrenia: A neurodevelopmental model. In M. F. Lenzenweger & R. H. Dworkin (Eds.), *Origins and development of schizophrenia* (pp. 67–92). Washington, DC: American Psychological Association.

Cannon, T. D., Hollister, J. M., Bearden, C. E., & Hadley, T. (1997). A prospective cohort study of genetic and perinatal influences in schizophrenia. *Schizophrenia Research*, *24*, 248.

Cardno, A. G., Rijsdijk, F. V., Sham, P. C., Murray, R. M., & McGuffin, P. (2002). A twin study of genetic relationships between psychotic symptoms. *American Journal of Psychiatry*, *159*, 539–545.

Carlsson A. (1988). The current status of the dopamine hypothesis of schizophrenia. *Neuropsychopharmacology*, *1*(3), 179–86.

Carlsson, A., Hansson, L. O., Waters, N., & Carlsson, M. L. (1997). Neurotransmitter aberrations in schizophrenia: New perspectives and therapeutic implications. *Life Sciences*, *61*(2), 75–94.

Carlsson, A., Hansson, L.O., Waters, N., & Carlsson, M.L. (1999). A glutamatergic deficiency model of schizophrenia. *British Journal of Psychiatry*, *37*, 2–6.

Carlsson, A., Waters, N., Holm-Waters, S., Tedroff, J., Nilsson, M., & Carlsson, M. L. (2001). Interactions between monoamines, glutamate, and GABA in schizophrenia: New evidence. *Annual Review of Pharmacology & Toxicology*, *41*, 237–260.

Carpenter, W. T., & Buchanan, R. W. (1994). Schizophrenia. *New England Journal of Medicine*, *330*, 681–690.

Dalman, C., Allebeck, P., Cullberg, J., Grunewald, C., & Koester, M. (1999). Obstetric complications and the risk of schizophrenia: A longitudinal study of a national birth cohort. *Archives of General Psychiatry*, *56*, 234–240.

Davidson, L., & McGlashan, T. H. (1997). The varied outcomes of schizophrenia. *Canadian Journal of Psychiatry*, *42*, 34–43.

DeLisi, L. E. (1992). The significance of age of onset for schizophrenia. *Schizophrenia Bulletin*, *18*, 209–215.

Dennert, J. W., & Andreasen N. C. (1983). CT scanning and schizophrenia: A review. *Psychiatric Developments*, *1*(1), 105–22.

Dickerson, F. B. (2000). Cognitive behavioral psychotherapy for schizophrenia: A review of recent empirical studies. *Schizophrenia Research*, *43*, 71–90.

Diforio, D., Kestler, L. & Walker, E. (2000). Executive functions in adolescents with schizotypal personality disorder. *Schizophrenia Research*, *42*, 125–134.

Done, D. J., Crow, T. J., Johnstone, E. C., & Sacker, A. (1994). Childhood antecedents of schizophrenia and affective illness: Social adjustment at ages 7 and 11. *British Medical Journal*, *309*, 699–703.

Ellis, A. (1986). Rational-emotive therapy and cognitive behavior therapy: Similarities and differences. In A. Ellis and R. Grieger (Eds), *Handbook of rational-emotive therapy* (Vol. 2, pp. 31–45). New York: Springer.

Feighner, J. P., Robins, E., & Guze, S. B. (1972). Diagnostic criteria for use in psychiatric research. *Archives of General Psychiatry*, *26*, 57–63.

Forster, P. L., Buckley, R., & Phelps, M. A. (1999). Phenomenology and treatment of psychotic disorders in the psychiatric emergency service. *Psychiatric Clinics of North America*, *22*, 735–754.

Fromm-Reichmann, F. (1948). Notes on the treatment of schizophrenia by psychoanalytic psychotherapy. *Psychiatry*, *11*, 263.

Goff, D. C., & Coyle, J. T. (2001). The emerging role of glutamate in the pathophysiology and treatment of schizophrenia. *American Journal of Psychiatry*, *158*, 1367–1377.

Goff, D. C., Heckers, S., & Freudenreich, O. (2001). Advances in the pathophysiology and treatment of psychiatric disorders: Implications for internal medicine. *Medical Clinics of North America*, *85*, 663–689.

Gottesman, I. I. (1991). *Psychiatric genesis: The origins of madness*. New York: W. H. Freeman.

Gottesman, I. I., & Bertelsen, A. (1989). Confirming unexpressed genotypes for schizophrenia: Risks in the offspring of Fischer's Danish identical and fraternal discordant twins. *Archives of General Psychiatry*, *46*, 867–872.

Grebb, J. A., & Cancro, R. (1989). Schizophrenia: Clinical features. In J. I. Kaplian & B. J. Sadock (Eds.), *Synopsis of psychiatry: behavioral sciences, clinical psychiatry* (5th ed., pp. 757–777). Baltimore: Williams & Wilkins.

Green, M. F., Kern, R. S., Braff, D. L., & Mintz, J. (2000). Neurocognitive deficits and functional outcome in schizophrenia: Are we measuring the "right stuff"? *Schizophrenia Bulletin*, *26*(1), 119–136.

Green, M. F., Nuechterlein, K. H., Breitmeyer, B., & Mintz, J. (1999). Backward masking in unmedicated schizophrenic patients in psychotic remission: Possible reflection of aberrant cortical oscillation. *American Journal of Psychiatry*, *156*, 1367–1373.

Harvey, P. D., & Walker, E. F. (Eds.). (1987). *Positive and negative symptoms of psychosis: Description, research, and future directions*. Hillsdale, NJ: Lawrence Erlbaum Associates.

Henn, F. A., & Braus, D. F. (1999). Structural neuroimaging in schizophrenia. An integrative view of neuromorphology. *European Archives of Psychiatry & Clinical Neuroscience, 249*(Suppl. 4), 48–56.

Heston, L. L. (1966). Psychiatric disorders in foster home reared children of schizophrenic mothers. *British Journal of Psychiatry, 112*, 819–825.

Howells, J. G. (1991). *The concept of schizophrenia: Historical perspectives.* Washington DC: American Psychiatric Press.

Huttunen, M. (1989). Maternal stress during pregnancy and the behavior of the offspring. In S. Doxiadis & S. Stewart (Eds.), *Early influences shaping the individual. NATO Advanced Science Institute Series: Vol. 160. Life sciences.* New York: Plenum.

Jentsch, J. D., Roth, R. H., & Taylor, J. R. (2000). Role for dopamine in the behavioral functions of the prefrontal corticostriatal system: Implications for mental disorders and psychotropic drug action. *Progress in Brain Research, 126*, 433–453.

Jones, P., Rodgers, B., Murray, R., & Marmot, M. (1994). Child developmental risk factors for adult schizophrenia in the British 1946 birth cohort. *Lancet, 344*, 1398–1402.

Kaplan, H. I., & Sadock, B. J. (1998). Kaplan and Sadock's synopsis of psychiatry: Behavioral sciences/clinical psychiatry (8th ed.). Baltimore, MD, US: Williams & Wilkins Co., 1401 pp.

Karayiorgou, M., Morris, M. A., & Morrow, B. (1995). Schizophrenia susceptibility associated with interstitial deletions of chromosome 22q11. *Proceedings of the National Academy of Science 92*, 7612–7616.

Keith, S. J., Regier, D. A., & Rae, D. S. (1991). Schizophrenic disorders. In L. N. Robins & D. A. Regier (Eds.), *Psychiatric disorders in America: The Epidemiologic Catchment Area study* (pp. 33–52). New York: Free Press.

Kendler, K. S., McGuire, M., Gruenberg, A. M., & Walsh, D. (1995b). Schizotypal symptoms and signs in the Roscommon Family Study: Their factor structure and familial relationship with psychotic and affective disorders. *Archives of General Psychiatry, 52*, 296–303.

Kendler, K. S., Neale, M. C., & Walsh, D. (1995). Evaluating the spectrum concept of schizophrenia in the Roscommon Family Study. *American Journal of Psychiatry, 152*, 749–754.

Kestler, L. P., Walker, E., & Vega, E. M. (2001). Dopamine receptors in the brains of schizophrenia patients: a meta-analysis of the findings. *Behavioural Pharmacology, 12*, 355–371.

Kety, S. S. (1988). Schizophrenic illness in the families of schizophrenic adoptees: Findings from the Danish national sample. *Schizophrenia Bulletin, 14*, 217–222.

Kraepelin, E. (1913). Psychiatrie (8th ed.). Translated by R. M. Barclay (1919) from Vol. 3, Pt. 2, as *Dementia praecox and paraphrenia.* Edinburgh, Livingstone.

Kringlen, E., & Cramer, G. (1989). Offspring of monozygotic twins discordant for schizophrenia. *Archives of General Psychiatry, 46*, 873–877.

Kulhara, P., Chakrabarti, S. (2001). Culture and schizophrenia and other psychotic disorders. *Psychiatric Clinics of North America, 24*, 449–464.

Kuperberg, G., & Heckers, S. (2000). Schizophrenia and cognitive function. *Current Opinion in Neurobiology, 10*, 205–210.

Larsen, T. K., Friis, S., Haahr, U., Joa, I., Johannessen, J. O., Melle, I., Opjordsmoen, S., Simonsen, E., & Vaglum, P. (2001). Early detection and intervention in first-episode schizophrenia: A critical review. *Acta Psychiatrica Scandinavic, 103*, 323–334.

Lawrie, S. M., & Abukmeil, S. S. (1998). Brain abnormality in schizophrenia: A systematic and quantitative review of volumetric magnetic resonance imaging studies. *British Journal of Psychiatry, 172*, 110–120.

Lehman, A. F. (1995). Vocational rehabilitation in schizophrenia. *Schizophrenia Bulletin, 21*(4), 64–56.

Lehman, A. F., Goldberg, R., Dixon, L., McNary, S., Postrado, L., Hackman, A., & McDonnell, K. (2002). Improving employment outcomes for persons with severe mental illnesses. *Archives of General Psychiatry, 59*, 165–172.

Lewis, D. A., Pierri, J. N., Volk, D. W., Melchitzky, D. S., Woo, T. U. (1999). Altered GABA neurotransmission and prefrontal cortical dysfunction in schizophrenia. *Biological Psychiatry, 46*, 616–626.

Lieberman, J. A., Perkins, D., Belger, A., Chakos, M., Jarskog, F., Boteva, K., & Gilmore, J. (2001). The early stages of schizophrenia: Speculations on pathogenesis, pathophysiology, and therapeutic approaches. *Biological Psychiatry, 50*, 884–897.

Lindstrom, L. H., Gefvert, O., Hagberg, G., Lundberg, T., Bergstrom, M., Hartvig, P., & Langstrom, B. (1999). Increased dopamine synthesis rate in medial prefrontal cortex and striatum in schizophrenia indicated by L-(beta-11C) DOPA and PET. *Biological Psychiatry, 46*, 681–688.

McNeil, T. F. (1988). Obstetric factors and prerinatal injuries. In M. T. Tsuang & J. C. Simpson (Eds.), *Handbook of schizophrenia: Nosology, epidemiology and genetics* (Vol. 3, pp. 319–343). Amsterdam: Elsevier Science.

McNeil, T. F., Cantor-Graae, E., & Weinberger, D. R. (2000). Relationship of obstetric complications and differences in size of brain structures in monozygotic twin pairs discordant for schizophrenia. *American Journal of Psychiatry, 157*, 203–212.

Meltzer, H. J. (2001). Treatment of suicidality in schizophrenia. In H. Hendin & J. J. Mann (Eds.), *The clinical science of suicide prevention. Annals of the New York Academy of Sciences* (Vol. 932, pp. 44–60). New York: New York Academy of Sciences.

Miller, T. J., McGlashan, T. H., Rosen, J. L., Somjee, L., Markovich, P. J., Stein, K., & Woods, S. W. (2002). Prospective diagnosis of the initial prodrome for schizophrenia based on the Structured Interview for Prodromal Syndromes: Preliminary evidence of interrater reliability and predictive validity. *American Journal of Psychiatry, 159,* 863–865.

Mowry, B. J., & Nancarrow, D. J. (2001). Molecular genetics of schizophrenia. *Clinical & Experimental Pharmacology & Physiology, 28,* 66–69.

Murray, R. M., Jones, P. B., O'Callaghan, E., & Takei, N. (1992). Genes, viruses and neurodevelopmental schizophrenia. *Journal of Psychiatric Research, 26,* 225–235.

Neumann, C., Walker, E. Lewine, R., & Baum, K. (1996). Childhood behavior and adult neuropsychological dysfunction in schizophrenia. *Neuropsychiatry, Neuropsychology and Behavioral Neurolog, 9,* 221–229.

Penn, D. L., Corrigan, P. W., Bentall, R. P., Racenstein, J. M., & Newman, L. (1997). Social cognition in schizophrenia. *Psychological Bulletin, 121*(1), 114–132.

Penn, D. L., & Mueser, K. T. (1996). Research update on the psychosocial treatment of schizophrenia. *American Journal of Psychiatry, 153,* 607–617.

Penn, D. L., Combs, D. R., Ritchie, M., Francis, J., Cassisi, J., Morris, S., & Townsend, M. (2000). Emotion recognition in schizophrenia: Further investigation of generalized versus specific deficit models. *Journal of Abnormal Psychology. 109*(3), 512–516

Potash, J. B., Willour, V. L., Chiu, Y. F., Simpson, S. G., MacKinnon, D. F., Pearlson, G. D., DePaulo, J. R., Jr., & McInnis, M. G. (2001). The familial aggregation of psychotic symptoms in bipolar disorder pedigrees. *American Journal of Psychiatry, 158,* 1258–1264.

Raine, A., & Mednick, S. (Eds.). (1995). *Schizotypal personality disorder.* London: Cambridge University press.

Regier, D. A., Farmer, M. E., Rae, D. S., Locke, B. Z., Keith, S. J., Judd, L. L., & Goodwin, F. K. (1990). Comorbidity of mental disorders with alcohol and other drug abuse. Results from the Epidemiologic Catchment Area (ECA) Study. *Journal of the American Medical Association, 264,* 2511–2518.

Riecher-Rossler, A., & Hafner, H. (2000). Gender aspects in schizophrenia: Bridging the border between social and biological psychiatry. *Acta Psychiatrica Scandinavica, 102*(Suppl.), 58–62.

Rosebush, P. I., & Mazurek, M. F. (2001). Identification and treatment of neuroleptic malignant syndrome. *Child and Adolescent Psychopharmacology News, 6*(3), p. 4.

Sadock, B. J., & Sadock, V. A. (Eds.). (2000). *Kaplan & Sadock's comprehensive textbook of psychiatry* (7th, ed., Vol. 1). New York: Lippincott Williams & Wilkins.

Schmajuk, N. A. (2001). Hippocampal dysfunction in schizophrenia. *Hippocampus, 11,* 599–613.

Schneider, K. (1959). *Clinical Psychopathology.* New York: Grune and Stratton.

Schwartz, R. C., & Cohen, B. N. (2001). Risk factors for suicidality among clients with schizophrenia. *Journal of Counseling & Development, 79,* 314–319.

Siris, S. G. (2001). Suicide and schizophrenia. *Journal of Psychopharmacology, 1*(2), 127–35.

Smythe, J. W., McCormick, C. M., Rochford, J., & Meaney, M. J. (1994). The interaction between prenatal stress and neonatal handling on nociceptive response latencies in male and female rats. *Physiology and Behavior, 55,* 971–974.

Soares, J. C., & Innis, R. B. (1999). Neurochemical brain imaging investigations of schizophrenia. *Biological Psychiatry, 46,* 600–615.

Spitzer, R. L., Endicott, J., & Robins, E. (1978). *Research diagnostic criteria (RDC) for a selected group of functional disorders.* New York: Biometrics Research.

Squires, R. F., & Saederup, E. (1991). A review of evidence for GABergic redominance/glutamatergic deficit as a common etiological factor in both schizophrenia and affective psychoses: More support for a continuum hypothesis of "functional" psychosis. *Neurochemical Research, 16,* 1099–1111.

Suddath, R. L., Christison, G. W., Torrey, E. F., Casanova, M. F., & Weinberger, D. R. (1990). Anatomical abnormalities in the brains of monozygotic twins discordant for schizophrenia. *New England Journal of Medicine, 322,* 789–794.

Susser, E. S., & Brown, A. S. (Eds.). (1999). *Prenatal exposures in schizophrenia. Progress in psychiatry.* Washington, DC: American Psychiatric Press.

Tienari, P., Wynne, L. C., Moring, J. & Lahti, I. (1994). The Finnish adoptive family study of schizophrenia: Implications for family research. *British Journal of Psychiatry, 164*(Suppl. 23), 20–26.

Torrey, E. F. (1987). Prevalence studies in schizophrenia. *British Journal of Psychiatry, 150,* 598–608.

Torrey, E. F., Bowler, A. E., & Taylor, E. H. (1994). *Schizophrenia and manic-depressive disorder: The biological roots of mental illness as revealed by the landmark study of identical twins.* New York: Basic Books.

Torrey, E. F., Miller, J., Rawlings, R., & Yolken, R. H. (1997). Seasonality of births in schizophrenia and bipolar disorder: A review of the literature. *Schizophrenia Research, 28,* 1–38.

Tsai, G., & Coyle, J. T. (2002). Glutamatergic mechanisms in schizophrenia. *Annual Review of Pharmacology & Toxicology, 42*, 165–179.

van Os, J., & Selten, J. (1998). Prenatal exposure to maternal stress and subsequent schizophrenia: The May 1940 invasion of The Netherlands. *British Journal of Psychiatry, 172*, 324–326.

Ventura, J., Nuechterlein, K. H., Hardesty, J. P., & Gitlin, M. (1992). Life events and schizophrenic relapse after withdrawal of medication. *British Journal of Psychiatry, 161*, 615–620.

Walker, E. (1994). Developmentally moderated expressions of the neuropathology underlying schizophrenia. *Schizophrenia Bulletin, 20*, 453–480.

Walker, E. (2002). Adolescent neurodevelopment and psychopathology. *Current Directions in Psychological Science, 11*, 24–28.

Walker, E., & Baum, K. (1998). Developmental changes in the behavioral expression of the vulnerability for schizophrenia. In M. Lenzenweger & R. Dworkin (Eds.), *Origins and development of schizophrenia: Advances in experimental psychopathology* (pp. 469–491). Washington, DC: American Psychological Association.

Walker E., & Diforio, D. (1997). Schizophrenia: A neural diathesis-stress model. *Psychological Review, 104*, 1–19.

Walker, E., Grimes, K., Davis, D., & Smith, A. (1993). Childhood precursors of schizophrenia; Facial expressions of emotion. *American Journal of Psychiatry, 150*, 1654–1660.

Walker, E., & Lewine, R. J. (1990). Prediction of adult-onset schizophrenia from childhood home movies of the patients. *American Journal of Psychiatry, 147*, 1052–1056.

Walker, E., Lewis, N., Loewy, R., Paylo, S. (1999) Motor functions and psychopathology [Special issue]. *Development and Psychopathology 11*, 509–523.

Walker, E., Marwit, S., & Emory, E. (1980). A cross-sectional study of emotion recognition in schizophrenics. *Journal of Abnormal Psychology.* 89(3), 428–436.

Walker, E., Savoie, T., & Davis, D. (1994). Neuromotor precursors of schizophrenia. *Schizophrenia Bulletin, 20*, 441–452.

Walker, E., Walder, D., & Reynolds, F. (2001). Developmental changes in cortisol secretion in normal and at-risk youth. *Development and Psychopathology, 13*, 719–730.

Weinstein, D., Diforio, D., Schiffman, J., Walker, E., & Bonsall, B. (1999). Minor physical anomalies, dermatoglyphic asymmetries and cortisol levels in adolescents with schizotypal personality disorder. *American Journal of Psychiatry, 156*, 617–623.

Weinstock, M. (1996). Does prenatal stress impair coping and regulation of hypothalamic-pituitary-adrenal axis? *Neuroscience and Biobehavioral Reviews, 21*, 1–10.

Welberg, L. A., & Seckl, J. R. (2001). Prenatal stress, glucocorticoids and the programming of the brain. *Journal of Neuroendocrinology, 2*, 113–28.

Yung, A. R., Phillips, L. J., McGorry, P. D., Hallgren, M. A., McFarlane, C. A., Jackson, H. J., Francey, S., Harrigan, S., Patton, G. C., & Jackson, H. J. (1998). Prediction of psychosis: A step towards indicated prevention of schizophrenia. *British Journal of Psychiatry, 172*(Suppl. 33), 14–20.

10

Personality Disorders

Linda Anne Coker and Thomas A. Widiger

University of Kentucky

In 1980, the American Psychiatric Association (APA) published the third edition of the Diagnostic and Statistical Manual of Mental Disorders (DSM–III; APA, 1980), introducing a multiaxial classification system. Axis II of this new manual was devoted primarily to personality dysfunction, because of the considerable prevalence of maladaptive personality traits in general clinical practice and the substantial impact of these traits on the course and treatment of other mental disorders (Frances, 1980).

In this chapter, we begin by discussing issues in the diagnosis of personality disorders as defined by DSM–IV-TR (APA, 2000). We also include an alternative model for the diagnosis and classification of maladaptive personality functioning, the five-factor model (FFM; Costa & McCrae, 1992). DSM–IV-TR includes ten individual personality disorders, organized into three clusters: (a) paranoid, schizoid, and schizotypal (the odd-eccentric cluster); (b) antisocial, borderline, histrionic, and narcissistic (dramatic-emotional-erratic cluster); and (c) avoidant, dependent, and obsessive-compulsive (anxious-fearful cluster) (APA, 2000). We present what is currently known about five of the more heavily researched personality disorders (i.e., antisocial, borderline, avoidant, schizoid, and dependent) and indicate how the FFM conceptualization of each of them extends our understanding of their diagnosis, epidemiology, etiology, and pathology. Space limitations prohibit detailed coverage of all of the DSM–IV-TR personality disorders, but information concerning these additional personality disorders is provided in the general discussion.

PERSONALITY DISORDER

Virtually all adults with psychological problems have a characteristic manner of thinking, feeling, behaving, and relating to others that was present before the onset of an Axis I disorder, and, for many of these persons, these personality traits are so maladaptive that they constitute a personality disorder. A *personality disorder* is defined in DSM–IV-TR as "an enduring pattern of inner experience and behavior that deviates markedly from the expectations of the individual's culture, is pervasive and inflexible, has an onset in adolescence or early adulthood, is stable over time, and leads to distress or impairment" (APA, 2000, p. 686).

The prevalence of personality disorders within clinical settings is estimated to be above 50% (Mattia & Zimmerman, 2001). Perhaps 60% of inpatients within some clinical settings are diagnosed with borderline personality disorder (APA, 2000; Gunderson, 2001). Antisocial personality disorder may be diagnosed in up to 50% of inmates within a correctional setting (Widiger & Corbitt, 1995). The course and treatment of most other disorders is substantially altered by the presence of a comorbid personality disorder (Dolan-Sewell, Krueger, & Shea, 2001), yet the prevalence of personality disorder is generally underestimated in clinical practice (Zimmerman & Mattia, 1999). This situation may be due to a lack of time to provide systematic or comprehensive evaluations of personality functioning (Widiger & Coker, 2001), or perhaps to a reluctance to diagnose them because insurance companies may consider personality disorders untreatable (Zimmerman & Mattia, 1999).

It is estimated that 10% to 15% of the general population would meet criteria for one of the ten DSM–IV personality disorders (Mattia & Zimmerman, 2001; Torgesen, Kringlen, & Cramer, 2001). Table 10.1 provides prevalence data reported by the best available studies to date for estimating the prevalence of individual personality disorders within the community. These prevalence estimates are generally close to those provided in DSM–IV-TR, although there is variation across studies due to differences in setting and assessment instruments.

A common misconception concerning personality disorders is that they are untreatable. This is not the case. Personality dysfunction can be the focus of treatment (Beck et al., 1990; Gabbard, 1994; Markovitz, 2001). Personality disorders are among the most difficult disorders to treat, however, because they involve well-established behaviors that may be integral to a client's self-image (Stone, 1993). Nevertheless, psychosocial and pharmalogic treatments can produce clinically and socially meaningful changes, (Perry, Banon, & Ianni, 1999; Sanislow & McGlashan, 1998), although the development of an ideal or fully healthy personality structure is unlikely. Given the considerable social, public health, and personal costs associated with some of the personality disorders, such as antisocial and borderline, even small improvements in functioning and reductions in symptomatology can be important.

There is considerable personality disorder diagnostic comorbidity (Bornstein, 1998; Lilienfeld, Waldman, & Israel, 1994; Oldham et al., 1992; Widiger & Trull, 1998). Patients who are diagnosed with one personality disorder are likely to meet the diagnostic criteria for at least one other personality disorder. Table 10.2 provides DSM–III-R (APA, 1987) co-occurrence statistics, obtained for the development of DSM–IV. Diagnostic co-occurrence is so common and so extensive that most personality disorder researchers believe that a dimensional description provides a clearer and more accurate picture of personality dysfunction (Cloninger, 2000; Livesley, 1998; Oldham & Skodol, 2000; Widiger, 2000).

One approach has been to apply a broader dimensional model of general personality functioning to the study of personality disorders. Five broad domains of personality functioning have been identified empirically through the study of the languages of a number of different cultures (de Raad, di Blas, & Perugini, 1999; John & Srivastava, 1999). Language can be understood as a sedimentary deposit of the observations of persons over the thousands of years of the language's development and transformation. The most important domains of personality functioning are those with the greatest number of terms to describe and differentiate their various manifestations and nuances, and the structure of personality is evident in the empirical relationship among the trait terms (Goldberg, 1993). Such lexical analyses of languages have typically identified five fundamental dimensions of personality: neuroticism (or negative affectivity) versus emotional stability, introversion versus extraversion, conscientiousness (constraint) versus undependability, antagonism versus agreeableness, and closedness versus

TABLE 10.1

Epidemiology of Personality Disorders

	Sample N	N	Int	DSM	PRN	SZD	STP	ATS	BDL	HST	NCS	AVD	DPD	OCP
Drake et al. (1988)	Men(47)	369	Clinical	III	1.1	4.1	2.4	0.8	0.5	3.8	3.5	1.6	10.3	0.5
Coryell et al. (1989)	R-HN	185	SIDP	III	0.5	1.6	2.2	1.6	1.1	1.6	0.0	1.6	0.5	3.2
Maier et al. (1992)	Comm	452	SCID-II	III-R	1.8	0.4	0.7	0.2	1.1	1.3	0.0	1.1	1.5	2.2
Black et al. (1993)	R-HN	127	SIDP	III	1.6	0.0	3.9	0.0	5.5	3.9	0.0	3.2	2.4	7.9
Black et al. (1993)	R-OCD	120	SIDP	III	1.7	0.0	2.5	0.8	0.8	2.5	0.0	0.8	0.8	10.8
Moldin et al. (1994)	HN	302	PDE	III-R	0.0	0.0	0.7	2.6	2.0	0.3	0.0	0.7	1.0	0.7
Samuels et al. (1994)	Comm	762	Clinical	III	0.0	0.0	0.1	1.5	0.4	2.1	0.0	0.0	0.1	1.7
Klein et al. (1995)	R-DP	258	PDE	III-R	1.7	0.9	0.0	2.2	1.7	1.7	3.9	5.2	0.4	2.6
Lenzenweger et al. (1997)	Stdts	1646	PDE	III-R	0.4	0.4	0.0	0.8	0.0	1.9	1.2	0.4	0.4	0.0
Torgersen et al. (2001)	Comm	2053	SIDP-R	III-R	2.4	1.7	0.6	0.7	0.7	2.0	0.8	5.0	1.5	2.0
Samuels et al. (2002)	Comm	742	IPDE	IV	0.7	0.7	1.8	4.5	1.2	0.4	0.1	1.4	0.3	1.2
Median					1.1	0.4	0.7	0.8	1.1	1.9	0.0	1.6	0.8	2.2
DSM-IV estimates					.5–2.5	uncm	3.0	2.0	2.0	2–3	<1	.5–1	—	1.0

Note: N = number of persons in study; Int = interview that was used; Edition of Diagnostic and Statistical Manual that was used (DSM–III or DSM–III–R); PRN = paranoid; SZD = schizoid; STP = schizotypal; ATS = antisocial; BDL = borderline; HST = histrionic; NCS = narcissistic; AVD = avoidant; DPD = dependent; OCP = obsessive-compulsive; R-HN = relatives of hypernormal (persons without history of mental disorder); R-OCD = relatives of persons with obsessive-compulsive anxiety disorder; Men(47) = males of approximate age of 47; R-DP = relatives of persons with depression; Stdts = students; Comm = community; IPDE = International Personality Disorder Examination; SIDP = Structured Interview for Personality Disorder [Pfohl et al., 1997]; SCID–II = Structured Clinical Interview for DSM personality disorder [First et al., 1997]; Clinical = unstructured or unspecified semistructured interview; uncm = uncommon.

TABLE 10.2

DSM–III–R Personality Disorder Diagnostic Co-Occurrence Aggregated Across Six Research Sites

	PRN	SZD	SZT	ATS	BDL	HST	NCS	AVD	DPD	OCP
Paranoid (PRN)	—	8	19	15	41	28	26	44	23	21
Schizoid (SZD)	38	—	39	8	22	8	22	55	11	20
Schizotypal (SZT)	43	32	—	19	44	17	26	68	34	19
Antisocial (ATS)	30	8	15	—	59	39	40	25	19	9
Borderline (BDL)	31	6	16	23	—	30	19	39	36	12
Histrionic (HST)	29	2	7	17	41	—	40	21	28	13
Narcissistic (NCS)	41	12	18	25	38	60	—	32	24	21
Avoidant (AVD)	33	15	22	11	39	16	15	—	43	16
Dependent (DPD)	26	3	16	16	48	24	14	57	—	15
Obs-Compulsive (OCP)	31	10	11	4	25	21	19	37	27	—

Note: Sites used DSM–III–R criterion sets. Data obtained for purposes of informing the development of the DSM–IV personality disorder diagnostic criteria (Widiger & Trull, 1998). Read table as follows: 8% of persons diagnosed with paranoid personality disorder met DSM–III–R criteria for schizoid; 38% of persons diagnosed with schizoid personality disorder met DSM–III–R criteria for paranoid.

openness to experience (Costa & McCrae, 1992). Each of these five broad domains can be differentiated further in terms of underlying facets. For example, the facets of antagonism versus agreeableness include suspiciousness versus trusting gullibility, callous tough-mindedness versus tender-mindedness, confidence and arrogance versus modesty and meekness, exploitation versus altruism and sacrifice, oppositionalism and aggression versus compliance, and deception and manipulation versus straightforwardness and honesty (Costa & McCrae, 1992).

Each of the DSM–IV personality disorders can be readily understood as maladaptive and extreme variants of these personality dimensions that are present in all persons to differing degrees (Widiger, Trull, Clarkin, Sanderson, & Costa, 1994/2002). Table 10.3 provides two descriptions of the DSM–IV-TR personality disorders in terms of this five-factor model. Widiger et al. (1994/2002) used the DSM–IV diagnostic criteria sets to develop their hypothetical FFM profiles. Lynam and Widiger (2001) obtained FFM ratings of prototypic cases by researchers of each personality disorder. From the perspective of DSM–IV-TR, paranoid personality disorder (PPD) is comprised of high angry hostility and low levels of trust, straightforwardness, compliance, and modesty. Researchers describe PPD similarly, but also add low levels of warmth, gregariousness, openness to actions, openness to values, altruism, and tender-mindedness.

The divergence between the DSM–IV-TR and researcher FFM descriptions is particularly evident for the histrionic and obsessive-compulsive personality disorders. The researchers rated individuals with obsessive-compulsive personality dysfunction as being extremely low in impulsiveness and excitement seeking, two aspects that are not included in DSM–IV-TR criteria. They also rated individuals with histrionic personality dysfunction as very low in self-consciousness and high in impulsivity, aspects also not included in DSM–IV-TR. Lynam and Widiger (2001) concluded that the expert consensus FFM profiles may provide a more complete description than is provided by DSM–IV-TR.

FIVE PERSONALITY DISORDERS AND THEIR FIVE-FACTOR FORMULATIONS

We now turn our attention to five DSM–IV-TR personality disorders: antisocial, schizoid, borderline, avoidant, and dependent. We describe for each of them what is known about their

TABLE 10.3

DSM–IV Personality Disorders From the Perspective of the Five-Factor Model of General Personality Functioning

	PRN	*SZD*	*SZT*	*ATS*	*BDL*	*HST*	*NCS*	*AVD*	*DPD*	*OCP*
Neuroticism										
Anxiousness			H *H*	*L*	H *H*			H *H*	H *H*	*H*
Angry hostility	H *H*			H *H*	H *H*		H *H*			
Depressiveness					H *H*	H		H		
Self-consciousness			H *H*	*L*		H *L*	H *L*	H *H*	H *H*	
Impulsivity				*H*	H *H*	*H*		*L*		*L*
Vulnerability					H *H*			H *H*	H *H*	
Extraversion										
Warmth	*L*	L *L*	L *L*			H			H	
Gregariousness	*L*	L *L*	L *L*			H *H*	*L*	L *L*		
Assertiveness		*L*		*H*			*H*	L *L*	L *L*	*H*
Activity		*L*		*H*		*H*				
Excitement-seeking		*L*		H *H*		H *H*	*H*	L *L*		*L*
Positive emotionality		L *L*	L *L*			H *H*		*L*		
Openness										
Fantasy			H			H *H*	*H*			
Aesthetics										
Feelings		L *L*				H *H*	*L*			*L*
Actions	*L*	*L*	H	*H*		*H*	*H*	*L*		*L*
Ideas			H *H*							*L*
Values	*L*									L *L*
Agreeableness										
Trust	L *L*		*L*	*L*	*L*	H *H*	*L*		H *H*	
Straightforwardness	L *L*			L *L*			*L*			
Altruism	*L*			L *L*			L *L*	*H*		
Compliance	L *L*			L *L*	*L*		*L*		H *H*	*L*
Modesty				*L*			L *L*	*H*	H *H*	
Tender-mindedness	*L*			L *L*			L *L*			
Conscientiousness										
Competence					*L*					H *H*
Order			*L*							H *H*
Dutifulness				L *L*						H *H*
Achievement-striving							*H*			H *H*
Self-discipline				L *L*	*L*					*H*
Deliberation				L *L*	*L*	*L*				*H*

Note: H and L indicate DSM–IV descriptions by Widiger et al., 1994/2002. *H* and *L* indicate researcher ratings from Lynam & Widiger, 2001.

etiology, pathology, differential diagnosis, comorbidity, course, and treatment. We also indicate how each of them can be understood from the perspective of the FFM of general personality functioning and how this conceptualization helps to address one or more of the issues that has been problematic for that personality disorder.

Antisocial Personality Disorder

Definition. DSM–IV-TR defines *antisocial personality disorder* (ASPD) as a pervasive pattern of disregard for and violation of the rights of others (APA, 2000). This disorder has also been referred to as psychopathy (Hare et al., 1991), sociopathy, or dissocial (World Health

Organization, 1992) personality disorder. Its primary diagnostic criteria include criminal activity, deceitfulness, impulsivity, aggression, reckless irresponsibility, and indifference to the mistreatment of others.

Etiology and Pathology.   Twin, family, and adoption studies have provided substantial support for a genetic contribution to the etiology of the criminal, delinquent tendencies of persons meeting criteria for ASPD (Nigg & Goldsmith, 1994; Stoff, Breiling, & Maser, 1997). Exactly what is inherited in ASPD, however, is not known; it could be impulsivity, antagonistic callousness, or abnormally low anxiousness.

One influential theory for the etiology of ASPD is that it results from abnormally low levels of behavioral inhibition and high levels of behavioral activation systems that are important for normal, adaptive functioning (Fowles, 2001; Widiger & Lynam, 1998). The behavioral inhibition system (BIS) is said to inhibit behavior in response to punishment, in opposition to a behavioral activation system (BAS) that activates behavior in response to reward. The observed symptoms of ASPD could be evidence of a malfunctioning BIS acting in concert with a normal or strong BAS. In this manner, normal sensitivity and anxiety in response to threatening and stressful situations may be reduced or altogether absent. Low arousal would also help minimize feelings of guilt or remorse and increase resistance to aversive conditioning. An electrodermal response hyporeactivity in psychopaths may be particularly associated with a deficit in anticipatory anxiety and worrying, though the alarm reactions of flight versus fight are intact (Fowles, 2001; Stoff et al., 1997).

Substantial research also supports the contributions of environmental factors such as modeling by family members and peers (Stoff et al., 1997), though no one environmental factor appears to be specific to its development. Excessively harsh or erratic discipline, and an environment in which feelings of empathy are discouraged (if not punished) and tough-mindedness, aggressiveness, and exploitation are encouraged (if not reinforced), have each been associated with the development of ASPD (Sutker & Allain, 2001). It is possible that persons with ASPD may have had any feelings of anxiety, guilt, and remorse extinguished through progressive, cumulative experiences of harsh aggression, abuse, and exploitation.

Some distress-proneness (FFM anxiousness or neuroticism) and attentional self-regulation (FFM constraint or conscientiousness) may be necessary to develop an adequate sense of guilt or conscience. Normal levels of neuroticism promote the internalization of a conscience by associating wrongdoing or misbehavior with distress and anxiety, and the temperament of self-regulation helps modulate impulses into socially acceptable channels (e.g., counting to 100 when angry) (Clark, Kochanska, & Ready, 2000; Fowles & Kochanska, 2000; Kochanska & Murray, 2000; Rothbart & Ahadi, 1994). High levels of arousal at age 15 have been shown to serve as a protective factor against criminal activities at age 30 in persons at high risk for becoming criminals (Raine, Lencz, & Mednick, 1995; Raine, Reynolds, Venables, Mednick, & Farrington, 1998). Additional factors, such as high intelligence, may also help to avoid the development of ASPD by offering the possibility of alternative life paths. In sum, ASPD appears to be the result of a constellation of factors, including genetic predisposition, experiences within the family environment, and sociological factors, coupled with a lack of preventive factors (Stoff et al., 1997; Sutker & Allain, 2001).

Differential Diagnosis.   The predominant instrument for the assessment of the antisocial/psychopathic personality disorder is the Psychopathy Checklist–Revised (PCL–R; Hare, 1991). The PCL–R assesses a few additional psychopathic personality traits such as glibness, superficial charm, callousness, and arrogance, beyond the criminal, exploitative, remorseless, and irresponsible behaviors that define DSM–IV antisocial personality.

At times, ASPD is difficult to differentiate from a substance-dependence disorder because many persons with ASPD develop a substance-related disorder, and many persons with substance dependence engage in antisocial acts. However, the requirement that conduct disorder be present before the age of 15 usually ensures the onset of ASPD before the onset of a substance-related disorder. If both were evident before the age of 15, then it is likely that both disorders are now present and both diagnoses should be given. Often, ASPD and substance dependence interact, exacerbating each other's development (Myers, Stewart, & Brown, 1998; Sher & Trull, 1994; Stoff et al., 1997; Sutker & Allain, 2001).

Epidemiology and Comorbidity.   The National Institute of Mental Health Epidemiologic Catchment Area (ECA) study estimated that 3% of males and 1% of females meet DSM criteria for ASPD (Robins, Tipp, & Przybeck, 1991). Subsequent studies have replicated this rate, but it has also been suggested that the ECA finding may have underestimated the prevalence in males, because of failure to consider the full range of ASPD features. Other estimates have been as high as 6% in males (Kessler et al., 1994; Robins et al., 1991). Within prison and forensic settings, the rate of ASPD has been estimated to be 50% (Hare, Hart, & Harpur, 1991; Robins et al., 1991). However, the ASPD criteria may inflate the prevalence within such settings because of the emphasis on overt acts of criminality, delinquency, and irresponsibility (Sutker & Allain, 2001; Widiger et al., 1996). More specific criteria for psychopathy provided by the PCL–R obtain a more conservative estimate of 20% to 30% of male prisoners meeting criteria for ASPD (Hare et al., 1991), by placing relatively less emphasis on the history of criminal behavior and more emphasis on personality traits associated with this criminal history (e.g., callousness and arrogance).

ASPD is much more common in men than in women (Corbitt & Widiger, 1995; Robins et al., 1991). A sociobiological explanation for the differential sex prevalence is the presence of a genetic advantage for social irresponsibility, infidelity, superficial charm, and deceit in males that contributes to a higher likelihood of developing features of ASPD (i.e., males with these traits are more likely to have offspring than males without these traits) (Stoff et al., 1997; Sutker & Allain, 2001). ASPD and histrionic personality disorder (HPD) may also share a biogenetic disposition (possibly toward impulsivity or sensation seeking) that is mediated by gender-specific biogenetic and sociological factors toward respective gender variants (Hamburger, Lilienfeld, & Hogben, 1996; Lilienfeld & Hess, 2001). ASPD and HPD share a variety of behavioral and personality characteristics (e.g., superficial charm, shallow emotions, manipulativeness, and self-centeredness) that may be expressed as antisocial personality disorder in males and histrionic personality disorder in females.

Five-Factor Model Reformulation.   Antisocial PD can be understood primarily as excessive, maladaptively low conscientiousness and low agreeableness (see Table 10.3). Specifically, these individuals would be described as aimless, unreliable, lax, negligent, and hedonistic (low in the facets of self-discipline and deliberation; Costa & McCrae, 1985), as well as manipulative, exploitative, and ruthless (low in straightforwardness, altruism, compliance, and tender-mindedness).

One issue surrounding the DSM diagnosis of ASPD has been the failure to include all of the personality traits of psychopathy identified originally by Cleckley (1941/1988), emphasizing instead those traits that could most easily be identified by objectively observed behaviors (e.g., irresponsible and/or illegal acts). Psychopathy researchers (Harpur, Hart, & Hare, 2002; Patrick et al., 1993) have argued that an emotionally detached interpersonal style is integral to the diagnosis of the disorder, that the DSM definition of ASPD fails to capture these features in the diagnostic criteria, and that these features are relevant and important to clinical treatment.

Table 10.3 illustrates the differences between the DSM–IV and PCL–R conceptualizations of this disorder. The FFM description of antisocial personality disorder by the researchers (Lynam & Widiger, 2001) includes the PCL–R components of glib charm (abnormally low self-consciousness), arrogance (low modesty), and callous lack of empathy (tough-mindedness) that are not represented within the DSM–IV diagnostic criteria for this disorder. In fact, the researchers' FFM description also includes the absence of anxiousness that was included in the original conceptualization of this disorder by Cleckley (1941/1988) but was excluded from the PCL–R (Lilienfeld, 1994). Considerable evidence supports the FFM conceptualization of ASPD (Forth, Brown, Hart, & Hare, 1996; Hart & Hare, 1994; Lynam, 2002; Miller, Lynam, Widiger, & Leukefeld, 2001; Widiger & Lynam, 1998). These studies have shown that the FFM does provide a comprehensive and clinically valid description of the antisocial or psychopathic personality, and that the FFM conceptualization of ASPD maps well onto measures of psychopathy and ASPD.

The five-factor conceptualization of this disorder also clarifies other issues surrounding this diagnosis. PCL–R psychopathy is conceptualized as encompassing two broad factors (Hare, 1991; Harpur et al., 2002). The first factor, considered by some to represent the core of the disorder, includes items describing a callous and remorseless use of others; the second includes items describing deviant and impulsive behaviors. The two-factor structure has often been used in research, but has been criticized for the failure to offer a psychological conceptualization of the second factor and for relegating it to an undeserved secondary status (Lilienfeld, 1994; Rogers & Bagby, 1994). "This overlooks the fact that [the second factor] includes several personality dimensions, such as impulsivity, irresponsibility, and sensation-seeking" (Lynam, 2002, p. 337). A reinterpretation of the PCL–R in terms of the FFM allows the first factor to be understood as almost pure antagonism; the more confusing nature of the second factor occurs because it is a mixture of low conscientiousness with some antagonism, neuroticism, and extraversion (Lynam, 2002).

Researchers have for many years been attempting to identify the single, core pathology of psychopathy, and a variety of compelling but inconsistent models have been proposed. These alternative conceptualizations can be integrated and their inconsistencies addressed by the FFM. Their apparent inconsistency may reflect that each alternative model of pathology focuses on a different facet and at times even a different domain of the FFM. Lykken (1957), Fowles (1993), and Patrick, Bradley, and Lang (1993) have argued that the primary deficit of psychopathy lies in poor fear conditioning and electrodermal hypoarousal, a focus of research that places particular emphasis on low neuroticism (i.e., low anxiousness or low vulnerability). Others have argued that a lack of response modulation is the primary deficit, an inability to refrain from acting on first impulse (Newman, Patterson, Howland, & Nichols, 1990; Patterson & Newman, 1993), represented in the FFM domain of conscientiousness/constraint by the facet of deliberation. Cleckley (1941/1988) described the core of psychopathy as "semantic dementia," referring to a deficit in processing affective language. This deficit can be understood in terms of the antagonism facet of tough-mindedness. It has also been argued that the primary deficit of psychopathic individuals lies in an inability or impairment in processing social information cues (Dodge, 1980; Dodge & Crick, 1990). In an FFM profile of these persons, this feature would be described as extremely high antagonism, particularly deception, aggression, and exploitation. In sum, the personality profile for the prototypic psychopath involves a constellation of personality traits that together provides a quite virulent and at times even lethal mix (i.e., high antagonism, low conscientiousness, low vulnerability, low anxiousness, high assertiveness, high gregariousness, and high excitement seeking).

An FFM conceptualization of ASPD also provides some clarity in regard to the "successful" psychopath. Systematic research has been confined largely to the study of the "unsuccessful" psychopath, which typically means the incarcerated criminal (Sutker & Allain, 2001). However, there is also considerable social and theoretical interest in understanding the psychopath who is equally exploitative, callous, and ruthless, but either manages never to get arrested or convicted, or who pursues a white-collar career that only flirts with the edges of the legal system (Hare, 1993). From the perspective of the FFM, these persons would share many of the traits of the prototypic psychopath (i.e., low anxiousness, high fearlessness, high in assertiveness and gregariousness, and high in the exploitativeness and callousness of antagonism), but would be high rather than low in the facets of conscientiousness (Lynam, 2002). Such persons can be even more dangerous than most of the incarcerated psychopaths because they share the disposition to engage in behavior harmful to others, but also possess the traits (deliberation, competence, and self-discipline) that would contribute to a more "successful" outcome.

The FFM also provides an explanation of the comorbidity of ASPD. Antisocial features are commonly evident in the histrionic and borderline personality disorders, as persons with these disorders display impulsivity, excitement seeking, self-centeredness, manipulativeness, irresponsibility, and a low frustration tolerance. However, the histrionic and borderline diagnoses are not typically characterized by a cold, calculating violation of others' rights through criminal activity (low altruism and tender-mindedness). Persons with narcissistic personality disorder are characterized by an antisocial lack of empathy and may often exploit and use others (low in altruism). In fact, many of the traits of narcissistic personality disorder are evident in psychopathy, including a lack of empathy, glib and superficial charm, and arrogant self-appraisal (low modesty) (Widiger et al., 1996). However, prototypic narcissistic personality disorder is not characterized by being low in the agreeableness facets of compliance and straightforwardness, nor by being low in the conscientiousness facet of dutifulness.

Treatment. ASPD is considered the most difficult personality disorder to treat (Stoff et al., 1997; Stone, 1993). Individuals with ASPD may be seductively charming and declare their commitment to change, though they usually lack a motivation to change. They do not see the costs associated with antisocial acts (e.g., imprisonment and lack of meaningful interpersonal relationships), and may stay in treatment only as required by an external source, such as a parole officer. Residential programs that provide a carefully controlled environment of structure and supervision, combined with peer confrontation, have been recommended (Gabbard, 1994). However, it is unknown what benefits may be sustained after the ASPD individual leaves this environment. When in inpatient treatment, individuals with ASPD are likely to manipulate and exploit staff and fellow patients (Gabbard, 1994). Studies have indicated that outpatient therapy is not likely to be successful, but the extent to which persons with ASPD are unresponsive to treatment may have been somewhat exaggerated. Salekin (2002) indicates that the heterogeneity of the definitions of psychopathy (e.g., Cleckley's vs. Hare's conceptualization or psychoanalytic vs. behavioral), as well as the polythetic nature of a diagnosis of ASPD, may be significant factors in a therapist's assessment of the amenability to treatment of an ASPD or psychopathic client. Furthermore, several therapeutic approaches (cognitive-behavioral, psychoanalytic, and a combination of the two) have shown some success in reduction of the severity of psychopathic traits (Salekin, 2002).

Identification and intervention in early childhood is likely to be the most effective treatment for ASPD (Stoff et al., 1997). In adulthood, lengthy incarceration may be the most effective "treatment." It is known that antisocial behaviors tend to lessen as the individual ages (Sutker & Allain, 2001). A peer may be able to develop a better rapport with an ASPD individual, because of a greater mutual sense of trust and respect. Because there is some evidence that the ability to form a therapeutic alliance is an important indicator of treatment success, factors such as demographic similarity between therapist and client and the therapist's positive regard for the client should be considered before attempting treatment (Gertsley et al., 1989; Stoff et al., 1997).

Therapists of individuals with ASPD should also bear in mind that they may have considerable negative feelings toward clients with extensive histories of aggressive, exploitative, and abusive behaviors toward others. Rather than attempting to develop a sense of conscience in these individuals, therapeutic techniques should be focused on rational and utilitarian arguments against repeating past behavior. These approaches would focus on the tangible, material value of prosocial behavior (Beck et al., 1990). Some research has indicated that impulsive aggression might be treated with lithium, though its effect on other ASPD symptomatology remains to be seen (Markovitz, 2001).

Schizoid Personality Disorder

Definition.   Schizoid personality disorder (SZPD) is defined in DSM–IV as a pervasive pattern of social detachment and restricted emotional expression (APA, 2000). Its primary diagnostic criteria include a lack of desire for close relationships, consistent preference for solitary activities, lack of interest in sexual contact with others, anhedonia, and emotional detachment.

Etiology and Pathology.   There has been little systematic research on the etiology and pathology of schizoid personality disorder. There are theoretical speculations that it might be the result of a sustained history of modeling and reinforcement by parental figures of interpersonal withdrawal, indifference, and detachment (Bernstein & Travaglini, 1999), but no studies have been conducted to assess the validity of these theories.

Schizoid personality disorder has also been conceptualized as a subthreshold or characterologic variant of a spectrum of schizophrenic pathology. A fundamental distinction of schizophrenic symptomatology is between positive and negative symptoms. Positive symptoms include hallucinations, delusions, inappropriate affect, and loose associations; negative symptoms include flattened affect, alogia, anhedonia, and avolition. Subthreshold variants of the positive symptoms might include the cognitive and perceptual aberrations that are relatively specific to the schizotypal personality disorder, which is conceptualized by most researchers to be a characterologic variant of schizophrenia (Miller, Useda, Trull, Burr, & Minks-Brown, 2001). Schizoid personality disorder might likewise involve subthreshold variants of the negative symptoms of schizophrenia, including flattened affectivity, anhedonia (takes pleasure in few, if any, activities), and avolition (social withdrawal and isolation). There is strong support for a genetic relationship between schizotypal personality disorder and schizophrenia, which is not surprising as its diagnostic criteria were developed on the basis of interviews with biological relatives of persons with schizophrenia (Miller, M. B., et al., 2001). However, the evidence for a genetic relationship between schizoid personality disorder and schizophrenia is not strong (Bernstein & Travaglini, 1999; Miller, M. B., et al., 2001).

Epidemiology and Comorbidity.   Approximately half of the general population exhibits introversion within the normal range of functioning. Only a small minority of the population meets criteria for schizoid personality disorder (Mattia & Zimmerman, 2001). Estimates of the prevalence of SZPD within the general population have been less than 1% (see Table 10.2) and SZPD is among the least frequently diagnosed personality disorders within clinical settings. Many of the persons who were diagnosed with SZPD before DSM–III are probably now diagnosed with either the avoidant or the schizotypal personality disorders (Widiger, Frances, & Spitzer, 1988), and prototypic (pure) cases of SZPD are likely to be quite rare within the population.

Course. Individuals with SZPD will have been socially isolated and withdrawn as children and adolescents. They may not have been accepted well by their peers, and may have even been ostracized (APA, 2000). As adults, they will have few friendships. Those friendships that do develop are likely to have been initiated by their peers or colleagues. They will have had few sexual or intimate relationships (if any) and may never marry. The extent to which the other person desires or needs emotional support, warmth, and intimacy will likely determine the success of a relationship. Persons with SZPD may do well and even excel within an occupation, as long as substantial social interaction is not required. These individuals may eventually find employment and a relationship that is relatively comfortable, but they could also drift from one job to another and remain isolated throughout much of their life. If they become a parent, they are likely to have considerable difficulty providing warmth and emotional support, and may appear detached and disinterested.

Five-Factor Model Reformulation. Conceptualizing schizoid personality disorder as a maladaptive variant of normal introversion provides empirical support for genetic contributions to its etiology (Plomin & Caspi, 1999) and an empirically supported neuropathology (Depue, 1996). FFM extraversion versus introversion is characterized by some researchers as a domain of positive affectivity (Watson & Clark, 1997). Positive affectivity is aligned with extraversion, just as negative affectivity is aligned with neuroticism. Positive emotionality is included as one of the FFM facets of extraversion. Watson and Tellegen (1985) emphasize the positive emotional component of extraversion, as they hypothesize that it provides the motivating force of extraverted behavior. Depue (1996) and his colleagues have conducted considerable research to support the hypothesis that the BAS (or what he refers to as the behavioral facilitation system) is a fundamental domain of personality functioning governed by dopaminergic activity within the mesolimbic system. The BAS may provide the general motivation or incentive to engage in goal-directed behavior and the physical and mental energy, self-confidence, and optimism to sustain necessary expectations for eventual successful outcomes (Depue, 1996; Rothbart & Ahadi, 1994). There are considerable individual differences in the level of activity along the pathways of the behavioral activation system, providing the neurological substrate for the broad personality domain of extraversion versus introversion (Watson & Clark, 1997). Persons at the lowest levels will experience little pleasure in activities (i.e., experience anhedonia), will be indifferent to the praise of others, will be socially withdrawn and inactive, will lack close friends, will show an emotional coldness, detachment, and flattened affectivity, and will likely be diagnosed as having schizoid personality disorder.

Considerable research supports the use of the FFM to describe schizoid personality disorder (Clark & Livesley, 1994; Costa & McCrae, 1990; Dyce & O'Connor, 1998; Lynam & Widiger, 2001; Soldz, Budman, Demby, & Merry, 1993; Trull et al., 1998; Widiger & Costa, 2002; Wiggins & Pincus, 1989). Most studies have found that low scores on the domain of extraversion are associated with and characteristic of schizoid personality dysfunction.

A five-factor formulation of schizoid personality disorder can provide clinicians with information necessary for differential diagnosis of the disorder. SZPD can be confused with the schizotypal and avoidant personality disorders, as both involve social isolation and withdrawal (Kalus, Bernstein, & Siever, 1993). Schizotypal personality disorder, however, includes cognitive-perceptual aberrations and could be best described by the facets of high anxiousness, high openness to fantasy, and high self-consciousness. The major distinction with avoidant personality disorder is the absence of an intense desire for intimate social relationships. Avoidant persons can also be described as high in anxiousness and self-consciousness, whereas the schizoid person is largely indifferent to the reactions or opinions of others.

Treatment.   It is rare for prototypic cases of SZPD to enter treatment, whether for their schizoid traits or an Axis I disorder. Their lack of social interaction is likely to be more worrisome to relatives or colleagues than it is to themselves, and their lack of interest in interpersonal contact will often prevent treatment entry. If a person with schizoid personality disorder presents for treatment of an Axis I disorder (substance dependence, for example), an effective therapist will likely provide treatment in a businesslike (versus interpersonally engaging) style (Stone, 1993). An approach that includes education and feedback concerning others' perceptions of them is likely to be acceptable to those with SZPD. In this respect, group therapy may be useful for these individuals, though the group may need to be especially patient with and accepting of schizoid detachment and flat affect.

Borderline Personality Disorder

Definition.   Borderline personality disorder (BPD) is a pervasive pattern of impulsivity and instability in interpersonal relationships and self-image (APA, 2000). Its primary diagnostic criteria include extreme efforts to avoid abandonment; instability in relationships, affect, and identity; and reckless impulsivity.

Etiology and Pathology.   There are studies supportive of BPD as a disorder with a genetic disposition that cannot be accounted for by other comorbid disorders. Many studies have also suggested a genetic history comorbid with mood and impulse control disorders (Silk, 2000; Torgesen, 2000). There is also substantial empirical support for a childhood history of physical and/or sexual abuse, parental conflict, loss, and neglect (Johnson, Cohen, Brown, Smalles, & Bernstein, 1999; Zanarini, 2000). Past traumatic events are present in many (if not most) cases of BPD, contributing to the comorbidity with posttraumatic stress and dissociative disorders (Brodsky, Cloitre, & Dulit, 1995; Gunderson, 2001; Hefferman & Cloitre, 2000), but the nature of these events and the age at which they occurred appear to vary. BPD may involve the interaction of a genetic disposition toward an emotionally unstable temperament with a cumulative and evolving series of intensely pathogenic relationships (Gunderson, 2001; Morey & Zanarini, 2000).

The pathogenic mechanisms of BPD are addressed in numerous theories. Most concern issues regarding abandonment, separation, and/or exploitative abuse; thus, "frantic efforts to avoid abandonment" is the first item in the DSM–IV-TR diagnostic criterion set (Gunderson, Zanarini, & Kisiel, 1991; Mattia & Zimmerman, 2001). Intense, disturbed, and/or abusive relationships with the significant persons of their past will have been a constant in the life of persons with BPD (Gunderson, 2001). Therefore, the development of malevolent perceptions and expectations of others (Ornduff, 2000) is not surprising. These expectations, along with an impairment in the ability to regulate affect (Linehan, 1993), may contribute to the perpetuation of intense, hostile, and unstable relationships. Neurochemical dysregulation is evident in individuals with BPD, but whether this dysregulation is a result, cause, or correlate of prior interpersonal traumas (Gunderson, 2001; Silk, 2000) remains unclear.

Differential Diagnosis.   Zanarini, Gunderson, Frankenburg, and Chauncey (1989) developed a semistructured interview for the assessment of borderline personality disorder, the Diagnostic Interview for Borderlines–Revised (DIB–R). The DIB–R provides a thorough evaluation of the components of borderline personality, covering the affective dysregulation and perceptual aberrations of the disorder that might not be assessed as well in more general personality disorder interviews (Widiger & Coker, 2001).

Most persons with BPD develop mood disorders (Links, Heslegrave, & van Reekum, 1998), and it can be difficult to differentiate BPD from a mood disorder if the assessment is confined to the current symptomatology (Gunderson, 2001; Widiger & Coker, 2001). The diagnostic criteria of BPD require that the borderline symptomatology be evident since adolescence, which should differentiate BPD from a mood disorder in all cases other than a chronic mood disorder. If a chronic mood disorder is present, then the additional features of transient, stress-related paranoid ideation, dissociative experiences, impulsivity, and anger dyscontrol that are evident in BPD should be emphasized in the diagnosis (Gunderson, 2001).

Epidemiology and Comorbidity.   It is estimated that 1% to 2% of the general population would meet the DSM–IV criteria for BPD (see Table 10.1). BPD is the most prevalent personality disorder within most clinical settings (although perhaps not the most prevalent in community settings; see Table 10.1). Approximately 15% of all inpatients (51% of inpatients with a personality disorder) and 8% of all outpatients (27% of outpatients with a personality disorder) will meet criteria for borderline personality disorder. Approximately 75% of persons with BPD will be female (Corbitt & Widiger, 1995; Gunderson, 2001). Persons with BPD will meet DSM–IV-TR criteria for at least one Axis I disorder, ranging from mood (major depressive disorder), anxiety (posttraumatic stress disorder), eating (bulimia nervosa), and substance (alcohol dependence) disorders to dissociative (dissociative identity disorder) or psychotic (brief psychotic) disorders (Gunderson, 2001; Links et al., 1998; Zanarini et al., 1998a).

Course.   Individuals with BPD are likely to have been emotionally unstable, impulsive, and hostile as children. As adolescents, their intense affectivity and impulsivity may contribute to involvement with rebellious groups, along with a variety of Axis I disorders, including eating disorders, substance abuse, and mood disorders. BPD is often diagnosed in children and adolescents. However, considerable caution should be used when doing so, as some of the symptoms of BPD (e.g., identity disturbance, hostility, and unstable relationships) could be confused with a normal adolescent rebellion or identity crisis (Ad-Dab'bagh & Greenfield, 2001; Gunderson, 2001).

As adults, persons with BPD may be repeatedly hospitalized, because of their affect and impulse dyscontrol, psychotic-like and dissociative symptomatology, and risk of suicide and suicide attempts (Gunderson, 2001; Zanarini et al., 1998a). These individuals are at a high risk for developing depressive, substance-related, bulimic, and posttraumatic stress disorders. The risk of suicide is increased with a comorbid mood disorder and substance-related disorder. It is estimated that 3% to 10% of persons with BPD will have committed suicide by the age of 30 (Gunderson, 2001). Intimate relationships tend to be very unstable and explosive, and employment history is generally poor (Daley, Burge, & Hammen, 2000; Stone, 2001). As the person reaches the age of 30, affective lability and impulsivity may begin to diminish. These symptoms may lessen earlier if the person becomes involved with a supportive and patient sexual partner (Stone, 2001). Some, however, may obtain stability by abandoning the effort to obtain a relationship, opting instead for a lonelier but less volatile life. Occurrence of a severe stressor, however, can easily disrupt the lessening of symptomatology, resulting in a brief psychotic, dissociative, or mood disorder episode.

Five-Factor Model Reformulation.   Borderline PD is primarily composed of excessively high neuroticism. In particular, these individuals are at the very highest range of anxiousness, angry hostility, depressiveness, impulsiveness, and vulnerability. Borderline clients will also likely be low in the agreeableness facets of trust and compliance and low on the conscientiousness facet of competence.

Table 10.4 provides 22 correlations between the domains of the FFM and BPD symptomatology reported across 13 studies. The median correlations are .47 (neuroticism), .00 (extraversion), .00 (openness), .26 (antagonism), and −.21 (conscientiousness), consistent with the expectations (Lynam & Widiger, 2001; Widiger et al., 1994/2002). A median correlation of only .47 with neuroticism might appear to be lower than what should be obtained. However, it is useful to compare this correlation with the convergent validity of alternative measures of borderline personality disorder. Widiger and Coker (2001) reported a median convergent validity coefficient for borderline personality disorder of .53 across forty-five studies. In other words, FFM neuroticism is correlated with borderline personality disorder symptomatology almost as high as any two measures of borderline symptomatology are correlated with one another.

Two studies have focused specifically on the FFM conceptualization of borderline personality disorder. Clarkin, Hull, Cantor, and Sanderson (1993) explored empirically the FFM conceptualization of BPD in a sample of sixty-two female inpatients with BPD diagnoses provided by clinicians at Cornell University Medical Center using the Structured Clinical Interview for DSM personality disorder (SCID–II), a semistructured interview for the assessment of personality disorders (First, Spitzer, Gibbon, & Williams, 1995). Despite the restrictions in range on borderline symptomatology within this sample (i.e., all participants met criteria for BPD), Clarkin et al. confirmed a close correspondence between the facets of the five-factor model and borderline symptomatology. The findings of Clarkin et al. (1993) were subsequently replicated by Wilberg, Urnes, Friis, Pederson, and Karterud (1999). Wilberg et al. administered the Revised NEO Personality Inventory (NEO–PI–R; Costa & McCrae, 1992) to a sample of sixty-three persons participating in a day hospital group psychotherapy program for poorly functioning outpatients with personality disorders. Wilberg et al. obtained assessments of the diagnostic criteria for BPD after the 18-week treatment ended, based in part on data obtained from an administration of the SCID–II at the time of admission, as well as the impressions of the clinicians during the course of treatment. Wilberg et al. (1999) confirmed the predicted relations with neuroticism, as well as low conscientiousness, low trust, and low straightforwardness.

The FFM conceptualization of BPD is helpful in explaining its substantial prevalence and diagnostic comorbidity. Persons with BPD are likely to meet DSM–IV criteria for at least one other personality disorder, particularly histrionic, dependent, antisocial, schizotypal, and passive-aggressive (see Table 10.3; Links et al., 1998; Zanarini et al., 1998b). Researchers and clinicians have at times responded to this extensive co-occurrence by imposing a diagnostic hierarchy whereby other disorders are not diagnosed in the presence of BPD because BPD is generally the most severely dysfunctional personality disorder (Gunderson et al., 2000). A potential limitation of this approach is that it "resolves" the complexity of personality by largely ignoring it. This approach fails to recognize the presence of maladaptive personality traits that could be important for understanding a patient's dysfunctions and for developing an optimal treatment plan (Zimmerman & Mattia, 1999). Neuroticism, as a characteristic level of emotional instability (i.e., vulnerability to stress, impulse dyscontrol, anxiousness, depressiveness, and other components of negative affectivity) is almost ubiquitous within clinical populations. A diagnostic category defined primarily by and including essentially all of the facets of neuroticism should be highly prevalent within clinical settings. In addition, all of the other DSM–IV-TR personality disorders include at least some components of neuroticism, and the variants in symptomatology accounted for by neuroticism explain much of the comorbidity of BPD with other personality disorders (Lynam & Widiger, 2001).

The five-factor model can also help shed light on the controversy over the pathology and etiology of borderline personality disorder. Zanarini (2000) has argued that the central

TABLE 10.4

Correlations of Borderline Personality Disorder With Domains of the FFM

| Study | Sample | Measures | | | | | | | |
		BPD	FFM	N	E	O	A	C
Wiggins & Pincus (1989)	550 stdts	MMPI	NEOPI	.66***	.00	.13**	−.21***	−.20***
Costa & McCrae (1990)	274 comm	MMPI	NEOPI	.47***	.19**	.09	−.21***	−.32***
Costa & McCrae (1990)	207 comm	MCMI-I	NEOPI	.52***	−.22***	−.10	.14*	−.10
Costa & McCrae (1990)	62 comm	MCMI-II	NEOPI	.46**	−.09	−.16	−.22	−.22
Trull (1992)	54 pts	MMPI	NEOPI	.61***	.13	.18	−.45***	−.24
Trull (1992)	54 pts	PDQR	NEOPI	.60***	.19	.28*	−.39***	−.17
Trull (1992)	54 pts	SIDPR	NEOPI	.48***	.04	−.08	−.46***	−.31*
Soldz et al. (1993)	102 pts	MCMI-II	50-BSRS	.56***	.04	−.02	−.26*	−.34***
Soldz et al. (1993)	102 pts	PDE	50-BSRS	.42***	.06	.20*	−.13	−.10
West (1993)	457 stdts	MMPI	NEOPI	.43***	.09	.02	−.21***	−.15
West (1993)	457 stdts	PDQR	NEOPI	.49***	−.20**	−.01	−.34***	−.22*
Yeung et al. (1993)	224 comm	SIDP	NEOFFI	.23***	−.03	−.01	−.28***	−.18**
Coolidge et al. (1994)	233 stdts	CATI	NEOPI	.66***	−.16*	.16*	−.29**	−.22**
Hyer et al. (1994)	80 pts	MCMI-II	NEOPI	.36***	−.10	.00	−.07	−.08
Duijsens & Diekstra (1996)	450 comm	VKP	23BB5	.29***	−.16	.10	−.33***	−.12
Duijsens & Diekstra (1996)	210 comm	VKP	5PFT	.46***	.01	−.14	−.30***	−.24***
Ball et al. (1997)	363 pts	SCID-II	NEOFFI	.41***	−.02	.08	−.19***	−.20***
Blais (1997)	100 pts	Clinician	Adjectives	.37***	.04	.00	−.09	−.21**
Dyce & O'Connor (1998)	614 stdts	MCMI-III	NEOPIR	.64***	−.27***	.01	−.31***	−.35***
Trull et al. (2003)	232 mixed	PDQR	SIFFM	.62***	−.25**	.28**	−.12	−.35***

* $p < .05$; ** $p < .01$; *** $p < .001$

Note: BPD = borderline personality disorder; FFM = five-factor model; N = neuroticism; E = extraversion; O = openness; A = agreeableness; C = conscientiousness; stdts = students; comm = community; pts = patients; MMPI = Minnesota Multiphasic Personality Inventory; MCMI = Millon Clinical Multiaxial Inventory; PDQR = Personality Diagnostic Questionnaire–Revised; SIDPR = Structured Interview for Personality Disorders–Revised; PDE = Personality Disorder Examination; CATI = Coolidge Axis II Inventory; VKP = Vragenlijst voor Kenmerken van de Persoonlijkheid; SCID–II = Structured Clinical Interview for DSM–IV Personality Disorders; Clinician = ratings by unstructured clinical interviews; NEOPIR = NEO Personality Inventory Revised; 50-BSRS = 50-Bipolar Self-Rating Scale; NEOFFI = NEO Five Factor Inventory; 23BB5 = 23 Bipolar Big Five Questionnaire; Five Personality Factor Test; SIFFM = Structured Interview for the Five Factor Model.

pathology of BPD is equivalent to an excessively high level of impulsivity (a facet of neu-roticism), leading those with the disorder to make one disastrously impulsive decision after another. Linehan (1993) has argued that the central pathological feature of the borderline pa-tient is an excessively high level of vulnerability (also a facet of neuroticism), which leaves the patient with no "emotional skin" (p. 44) to deal with problems. In contrast to the current DSM diagnostic criteria hierarchy, a five-factor view does not necessitate a single, central pathol-ogy or feature. Rather, the entire domain of neuroticism is important in the consideration of borderline personality disorder, and the patient's level on each facet is related to its clinical importance.

Treatment. Clients with BPD tend to form relationships with therapists that are similar to their other relationships, insofar as the relationships have the potential for being tremendously intense, volatile, and disruptive. The American Psychiatric Association (2001) has published practice guidelines for the psychotherapeutic and pharmacologic treatment of persons with bor-derline personality disorder. Because borderline patients can present with significant suicide risk, a thorough evaluation of the potential for suicidal ideation and activity should have the initial priority. Also, many patients with borderline personality disorder have comorbid Axis I disorders, some of which might take priority (e.g., major depressive disorder, substance depen-dence, or dissociative disorder). Borderline patients are often highly motivated for treatment, but their relationship with the therapist might become as intense as his or her relationships with other significant persons. Ongoing consultation with colleagues is recommended to address the therapist's negative reactions (e.g., distancing, rejecting, or abandoning the patient in response to feelings of anger or frustration) as well as positive reactions (e.g., fantasies of being the therapist who in fact rescues or cures the patient, romantic or sexual feelings in response to a seductive patient). Immediate and historical issues should be addressed in therapy, and the client should feel safe expressing and addressing anger, bitterness, and depression. Weekly meetings should be provided. Sessions should emphasize the building of a strong therapeutic alliance, monitoring self-destructive and suicidal behaviors, validation of suffering and abusive experience (but also help the client take responsibility for actions), promotion of self-reflection rather than impulsive action, and setting limits on self-destructive behavior (APA, 2001). The tendency of borderline patients to engage in "splitting" (polarization of an emotional response) should also be carefully monitored and addressed (e.g., devaluation of prior therapists, coupled with idealization of current therapist).

Dialectical behavior therapy (DBT; Linehan, 1993) has been shown empirically to be an effective treatment of BPD. The dialectical component of DBT was derived largely from Zen Buddhist principles of overcoming suffering through acceptance. Mastery of conflict is achieved in part through no longer struggling or fighting adversity; pain is overcome when it is no longer fought. DBT initially focuses on reducing self-harm and suicidal urges and behaviors that disrupt treatment (substance abuse, avoidance). After mastery of these issues, DBT teaches individuals with BPD a new set of coping skills focused on emotional control and interpersonal issues. Individuals in DBT attend regular sessions with an individual therapist and discuss problems in using the skills. These sessions are augmented with a didactic skills-training group. The APA (2001) concluded that psychodynamic psychotherapy has obtained empirical support for the treatment of BPD that is equal to DBT, but this conclusion has since been disputed (Sanderson, Swenson, & Bohus, 2002).

Avoidant Personality Disorder

Definition. Avoidant personality disorder (AVPD) involves a pervasive pattern of timid-ity, inhibition, inadequacy, and social hypersensitivity (APA, 2000). Its primary diagnostic criteria include avoiding interpersonal contact and activities due to fear of criticism and viewing oneself as inept and inferior to others.

Etiology and Pathology. There have not been any systematic studies on the heritability or psychosocial etiology of AVPD (Bernstein & Travaglini, 1999; Nigg & Goldsmith, 1994). There are a number of theoretical models for its etiology and pathology. AVPD may involve elevated peripheral sympathetic activity and adrenocortical responsiveness, resulting in excessive autonomic arousal, fearfulness, and inhibition (Siever & Davis, 1991). Cognitive models emphasize an excessive self-consciousness and cognitive schemas of inadequacy and inferiority (Beck et al., 1990; Dreessen, Arntz, Hendriks, Keune, & van den Hout, 1999).

Differential Diagnosis. The most difficult differential diagnosis for AVPD is with generalized social phobia (Tillfors, Furmak, Ekselius, & Fredrikson, 2001; van Velzen, Emmelkamp, & Scholing, 2000; Widiger, 2001). Both disorders involve timidity, anxiety, and an avoidance of social situations, and both may have been present since late childhood or adolescence. In fact, many persons with AVPD initially seek treatment for social phobia. To the extent that the behavior pattern pervades the person's everyday functioning and has been evident since childhood, the diagnosis of a personality disorder would be more accurate.

Epidemiology and Comorbidity. Timidity, shyness, and social anxiety are not uncommon problems (Crozier & Alden, 2001), and AVPD is one of the more prevalent personality disorders within clinical settings. Approximately 5% to 25% of all patients would meet criteria for AVPD (APA, 2000; Mattia & Zimmerman, 2001). However, only 1% to 2% of the general population would meet criteria for avoidant personality disorder (see Table 10.2). It appears to occur equally among males and females, with some studies reporting more males and others reporting more females (Corbitt & Widiger, 1995).

Course. Adolescence is a particularly difficult developmental period for persons with AVPD, because of the emphasis on peer relationships and popularity. Avoidance of social situations inhibits the development of adequate social skills, further handicapping any eventual efforts to develop relationships. Persons with AVPD may enjoy occupational success, finding considerable gratification and esteem through a job or career that requires little interaction or public performance. A job may serve as a distraction from intense feelings of loneliness and insecurity. Persons with AVPD may be very responsible, empathic, and affectionate parents, but may unwittingly impart feelings of social anxiousness and awkwardness. As the person ages, symptoms of AVPD lessen in intensity.

Five-Factor Model Reformulation. AVPD is conceptualized in terms of the FFM as being a maladaptive variant of the domain and facets of neuroticism (particularly the facets of anxiousness, self-consciousness, and vulnerability) and introversion (abnormally low gregariousness, low assertiveness, and low excitement seeking; see Table 10.3). Widiger (2001) presented data from thirteen studies supportive of this conceptualization of AVPD, and noted that similar patterns of findings have been obtained in clinical, community, and college populations. Avoidant personality traits, assessed by a variety of methods, are consistently and often highly correlated with neuroticism and introversion, but are rarely correlated with any of the other domains of personality. Two of the studies reported results for the facets of neuroticism and introversion. Dyce and O'Connor (1998) reported correlations of .49, .62, and .46 (respectively) with the neuroticism facets of anxiousness, self-consciousness, and vulnerability ($p < .001$); $-.37$, $-.29$, and $-.24$ with the extraversion facets of gregariousness, activity, and excitement seeking ($p < .001$). Trull, Widiger, and Burr (2001) reported correlations of .43, .70, and .56 (respectively) with the neuroticism facets of anxiousness, self-consciousness, and vulnerability ($p < .001$); $-.33$, $-.45$, and $-.40$ with the extraversion facets of gregariousness, activity, and excitement seeking ($p < .001$).

Conceptualizing avoidant personality disorder as a maladaptive variant of introversion also provides an empirically based understanding of its etiology. There is considerable empirical support for the heritability of introversion and neuroticism (Plomin & Caspi, 1999). In childhood, neuroticism appears as a distress-prone or inhibited temperament (Rothbart & Ahadi, 1994). Parents may exacerbate shyness, timidity, and interpersonal insecurity through overprotection and excessive cautiousness (Schmidt, Polak, & Spooner, 2001). Overprotective parental behavior, coupled with a distress-prone temperament, has been shown to contribute to the development of social inhibition and timidity (Burgess, Rubin, Chea, & Nelson, 2001; Rothbart & Ahadi, 1994). The neuropathology of AVPD may also be clarified if it is understood as being a maladaptive variant of general neuroticism and introversion. Just as ASPD may involve deficits in the functioning of a behavioral inhibition system, AVPD may involve excessive functioning of this same system (Depue, 1996). The pathology of AVPD, however, may also be more psychological than neurochemical, with the timidity, shyness, and insecurity being a natural result of a cumulative history of embarrassing, denigrating, and devaluing experiences (Schmidt et al., 2001).

A five-factor formulation of this disorder can also aid the clinician in differential diagnosis of avoidant personality. For example, many persons with AVPD may also meet criteria for dependent personality disorder (DPD, see below). This diagnosis might appear contradictory, given that AVPD involves social withdrawal whereas DPD involves excessive social attachment. However, if an individual with AVPD is able to obtain a relationship, he or she will often cling to this relationship in a dependent manner. Both disorders include abnormally high levels of the neuroticism facets of anxiousness, self-consciousness, and vulnerability. A distinction between AVPD and DPD is best made when the person is seeking a relationship. Avoidant individuals tend to be very shy and inhibited (and are therefore slow to get involved with someone), whereas dependent individuals desperately seek another relationship as soon as one ends (i.e., avoidant persons are high in introversion whereas dependent persons are high in extraversion).

Treatment.   Many persons with AVPD present for treatment of social phobia or other anxiety disorders related to their avoidant traits. A thorough initial assessment will indicate that the individual suffers not simply from shyness or dyscontrolled anxiousness, but rather from a pattern of interpersonal insecurity, low self-esteem, and feelings of inadequacy.

Social skills training, systematic desensitization, and a hierarchy of in vivo exposure to feared social situations have been shown to be useful in the treatment of AVPD (Beck et al., 1990; Stone, 1993). It is also important for the therapist to address insecurities concerning attractiveness, rejection, and intimacy (Gabbard, 1994). Individuals with AVPD may be hesitant to discuss these issues, feeling that they may "waste the therapist's time with stupid concerns." Therapists should be especially empathic with such individuals, and use of cognitive techniques to address such insecurities may be useful. Supportive groups may be helpful for individuals with AVPD. A group environment may provide an understanding of the irrationality of their expectations and perceptions concerning interpersonal contact.

Pharmacologic treatment of AVPD may include anxiolytic and/or antidepressant medication. Though AVPD clients should be monitored for dependence on anxiolytic medication, these medications may be especially useful in initial attempts to overcome social anxiety (e.g., in vivo exposures).

Dependent Personality Disorder

Definition. Dependent personality disorder (DPD) involves a pervasive and excessive need to be taken care of that leads to submissiveness, clinging, and fears of separation (APA, 2000; Bornstein, 1999; Pincus & Wilson, 2001). Its primary diagnostic criteria include extreme difficulty making decisions without others' input, need for others to assume responsibility for most aspects of daily life, extreme difficulty disagreeing with others, inability to initiate projects due to lack of self-confidence, and going to excessive lengths to obtain the approval of others.

Etiology and Pathology. Insecure interpersonal attachment (Bornstein, 1999; Pincus & Wilson, 2001; Stone, 1993) is central to the etiology and pathology of DPD. Insecure attachment and helplessness may be generated through a parent–child relationship, perhaps by a clinging parent or a continued infantilization during a time in which individuation and separation normally occurs (Gabbard, 2000; Thompson & Zuroff, 1998). However, the combination of an anxious and/or inhibited temperament with inconsistent or overprotective parenting may also generate or exacerbate dependent personality traits (Bornstein, 1999; O'Neill & Kendler, 1998; Rothbart & Ahadi, 1994). Unable to generate feelings of security and confidence for themselves, dependent persons may rely on a parental figure or significant other for constant reassurance of their worth. Eventually, persons with DPD may come to believe that their self-worth is defined by their importance to another person (Beck et al., 1990).

Differential Diagnosis. Excessively dependent behavior may be seen in persons who have developed debilitating mental and physical conditions, such as agoraphobia, schizophrenia, severe injuries, or dementia. However, a diagnosis of DPD requires the presence of the dependent traits since late childhood or adolescence (APA, 2000). One can diagnose the presence of a personality disorder at any age during a person's lifetime, but if (for example) a DPD diagnosis is given to a person at the age of 75, this presumes that the dependent behavior was evident since the age of approximately 18 (i.e., predates the onset of a comorbid mental or physical disorder).

Differences in personality due to differing cultural norms should not be confused with the presence of a personality disorder (Alarcon, 1996; Alarcon & Foulks, 1997; Bornstein, 1999). Cultural groups differ greatly in the degree of importance attached to deferent behavior, politeness, and passivity. The diagnosis of DPD requires that the dependent behavior result in clinically significant functional impairment or distress.

Epidemiology and Comorbidity. DPD is estimated to occur in 5% to 30% of patients and 2% to 4% of the general community (Mattia & Zimmerman, 2001) and is one of the most prevalent personality disorders (APA, 2000). Studies have indicated that dependent personality traits are a risk factor for the development of depression in response to interpersonal loss (Hammen et al., 1995; Robins, Hayes, Block, Kramer, & Villena, 1995; Widiger, Verheul, & van den Brink, 1999).

Course. To the extent that independent responsibility and initiative are required, job functioning will be impaired or unsatisfactory. Individuals with DPD are prone to mood disorders throughout life, particularly major depression and dysthymia, and to anxiety disorders, particularly agoraphobia, social phobia, and panic disorder. However, the severity of the symptomatology tends to lessen with age, particularly if the person has obtained a reliable, empathic partner.

Five-Factor Model Reformulation. The dependent personality can primarily be characterized by maladaptively high levels of agreeableness and the neuroticism facets of anxiousness, self-consciousness, and vulnerability. Persons with DPD will have been excessively submissive as children and adolescents, and some may have had a chronic physical illness or a separation anxiety disorder during childhood (APA, 2000). Persons with DPD fear intensely the loss of care and support from others, particularly a person to whom they have an emotional attachment (Bornstein, 1999; Stone, 1993). They are unable to be alone, as their sense of self-worth, value, or meaning is obtained through the presence of a relationship. They have few other sources of self-esteem and experience perpetual doubts and insecurities regarding the current source of support. Persons with DPD require constant reassurance that any particular relationship will continue, fearing that at some point they may again be alone (Overholser, 1996). As well, persons with dependent symptomatology would likely be described as maladaptively low in the facet of assertiveness and abnormally high in warmth. Persons with DPD may become quickly attached to persons who are unreliable, unempathic, and even exploitative or abusive. More desirable partners may be driven away by excessive clinging and constant demands for reassurance.

Researchers have found an association between the FFM domain of agreeableness and dependent personality disorder symptomatology (Costa & McCrae, 1990; Dyce & O'Connor, 1998; Hyer et al., 1994). McCrae and Costa (1987) state that extremely high scores on agreeableness may describe a "dependent and fawning" (p. 88) person. Some studies have not confirmed the association (Bornstein & Cecero, 2000) between maladaptive agreeableness and dependent symptomatology. However, it appears that the few anomalous results reflect the fact that the most common measure of the FFM, the NEO–PI–R, does not represent maladaptively high agreeableness sufficiently to obtain consistent confirmation of this relationship (Haigler & Widiger, 2001).

A controversial issue in the diagnosis of dependent personality disorder is its differential sex prevalence (Bornstein, 1999; Widiger, 1998). DPD is diagnosed more frequently in females. Some researchers have argued that the more frequent diagnosis of dependent personality disorder in women reflects a bias in Western culture, and that the disorder pathologizes normal female behavior. The FFM offers a possible resolution to this issue. Researchers have consistently found that women tend to score higher than men on the domain of agreeableness, higher than men on the anxiousness facet of neuroticism, and lower than men on the assertiveness facet of extraversion (Costa & McCrae, 1988, 1992; Feingold, 1994; Trapnell & Wiggins, 1990). Costa, Terracciano, and McCrae (2001) found these differences to be consistent across twenty-six cultures, ranging from very traditional (Pakistan) to modern (The Netherlands). Thus, it is perhaps to be expected that a differential sex prevalence would be observed. This is not to suggest, however, that no gender bias operates in clinical decision making. Gender stereotyping could occur in clinical settings, because of the relation of the personality disorder to common gender differences. In other words, it is the existence of the gender-related traits that contributes to the occurrence of stereotypic perceptions and gender-biased assessments (Widiger, 1998).

Many persons with DPD meet the criteria for histrionic and borderline personality disorders (see Table 10.2). Persons with DPD and HPD may both display high scores on the neuroticism facet of self-consciousness and the agreeableness facet of trust, displaying strong needs for reassurance and approval. However, persons with DPD tend to score higher on the agreeableness facets of altruism, modesty, and compliance. Persons with HPD tend to be more flamboyant, assertive, and self-centered (high on the facet of gregariousness and low in modesty and altruism), and persons with BPD tend to be much more dysfunctional and emotionally dysregulated (higher in all facets of neuroticism) (Bornstein, 1999).

Treatment. Persons with DPD are often in treatment for one or more Axis I disorders, particularly a mood (depressive) or anxiety disorder. These individuals tend to be very agreeable, compliant, and grateful clients, at times to excess. Many individuals with DPD find that the therapeutic relationship satisfies their need for support and concern. The therapist can be perceived as a caring partner who will always be available for the patient. The dependent client may fear successful treatment, because termination may shortly follow. Thus, the client may remain excessively compliant and agreeable to be a patient that the therapist will continue to treat. Therapists should be careful not to unwittingly encourage this submissiveness, nor to reject the client to be rid of their clinging dependency. Individuals with DPD may have unrealistic expectations of their therapist, making unrealistic demands on the therapist's time.

An important component of treatment is often a thorough exploration of the need for support and its root causes. Cognitive-behavioral techniques can be useful to address feelings of inadequacy and helplessness and to provide training in assertiveness and problem-solving techniques. Group therapy may be useful for persons with DPD, providing interpersonal feedback and modeling autonomous behavior. DPD is not known to respond to pharmacotherapy.

CONCLUSIONS

Maladaptive personality traits can be the focus of clinical treatment and often impair or impede the treatment of other mental disorders. Chart reviews of practitioners suggest that they are not being diagnosed as frequently as they occur, perhaps because it can be difficult to obtain coverage for their treatment. This is regrettable because some maladaptive personality traits (e.g., borderline and antisocial) have substantial social and public health care costs.

The five-factor model offers a compelling alternative to the categorical diagnosis of personality disorders as provided in DSM–IV-TR. Advantages of understanding personality disorders in terms of this dimensional model are the provision of more specific descriptions of individual patients (including adaptive as well as maladaptive personality functioning), the avoidance of arbitrary categorical distinctions, and the ability to bring to bear the extensive amount of research on the heritability, temperament, development, and course of general personality functioning to an understanding of personality disorders.

REFERENCES

Ad-Dab'bagh, Y. & Greenfield, B. (2001). Multiple complex developmental disorder: The "multiple and complex" evolution of the "childhood borderline syndrome" construct. *Journal of American Academic Child and Adolescent Psychiatry, 40*, 954–964.

Alarcon, R. D. (1996). Personality disorders and culture in DSM-IV: A critique. *Journal of Personality Disorders, 10*, 260–270.

Alarcon, R. D., & Foulks, E. F. (1997). Cultural factors and personality disorders: A review of the literature. In T. A. Widiger, A. J. Frances, H. A. Pincus, R. Ross, M. B. First, W. W. Davis, & M. Klein (Eds.), *DSM-IV sourcebook* (Vol. 3, pp. 975–982). Washington, DC: American Psychiatric Association.

American Psychiatric Association (1980). *Diagnostic and statistical manual of mental disorders* (3rd ed.). Washington, DC: Author.

American Psychiatric Association (1987). *Diagnostic and statistical manual of mental disorders* (3rd ed., rev.). Washington, DC: Author.

American Psychiatric Association (2000). *Diagnostic and statistical manual of mental disorders.* Text Revision (4th ed., rev. ed.). Washington, DC: Author.

American Psychiatric Association (2001). *Practice guidelines for the treatment of patients with borderline personality disorder.* Washington, DC: Author.

Ball, S. A., Tennen, H., Poling, J. C., Kranzler, H. R., & Rounsaville, B. J. (1997). Personality, temperament, and character dimensions and the DSM-IV personality disorders in substance abusers. *Journal of Abnormal Psychology*, *106*, 545–553.

Beck, A. T., Freeman, A., and Associates (1990). *Cognitive therapy of personality disorders*. New York: Guilford Press.

Bernstein, D. P., & Travaglini, L. (1999). Schizoid and avoidant personality disorders. In T. Millon, P. H. Blaney, & R. D. Davis (Eds.), *Oxford textbook of psychopathology* (pp. 523–534). New York: Oxford University Press.

Black, D. W., Noyes, R., Pfohl, B., Goldstein, R. B., & Blum, N. (1993). Personality disorder in obsessive-compulsive volunteers, well comparison subjects, and their first degree relatives. *American Journal of Psychiatry*, *150*, 1226–1232.

Blais, M. (1997). Clinician ratings of the five-factor model of personality and the DSM-IV personality disorders. *Journal of Nervous and Mental Disease*, *185*, 388–393.

Bornstein, R. F. (1998). Reconceptualizing personality disorder diagnoses in the DSM-V: The discriminant validity challenge. *Clinical Psychology: Science and Practice*, *5*, 333–343.

Bornstein, R. F. (1999). Dependent and histrionic personality disorders. In T. Millon, P. Blaney, & R. Davis (Eds.), *Oxford textbook of psychopathology* (pp. 535–554). Oxford, United Kingdom: Oxford University Press.

Bornstein, R. F., & Cecero, J. J. (2000). Deconstructing dependency in a five-factor world: A meta-analytic review. *Journal of Personality Assessment*, *74*, 324–343.

Brodsky, B. S., Cloitre, M., & Dulit, R. A. (1995). Relationship of dissociation to self-mutilation and childhood abuse in borderline personality disorder. *American Journal of Psychiatry*, *152*, 1788–1792.

Burgess, K. B., Rubin, K. H., Chea, C. S. L., & Nelson, L. J. (2001). Behavioral inhibition, social withdrawal, and parenting. In W. R. Crozier & L. E. Alden (Eds.), *International handbook of social anxiety: Concepts, research, and interventions relating to the self and shyness* (pp. 137–158). New York: Wiley.

Clark, L. A., Kochanska, G., & Ready, R. (2000). Mothers' personality and its interaction with child temperament as predicting parenting behavior. *Journal of Personality and Social Psychology*, *79*, 274–285.

Clark, L. A., & Livesley, W. J. (1994). Two approaches to identifying the dimensions of personality disorder: Convergence on the five-factor model. In P. T. Costa, Jr. & T. A. Widiger (Eds.), *Personality disorders and the five-factor model of personality* (pp. 261–277). Washington, DC: American Psychological Association.

Clarkin, J. F., Hull, J. W., Cantor, J., & Sanderson, C. (1993). Borderline personality disorder and personality traits: A comparison of SCID-II BPD and NEO-PI. *Psychological Assessment*, *5*, 472–476.

Cleckley, H. (1941/1988). *The mask of sanity*. St. Louis, MO: Mosby.

Cloninger, C. R. (2000). A practical way to diagnose personality disorders: A proposal. *Journal of Personality Disorders*, *14*, 99–108.

Coolidge, F. L., Becker, L. A., Dirito, D. C., Durham, R. L., Kinlaw, M. M., & Philbrick, P. B. (1994). On the relationship of the five-factor personality model to personality disorders: Four reservations. *Psychological Reports*, *75*, 11–21.

Corbitt, E. M., & Widiger, T. A. (1995). Sex differences among the personality disorders: An exploration of the data. *Clinical Psychology: Science and Practice*, *2*, 225–238.

Coryell, W. H., & Zimmerman, M. (1989). Personality disorder in the families of depressed, schizophrenic, and never-ill probands. *American Journal of Psychiatry*, *146*, 496–502.

Costa, P. T. Jr., & McCrae, R. R. (1985). *The NEO Personality Inventory manual*. Odessa, FL: Psychological Assessment Resources.

Costa, P. T. Jr., & McCrae, R. R. (1988). Personality in adulthood: A six-year longitudinal study of self-reports and spouse ratings on the NEO Personality Inventory. *Journal of Personality Assessment*, *54*, 853–863.

Costa, P. T. Jr. & McCrae, R. R. (1990). Personality disorders and the five-factor model of personality. *Journal of Personality Disorders*, *4*, 362–371.

Costa, P. T., Jr. & McCrae, R. R. (1992). Revised NEO Personality Inventory (NEO-PI-R) and NEO Five Factor Inventory (NEO-FFI) professional manual. Odessa, FL: Psychological Assessment Resources.

Costa, P. T., Jr., Terracciano, A., & McCrae, R. R. (2001). Gender differences in personality traits across cultures: Robust and surprising findings. *Journal of Personality and Social Psychology*, *81*, 322–331.

Crozier, W. R., & Alden, L. E. (Eds.) (2001). *International handbook of social anxiety: Concepts, research, and interventions relating to the self and shyness*. New York: Wiley.

Daley, S. E., Burge, D., & Hammen, C. (2000). Borderline personality disorder symptoms as predictors of 4-year romantic relationship dysfunction in young women: Addressing issues of specificity. *Journal of Abnormal Psychology*, *109*, 451–460.

Depue, R. A. (1996). A neurobiological framework for the structure of personality and emotion: Implications for personality disorders. In J. C. Clarkin & M. F. Lenzenweger (Eds.), *Major theories of personality disorder*. New York: Guilford Press.

De Raad, B., di Blas, L., & Perugini, M. (1999). Two independently constructed Italian trait taxonomies: Comparisons among Italian and between Italian and Germanic languages. *European Journal of Personality*, *12*, 19–41.

Dodge, K. A. (1980). Social cognition and children's aggressive behavior. *Child Development*, *53*, 620–635.

Dodge, K. A., & Crick, N. R. (1990). Social information processing bases of aggressive behavior in children. *Personality and Social Psychology Bulletin, 16,* 8–22.

Dolan-Sewell, R. G., Krueger, R. F., & Shea, M. T. (2001). Co-occurrence with syndrome disorders. In W. J. Livesley (Ed.), *Handbook of personality disorders* (pp. 84–104). New York: Guilford Press.

Drake, R. E., Adler, D. A., & Vaillant, G. E. (1988). Antecedents of personality disorders in a community sample of men. *Journal of Personality Disorders, 2,* 60–68.

Dreessen, L., Arntz, A., Hendriks, T., Keune, N., & van den Hout, M. (1999). Avoidant personality disorder and implicit schema-congruent information processing bias: A pilot study with a pragmatic inference task. *Behavioral Research and Therapy, 37,* 619–632.

Duijsens, I., & Diekstra, R. F. W. (1996). DSM-III-R and ICD-10 personality disorders and their relationship with the Big Five dimensions of personality. *Personality and Individual Differences, 21,* 119–133.

Dyce, J. A., & O'Connor, B. P. (1998). Personality disorders and the five-factor model: A test of facet-level predictions. *Journal of Personality Disorders, 12,* 31–45.

Feingold, A. (1994). Gender differences in personality: A meta-analysis. *Psychological Bulletin, 116,* 429–456.

First, M., Gibbon, M., Spitzer, R. L., Williams, J. B. W., & Benjamin, L. S. (1997). *User's guide for the structured clinical interview for DSM–IV Axis II personality disorders.* Washington, DC: American Psychiatric Press.

First, M. B., Spitzer, R. L., Gibbon, M., & Williams, J. B. W. (1995). The Structured Clinical Interview for DSM-III-R Personality Disorders (SCID-II): Part I. Description. *Journal of Personality Disorders, 9,* 83–91.

Forth, A. E., Brown, S. L., Hart, S. D., & Hare, R. D. (1996). The assessment of psychopathy in male and female noncriminals: Reliability and validity. *Personality and Individual Differences, 20,* 531–543.

Fowles, D. C. (2001). Biological variables in psychopathology: A psychobiological perspective. In H. E. Adams & P. B. Sutker (Eds.), *Comprehensive handbook of psychopathology* (3rd ed., pp. 85–104). New York: Plenum.

Fowles, D. C., & Kochanska, G. (2000). Temperament as a moderator of pathways to conscience in children: The contribution of electrodermal activity. *Psychophysiology, 37,* 788–795.

Frances, A. J. (1980). The DSM-III personality disorders section: A commentary. *American Journal of Psychiatry, 137,* 1050–1054.

Gabbard, G. O. (1994). *Psychodynamic psychiatry in clinical practice. The DSM–IV edition.* Washington, DC: American Psychiatric Press.

Gabbard, G. O. (2000). Psychodynamic psychotherapy of borderline personality disorder: A contemporary approach. *Bulletin of Menninger Clinic, 65,* 41–57.

Gertsley, L, McLellan, T., Alterman, A., Woody, G., Luborsky, L, & Prout, M. (1989). Ability to form an alliance with the therapist: A possible marker of prognosis for patients with antisocial personality disorder. *American Journal of Psychiatry, 146,* 508–512.

Goldberg, L. R. (1993). The structure of phenotypic personality traits. *American Psychologist, 48,* 26–34.

Gunderson, J. G. (2001). Borderline personality disorder: A clinical guide. Washington, DC: American Psychiatric Press.

Gunderson, J. G., Shea, T., Skodol, A. E., McGlashan, T. H., Morey, L. C., Stout, R. L., Zanarini, M. C., Grilo, C. M., Oldham, J. M., & Keller, M. B. (2000). The Collaborative Longitudinal Personality Disorders Study: Development, aims, design, and sample characteristics. *Journal of Personality Disorders, 14,* 300–315.

Gunderson, J. G., Zanarini, M. C., & Kisiel, C. L., (1991). Borderline personality disorder: A review of data on DSM-III-R descriptions. *Journal of Personality Disorders, 5,* 340–352.

Haigler, E. D., & Widiger, T. A. (2001). Experimental manipulation of NEO-PI-R items. *Journal of Personality Assessment, 77,* 339–358.

Hamburger, M. E., Lilienfeld, S. O., & Hogben, M. (1996). Psychopathy, gender, and gender roles: implications for antisocial and histrionic personality disorder. *Journal of Personality Disorders, 10,* 41–55.

Hammen, C. L., Burge, D., Daley, S. E., Davila, J., Paley, B., & Rudolph, K. D. (1995). Interpersonal attachment cognitions and predictions of symptomatic responses to interpersonal stress. *Journal of Abnormal Psychology, 104,* 436–443.

Hare, R. D. (1991). The Hare Psychopathy Checklist-Revised Manual. North Tonawanda, New York: Multi-Health Systems.

Hare, R. D. (1993). *Without conscience: The disturbing world of the psychopaths among us.* New York: Pocket Books.

Hare, R. D., Hart, S. D., & Harpur, T. J. (1991). Psychopathy and the DSM-IV criteria for antisocial personality disorder. *Journal of Abnormal Psychology, 100,* 391–398.

Harpur, T. J., Hart, S. D., & Hare, R. D. (2002). Personality of the psychopath. In P. T. Costa, Jr., & T. A. Widiger, (Eds.), *Personality disorders and the five factor model of personality* (2nd ed.). Washington, DC: American Psychological Association.

Hart, S., & Hare, R. (1994). Psychopathy and the Big Five: Correlations between observers' ratings of normal and pathological personality. *Journal of Personality Disorders, 8,* 32–40.

Hefferman, K., & Cloitre, M. (2000). A comparison of posttraumatic stress disorder with and without borderline personality disorder among women with a history of childhood sexual abuse: Etiological and clinical characteristics. *Journal of Nervous and Mental Disorder, 188*, 589–595.

Hyer, L., Brawell, L., Albrecht, B., Boyd, S., Boudewyns, P., & Talbert, S. (1994). Relationship of NEO-PI to personality styles and severity of trauma in chronic PTSD victims. *Journal of Clinical Psychology, 50*, 699–707.

John, O. P., & Srivastava, S. (1999). The Big Five trait taxonomy: History, measurement, and theoretical perspectives. In L. A. Pervin & O. P. John (Eds.), *Handbook of personality: Theory and research* (pp. 102–138). New York: Guilford Press.

Johnson, J. G., Cohen, P., Brown, J., Smalles, E. M., & Bernstein, D. P. (1999). Childhood maltreatment increases risk for personality disorders during early adulthood. *American Journal of Psychiatry, 56*, 600–606.

Kalus, O., Bernstein, D. P., & Siever, L. J. (1993). Schizoid personality disorder: A review of current status and implications for DSM-IV. *Journal of Personality Disorders, 7*, 43–52.

Kessler, R. C., McGonagle, K. A., Zhao S., Nelson, C. B., Hughes, M., & Muiphy, C. (1994). Lifetime and 12-month prevalence of DSM-III-R psychiatric disorders in the United States: Results from the national comorbidity survey. *Archives of General Psychiatry, 51*, 8–19.

Klein, D. N., Riso, L. P., Donaldson, S. K., Schwartz, J. E., Anderson, R. L., Oiumette, P. C., Lizardi, H., & Aronson, T. A. (1995). Family study of early-onset dysthymia: Mood and personality disorders in a relatives of outpatients with dysthymia and episodic major depressive and normal controls. *Archives of General Psychiatry, 52*, 487–496.

Kochanska, G., & Murray, K. T. (2000). Mother-child responsive orientation and conscience development: From toddler to early school age. *Child Development, 71*, 417–431.

Lenzenweger, M. F., Loranger, A. W., Korfine, L., & Neff, C. (1997). Detecting personality disorders in a nonclinical population. *Archives of General Psychiatry, 54*, 345–351.

Lilienfeld, S. O. (1994). Conceptual problems in the assessment of psychopathy. *Clinical Psychology Review, 14*, 17–38.

Lilienfeld, S. O., & Hess, T. H. (2001). Psychopathic personality traits and somatization: Sex differences and the mediating role of negative emotionality. *Journal of Psychopathology and Behavioral Assessment, 23*, 11–24.

Lilienfeld, S. O., Waldman, I. D., & Israel, A. C. (1994). A critical examination of the use of the term "comorbidity" in psychopathology research. *Clinical Psychology: Science and Practice, 1*, 71–83.

Linehan, M. M. (1993). Cognitive-behavioral treatment of borderline personality disorder. New York: Guilford Press.

Links, P. S., Heslegrave, R., & van Reekum, R. (1998). Prospective follow-up study of borderline personality disorder: Prognosis, prediction of outcome, and Axis II comorbidity. *Canadian Journal of Psychiatry, 43*, 265–270.

Livesley, W. J. (1998). Suggestions for a framework for an empirically based classification of personality disorder. *Canadian Journal of Psychiatry, 43*, 137–147.

Lykken, D. T. (1957). A study of anxiety in the sociopathic personality. *Journal of Abnormal and Clinical Psychology, 55*, 6–10.

Lynam, D. R. (2002). Psychopathy from the perspective of the five-factor model of personality. In P. T. Costa, Jr. & T. A. Widiger (Eds.), *Personality disorders and the five-factor model of personality* (pp. 325–348). Washington, DC: American Psychological Association.

Lynam, D. R., & Widiger, T. A. (2001). Using the five-factor model to represent the personality disorders. *Journal of Abnormal Psychology, 110*, 401–412.

Maier, W., Lichtermann, D., Klinger, T., & Heun, R. (1992). Prevalences of personality disorders (DSM-III-R) in the community. *Journal of Personality Disorders, 6*, 187–196.

Markovitz, P. (2001). Pharmacotherapy. In W. J. Livesley (Ed.), *Handbook of personality disorders* (pp. 475–493). New York: Guilford Press.

Mattia, J. I. & Zimmerman, M. (2001). Epidemiology. In W. J. Livesley (Ed.), *Handbook of personality disorders* (pp. 107–123). New York: Guilford.

McCrae, R. R., & Costa, P. T., Jr. (1987). Validation of the five-factor model of personality across instruments and observers. *Journal of Personality and Social Psychology, 52*, 81–90.

Miller, J. D., Lynam, D. R., Widiger, T. A., & Leukefeld, C. (2001). Personality disorders as extreme variants of common personality dimensions: Can the five-factor model adequately represent psychopathy? *Journal of Personality, 69*, 253–276.

Miller, M. B., Useda, J. D., Trull, T. J., Burr, R. M., & Minks-Brown, C. (2001). Paranoid, schizoid, and schizotypal personality disorders. In H. E. Adams & P. B. Sutker (Eds.), *Comprehensive handbook of psychopathology* (3rd ed., pp. 535–558). New York: Plenum.

Moldin, S. O., Rice, J. P., Erlenmeyer-Kimling, L., & Squires-Wheeler, E. (1994). Latent structure of DSM-III-R Axis II psychopathology in a normal sample. *Journal of Abnormal Psychology, 103*, 259–266.

Morey, L. C., & Zanarini, M. C. (2000). Borderline personality: Traits and disorder. *Journal of Abnormal Psychology, 109*, 733–737.

Myers, M. G., Stewart, D. G., & Brown, S. A. (1998). Progression from conduct disorder to antisocial personality following treatment for adolescent substance abuse. *American Journal of Psychiatry, 155*, 479–485.

Newman, J. P., Patterson, C., Howland, E., & Nichols, S. (1990). Passive avoidance in psychopaths: The effects of reward. *Personality and Individual Differences, 11*, 1101–1114.

Nigg, J. T., & Goldsmith, H. H. (1994). Genetics of personality disorders: Perspectives from personality and psychopathology research. *Psychological Bulletin, 115*, 346–380.

Oldham, J. M., & Skodol, A. E. (2000). Charting the future of Axis II. *Journal of Personality Disorders, 14*, 17–29.

Oldham, J. M., Skodol, A. E., Kellman, H. D., Hyler, S. E., Rosnick, L., & Davies, M. (1992). Diagnosis of DSM-III-R personality disorders by two semistructured interviews: Patterns of comorbidity. *American Journal of Psychiatry, 149*, 213–220.

O'Neill, F. A., & Kendler, K. S. (1998). Longitudinal study of interpersonal dependency in female twins. *British Journal of Psychiatry, 172*, 154–158.

Ornduff, S. R. (2000). Childhood maltreatment and malevolence: Quantitative research findings. *Clinical Psychology Review, 20*, 991–1018.

Overholser, J. C. (1996). The dependent personality and interpersonal problems. *Journal of Nervous and Mental Disorder, 184*, 8–16.

Patrick, C. J., Bradley, M. M., & Lang, P. J. (1993). Emotion in the criminal psychopath: Startle reflex modulation. *Journal of Abnormal Psychology, 102*, 82–92.

Patterson, M. C., & Newman, J. P. (1993). Reflectivity and learning from aversive events: Toward a psychological mechanism for the syndromes of disinhibition. *Psychological Review, 100*, 716–736.

Perry, J. C., Banon, E., & Ianni, F. (1999). Effectiveness of psychotherapy for personality disorders. *American Journal of Psychiatry, 156*, 1312–1321.

Pfohl, B., Blum, N., & Zimmerman, M. (1997). *Structured interview for DSM–IV personality*. Washington, DC: American Psychiatric Press.

Pincus, A. L., & Wilson, K. R. (2001). Interpersonal variability in dependent personality. *Journal of Personality, 69*, 223–252.

Plomin, R., & Caspi, A. (1999). Behavioral genetics and personality. In L. Pervin & O. John (Eds.), *Handbook of personality* (2nd ed., pp. 251–276). New York: Guilford Press.

Raine, A., Lencz, T., Mednick, S. A. (Eds.) (1995). *Schizotypal personality*. New York: Cambridge University Press.

Raine, A., Reynolds, C., Venables, P. H., Mednick, S. A., & Farrington, D. P. (1998). Fearlessness, stimulus-seeking, and large body size at age 3 as early predispositions to childhood aggression at age 11 years. *Archives of General Psychiatry, 55*, 745–751.

Robins, C. J., Hayes, A. H., Block, P., Kramer, R. J., & Villena, M. (1995). Interpersonal and achievement concerns and the depressive vulnerability and symptom specificity hypothesis: A prospective study. *Cognitive Therapy and Research, 19*, 1–20.

Robins, L. N., Tipp, J., & Przybeck, T. (1991). Antisocial personality. In L. N. Robins & D. A. Regier (Eds.), *Psychiatric disorders in America* (pp. 258–290). New York: Free Press.

Rogers, R., & Bagby, R. M. (1994). Dimensions of psychopathy: A factor analytic study of the MMPI Antisocial Personality Disorder scale. *International Journal of Offender Therapy and Comparative Criminology, 38*, 297–308.

Rothbart, M. K., & Ahadi, S. A. (1994). Temperament and the development of personality. *Journal of Abnormal Psychology, 103*, 55–66.

Salekin, R. T. (2002). Psychopathy and therapeutic pessimism: Clinical lore or clinical reality? *Clinical Psychology Review, 22*, 79–112.

Samuels J., Eaton, W. W., Bienvenu, O. J. Brown, C. H., Costa, P. T., & Nestadt, G. (2002). Prevalence and correlates of personality disorders in a community sample. *British Journal of Psychiatry, 180*, 536–542.

Samuels, J. F., Nestadt, G., & Romanoski, A. J. (1994). DSM-III personality disorders in the community. *American Journal of Psychiatry, 151*, 1055–1062.

Sanderson, C. J., Swenson, C. & Bohus, S. (2002). A critique of the American Psychiatric Practice guidelines for the treatment of patients with borderline personality disorder. *Journal of Personality Disorders, 16*, 122–129.

Sanislow, C. A., & McGlashan, T. H. (1998). Treatment outcome of personality disorders. *Canadian Journal of Psychiatry, 43*, 237–250.

Schmidt, L. A., Polak, C. P., & Spooner, A. L. (2001). Biological and environmental contributions to childhood shyness: A diathesis-stress model. In W. R. Crozier & L. E. Alden, (Eds.), *International handbook of social anxiety: Concepts, research, and interventions relating to the self and shyness* (pp. 29–51). New York: Wiley.

Sher, K. J., & Trull, T. J. (1994). Personality and disinhibitory psychopathology: Alcoholism and antisocial personality disorder. *Journal of Abnormal Psychology, 103*, 92–102.

Siever, L. J., & Davis, K. L. (1991). A psychobiological perspective on the personality disorders. *American Journal of Psychiatry, 148*, 1647–1658.

Silk, K. R. (2000). Borderline personality disorder: Overview of biologic factors. *Psychiatric Clinics of North America*, *23*, 61–75.

Soldz, S., Budman, S., Demby, A., & Merry, J. (1993). Representation of personality disorders in circumplex and five-factor space: Explorations with a clinical sample. *Psychological Assessment, 5*, 41–52.

Stoff, D. M., Breiling, J., & Maser, J. D. (Eds.) (1997). *Handbook of antisocial behavior*. New York: Wiley.

Stone, M. H. (1993). Abnormalities of personality: Within and beyond the realm of treatment. New York: W. W. Norton.

Stone, M. H. (2001). Natural history and long-term outcome. In W. J. Livesley (Ed.), *Handbook of personality disorders* (pp. 259–273). New York: Guilford Press.

Sutker, P. B., & Allain, A. N. (2001). Antisocial personality disorder. In P. B. Sutker & H. E. Adams (Eds.), *Comprehensive textbook of psychopathology* (3rd ed., pp. 445–490). New York: Plenum.

Thompson, S., & Zuroff, D. C. (1998). Dependent and self-critical mothers' responses to adolescent autonomy and competence. *Personality and Individual Differences, 24*, 311–324.

Tillfors, M., Furmark, T., Ekselius, L., & Fredrikson, M. (2001). Social phobia and avoidant personality disorder as related to parental history of social anxiety: A general population study. *Behavioral Research and Therapy, 39*, 289–298.

Torgesen, S. (2000). Genetics of patients with borderline personality disorder. *Psychiatric Clinics of North America*, *23*, 1–9.

Torgesen, S., Kringlen, E., & Cramer, V. (2001). The prevalence of personality disorders in a community sample. *Archives of General Psychiatry, 58*, 590–596.

Trapnell, P. D., & Wiggins, J. S. (1990). Extension of the Interpersonal Adjective Scales to include the Big Five dimensions of personality. *Journal of Personality and Social Psychology, 59*, 781–790.

Trull, T. J. (1992). DSM-III-R personality disorders and the five-factor model of personality: An empirical comparison. *Journal of Abnormal Psychology, 101*, 553–560.

Trull, T. J., Widiger, T. A., & Burr, R. (2001). A structured interview for the assessment of the five-factor model of personality:2. Facet-level relations to the Axis II personality disorders. *Journal of Personality, 69*, 175–198.

Trull, T. J., Widiger, T. A., Lynam, D. R., & Costa, P. T. (2003). Borderline personality disorder from the perspective of general personality functioning. *Journal of Abnormal Psychology, 112*, 193–202.

Trull, T. J., Widiger, T. A., Useda, J. D., Holcomb, J., Doan, B-T, Axelrod, S. R., Stern, B. L., & Gershuny, B. S. (1998). A structured interview for the assessment of the five-factor model of personality. *Psychological Assessment, 10*, 229–240.

van Velzen, C. J., Emmelkamp, P. M., & Scholing, A. (2000). Generalized social phobia versus avoidant personality disorder: Differences in psychopathology, personality traits, and social and occupational functioning. *Journal of Anxiety Disorders, 14*, 395–411.

Watson, D., & Clark, L. A. (1997). Extraversion and its positive emotional core. In R. Hogan, J. Johnson, & S. Briggs (Eds.), *Handbook of personality psychology* (pp. 767–793). New York: Academic Press.

Watson, D., & Tellegen, A. (1985). Toward a consensual structure of mood. *Psychological Bulletin, 98*, 219–235.

West, K. Y. (1993). Schizotypal personality disorder: The placement of cognitive and perceptual aberrations within the five-factor model. Unpublished master's thesis. University of Kentucty, Lexington, Ky.

Widiger, T. A. (1998). Sex biases in the diagnosis of personality disorders. *Journal of Personality Disorders, 12*, 95–118.

Widiger, T. A. (2000). Personality disorders in the 21st century. *Journal of Personality Disorders, 14*, 3–16.

Widiger, T. A. (2001). Social anxiety, social phobia, and avoidant personality disorder. In W. R. Crozier & L. E. Alden (Eds.), *International handbook of social anxiety* (pp. 335–356). New York: Wiley.

Widiger, T. A., Cadoret, R., Hare, R., Robins, L., Rutherford, M., Zanarini, M., Alterman, A., Apple, M., Corbitt, E., Forth, A., Hart S., Kultermann, J., Woody, G., & Frances, A. (1996). DSM-IV antisocial personality disorder field trial. *Journal of Abnormal Psychology, 105*, 3–16.

Widiger, T. A., & Coker, L. A. (2001). Assessing personality disorders. In J. N. Butcher (Ed.), *Clinical personality assessment: Practical approaches* (2nd ed., pp. 407–434). New York: Oxford University Press.

Widiger, T. A., & Corbitt, E. M. (1995). Antisocial personality disorder in DSM-IV. In W. J. Livesley (Ed.), *The DSM-IV personality disorders* (pp. 103–126). New York: Guilford Press.

Widiger, T. A., & Costa, P. T., Jr. (2002). FFM personality disorder research. In P. T. Costa, Jr. & T. A. Widiger (Eds.), *Personality disorders and the five-factor model of personality* (pp. 59–87). Washington, DC: American Psychological Association.

Widiger, T. A., Frances, A. J., Spitzer, R. L. (1988). The DSM-III-R personality disorders: An overview. *American Journal of Psychiatry, 145*, 786–795.

Widiger, T. A. & Lynam, D. R. (1998). Psychopathy from the perspective of the five-factor model of personality. In T. Millon, E. Simonson, M. Birket-Smith, & R. D. Davis (Eds.), *Psychopathy: Antisocial, criminal, and violent behaviors* (pp. 171–187). New York: Guilford Press.

Widiger, T. A., & Trull, T. J. (1998). Performance characteristics of the DSM-III-R personality disorder criteria sets. In T. A. Widiger, A. J. Frances, H. A. Pincus, R. Ross, M. B. First, W. W. Davis, & M. Klein (Eds.), *DSM-IV sourcebook* (Vol. 4, pp. 357–373). Washington, DC: American Psychiatric Association.

Widiger, T. A., Trull, T. J., Clarkin, J. F., Sanderson, C., & Costa, P. T., Jr. (1994/2002). A description of the DSM-IV personality disorders with the five-factor model of personality. In P. T. Costa, Jr. & T. A. Widiger (Eds.), *Personality disorders and the five-factor model of personality* (pp. 89–99). Washington, DC: American Psychological Association.

Widiger, T. A., Verheul, R., & van den Brink, W. (1999). Personality and psychopathology. In L. Pervin & O. John (Eds.), *Handbook of personality* (2nd ed., pp. 347–366). New York: Guilford Press.

Wiggins, J. S., & Pincus, A. L. (1989). Personality: Structure and assessment. *Annual Review of Psychology, 43,* 473–504.

Wilberg, T., Urnes, O., Friis, S., Pederson, G., & Karterud, S. (1999). Borderline and avoidant personality disorders and the five-factor model of personality: A comparison between DSM-IV diagnoses and NEO-PI-R. *Journal of Personality Disorders, 13,* 226–240.

World Health Organization (1992). The ICD-10 Classification of mental and behavioural disorders: Clinical descriptions and diagnostic guidelines. Geneva, Switzerland: World Health Organization.

Yeung, A. S., Lyons, M. J., Waternaux, C. M., Faraone, S. V., & Tsuang, M. T. (1993). The relationship between DSM-III personality disorders and the five-factor model of personality. *Comprehensive Psychiatry, 34,* 227–234.

Zanarini, M. C. (2000). Childhood experiences associated with the development of borderline personality disorder. *Psychiatric Clinics of North America, 23,* 89–101.

Zanarini, M. C., Frankenburg, F. R., Dubo, E. D., Sickel, A. E., Trikha, A., Levin, A., & Reynolds, V. (1998a). Axis I comorbidity of borderine personality disorder. *American Journal of Psychiatry, 155,* 1733–1739.

Zanarini, M. C., Frankenburg, F. R., Dubo, E. D., Sickel, A. E., Trikha, A., Levin, A., & Reynolds, V. (1998b). Axis II comorbidity of borderine personality disorder. *Comprehensive Psychiatry, 39,* 296–302.

Zanarini, M. C., Gunderson, J. G., Frankenburg, F. R., and Chauncey, D. L. (1989). The Revised Diagnostic Interview for Borderlines: Discriminating BPD from other Axis II disorders. *Journal of Personality Disorders, 3,* 10–18.

Zimmerman, M. & Mattia, J. I. (1999). Differences between clinical and research practices in diagnosing borderline personality disorder. *American Journal of Psychiatry, 156,* 1570–1574.

11

Eating Disorders

Janet Polivy
C. Peter Herman
Michele Boivin
University of Toronto

Until the 1960s and 70s, few people had heard of anorexia nervosa (AN), but it soon began to be reported with increasing frequency in western societies. Young females from middle- and upper-class families were voluntarily starving themselves and losing weight to the point of emaciation and sometimes death. A decade later, a new eating disorder was recognized; in bulimia nervosa (BN),[1] young women alternate between starving and eating prodigious amounts of food, often followed by purging. Although these eating disorders have flourished recently in Westernized societies during periods of relative affluence and enhanced social opportunities for women (Bemporad, 1996; 1997), voluntary self-starvation and periods of binge eating and purging have been reported throughout history. Eating disorders that would be recognizable today as anorexia nervosa and bulimia nervosa have existed since ancient times (Bemporad, 1997). Eating disorder not otherwise specified (or EDNOS, which will not be discussed in this chapter, as it is not a clear diagnostic category) and binge eating disorder (BED) were added in the recent version of the *Diagnostic and Statistical Manual of Mental Disorders*, or DSM–IV [American Psychiatric Association (APA), 1994].

Whether the various eating disorders are fundamentally different is debatable (see e.g., Joiner, Vohs, & Heatherton, 2000); core symptoms (e.g., preoccupation with food, disturbed body perception, and inadequate sexual behavior) do not differ between AN and BN patients. Bulimic eating disorders appear to exist on a continuum of clinical severity, from BED (least severe), through nonpurging-type BN (intermediate severity), to purging-type BN (most severe) (Hay & Fairburn, 1998). The spectrum hypothesis considers all eating disorders as different manifestations of a single disorder or syndrome (VanderHam, Meulman, VanStrien, & vanEngeland, 1997). In this chapter, we will discuss the major eating disorders, using the DSM to describe the primary features of AN, BN, and the newer BED (about which substantially less is known). We will then review the prevalence and prognosis of eating disorders and provide an overview of the main hypotheses concerning what causes them to occur in a given individual. Finally, we will discuss the principal treatments for eating disorders.

---

[1]Bulimia comes from the Greek word *bulimos* meaning "ox hunger." Bulimics thus act as if they are "as hungry as an ox."

DIAGNOSTIC CRITERIA AND CORE PATHOLOGICAL FEATURES OF EATING DISORDERS

The DSM–IV-TR (APA, 2000) is the most widely accepted set of criteria for psychological/ psychiatric disorders in North America. The symptoms of eating disorders were compiled by a panel of experts who treat these problems, and the symptoms were then sent to others in the field for comments and corrections. In this version of the DSM, all symptoms are supposed to be empirically supported and to reflect a consensus among those who treat and study the disorders. For eating disorders, this is a difficult proposition, as we shall see. Not all criteria for the disorder are easy to define (for example, exactly what behaviors constitute binge eating?); the criteria as listed have some ambiguities. Moreover, there are controversies concerning just how universal some symptoms are (e.g., amenorrhea). Finally, many psychologists object to the medicalization of abnormal behavior implied by a diagnosis. Despite these debates about the utility of the DSM, many researchers use the DSM criteria for eating disorders to facilitate communication across research settings, to ennsure that all are studying the same phenomena. For clinicians treating the problems, diagnostic criteria can point to symptoms that need to be treated and methods of treating them, and also can allow for assessment of successful change. For these reasons, we will use the criteria for eating disorders as set out in the DSM, but we will point out where these criteria have been questioned.

The DSM–IV diagnostic criteria for AN are refusal to maintain body weight at or above a minimum of 85% of normal weight for age and height, accompanied by an intense fear of fatness, disturbed experience of one's body weight or shape, and amenorrhea (for at least three consecutive menstrual cycles). In addition, bulimic-type anorexia includes regular episodes of binge eating or purging, but restrictor-type anorexia entails only starving (and both types may involve compulsive exercising). Although amenorrhoea has been an important criterion for AN for some time, women with AN and women with all the features of AN except amenorrhoea are otherwise indistinguishable, leading some to question the utility of amenorrhoea as a diagnostic criterion (Cachelin & Maher, 1998; Garfinkel et al., 1996).

Usually, the early (preadolescent) onset of an eating disorder predicts a better outcome. Extremely early onset of AN seems to occur more frequently in boys than in girls. There is a risk of permanent side effects, such as short stature, if those with early-onset AN experience lengthy or chronic malnutrition (Theander, 1996).

The DSM–IV describes BN as recurrent episodes of binge eating (i.e., eating more food than most people would eat in a similar time period and situation and feeling out of control of one's eating during the episode) accompanied by compensatory behaviors (such as purging, exercising, or fasting) to prevent a corresponding weight gain. These behaviors must occur at least twice a week for at least 3 months. Also, the individual's self-evaluation relies excessively on body weight and shape. If any of these symptoms occur in the context of an episode of AN, then AN becomes the primary diagnosis. The purging type of BN features self-induced vomiting or laxative, diuretic, or enema abuse; nonpurging BN involves fasting, exercising, or other (nonpurging) means of compensating for binge eating (APA, 1994). Impulsive behaviors such as sexual promiscuity, suicide attempts, drug abuse, and stealing or shoplifting are common among people with BN (e.g., Goldner, Geller, Birmingham, & Remick, 2000; Matsunaga, Kiriike et al., 2000).

Both AN and BN often emerge during late adolescence, with a female-to-male ratio between 10:1 and 15:1 (Bramon-Bosch, Troop, & Treasure, 2000; Braun, Sunday, Huang, & Halmi, 1999). Although the disorders are more prevalent in females, the nature of the disorders is the same in the two sexes. For individuals with eating disorder, a negative body image and a variety of psychological problems appear to emerge during puberty (see e.g., Polivy &

Herman, 2002, for a review). Even before the onset of their disorder, adolescents with BN report various problems such as weight-related concerns, attitudes of withdrawal and social isolation, and deterioration of body-image, self-image, and relationships with siblings and peers. The prevalence of these problems among adolescents with BN suggests that early psychological distress may precede the onset of an eating disorder (Corcos et al., 2000).

Binge eating disorder (BED) is described by DSM–IV (in the research appendix) as similar to BN in that it entails recurrent binge eating episodes accompanied by subjective feelings of lack of control over one's eating. The difference between BN and BED is that the purging and compensatory behaviors that occur regularly in BN are infrequent in BED (APA, 1994). The binge eating typically begins in late adolescence or the early 20s and frequently follows dieting and weight loss. Typically, individuals with BED are overweight and do not exhibit the chronic weight and shape concerns that characterize people with AN and BN. Eating disorder not otherwise specified (EDNOS) is a catchall category for syndromes that do not quite fit the diagnostic criteria for the other eating disorders (e.g., binge eating occurring with some regularity, but less than twice a week) (APA, 1994).

Despite the primacy of binge eating as a diagnostic feature of BN, BED, and bulimic-type AN, attempts to define binge eating have been unsatisfactory, and there is considerable variability in what sorts of eating episodes individuals label as binges (Johnson, Carr-Nangle, Nangle, Antony, & Zayfert, 1997). What, for instance, is a larger than normal amount of food? Commonly noted triggers for binge eating include negative affect or stress, the presence of attractive fattening food, abstinence violation (i.e., having already eaten something fattening or diet-breaking), ingestion of alcohol, and being alone (Polivy & Herman, 1993). Examination of videotaped eating episodes indicates that feelings of loss of control and violation of dietary strictures are critical in leading people to construe a particular episode as a binge (Johnson, Boutelle, Torgrud, Davig, & Turner, 2000). Laxative abuse among women with eating disorders is an indicator of greater psychopathology, irrespective of other features such as eating disorder diagnostic category, age, body weight, impulsive behaviors, or personality features (Pryor, Wiederman, & McGilley, 1996).

INCIDENCE AND PREVALENCE OF EATING DISORDERS

Since the 1950s, the incidence of AN in females aged 15 to 24 has increased markedly; it is currently estimated at 8.1 per 100,000 population per year (or .008%, with BN even higher at 11.4 per 100,000, or .011%) (Hoek, 1993), and some estimate that the number is as high as 19.2 (or .019%) (Rooney, McClelland, Crisp & Sedgwick, 1995). Of course, this increase may represent a combination of a true increase in incidence as well as increased recognition of cases that formerly would not have been acknowledged (Wakeling, 1996). Nevertheless, these incidence figures may well be significant underestimates; the disorders still often escape detection or diagnosis (Rooney et al., 1995) because dieting and the pursuit of thinness are so ubiquitous and socially acceptable in western culture. Indeed, more recent studies find incidence rates as high as 300 per 100,000 (.30%) for females and 20 per 100,000 (.02%) for males (Striegel-Moore, Garvin, Dohm, & Rosenheck, 1999). In a recent national study, 5% of the 700 women sampled reported binge eating within the past 30 days, 29% reported intense dieting or fasting in the past 3 months, 43% claimed that their weight and shape were very important or more important than anything else, and 1.5% of the women met criteria for nonpurging BN (Vogeltanz-Holm et al., 2000). Some of these reports, however, may be unreliable because of changes in diagnostic and referral practices (Fombonne, 1996). Changing diagnostic and referral practices make it virtually impossible to know the true rate of increase in the incidence of eating disorders. More ominously, however, the prevalence of partial or subclinical eating disorders is at least twice that of full-syndrome eating disorders (Shisslak, Crago, & Estes, 1995). Longitudinal studies also provide evidence of progression from less to more severe disturbances in eating behavior in a small number of individuals; some normal dieters become pathological dieters, who in turn progress to partial- or full-syndrome eating disorders (Shisslak et al., 1995). Of course, we do not claim that this is the normal course of events; but some evidence suggests that eating disorders often begin with the normal dieting found in a majority of young females (Polivy & Herman, 1987).

CONCOMITANT PSYCHOLOGICAL PROBLEMS

People with eating disorders often engage in obsessive-compulsive behaviors such as calorie counting, body preoccupation, ruminations about food, ritualism, perfectionism, and meticulousness (Kaye, 1997). The lifetime prevalence of obsessive-compulsive disorder has been estimated to be 30% among people with eating disorders (e.g., Hudson, Pope, & Jonas, 1983) but only 2.5% to 3% among the general population. Obsessive-compulsive disorders are three times more common among people with AN than among people with BN (Hudson et al., 1983).

Several other disorders are frequently found in conjunction with eating disorders. Alcohol abuse is commonly found in BN, and anxiety disorders and depression are prevalent in both AN and BN (e.g., Dansky, Brewerton, & Kilpatrick, 2000; Hudson et al., 1983). A follow-up of a large sample of AN patients found that 10 years later, 51% still met criteria for an Axis I psychiatric disorder (especially anxiety disorder), and 23% met the criteria for a personality disorder (most often avoidant-dependent and obsessive-compulsive) (Herpertz-Dahlman et al., 2001). Depression is also frequently observed among people with eating disorders (Hudson et al., 1983).

Axis II personality disorders are frequently observed among people with eating disorders (e.g., Wilfley et al., 2000; Wonderlich, 1995; Wonderlich & Mitchell, 2001). Obsessive-compulsive personality disorder, like obsessive-compulsive disorder, is common in AN. Disorders related to impulsive personality, as well as borderline personality disorders, are more often present in BN and BED (e.g., Wonderlich & Mitchell, 2001). Because malnutrition can exaggerate symptoms of personality disorders, Matsunaga, Kaye, and colleagues (2000) studied individuals who had recovered from eating disorders for at least a year to be certain that the measurement of personality disorders was not distorted by malnutrition and eating disorder symptomatology. They found that 25% of their participants met the criteria for at least one personality disorder.

PROGNOSIS FOR EATING DISORDERS

Eating disorders are serious problems. Mortality-rate estimates range from just over 5% (Casper & Jabine, 1996; Herzog, Greenwood, Dorer et al., 2000; Sullivan, 1995) to 8.3% (Steinhausen, Seidel, & Metzke, 2000). Nevertheless, approximately 50% to 60% of patients have a good outcome, with significant reduction of symptoms 5 years after beginning treatment (Casper & Jabine, 1996; Herpertz-Dahlman et al., 2001; Steinhausen et al., 2000). Unfortunately, about one-third of patients continue to meet diagnostic criteria 5 years or more after initial treatment (Fairburn, Cooper, Doll, Norman, & OConnor, 2000; Keel, Mitchell, Miller, Davis, & Crow, 1999). A history of substance-use problems and a longer duration of the disorder at presentation are predictors of worse outcome (Keel et al., 1999). The long-term prognosis for bulimics is generally poor, with about one-third of those assessed remitting each year, but another one-third relapsing each year over 5 years; those with BED are likely to improve on their own, with only 18% still meeting diagnostic criteria after 5 years (Fairburn et al., 2000).

CAUSAL THEORIES OF EATING DISORDERS

Eating disorders are not uniform conditions; there is no single cause or even invariable symptom. The DSM definition (using words such as "refusal" to maintain one's weight, and "fear of fatness") strongly implies that eating disorders have a psychological foundation, though biological/genetic formulations have been offered. Hilde Bruch, one of the first modern theorists to discuss eating disorders, described AN as "a complex condition determined by many simultaneously interacting factors" (1975, p. 159). She was the first to point out that these patients use eating to fulfill a variety of nonnutritional needs. Moreover, despite the characteristic preoccupation with food and eating accompanying eating disorders, patients are "unable to recognize hunger or distinguish it from other states of bodily tension or emotional arousal" (p. 160). Bruch posited that patients interpret all tension states as a "need to eat" instead of identifying the correct source (Bruch, 1975).

Fairburn (e.g., Fairburn, Welch, Doll, Davies, & OConnor, 1997) hypothesizes that there are two broad classes of risk factors for eating disorders: those enhancing the general risk for psychiatric disorder and those that specifically increase the risk for dieting and eating problems. With respect to exposure to most potential risk factors, BN patients resemble patients with other psychiatric disorders more than they resemble people without diagnosable psychological problems. BN patients, however, show a distinctive pattern of exposure to factors likely to elevate the risk of dieting and negative self-evaluation, supporting the hypothesis that BN is the result of exposure to both general risk factors for psychiatric disorder and specific risk factors for dieting.

The addiction model (Davis & Claridge, 1998; Wilson, 1991) posits an addictive process operating in eating disorders. Conditioned physiological responses to food produce anticipatory secretion of insulin (Booth, 1988; Woods & Brief, 1988), which causes both craving and overeating (if only through increased tolerance to food (e.g., Booth, 1988; Wilson, 1991; Woods & Brief, 1988)). Some argue that self-starvation accompanied by excessive exercising reflects an addiction to the body's endogenous opioids (Davis & Claridge, 1998), citing both high scores by AN and BN patients on the Addiction Scale of the Eysenck Personality Questionnaire and correlations between the addiction scale and, weight preoccupation and excessive exercising. Wilson, however, dismisses the addiction model for three reasons. First, evidence for an addictive personality is lacking. Second, the model does not address the core clinical characteristics of eating disorders (e.g., the role of dietary restraint and abnormal attitudes about the importance of body shape) or the identified concomitant psychopathology (e.g., extremely low self-esteem, interpersonal distrust, and feelings of ineffectiveness). Third, it fails to account for psychobiological connections between dieting and eating disorders. Wilson notes that bulimic behavior does not meet the criteria for an addictive disorder (i.e., tolerance, physical dependence, or craving), and therefore he sees the addiction model as a conceptual dead end (Wilson, 1991).

Cognitive theories of eating disorders emphasize the biases in people's beliefs, expectancies, and information processing pertaining to body size and eating. Some research has supported predictions derived from these cognitive theories (Williamson, Muller, Reas, & Thaw, 1999). As we shall discuss later, these theories dominate current treatment strategies. Information-processing biases, such as a focus on food and weight to the exclusion of other information, may explain several psychopathological features of AN and BN, including denial, resistance to treatment, and misinterpretation of therapeutic interventions.

Personality factors are also thought to contribute to susceptibility to eating disorders. Some assessment instruments such 'as the Eating Disorders Inventory (EDI; Garner, Olmsted, & Polivy, 1983) were specifically designed to measure underlying personality dispositions theoretically linked to eating disorders. Investigations using this scale have found that personality factors such as perfectionism, feelings of ineffectiveness (or low self-esteem), reduced interoceptive awareness (or sensitivity to internal signals such as hunger and satiety), and interpersonal distrust are characteristic of those with eating disorders (e.g., Garner, Olmsted, Polivy, & Garfinkel, 1984; Leon, Fulkerson, Perry, & Early-Zald, 1995). Strober (1980) found evidence of obsessive personality traits, extraversion, and need for social approval before the development of the disorder in anorexic adolescents who had returned to normal weight.

A recent investigation took the innovative step of simply asking the patients what caused the emergence of their eating disorder (Nevonen & Broberg, 2000). Interpersonal and weight-related problems were the most commonly reported causes, and dieting or dieting plus purging was the most commonly reported response to these stresses. Thus, interpersonal and weight-related distress, together with dieting behavior, are what people see as responsible for the emergence of their eating disorders. Self-report—in response to oral or written questions—is one of the main sources of data in research on eating disorders; unfortunately, self-report is notoriously unreliable (Nisbett & Wilson, 1977). Eating disorder researchers by and large are too eager to take patients' self-descriptions at face value, if only because such descriptions are easy to elicit. It is not likely that people with eating disorders would be able to identify the source of their disorder with such ease when the research of several decades has not been able to do so. A full understanding of the causes of eating disorders will require more work and more sophisticated research designs than are currently being used.

Sociocultural models suggest that the idealization of thinness and unremitting portrayals of slim role models in the media contribute to widespread body dissatisfaction, which in some susceptible individuals produces pathological dieting and ultimately eating disorders (see e.g., Heatherton & Polivy, 1992; Stice, 2001; Striegel-Moore, 1993). Some research (Mills, Polivy, Herman, & Tiggemann, 2002) suggests that exposure to idealized models may promote dieting not by causing body dissatisfaction but rather by inspiring young women to work toward a fantasized, thinner future self. The sociobiological position posits that eating disorders and the societal pursuit of thinness reflect sexual competition among women (Abed, 1998). Thinness may either enhance women's reproductive prospects by making them more attractive to males or, in a contrary version, delay reproduction (by impairing fertility through emaciation) until a more propitious time.

Speculation about the cause(s) of eating disorders has thus gone through many phases over the last three decades, variously favoring biological, familial, and psychosocial factors, which are hypothesized to interact in complex ways to produce the disorders (Ward, Tiller, Treasure, & Russell, 2000). For at least the last decade, the biopsychosocial model, positing an interplay between the organism, its past behavior, and its environment (biological, psychological, and environmental variables) has been the primary explanatory model of eating disorders (e.g., Schlundt & Johnson, 1990). For example, in binge eating, environmental (e.g., situational influences, sociorelationship systems), behavioral (e.g., previous eating or dieting, ongoing activity), cognitive (e.g., knowledge of dieting, expectations, body image), emotional (e.g., mood, psychopathology), and physiological (e.g., blood levels of nutrients, hormones, neurochemicals) antecedents affect behaviors such as binge eating, purging, and dieting, which then themselves have consequences for behavior, cognition, emotion, and physiology.

RISK FACTORS FOR EATING DISORDERS

Current theories of eating disorders—what causes them, why they afflict women, and why there has been such an increase in recent times—thus range widely. The basic question of what goes wrong to produce AN and BN has been addressed at the broad level of sociocultural influences, at the narrow level of familial effects, and at the even narrower level of individual risk factors related to personality, cognition, or physiology (e.g., Leung, Geller, & Katzman, 1996; Polivy & Herman, 2002; Polivy, Herman, Mills, & Wheeler, 2003). One might expect that the research on specific risk factors would be derived from one or another of the causal theories, but such is not the case. The voluminous literature on risk factors is to a great extent independent of and uninformed by the causal theories outlined previously. Whereas some self-report questionnaires (such as the EDI) are based on theoretical models (such as Bruch, 1975), research on risk factors for eating disorders seems to be, for the most part, atheoretical. Many studies in this area merely report correlations among self-report inventories and make no attempt to tie the particular measures chosen to any particular theory of how eating disorders develop. In part, this situation no doubt reflects the difficulty of measuring preclinical pathological processes with paper-and-pencil self-report devices, as well as the problem of operationalizing theoretical constructs. Despite these drawbacks, literally thousands of studies have attempted to specify the risk factors for eating disorders, and numerous chapters and books have addressed these questions. It is crucial to remember, however, that the risk-factor approach is essentially correlational, and that risk factors are really just variables associated with eating disorders, usually in an unspecified fashion. While the reader would no doubt like us to provide an in-depth review of these risk factors here, space limitations permit only a brief overview of prominent research trends examining risk factors associated with eating disorders.

Sociocultural Factors

For several decades, an unrealistically thin body shape has been the cultural ideal for women in Western society. To attain this physique, women have become increasingly likely to diet and/or exercise (e.g., Polivy & Herman, 1987; Stice, 2001), but are unlikely to succeed in this quest. This societal obsession with a slim female body has been blamed for women's widespread dissatisfaction with their bodies and a concomitant rise in the prevalence of eating disorders (Stice, 2001). These sociocultural pressures have long been targeted as causes (or at least contributors) to eating disorders (e.g., Striegel-Moore, 1993). The chief promoters of this sociocultural pressure to be thin are the media, sex-role expectations, and particular economic, racial, and ethnic contexts.

Peer and Media Influences. To no one's surprise, it has been shown that adolescents watch more television, read more magazines, and in general appear to attend more to the media than any other age group, and are thus bombarded with messages about thinness and dieting (Polivy & Herman, 2002; Polivy et al., 2003). These messages are directed primarily at girls, who are presented with thin, attractive models, an insistence that thinness will bring success and happiness in all spheres of life (no matter how unrelated to appearance), and a blatant derogation of fat or even normal-weight physiques (Polivy & Herman, 2002; Polivy et al., 2003). Many studies have demonstrated an increase in depression and negative self-image in young women following exposure to thin media images (Pinhas, Toner, Ali, Garfinkel, & Stuckless, 1999), and those with greater eating disorder symptomatology tend to expose themselves to larger doses of these media images than do most women their age (Stice & Shaw, 1994).

Recent data, however, suggest that it would be premature to blame the media for the increase in eating disorder. Mills et al. (2002) found that looking at pictures of thin models actually made chronic dieters feel thinner and better about themselves, possibly by inspiring them to fantasize about emulating the models. This outcome should not be so surprising—after all, why would women voluntarily buy and read fashion magazines if looking at them induced depression and self-derogation? More important, eating disorders have been reliably documented for centuries, without the benefit of twentieth-century media exposure. Media idealization of an unrealistically thin female shape may be a contributor to the increased prevalence of eating disorder, but it is clearly not the primary cause. After all, this "cause" is so prevalent in our culture that if it were as important as is sometimes claimed, we would be hard-pressed to explain why fewer than 10% of young women have eating disorders.

Gender. "Why women?" and "Why now?" are the two most frequently asked questions about the recent increase in the prevalence of eating disorders (e.g., Polivy et al., 2003; Striegel-Moore, 1993). Around the time that eating disorders began to proliferate, the social role of women was undergoing drastic changes. Instead of enacting the role of homemaker and mother, women were expected to fulfill the "superwoman ideal," requiring them to be smart, beautiful, have a successful career, and still maintain a perfect house, perfect children, and a perfect relationship with the perfect man. The stress of trying to be all things to all people may drive some young women to focus on one thing that they think they can control, their weight. The societal preference for thin female shapes may provide a goal that seems more attainable than becoming a superwoman, or perhaps even a means of becoming a superwoman. This role change may help to explain "Why women?" and "Why now?"

In addition, the pressure to be thin makes women dissatisfied with their bodies. When dissatisfied with their bodies, men tend to turn to healthy eating (Nowak, 1998) and exercise, but women turn to dieting (Drewnowski, Kurth, & Krahn, 1995). Dieting, however, is more likely to produce eating disorder symptomatology than sustained weight loss (e.g., Polivy & Herman, 1993; Stice, 2001). The thin ideal thus produces body dissatisfaction in women, which elicits dieting, which encourages pathological eating. But if this were the whole story, all female adolescents who are unable to achieve thinness (or at least all who diet) would be eating disordered, which is clearly not the case. Therefore we must look further for an explanation.

Race, Ethnicity, and Social Class. Until about 20 years ago, eating disorders were restricted primarily to Western, middle- and upper-class, white adolescent females. Now, however, they have penetrated all social classes, races, and even some non-Western venues such as Japan. Although the prevalence is still lower in most non-White groups and nonindustrial countries (Polivy et al., 2003), Black women in the United States are as likely as are White women to display eating disorder symptoms (Mulholland & Mintz, 2001). In addition, they are quickly becoming comparable to their White counterparts with respect to body-image dissatisfaction (Grant et al., 1999), vomiting, and abuse of laxatives or diuretics, and they are more likely to report binge eating (Striegel-Moore et al., 2000). Among the several potential explanations for the globalization of eating disorders, the most obvious is the influence of the media (Nasser, 1997).

Young minority-group females who are heavier, better educated, and who identify more closely with White, middle-class values have an increased risk of eating disorder. Assimilation into White culture thus carries with it an associated risk of developing eating disorders (Cachelin, Veisel, Barzegarnazari, & Streigel-Moore, 2000). After acculturation, non-White women appear to have eating attitudes similar to those of Western Whites, although some studies do not find this (e.g., Ogden & Elder, 1998).

The expression of eating disorders among non-White groups differs in some ways from what is found with White women. Minority women with eating problems are usually truly overweight, whereas White women with disordered eating may only feel overweight, but actually be normal weight (Striegel-Moore et al., 2000). Body dissatisfaction and fear of fatness occur less frequently, if at all, among non-White groups, but Black adolescents are more likely to binge and use laxatives than are Whites, who are more likely to restrict their eating (Striegel-Moore et al., 2000). Black adolescent girls may experience less pressure to conform to the thin ideal plaguing White girls and seem less inclined to derive their self-esteem, identity, and perception of self-control from their weight and appearance (Polivy et al., 2003). When eating disorder symptoms do occur among non-Whites, however, they seem to be related to the same risk factors and precipitants—including low family connectedness, perfectionism, emotional distress, body dissatisfaction, and sometimes serious depression and anxiety (e.g., Davis & Katzman, 1999)—as they are among Whites. Race and social class thus do not seem to be significant factors in the development of an eating disorder in any given individual.

Familial Influences

If societal values and pressures can have enough impact on an individual to constitute a risk factor for the development of an eating disorder, how much more influential are familial interactions? The family can be a source of cultural transmission of pathological values or a stressor on its own (through miscommunication, lack of emotional support, or internal conflict). It can also be a protective factor.

Family influences, such as how the family mediates cultural ideas about thinness and how family members convey these messages to each other, have been implicated as causes of eating disorders (Haworth-Hoeppner, 2000; Laliberte, Boland, & Leichner, 1999; Strober, Freeman, Lampert, Diamond, & Kaye, 2000; Strober & Katz, 1988). A critical family environment, coercive parental control, and a dominating discourse on weight in the household appear to increase the risk of eating disorders (Haworth-Hoeppner, 2000). Even during treatment, family influences are important. For example, mothers' expressed emotion (especially critical comments) predicted an adverse outcome for eating disorder patients (Vanfurth et al., 1996).

Both mothers and fathers contribute to the development of eating disorders. For example, AN patients complain that their mothers do not care about them. Mothers who themselves have an eating disorder transmit pathological behaviors to their daughters by the time the girls are 5 years old. Even when the mothers do not have eating disorders, mothers of daughters with eating disorder symptoms find their daughters less attractive and more in need of weight loss than do mothers whose daughters are asymptomatic. Mothers' comments about weight and shape convey their attitudes and behaviors to their daughters. Daughters of mothers who diet are more likely to do so themselves, and to use more extreme weight-loss techniques if mothers encourage them to or are dissatisfied with their own bodies (Polivy & Herman, 2002; Polivy et al., 2003).

Critical comments and expression of negative emotions by either parent predict both the development of AN and worse outcome for AN patients. Mothers' complaints about a lack of family cohesion also foretell daughters' increased eating pathology 2 years later. High parental expectations for achievement that ignore the daughter's needs and goals have also been detected in girls with eating disorders; these extrinsic goals force these girls to struggle to please others at the expense of their own autonomy. Parents of both AN and BN patients appear to discourage autonomy, negating their daughters' needs and self-expression. The patients feel that their parents are overcontrolling in an affectionless manner. The fact that these sorts of parent–adolescent conflicts over autonomy and identity tend to be more intense among girls than among boys may help to explain why eating disorders are so much more common among females than among males (Polivy et al., 2003).

Individual Factors

If sociocultural influences on pathogenesis were very powerful, AN and BN would presumably be more common than they are. In addition, the numerous clear descriptions of AN from at least the middle of the nineteenth century and possibly earlier suggest that factors other than our current culture cause the disorders. Moreover, although there is some evidence that the disorders may afflict more than one offspring in a family, if the family were responsible for the development of an eating disorder, we would expect to see greater concurrence among the female offspring in a family. Thus, whereas culture and family contribute to the development of eating disorders, they are not sufficient to explain the appearance of a disorder in a given person. In light of the causal models discussed earlier, perhaps we may find the missing piece of the puzzle in factors specific to the individual, such as biological, identity, personality, or cognitive determinants.

Genetic and Physiological Factors.   The reasonably stereotypic and reliable clinical presentation of AN and BN, with a consistent sex distribution and age of onset, suggests a biological substrate for the disorders. Twin studies, family studies, and recent molecular-genetic findings point to a potential genetic factor (e.g., Klump, Kaye, & Strober, 2001), especially for AN. Females with a first-degree relative who has an eating disorder are two to three times more likely to develop one themselves (Polivy et al., 2003).

A genetic predisposition to eating disorder may operate through faults in neurotransmitters, of which serotonin is the most frequently studied, possibly because it inhibits feeding, stimulus reactivity, and sexual activity. A disturbance of serotonergic activity is consistent with descriptions of anorectic patients as constrained, perfectionistic, and needing order even after weight restoration (Kaye, Weltzin, & Hsu, 1993). Moreover, anorexics who have returned to normal weight still have elevated levels of brain serotonin metabolites. Women who develop AN might have intrinsic vulnerabilities for perfectionistic, anxious, and obsessional behavior as a result of elevated serotonin levels, and these tendencies could become increasingly dysfunctional as a result of stress or other psychosocial stimuli (Kaye et al., 1993).

Patients with BN also show signs of serotonin dysregulation, which may contribute to their symptoms, including binge eating (Steiger et al., 2001; Wolfe, Metzger, & Jimerson, 1997). Serotonin may be associated with impulsivity, which may relate to the binge eating behavior and other impulsive behaviors exhibited by BN patients (Steiger et al., 2001). Because the evidence for the influence of elevated serotonin on eating disorders is strictly correlational, it is not possible to conclude that elevated serotonin causes eating disorder. Indeed, it may instead be a consequence of the disorder.

Hormonal changes associated with puberty may also increase susceptibility to eating disorder. Puberty in females is accompanied by increased body fat and a drastically different body shape—the curves that develop in pubescent girls definitely subvert the thin ideal to which girls aspire. This new, curvy shape may give rise to the increased body dissatisfaction and accompanying dieting that become normative in adolescent females and that are themselves potential risk factors for eating disorders (e.g., Polivy et al., 2003; Striegel-Moore, 1993). At the same time, hormonal development pushes girls into heterosexual interactions, which girls appear to find more stressful than do boys (Striegel-Moore, 1993).

Self-Esteem and Identity.   Among dieters who do not have eating disorders, depression scores are elevated and self-esteem scores are reduced; these scores are even more extreme among those with eating disorders (e.g., Polivy & Herman, 2002; Polivy et al., 2003), as they are in certain other psychological syndromes. Negative emotions are linked to disruptive eating behaviors, in a cyclic or spiral pattern (e.g., Polivy et al., 2003). Negative self-evaluation is possibly the most ubiquitous risk factor among eating disorder patients (Fairburn, Cooper, Doll, & Welch, 1999); feelings of ineffectiveness and lack of a strong sense of self were recognized as hallmarks of eating disorders as early as the 1970s (e.g., Bruch, 1975). The lower self-esteem among those with eating disorders also seems to be connected to a lack of a cohesive identity and distrust of one's body's ability to function on its own, both of which appear to be distinctively related to eating disorders.

The low self-esteem of those with eating disorders may reflect negative life experiences such as sexual or emotional abuse, which may also interfere with formation of a stable identity. Constructing an identity based on eating, weight, and shape may mask more basic problems with one's sense of self and create a sense of control that is otherwise lacking (Polivy & Herman, 2002). Threats to a precarious identity may exacerbate eating problems. For example, chronic dieters (restrained eaters), who resemble eating disorder patients in many ways, have been studied in the laboratory to learn about processes in eating disorder. Restrained eaters exposed to false feedback (from an inaccurate scale) indicating that they have gained weight react by overeating (McFarlane, Polivy, & Herman, 1998). Similarly, when allowed to eat after reporting about ways in which they have failed to meet their life goals, restrained eaters responded by overeating (Wheeler, Polivy, & Herman, 2002). Threats to one's identity seem to elicit disordered eating behavior.

Body Dissatisfaction and Dieting. The negative self-perception and low self-esteem characterizing eating disorders crystallize in negative feelings about one's body and an investment in improving it as a means of self-redemption (Polivy & Herman, 2002). Body dissatisfaction is a diagnostic criterion for eating disorder, according to the DSM–IV (APA, 1994). Stice's dual-pathway model (e.g., Stice, 2001) posits that it is the thin ideal that produces body image dissatisfaction, which then produces dieting, and eventually eating disorder symptomatology. Adolescent girls do have greater body dissatisfaction than do boys or older women, and those who place more emphasis on their bodies and are more dissatisfied with them tend to exhibit greater eating pathology (Polivy et al., 2003). Moreover, dieting has been implicated as a cause of binge eating and is thought to be a primary contributor to the "dieting disorders," as eating disorders are often called (Polivy & Herman, 2002). But if all the girls who embraced the thin ideal, dieted, and were dissatisfied with their bodies became eating disordered, much of the adolescent female population would be incapacitated! Thus, although most models of eating disorder include a role for body dissatisfaction and dieting, it is clear that these risk factors must interact with other factors such as extremely low self-esteem and identity deficiencies, other personality factors, and the familial and cultural issues discussed earlier.

Personality Factors. Those with eating disorders exhibit a consistent pattern of personality traits before, during, and after the disordered eating phase. Converging evidence from clinical reports, psychometric studies, and family or collateral sources presents the premorbid (i.e., before the onset of the disorder) personality of AN patients as perfectionistic, obsessive, socially inhibited, compliant, and emotionally restrained (e.g., Strober & Humphrey, 1987; Wonderlich, 1995). Bulimics are not only compliant and perfectionistic, but also tend to be impulsive, emotional, lacking in interoceptive awareness, and extraverted (e.g., Lilenfeld et al., 2000; Steiger et al., 2001). Perfectionism and negative self-evaluation characterize AN and BN patients before, during, and after recovery from the disorder (Fairburn et al., 1999). Negative affect, behavioral inhibition, and obsessiveness also continue after recovery from AN (Kaye, Gendall, & Strober, 1998). Moreover, perfectionism, ineffectiveness and interpersonal distrust are found in family members of eating disorder patients who do not themselves show symptoms of eating disorders (Lilenfeld et al., 2000). There are thus a number of personality traits linked to eating disorders. Although the evidence is correlational, the persistence of such traits before and after the disorder and their presence in nondisordered family members suggest that they could interact with adverse familial and social experiences and render an individual more likely to develop an eating disorder (e.g., Lilenfeld et al., 2000; Strober & Humphrey, 1987).

Cognitive Factors. People with eating disorders display several cognitive aberrations such as obsessive thoughts, distortions of attention and memory (reflecting a focus on food, weight, and shape), and rigid, all-or-nothing thinking (Polivy & Herman, 2002). Obsessing about weight and shape, and using these characteristics to determine one's self-worth, are central (and defining) features of eating disorders. The tendency to see the world through weight and shape schemata, which affect attention and memory, reflects an obsessive preoccupation with these issues. Experimental techniques such as the Stroop color-naming task demonstrate biased attention to weight and shape in eating disorder patients. All-or-nothing, black-and-white thinking makes them see themselves as failures if they eat so much as one bite of a "forbidden" food, and may promote binges in BN patients (Polivy & Herman, 2002). The prominent role of cognitive features in eating disorder has encouraged the use of cognitive therapies (see later) to normalize the cognitions that are presumed to underlie the eating disorder.

Combining Risk Factors

Because risk factor research is of necessity correlational, it cannot determine cause and effect. Furthermore, no single risk factor alone is capable of producing an eating disorder, and it would be simplistic to suppose that a disorder as complex as eating disorders are would have a single cause. In 1987, Johnson and Connors proposed a biopsychosocial model of eating disorder development. This model posits that biological predispositions (from genetic, hormonal, and pubertal influences), family factors, and cultural pressures to be thin and to fulfill a demanding social role interact to produce an identity-conflicted, vulnerable dieter. Those dieters with low self-esteem and affective instability are most susceptible to an eating disordered identity, particularly in response to stress or failure. Striegel-Moore (1993) has suggested that the number of simultaneous life challenges faced by an individual is related to her susceptibility to eating disorder. Girls who mature early and begin dating at the same time report more disturbed attitudes about eating and shape. Striegel-Moore also posits that early maturation is a source of adjustment difficulties, which, along with body dissatisfaction, dieting, and conflict with parents is sufficiently stressful to increase risk for an eating disorder. A related theory proposes that the many transitions that occur in adolescence (e.g., moving to junior high or high school, puberty, dating, disruptions in friendships, increased academic and sex role demands) and the restructuring of personality and behavior demanded by these transitions may overwhelm an adolescent who is already vulnerable because of familial or personal problems (e.g., Smolak & Levine, 1996).

The combination of (a) the contextual background of sociocultural expectations to look and act a certain way, (b) familial interaction patterns that negate the individual's attempts to achieve autonomy, (c) individual vulnerabilities based on genetics and personality, self-esteem, and identity deficits, and (d) the stresses required by transitional adjustments offers a potential starting point for identifying individuals most likely to develop an eating disorder. Although these combinatory models attempt to incorporate the complexity of eating disorders and the many identified risk factors, they have not yet provided predictive power sufficient to identify individuals most likely to succumb to the pressures and develop eating disorders.

TREATMENT OF EATING DISORDERS

Although the causes of eating disorders remain obscure, clinicians must nevertheless treat them. Here we review the basic rationale and techniques of the major therapies used in the treatment of eating disorder. We start with treatments targeting the most focal eating disorder symptoms and then discuss treatments that modify symptoms indirectly, by altering other internal or external processes. Next, we review the empirical literature on therapeutic efficacy. Finally, we discuss the factors contributing to relapse.

Cognitive-Behavioral Therapy

The most widely used and presumably most effective therapeutic technique for treating eating disorders continues to be cognitive-behavior therapy. The basic ideas underlying this therapy were initially described by Beck and his colleagues, who applied them to depression (see Beck, Rush, Shaw, and Emery, 1979, for a review). Soon thereafter, it was modified and extended to the treatment of the eating disorders. In 1981, Fairburn was the first to outline a cognitive-behavioral approach to the management of BN, and in 1982 Garner and Bemis applied cognitive behavior therapy to AN. Inevitably, this treatment has now been proposed for use with BED (e.g., Wilson & Fairburn, 2000). Although identifying, modifying, and replacing maladaptive thoughts and behaviors are central to therapy in all of these cases, the distinctive symptomatology of each disorder means that treatment must be adapted accordingly.

Cognitive-Behavior Therapy for AN. The rationale for the use of cognitive-behavior therapy for AN is that irrational and recalcitrant beliefs about the importance of body weight and shape support relentlessly pursued maladaptive behavior (especially weight loss). That these patients also suffer from deficiencies of identity and self-worth makes treatment even more difficult. Cognitive-behavior therapy for AN focuses both on specific symptoms and on underlying difficulties. According to Vitousek (1995), this therapy for AN targets four main areas. The first is the ego-syntonic nature of the disorder (i.e., seeing the disorder as positive or desirable); because individuals with AN prize slenderness, they must first acknowledge that the pursuit of slimness has a negative impact on their lives. Vitousek proposes asking the client to list both the positive and negative aspects of her anorexia; in turn, "each claimed advantage and disadvantage is cast as a hypothesis that can be examined for its validity and adaptiveness" (1995, p. 326), an exercise effectively constituting the first steps toward modifying cognitions. The second focus involves setting behavioral goals for normalized eating and weight gain and implementing cognitive coping strategies to deal with these changes. For instance, the myth that certain "forbidden" foods cause drastic weight gain may be debunked by having patients try these foods in controlled exposures. The third, related focus of treatment is modifying beliefs about weight and food. Clients are taught to challenge their self-defeating thoughts by learning to examine them rationally and replace them with more realistic possibilities (e.g., "there are no forbidden foods per se; it is excess caloric intake that leads to weight gain"). Once these most urgent aspects of the disorder have been addressed, treatment can then focus on the underlying self-concept issues that may be maintaining the disorder; ideally, other more attainable and adaptive goals may be identified to replace slenderness as the basis of identity.

In contrast to this traditional approach incorporating general issues such as self-esteem, Fairburn, Shafran, and Cooper (1998) have proposed a more focused cognitive-behavioral program for AN, targeting the patient's need for control and the attempt to attain this control through dieting. Treatment involves helping the client to achieve success and fulfillment from pursuits unrelated to weight and shape. They suggest that this streamlined treatment should be used first and broadened only if other issues prove to be obstacles to change (Fairburn et al., 1998).

Cognitive-Behavior Therapy for BN. Because BN is less ego-syntonic (i.e., acceptable to one's self-image) than is AN—the binge–purge cycle is often extremely distressing to the individual—cognitive behavior therapy for BN has a narrower focus, typically limited to eating behavior and thoughts about food, weight, and shape. Thus, as in AN, BN clients are taught to establish a normalized eating pattern consisting of regularly scheduled meals. (Skipping meals is avoided to prevent the extreme hunger that may foster a binge.) In addition, clients work on the reduction or elimination of bingeing and purging (through behavioral contracts with the therapist) and the development of coping techniques to prevent binges and associated compensatory behaviors. They are taught to identify the usual precipitants to bingeing (often with the help of a daily food diary), and to use distraction techniques (alternatives to binges such as taking a walk, calling a supportive friend, or delaying eating) or coping mechanisms (such as self-talk). Compensatory behaviors after lapses—such as purging, laxative use, excessive exercise or dietary restraint—are discouraged, in an attempt to break the binge–purge cycle; this technique is akin to the behavioral technique of exposure with response prevention. Finally, as with AN, excessive concern with body weight and shape is challenged through cognitive restructuring (e.g., Wilson, 1996; 1999).

Cognitive-Behavior Therapy for BED. Because BED involves bingeing without purging or any other form of compensatory behavior, individuals with BED are more often overweight than are those with BN. Thus, behavioral weight-loss strategies (e.g., an exercise plan) may be required, and the individual's societally induced prejudices against overweight must be eliminated in addition to merely challenging the importance of slenderness. It has been suggested (Wilson & Fairburn, 2000) that "the treatment of choice [for BED] would appear to be cognitive behavioral self-help" (p. 352). Indeed, no difference in outcome between therapist-led versus self-help format cognitive-behavior therapy has been found, and there were significant improvements over wait-list controls in the latter, suggesting that it may be a cost-effective, accessible alternative for patients with BED (Loeb, Wilson, Gilbert, & Labouvie, 2000).

It should be noted that these descriptions of cognitive-behavior therapy for eating disorders reflect either how it is carried out in experimental tests or in the ideal clinical setting, neither of which necessarily corresponds to clinical reality. Individual clinicians often tailor the technique as they see fit for individual clients, or they may combine cognitive-behavior therapy with other treatment strategies in an eclectic treatment plan.

Nutritional Counseling and Psychoeducation

As its name implies, nutritional or dietary counseling involves educating the patient about normal caloric needs and physiological processes. Kahm (1994) explained that while people with eating disorders may have a wealth of knowledge regarding the calorie content of most foods, this knowledge is usually used to achieve drastic weight loss rather than to maintain a healthy body. In fact, Beumont and Touyz (1995) suggested that failing to address nutritional issues in eating disorders "is as ridiculous as prohibiting the discussion of drinking behavior with patients with alcohol related disease" (p. 306). They also stated that this therapy is intended to change attitudes about food and eating, and then eating behavior, by arming people with accurate knowledge.

Psychoeducation provides accurate nutritional information, but also educates patients about the nature of their disorder. Olmsted and Kaplan (1995) advocated addressing four main topics beyond dietary information: the complex etiology of eating disorders, the often serious medical consequences of severe food restriction or continual bingeing and vomiting, the sociocultural idealization of the thin female body, and cognitive and behavioral strategies that one may use to modify eating problems. Although nutritional counseling and psychoeducation are rarely used as stand-alone therapies, Olmsted and Kaplan claimed that educational information is incorporated in up to 75% of studies of treatment for BN.

Interpersonal Therapy

In contrast to psychoeducation and cognitive-behavioral therapy, which are entirely focused on weight-related behaviors and, in the latter case, cognitions, interpersonal therapy does not touch on these issues in the treatment of eating disorders. Instead, it targets maladaptive personal relationships and relational styles because difficulties in these areas are seen as contributing to the development and maintenance of eating disorders (Birchall, 1999). Thus, the fundamental task of the interpersonal therapist is to identify one of Birchall's "problem areas—Grief, Role Transitions, Interpersonal Role Disputes (or) Interpersonal Deficits" (p. 315), and to work to improve the client's functioning in that area. Improved interpersonal relationships might reduce eating disorder symptoms in a number of ways. Enhanced control in relationships may generalize to enhanced control of eating in BN or BED. Furthermore, interpersonal therapy may reduce or eliminate common interpersonal triggers to bingeing. For example, depressed mood and interpersonal stress may be alleviated, and more frequent, positive social interactions may reduce boredom. Decreasing interpersonal stress may also improve anorectic behavior by providing a greater sense of control in areas of one's life other than eating.

Family Therapy

Family therapy focuses on interpersonal relationships, emphasizing the importance of stresses within the family as a whole rather than on individuals. It postulates that change by one member affects every other member in turn (Minuchin, Rosman, & Baker, 1978; Thode, 1990). The eating disorder patient is seen in conjunction with her parents and siblings (or with her spouse and children, as the case may be), and the goal becomes reducing family stressors and miscommunications to bring about a reduction in eating disorder symptoms. Thus, family therapy places responsibility for recovery on both the patient and her relatives. Geist, Heinmaa, Stephens, Davis, and Katzman's (2000) description of treatment provides a good example of the specific content of family therapy: (a) recruiting parents to actively engage in managing the patient's weight gain and eating, (b) ameliorating maladaptive communication within the family and particularly between the parents, and (c) elucidating the difference between normal methods of coping with family conflict and the symptoms the patient is currently exhibiting.

Psychoanalytic Therapy

Psychoanalytic or psychodynamic therapy may encompass a wide variety of specific techniques or foci. Herzog (1995) defines it broadly as "all long-term therapies that explicitly use the relationship between the patient and therapist as the primary treatment tool and that attend to transference and countertransference reactions" (p. 330). This therapy assumes that eating disorder symptoms are merely the overt pathological manifestations of underlying conflicts that the client has been unable to resolve adaptively. The psychoanalyst's task is to determine the unique meanings of these symptoms for each client. Many theorists suggest that establishing a strong therapeutic alliance is the first (and perhaps most crucial) step (Gonzalez, 1988;

Herzog, 1995). Establishing such an alliance may be particularly difficult and take longer in AN, because the patient will perceive the therapist as someone who wants her to give up her ego-syntonic dietary restriction. Once trust has developed, the psychoanalyst establishes a neutral stance toward the patient, who then free associates: "the hope is that the patients will project upon this 'blank screen' their characteristic thoughts and behaviors (transference)" (Johnson, 1995, p. 351). Much of therapy is then devoted to analyzing these transference reactions in the context of a thorough developmental history. Another strategy used in identifying the roots of the eating disorder is the analysis of dreams to determine their symbolic meaning. The countertransference relationship also constitutes an important source of information about the client; therapists interpret their own reactions to the client to further elucidate the quality of the client's interpersonal relationships. A nonjudgmental relationship between the therapist and client is said to serve a further purpose, providing the patient with an opportunity to relate appropriately on an interpersonal level, allowing the patient to resolve dependent or otherwise pathological relations with others (Herzog, 1995).

Contemporary psychoanalytic writers acknowledge that psychoanalysis may not be appropriate for all eating disorder patients. Herzog (1995) maintains that the treatment is appropriate for those patients presenting with character pathology; both Herzog and Johnson recommend psychoanalysis for prior-treatment nonresponders (i.e., for those patients whose symptoms linger after a course of cognitive or interpersonal therapy). Finally, Gonzalez (1988) cautions against using psychoanalysis for suicidal patients or for those whose extremely low weight makes hospitalization necessary; in these cases, the long-term focus of psychoanalysis would leave the patient at immediate risk of harm.

Pharmacotherapy

Pharmacotherapy departs significantly from other treatments by postulating some sort of organic cause for the disorder—or at least that the symptoms can be controlled pharmacologically—and attempting to treat symptoms accordingly, with drugs. By far the most common drugs are tricyclic antidepressants and selective serotonin reuptake inhibitors (SSRIs). Their use is based on the fact that depressive symptoms are prominent in both AN and BN and that some symptoms of both of these disorders resemble the clinical features of other disorders that respond favorably to these medications (e.g., Kruger & Kennedy, 2000; Mayer & Walsh, 1998). Other drugs that have been tried include antipsychotics (to treat the delusion-like obsessions with weight and shape), anxiolytics (to target the anxiety associated with eating disordered behavior and weight restoration in AN), mood stabilizers such as lithium (which may promote weight gain in AN and regulate affective lability in BN), and antiserotonergics (assumed to increase food intake and lead to weight gain in AN as it does in general medical usage). See Kruger and Kennedy, 2000, for a review.

Efficacy of Treatment

With a few exceptions (such as pharmacotherapy for AN), the efficacy of most of these treatments has been empirically validated; that is, they have been shown to lead to statistically significant improvements when compared to placebo or wait-list controls. We are left with the more interesting and useful question of which treatments are relatively more useful in treating eating disorders.

Treatment Recommendations for AN. Because of its low prevalence and its additional medical complications, there are significantly fewer controlled treatment trials for AN than there are for BN and BED. Furthermore, very few studies directly compare various forms of treatment for AN, making differences in efficacy somewhat difficult to gauge. Despite these limitations, there is a tenuous consensus that family therapy is the first-line treatment for most cases of AN (e.g., Wilson, 1999). On the basis of three available controlled trials of family therapy with AN, Russell, Dare, Eisler, and Le Grange (1992) concluded that family therapy is effective for anorectics with early onset (before age 18). It may be particularly effective for adolescents because they tend to express greater denial and less desire for help (Fisher, Schneider, Burns, Symons, & Mandel, 2001), making family involvement potentially more important. Most researchers (Kruger & Kennedy, 2000; Mayer & Walsh, 1998) recommend against the use of drugs in the acute treatment of AN, but some (e.g., Kaye et al., 1998) are now postulating a place for SSRIs in the maintenance of treatment gains. Psychoanalysis for AN has not been well studied, but Herzog (1995) stated that patients often require a minimum of 1 to 2 years of psychoanalysis, and maybe as much as 8 to 10 years for improvement to take place. A recently published long-term outcome study (Steinhausen et al., 2000) found that 80% of surviving AN patients recovered at 11-year follow-up regardless of the type of therapy received. In light of this finding, it is difficult to make a case for the use of long-term psychoanalysis in the treatment of AN. Further research is required to determine the efficacy of cognitive-behavior therapy for AN.

Treatment Recommendations for BN. Cognitive-behavior therapy is often considered the treatment of choice for BN (e.g., Wilson, 1996; 1999); it leads to reduction or remission of bingeing and purging in 50% of patients and improvements in dietary restraint, attitudes toward shape and weight, and associated psychopathology (Wilson, 1996). However, interpersonal therapy may be a suitable alternative; most studies comparing the two find them to be equally effective by the end of treatment and at follow-up, although cognitive-behavior therapy is faster-acting in the beginning (Birchall, 1999; Fairburn et al., 1995).

The efficacy of these first-line treatments is still somewhat limited (recall that only 50% of BN patients cease or significantly decrease binge eating and purging), so it is important to be aware of viable alternatives. Antidepressants are superior to placebos in reducing bingeing and purging (e.g., Goldstein, Wilson, Thompson, Potvin, and Rampey, 1995). On the other hand, a review of six controlled studies (Wilson, 1996) found cognitive-behavior therapy on its own to be superior to antidepressant drugs alone; moreover, cognitive-behavior therapy plus drugs was better than drugs alone, but no more effective than therapy alone or cognitive-behavior therapy plus placebo. Pharmacotherapy thus may not be a viable second choice if psychotherapy fails.

Family therapy for BN has not been well studied, though Dare and Eisler (2000) reported encouraging preliminary findings for their multifamily treatment program for adolescents with BN. Similarly, outcome data for psychodynamic treatment of BN are scarce, leading Johnson (1995) to recommend this approach only for those patients who do not respond to briefer forms of therapy.

Treatment Recommendations for BED. Because research on BED is fairly new, studies to date have focused primarily on cognitive-behavior therapy, interpersonal therapy, pharmacotherapy, and weight-loss treatments. Cognitive-behavior therapy seems to be effective in reducing binge eating (e.g., Loeb et al., 2000; Wilson & Fairburn, 2000). Interpersonal therapy has been shown to be as effective as cognitive-behavior therapy in reducing binges (and as ineffective at producing weight loss), and the rate of improvement for BED (unlike other eating disorders) is equal in both therapies (Wilson & Fairburn, 2000). In contrast, certain modes of pharmacotherapy have shown some promise in reducing not only binges but also weight. Many drugs, from appetite suppressants to antidepressants, have demonstrated efficacy in reducing binge eating (e.g., Shapira, Goldsmith, & McElroy, 2000, for appetite suppressants; McElroy et al., 2000 for antidepressants). Hudson, Carter, and Pope (1996) concluded from reviewing treatment trials that although tricyclic antidepressants are not effective for weight loss, SSRIs do produce weight loss among patients with BED. An important caveat is that this weight loss does not seem to be maintained (e.g., Devlin, Goldfein, Carino, & Wolk, 2000). Finally, behavioral weight-loss therapy has been suggested in the treatment of BED. One study found that although this was superior to weight-loss treatment in reducing binges in the short term (12 weeks), the difference disappeared at follow-up; neither cognitive-behavior therapy nor desipramine added to the efficacy of the behavioral weight-loss program in the long-term (Agras et al., 1994). Levine, Marcus, and Moulton (1996) found that 81% of women given an exercise-and-diet program were abstinent from bingeing at posttreatment, a significant improvement over those in a delayed-treatment control condition. This finding suggests that incorporating exercise in treatment for BED may assist in the remission of binge eating.

Conclusions About Treatment of Eating Disorders

Despite our poor understanding of the development of eating disorders, research into their treatment has made some progress. However, controlled trials comparing treatments may not reflect clinical reality, where therapists may sample from the available therapies and tailor treatments to specific clients. For instance, individual cognitive-behavior therapy might be paired with administration of drugs to help patients with BN, or interpersonal and family therapy might be bolstered with psychoeducation in the treatment of AN. These so-called multifaceted treatments (see Lansky & Levitt, 1992, for a review) may provide the best form of care, because the components of one therapy may enhance the effects of another or provide additional benefits beyond those available in the empirically established first-line treatment. Still, individually tailored treatments are difficult to evaluate systematically; although such tailoring makes some sense, it also makes it difficult for researchers to evaluate treatment efficacy.

RELAPSE

Defining relapse is difficult. A search of the literature on relapse in eating disorders yields a heterogeneous group of studies, none of which adequately define *relapse*. Theoretically, relapse signifies a return to disordered functioning following a period of symptom amelioration. Pike (1998) attempted to define relapse relative to initial treatment response, remission, and recovery. An initial satisfactory response for AN (before which relapse cannot occur) is operationalized as increasing body mass index (BMI) to at least 20, consuming significantly more calories (although not necessarily normalized eating), reducing fears about weight gain, a resumption of menses, and medical stabilization. Thus, complete symptom alleviation is not necessary for relapse to occur. According to Pike, relapse involves weight dropping to a BMI below 18.5, restrictive eating or bingeing with compensatory behavior, a return to overvaluing weight and shape, loss of menses, and in some cases a return of associated medical problems.

Unfortunately, many of the studies of relapse do not adopt a stringent operational definition. We will discuss relapse in all three forms of eating disorder as indexed by a return of disordered eating or a significant decline in functioning following some period of improvement.

Relapse in AN

Studies of relapse in AN place the risk at approximately 30% within 15 months after treatment, though a recent study followed forty patients for 1 year and found that thirty-one were readmitted in that time (e.g., Herzog et al., 1999; Strober, Freeman, & Morrell, 1997). AN patients seem particularly vulnerable to relapse soon after regaining weight and being discharged from the hospital and may need more attention then (Fennig & Roe, 2002).

Various factors have been found to predict relapse in AN, including later age of onset (Pike, 1998), duration of illness of longer than 6 years (Howard et al., 1999), increased duration of eating pathology before treatment (Herzog, Keller, Strober, Yeh, & Pei, 1992), amenorrhea lasting longer than 2.5 years, and a low BMI at hospitalization (Howard et al., 1999; Pike, 1998).

Personality and attitudinal variables also predict relapse. Greater obsessiveness before treatment predicts more severe dieting, higher eating disorder scores, and more frequent hospitalizations at 2-year follow-up (Zubieta, Demitrack, Fenick, & Krahn, 1995), at which time obsessionality is associated with lower weight and increased eating disorder symptomatology. It is unclear, however, whether obsessionality increases the risk of relapse or of a more negative course overall. In addition, a compulsive drive to exercise following discharge from treatment after initial improvement predicts relapse (Strober et al., 1997). Persistent anorexic attitudes (i.e., overvaluing weight and shape) and low desired weight (despite some weight restoration) predict relapse within 1 year of treatment termination (Pike, 1998); behavioral changes without corresponding cognitive changes increase the risk of relapse into anorexic symptoms.

Comorbidity (i.e., having more than one psychological problem) may pose an additional risk for relapse. A 10-year follow-up of anorexics discharged from hospital treatment found that those with a diagnosable eating disorder at follow-up had more and worse comorbid psychopathology, whereas those who "had no eating disorder at follow-up displayed essentially no general psychopathology" (Schork, Eckert, & Halmi, 1994, p. 113). However, Pike (1998) cautioned that the directionality of this relation is questionable; it is possible that more severe or longer-lasting eating disorder symptoms lead to other psychopathology rather than the reverse.

Few other predictors of relapse have been identified. One 7.5-year follow-up study found no significant predictors of relapse after recovery (Herzog et al., 1999). Similarly, although Strober et al. (1997) identified some predictors of postdischarge relapse following partial recovery, they were unable to identify any significant predictors of relapse following full recovery. This finding highlights an important practical distinction. Although AN is associated with a high rate (83%) of partial recovery, the rate of full recovery is much lower (33%; Herzog et al., 1999). Relapse may be more likely and more easily predicted following partial recovery, but it would be worthwhile to explore relapse following complete recovery.

Relapse in BN

Relapse rates for BN, as for AN, are typically around 30% (Herzog et al, 1999; Olmsted, Kaplan, & Rockert, 1994). Again, most relapses occur fairly quickly, usually within 6 months (Olmsted et al., 1994). Keller, Herzog, Lavori, Bradburn, and Mahoney (1992) found a cumulative probability of relapse of 63%, with 50% of those achieving complete recovery eventually relapsing into another episode of full-blown BN.

Contrary to AN, younger age was among the strongest predictors of relapse in BN (Olmsted et al., 1994). Higher vomiting frequency both before and following treatment was also associated with increased risk, indicating that severity of the disorder determines how intractable it is. Personality and attitudinal variables that have been shown to predict relapse in BN include impulsivity (Miller, 2000), obsessionality (Zubieta et al., 1995), poor body image (Freeman, Beach, Davis, & Solyom, 1985; Keller et al., 1992), more disordered attitudes toward eating before treatment, and greater interpersonal distrust following treatment (Olmsted et al., 1994). Factors that appear to decrease the risk of relapse include a reduced fear of maturity (Miller, 2000) and having a good support system (Keller et al., 1992).

Negative affect appears to play a significant role in relapse in BN. Bulimics who experience stressful situations (and anxiety, nervousness, and depression) are more likely to relapse after gaining control of their eating behavior than are those who do not (Mitchell, Davis & Goff, 1985). Because negative affect triggers disinhibited eating, it is not surprising that it too has been shown to trigger relapse among recovering bulimics. Fluvoxamine, an antidepressant, reduces the risk of relapse among BN patients, at least in the short term (Fichter, Krueger, Rief, Holland, & Doehne, 1996). Learning how to deal with negative affect is clearly a key to relapse prevention.

Relapse in BED

Current estimates of relapse rates in BED are somewhat more optimistic than are those observed in AN and BN. The only longitudinal study of BED to assess relapse rates (Fichter, Quadflieg, and Gnutzmann, 1998) found that at 6 years posttreatment, most participants did not have a diagnosable eating disorder, although approximately 15% had shifted to another diagnostic category (7.4% to BN and 7.4% to EDNOS), and approximately 6% met the criteria for BED once again.

Possibly because research into BED is in its infancy, all of the currently available studies of BED assess predictors of negative treatment outcome rather than predictors of relapse. These two categories may eventually be shown to overlap. As is the case with both AN and BN, the severity of the disorder appears to be a prime determinant of negative outcome in BED: the more frequent bingeing is at treatment intake, the more frequent it is following treatment (Peterson et al., 2000). Negative affect also predicts poorer treatment outcome for BED (Eldredge & Agras, 1997). Although BN and BED are distinct clinical syndromes, relapse factors in BN may well be fruitful guides to studying relapse factors in BED.

The fact that treatment for eating disorders has proceeded virtually independently of research on the causes of eating disorders should give us pause. Do we have to understand a problem to treat it, or can we simply tinker with different treatments until we find one (or some combination) that works, without necessarily understanding what caused the problem in the first place? If we did understand what caused the problem, would our treatments necessarily improve? Is it likely that we could therapeutically reverse the original causes? These are questions that pertain to all of psychopathology, but they are particularly salient in the domain of eating disorders. Moreover, they are not rhetorical questions. We really do not know how important the connection is between cause and treatment.

Even if treatment is not dependent on understanding causes, the question of what causes eating disorders remains important. Most of the interventions for eating disorders are therapeutic rather than preventative; that is, we tend to focus our efforts on treating eating disorders rather than preventing them from arising in the first place. An effective public health effort—stopping eating disorders before they get started—probably would be more valuable than effective therapy; but preventative interventions require a better understanding of what causes the disorder. Some efforts have been made in this area, but with limited success. For example, a program that provided girls as young as 10 or 11 with information on healthy eating and attitudes towards one's body changed only attitudes, not behavior (Smolak, Levine, & Schermer, 1998). Similarly, adolescents who participated in an 8-week eating disorder prevention program seemed to have improved both attitudes and behaviors immediately following the program. Within 6 months, however, they had not only reverted to their former behaviors but had become even more restrained in their eating than when they started. This result led the authors to conclude that prevention programs might do more harm than good! (Carter, Stewart, Dunn, & Fairburn, 1997).

Whether our interest in understanding what causes eating disorders is practical or just a matter of scientific curiosity, we must acknowledge that (a) we have not come a long way in the past 30 years toward a better understanding of why and how these disorders develop, and (b) the obstacles to making explanatory progress are significant. The most obvious obstacle is that the vast majority of studies examine correlates (or recollected precursors) of established eating disorders. This sort of research is inevitably inconclusive about causation. Path-analytic strategies (e.g., Stice, 2001) attempt to extract causal patterns from correlational data. There are severe limits, however, to the persuasiveness of such analyses. True experimentation is not likely to occur, and if it did, it would quickly be halted on ethical grounds. For example, it is difficult to get permission to study the bingeing of a BN patient in the lab. Although such patients binge all the time, it is regarded as unethical for researchers to actively induce a binge. Prospective research is more compelling than is retrospective research; but it too is correlational and therefore unsatisfying. Perhaps researchers will simply have to get used to the idea that they may never have a genuine understanding of eating disorders.

Of course, although many of us would be most pleased with a tight, experimentally based analysis of eating disorders, there are other satisfactions to be had. Decades ago, Hilde Bruch (1975, 1978) provided us with an account of eating disorders, based on her vast clinical experience and insight. The empirical research that has been conducted since Bruch first presented her elegant formulations has done little to undermine her analysis. Indeed, it may be argued that the empirical research enterprise has done little more than add some confirmation to her views, much as paleontology has been a footnote to Darwin. The reader who wants a clear understanding of eating disorders would be well-advised to skip the journal articles and go directly to Bruch, or if not to her, to her patients. As one of them concluded, "The main thing I've learned is that the worry about dieting, the worry about being skinny or fat, is just a smokescreen. This is not the real illness. The real illness has to do with the way you feel about yourself" (Bruch, 1978, p. 127).

REFERENCES

Abed, R. T. (1998). The sexual competition hypothesis for eating disorders. *British Journal of Medical Psychology, 71*, 525–547.

Agras, W. S., Telch, C. F., Arnow, B., Eldredge, K., Wilfley, D. E., Raeburn, S. D., Henderson, J., & Marnell, M. (1994). Weight loss, cognitive-behavioral, and desipramine treatments in binge eating disorder: An additive design. *Behavior Therapy, 25*, 225–238.

American Psychiatric Association. (1994). *Diagnostic and statistical manual of mental disorders* (4th ed.). Washington, DC: Author.

Beck, A. T., Rush, A. J., Shaw, B. F., & Emery, G. (1979). *Cognitive Therapy of Depression*. New York: Guilford.

Bemporad, J. R. (1996). Self-starvation through the ages: Reflections on the pre-history of anorexia nervosa. *International Journal of Eating Disorders, 19*, 217–237.

Bemporad, J. R. (1997). Cultural and historical aspects of eating disorders. *Theoretical Medicine, 18*, 401–420.

Beumont, P. J. V. & Touyz, S. W. (1995). The nutritional management of anorexia and bulimia nervosa. In K. D. Brownell & C. G. Fairburn (Eds.), *Eating disorders and obesity: A comprehensive handbook* (pp. 306–312). New York: Guilford.

Birchall, H. (1999). Interpersonal psychotherapy in the treatment of eating disorders. *European Eating Disorders Review, 7*, 315–320.

Booth, D. A. (1988). Culturally corralled into food abuse: The eating disorders as physiologically reinforced excessive appetites. In K. M. Pirke, W. Vandereycken, & D. Ploog (Eds.), *The psychobiology of bulimia nervosa* (pp. 18–32). Berlin: Springer-Verlag.

Bramon-Bosch, E., Troop, N., & Treasure, J. L. (2000). Eating disorders in males: A comparison with female patients. *European Eating Disorders Review, 8*, 321–328.

Braun, D. L., Sunday, S. R., Huang, A., & Halmi, K. A. (1999). More males seek treatment for eating disorders. *International Journal of Eating Disorders, 25*, 415–424.

Bruch, H. (1975). Obesity and anorexia nervosa: Psychosocial aspects. *Australia & New Zealand Journal of Psychiatry*, *9*, 159–161.

Bruch, H. (1978). The golden cage: The enigma of anorexia nervosa. Cambridge, MA: Harvard University Press.

Cachelin, F. M., & Maher, B. A. (1998). Is amenorrhea a critical criterion for anorexia nervosa? *Journal of Psychosomatic Research*, *44*, 435–440.

Cachelin, F. M., Veisel, C., Barzegarnazari, E., & Striegel-Moore, R. H. (2000). Disordered eating, acculturation, and treatment-seeking in a community sample of Hispanic, Asian, Black, and White women. *Psychology of Women Quarterly*, *24*, 244–253.

Carter, J. C., Stewart, D. A., Dunn, V. J., & Fairburn, C. G. (1997). Primary prevention of eating disorders: Might it do more harm than good? *International Journal of Eating Disorders*, *22*, 167–172.

Casper, R. C., & Jabine, L. N. (1996). An eight-year follow-up: outcome from adolescent compared to adult onset anorexia nervosa. *Journal of Youth and Adolescence*, *25*, 499–517.

Corcos, M., Flament, M. F., Giraud, M. J., Paterniti, S., Ledoux, S., Atger, F., & Jeammet, P. (2000). Early psychopathological signs in bulimia nervosa. A retrospective comparison of the period of puberty in bulimic and control girls. *European Child & Adolescent Psychiatry*, *9*,115–121.

Dansky, B. S., Brewerton, T. D., & Kilpatrick, D. G. (2000). Comorbidity of bulimia nervosa and alcohol use disorders: Results from the national women's study. *International Journal of Eating Disorders*, *27*, 180–190.

Dare, C. & Eisler, I. (2000). A multi-family group day treatment program for adolescent eating disorder. *European Eating Disorders Review*, *81*, 4–18.

Davis, C., & Claridge, G. (1998). The eating disorders as addiction: A psychobiological perspective. *Addictive Behaviors*, *23*, 463–475.

Davis, C., & Katzman, M. (1999). Perfectionism as acculturation: Psychological correlates of eating problems in Chinese male and female students living in the United States. *International Journal of Eating Disorders*, *25*, 65–70.

Devlin, M. J., Goldfein, J. A., Carino, J. S., & Wolk, S. L. (2000). Open treatment of overweight binge eaters with phentermine and fluoxetine as an adjunct to cognitive-behavioral therapy. *International Journal of Eating Disorders*, *28*, 325–332.

Drewnowski, A., Kurth, C. L., & Krahn, D. D. (1995). Effects of body image on dieting, exercise, and anabolic steroid use in adolescent males. *International Journal of Eating Disorders*, *17*, 381–386.

Eldredge, K. L., & Agras, W. S. (1997). The relationship between perceived evaluation of weight and treatment outcome among individuals with binge-eating disorder. *International Journal of Eating Disorders*, *22*, 43–49.

Fairburn, C. G. (1981). A cognitive behavioral approach to the management of bulimia. *Psychological Medicine*, *11*, 707–711.

Fairburn, C. G., Cooper, Z., Doll, H. A., Norman, P., & OConnor, M. (2000). The natural course of bulimia nervosa and binge eating disorder in young women. *Archives of General Psychiatry*, *57*, 659–665.

Fairburn, C. G., Cooper, Z., Doll, H. A., & Welch, S. L. (1999). Risk factors for anorexia nervosa: Three integrated case-control comparisons. *Archives of General Psychiatry*, *56*, 468–476.

Fairburn, C. G., Norman, P. A., Welch, S. L., O'Connor, M. E., Doll, H. A., & Peveler, R. C. (1995). A prospective study of outcome in bulimia nervosa and the long-term effects of three psychological treatments. *Archives of General Psychiatry*, *52*, 304–312.

Fairburn, C. G., Shafran, R., & Cooper, Z. (1998). A cognitive behavioral theory of anorexia nervosa. *Behavior Research and Therapy*, *37*, 1–13.

Fairburn, C. G., Welch, S. L., Doll, H. A., Davies, B. A., & OConnor, M. E. (1997). Risk factors for bulimia nervosa—A community-based case-control study. *Archives of General Psychiatry*, *54*, 509–517.

Fennig, S., & Roe, D. (2002). Physical recovery in anorexia nervosa: Is this the sole purpose of a child and adolescent medical-psychiatric unit? *General Hospital Psychiatry*, *24*, 87–92.

Fichter, M. M., Krueger, R., Rief, W., Holland, R., & Doehne, J. (1996). Fluvoxamine in prevention of relapse in bulimia nervosa: Effects on eating-specific psychopathology. *Journal of Clinical Psychopharmacology*, *16*, 9–18.

Fichter, M. M., Quadflieg, N., & Gnutzmann, A. (1998). Binge eating disorder: Treatment outcome over a 6-year course. *Journal of Psychosomatic Research*, *44*, 385–405.

Fisher, M., Schneider, M., Burns, J., Symons, H., & Mandel, F. S. (2001). Differences between adolescents and young adults at presentation to an eating disorders program. *Journal of Adolescent Health*, *28*, 222–227.

Fombonne, E. (1996). Is bulimia nervosa increasing in frequency? *International Journal of Eating Disorders*, *19*, 287–296.

Freeman, R. J., Beach, B., Davis, R. & Solyom, L. (1985). The prediction of relapse in bulimia nervosa. *Journal of Psychiatric Research*, *19*, 349–353.

Garfinkel, P. E., Lin, E., Goering, P., Spegg, C., Goldbloom, D., Kennedy, S., Kaplan, A., & Woodside, D. B. (1996). Should amenorrhoea be necessary for the diagnosis of anorexia nervosa? Evidence from a Canadian community sample. *British Journal of Psychiatry*, *168*, 500–506.

Garner, D. M., & Bemis K. M. (1982). A cognitive behavioral approach to the treatment of anorexia nervosa. *Cognitive Therapy and Research, 6*, 123–150.

Garner, D. M., Olmsted, M. P., & Polivy, J. (1983). Development and validation of a multidimensional eating disorder inventory for anorexia nervosa and bulimia. *International Journal of Eating Disorders, 2*, 15–34.

Garner, D. M., Olmstead, M., Polivy, J., & Garfinkel, P. E. (1984). Comparison between weight preoccupied women and anorexia nervosa. *Psychosomatic Medicine, 46*, 255–266.

Geist, R., Heinmaa, M., Stephens, D., Davis, R., & Katzman, D. K. (2000). Comparison of family therapy and family group psyhoeducation in adolescents with anorexia nervosa. *Canadian Journal of Psychiatry—Revue Canadienne de Psychiatrie, 45*, 173–178.

Goldner, E. M., Geller, J., Birmingham, C. L., & Remick, H. A. (2000). Comparison of shoplifting behaviours in patients with eating disorders, psychiatric control subjects, and undergraduate control subjects. *Canadian Journal of Psychiatry—Revue Canadienne de Psychiatrie, 45*, 471–475.

Goldstein, D. J., Wilson, M., Thompson, V. L., Potvin, J., & Rampey, A. H. (1995). Long term fluoxetine treatment of bulimia nervosa. *The British Journal of Psychiatry, 166*, 660–666.

Gonzalez, R. G. (1988). Bulimia and adolescence: Individual psychoanalytic treatment. In H. J. Schwartz (Ed.), *Bulimia: Psychoanalytic treatment and theory* (pp. 339–441). Madison, CT: International Universities Press.

Grant, K., Lyons, A., Landis, D., Cho, M., Scudiero, M., Reynolds, L., Murphy, J., & Bryant, H. (1999). Gender, body image, and depressive symptoms among low-income African American adolescents. *Journal of Social Issues, 55*, 299–315.

Haworth-Hoeppner, S. (2000). The critical shapes of body image: The role of culture and family in the production of eating disorders. *Journal of Marriage and the Family, 62*, 212–227.

Hay, P., & Fairburn, C. (1998). The validity of the DSM-IV scheme for classifying bulimic eating disorders. *International Journal of Eating Disorders, 23*, 7–15.

Heatherton, T. F., & Polivy, J. (1992). Chronic dieting and eating disorders: A spiral model. In J. Crowther, S. E. Hobfall, M. A. P. Stephens, & D. L. Tennenbaum (Eds.), *The etiology of bulimia: The individual and familial context* (pp. 133–155). Washington, DC: Hemisphere.

Herpertz-Dahlmann, B., Muller, B., Herpertz, S., Heusen, N., Hebebrand, J., & Remschmidt, H. (2001). Prospective 10-year follow-up in adolescent anorexia nervosa—Course, outcome, psychiatric comorbidity, and psychosocial adaptation. *Journal of Child Psychology and Psychiatry and Allied Disciplines, 42*, 603–612.

Herzog, D. B. (1995). Psychodynamic psychotherapy for anorexia nervosa. In K. D. Brownell & C. G. Fairburn (Eds.), *Eating disorders and obesity: A comprehensive handbook* (pp. 330–335). New York: Guilford.

Herzog, D. B., Dorer, D. J., Keel, P. K., Selwyn, S. E., Ekeblad, E. R., Flores, A. T., Greenwood, D. N., Burwell, R. A., & Keller, M. B. (1999). Recovery and relapse in anorexia and bulimia nervosa: A 7.5-year follow-up study. *Journal of the American Academy of Child and Adolescent Psychiatry, 38*, 829–837.

Herzog, D. B., Greenwood, D. N., Dorer, D. J., Flores, A. T., Ekeblad, E. R., Richards, A., Blais, M. A., & Keller, M. B. (2000). Mortality in eating disorders: A descriptive study. *International Journal of Eating Disorders, 28*, 20–26.

Herzog, D. B., Keller, M., Strober, M., Yeh, C., & Pai, S. (1992). Psychiatric comorbidity in treatment seeking anorexics and bulimics. *Journal of the American Academy of Child and Adolescent Psychiatry, 31*, 810–818.

Hoek, H. W. (1993). Review of the epidemiological studies of eating disorders. *International Review of Psychiatry, 5*, 61–74.

Howard, W. T., Evans, K. K., Quintero-Howard, C. V., Bowers, W. A., & Andersen, A. E. (1999). Predictors of success or failure of transition to day hospital treatment for inpatients with anorexia nervosa. *American Journal of Psychiatry, 156*, 1697–1702.

Hudson, J. I., Carter, W. P., & Pope, H. G. (1996). Antidepressant treatment of binge-eating disorder: Research findings and clinical guidelines. *Journal of Clinical Psychiatry, 57*(Suppl. 8), 73–79.

Hudson, J. I., Pope, H. G., and Jonas, J. M. (1983). Phenomenologic relationship of eating disorders to major affective disorder. *Psychiatry Research, 9*, 345–354.

Johnson, C. (1995). Psychodynamic treatment of bulimia nervosa. In K. D. Brownell & C. G. Fairburn (Eds.), *Eating disorders and obesity: A comprehensive handbook* (pp. 349–353). New York: Guilford.

Johnson, C., & Connors, M. E. (1987). *The etiology and treatment of bulimia nervosa*. New York: Basic Books.

Johnson, W. G., Boutelle, K. N., Torgrud, L., Davig, J. P., & Turner, S. (2000). What is a binge? The influence of amount, duration, and loss of control criteria on judgments of binge eating. *International Journal of Eating Disorders, 27*, 471–479.

Johnson, W. G., Carr-Nangle, R. E., Nangle, D. W., Antony, M. M., & Zayfert, C. (1997). What is binge eating? A comparison of binge eater, peer, and professional judgments of eating episodes. *Addictive Behaviors, 22*, 631–635.

Joiner, T. E., Vohs, K. D., & Heatherton, T. F. (2000). Three studies on the factorial distinctiveness of binge eating and bulimic symptoms among non-clinical men and women. *International Journal of Eating Disorders, 27*, 198–205.

Kahm, A. (1994). Recovery through nutritional counseling. In B. P. Kinoy (Ed.), *Eating disorders: New directions in treatment and recovery* (pp. 15–47). New York: Columbia University Press.

Kaye, W. H. (1997). Anorexia nervosa, obsessional behavior, and serotonin. *Psychopharmacological Bulletin, 33,* 335–344.

Kaye, W., Gendall, K., & Strober, M. (1998). Serotonin neuronal function and selective serotonin reuptake inhibitor treatment in anorexia and bulimia nervosa. *Biological Psychiatry, 44,* 825–838.

Kaye, W. H., Weltzin, T., & Hsu, L. G. (1993). Relationship between anorexia nervosa and obsessive and compulsive behaviors. *Psychiatric Annals, 23,* 365–373.

Keel, P. K., Mitchell, J. E., Miller, K. B., Davis, T. L., & Crow, S. (1999). Long-term outcome of bulimia nervosa. *Archives of General Psychiatry, 56,* 63–69.

Keller, M. B., Herzog, D. B., Lavori, P. W., Bradburn, I. S., & Mahoney, E. M. (1992). The naturalistic history of bulimia nervosa: Extraordinarily high rates of chronicity, relapse, recurrence, and psychosocial morbidity. *International Journal of Eating Disorders, 12,* 1–9.

Klump, K. L., Kaye, W. H., & Strober, M. (2001). The evolving genetic foundations of eating disorders. *Psychiatric Clinics of North America, 24,* 215–226.

Kruger, S., & Kennedy, S. H. (2000). Psychopharmacotherapy of anorexia nervosa, bulimia nervosa and binge-eating disorder. *Journal of Psychiatry and Neuroscience, 25,* 497–508.

Laliberte, M., Boland, F. J., & Leichner, P. (1999). Family climates: Family factors specific to disturbed eating and bulimia nervosa. *Journal of Clinical Psychology, 55,* 1021–1040.

Lansky, D. & Levitt, J. L. (1992). Multifaceted treatment of patients with severe eating disorders. In C. E. Stout, J. L. Levitt, & D. H. Ruben (Eds.), *Handbook for assessing and treating addictive disorders* (pp. 181–202). New York: Greenwood.

Leon, G., Fulkerson, J. A., Perry, C., & Early-Zald, M. B. (1995). Prospective analysis of personality and behavioral vulnerabilities and gender influences in the later development of disordered eating. *Journal of Abnormal Psychology, 104,* 140–149.

Leung, F., Geller, J., & Katzman, M. (1996). Issues and concerns associated with different risk models for eating disorders. *International Journal of Eating Disorder, 19,* 249–256.

Levine, M. D., Marcus, M. D., & Moulton, P. (1996). Exercise in the treatment of binge eating disorder. *International Journal of Eating Disorders, 19,* 171–177.

Lilenfeld, L. R. R., Stein, D., Bulik, C. M., Strober, M., Plotnicov, K., Pollice, C., Rao, R., Merikangas, K. R., Nagy, L., & Kaye, W. H. (2000). Personality traits among currently eating disordered, recovered and never ill first-degree female relatives of bulimic and control women. *Psychological Medicine, 30,* 1399–1410.

Loeb, K. L., Wilson, G. T., Gilbert, J. S., & Labouvie, E. (2000). Guided and unguided self-help for binge eating. *Behavior Research & Therapy, 38,* 259–272.

Matsunaga, H., Kaye, W. H., McConaa, C., Plotnicov, K., Pollice, C., & Rao, R. (2000). Personality disorders among subjects recovered from eating disorders. *International Journal of Eating Disorders, 27,* 353–357.

Matsunaga, H., Kiriike, N., Iwasaki, Y., Miyata, A., Matsui, T., Nagata, T., Yamagami, S., & Kaye, W. H. (2000). Multi-impulsivity among bulimic patients in Japan. *International Journal of Eating Disorders, 27,* 348–352.

Mayer, L. E. S., & Walsh, B. T. (1998). The use of selective serotonin reuptake inhibitors in eating disorders. *Journal of Clinical Psychiatry, 59*(Suppl. 15), 28–34.

McElroy, S. L., Casuto, L. S., Nelson, E. B., Lake, K. A., Soutullo, C. A., Keck, P. E., & Hudson, J. I. (2000). Placebo controlled trial of sertraline in the treatment of binge eating disorder. *The American Journal of Psychiatry, 157,* 1004–1006.

McFarlane, T., Polivy, J., & Herman, C. P. (1998). The effects of false feedback about weight on restrained and unrestrained eaters. *Journal of Abnormal Psychology, 107,* 312–318.

Miller, K. B. (2000). The long-term course of bulimia nervosa: Relapse, recovery, and comorbidity over time. *Dissertation Abstracts International, 61*(1-B), 542.

Mills, J., Polivy, J., Herman, C. P., & Tiggemann, M. (2002). Effects of media-portrayed idealized body images on restrained and unrestrained eaters. *Personality and Social Psychology Bulletin, 28,* 1687–1699.

Minuchin, S., Rosman, B. L., & Baker, L. (1978). *Psychosomatic families: Anorexia nervosa in context.* Cambridge, MA: Harvard University Press.

Mitchell, J. E., Davis, L. & Goff, G. (1985). The process of relapse in patients with bulimia. *International Journal of Eating Disorders, 4,* 457–463.

Mulholland, A. M., & Mintz, L. B., (2001). Prevalence of eating disorders among African American women. *Journal of Counseling Psychology, 48,* 111–116.

Nasser, M. (1997). *Culture and weight consciousness.* New York: Routledge.

Nevonen, L., & Broberg, A. G. (2000). The emergence of eating disorders: An exploratory study. *European Eating Disorders Review, 8,* 279–292.

Nisbett, R. E. & Wilson, T. D. (1977). Telling more than we can know: Verbal reportson mental processes. *Psychological Review, 84,* 231–259.

Nowak, M. (1998). The weight-conscious adolescent: Body image, food intake, and weight-related behavior. *Journal of Adolescent Health, 23,* 389–398.

Ogden, J., & Elder, C. (1998). The role of family status and ethnic group on body image and eating behavior. *International Journal of Eating Disorders, 23,* 309–315.

Olmsted, M. P., & Kaplan, A. S. (1995). Psychoeducation in the treatment of eating disorders. In K. D. Brownell & C. G. Fairburn (Eds.), *Eating Disorders and obesity: A comprehensive handbook* (pp. 299–305). New York: Guilford.

Olmsted, M. P., Kaplan, A. S., & Rockert, W. (1994). Rate and prediction of relapse in bulimia nervosa. *American Journal of Psychiatry, 151,* 738–743.

Peterson, C. B., Crow, S. J., Nugent, S., Mitchell, J. E., Engbloom, S., & Mussell, M. P. (2000). Predictors of treatment outcome for binge eating disorder. *International Journal of Eating Disorders, 28,* 131–138.

Pike, K. M. (1998). Long-term course of anorexia nervosa: Response, relapse, remission, and recovery. *Clinical Psychology Review, 18,* 447–475.

Pinhas, L., Toner, B. B., Ali, A., Garfinkel, P. E., & Stuckless, N. (1999). The effects of the ideal of female beauty on mood and body satisfaction. *International Journal of Eating Disorders, 25,* 223–226.

Polivy, J., & Herman, C. P. (1987). Diagnosis and treatment of normal eating. *Journal of Consulting & Clinical Psychology, 55,* 635–644.

Polivy, J., & Herman, C. P. (1993). Etiology of binge eating: Psychological mechanisms. In C. G. Fairburn and G. T. Wilson (Eds.), *Binge eating: Nature, assessment and treatment* (pp. 173–205). New York: Guilford.

Polivy, J., & Herman, C. P. (2002). Causes of eating disorders. *Annual Review of Psychology, 53,* 187–213.

Polivy, J., Herman, C. P., Mills, J., & Wheeler, H. B. (2003). Eating disorders in adolescence. In G. Adams & M. Berzonsky (Eds.), *The Blackwell handbook of adolescence.* Oxford: Blackwell, pp. 523–549.

Pryor, T., Wiederman, M. W., & Mcgilley, B. (1996). Laxative abuse among women with eating disorders: An indication of psychopathology? *International Journal of Eating Disorders, 20,* 13–18.

Rooney, B., Mcclelland, L., Crisp, A. H., & Sedgwick, P. M. (1995). The incidence and prevalence of anorexia nervosa in three suburban health districts in south west London, UK. *International Journal of Eating Disorders, 18,* 299–307.

Russell, G. F. M., Dare, C., Eisler, I., & Le Grange, P. D. F. (1992). Controlled trials of family treatments in anorexia nervosa. In K. A. Halmi (Ed.), *Psychobiology and treatment of anorexia nervosa and bulimia nervosa* (pp. 237–262). Washington, DC: American Psychiatric Press.

Schlundt, D. G., & Johnson, W. G. (1990). *Eating disorders: Assessment and treatment.* Boston: Allyn & Bacon.

Schork, E. J., Eckert, E. D., & Halmi, K. A. (1994). The relationship between psychopathology, eating disorder diagnosis, and clinical outcome at 10-year follow-up in anorexia nervosa. *Comprehensive Psychiatry, 35,* 113–123.

Shapira, N. A., Goldsmith, T. D., & McElroy, S. L. (2000). Treatment of binge eating disorder with topiramate: A clinical case series. *Journal of Clinical Psychiatry, 61,* 368–372.

Shisslak, C. M., Crago, M., & Estes, L. S. (1995). The spectrum of eating disturbances. *International Journal of Eating Disorders, 18,* 209–219.

Smolak, L., & Levine, M. P. (1996). Adolescent transitions and the development of eating problems. In L. Smolak, M. Levine, & R. Striegel-Moore (Eds.), *The developmental psychopathology of eating disorders: Implications for research, prevention, and treatment* (pp. 210–231). Mahwah, NJ: Lawrence Erlbaum Associates.

Smolak, L., Levine, M. P., & Schermer, F. (1998). A controlled evaluation of an elementary school primary prevention program for eating problems. *Journal of Psychosomatic Research, 44,* 339–353.

Steiger, H., Young, S. N., Kin, N. M. K., Koerner, N., Israel, M., Lageix, P., & Paris, J. (2001). Implications of impulsive and affective symptoms for serotonin function in bulimia nervosa. *Psychological Medicine, 31,* 85–95.

Steinhausen, H. C., Seidel, R., & Metzke, C. W. (2000). Evaluation of treatment and intermediate and long-term outcome of adolescent eating disorders. *Psychological Medicine, 30,* 1089–1098.

Stice, E. (2001). A prospective test of the dual-pathway model of bulimic pathology: Mediating effects of dieting and negative affect. *Journal of Abnormal Psychology, 110,* 1–12.

Stice, E., & Shaw, H. (1994). Adverse effects of the media portrayed thin-ideal on women and linkages to bulimic symptomatology. *Journal of Social and Clinical Psychology, 13,* 288–308.

Striegel-Moore, R. H. (1993). Etiology of binge eating: A developmental perspective. In C. G. Fairburn & G. T. Wilson (Eds.), *Binge eating: Nature, assessment and treatment* (pp. 144–172). New York: Guilford.

Striegel-Moore, R. H., Garvin, V., Dohm, F. A., & Rosenheck, R. A. (1999). Eating disorders in a national sample of hospitalized female and male veterans: Detection rates and psychiatric comorbidity. *International Journal of Eating Disorders, 25,* 405–414.

Striegel-Moore, R. H., Schreiber, G. B., Lo, A., Crawford, P., Obarzanek, E., & Rodin, J. (2000). Eating disorder symptoms in a cohort of 11 to 16-year-old black and white girls: The NHLBI growth and health study. *International Journal of Eating Disorders, 27*, 49–66.

Strober, M. (1980). Personality and symptomatological features in young, nonchronic anorexia nervosa patients. *Journal of Psychosomatic Research, 24*, 353–359.

Strober, M., Freeman, R., Lampert, C., Diamond, J., & Kaye, W. (2000). Controlled family study of anorexia nervosa and bulimia nervosa: Evidence of shared liability and transmission of partial syndromes. *American Journal of Psychiatry, 157*, 393–401.

Strober, M., Freeman, R., & Morell, W. (1997). The long-term course of anorexia nervosa in adolescents: Survival analysis of recovery, relapse, and outcome predictors over 10–15 years in a prospective study. *International Journal of Eating Disorders, 22*, 339–360.

Strober, M., & Humphrey, L. L. (1987). Familial contributions to the etiology and course of anorexia nervosa and bulimia. *Journal of Consulting and Clinical Psychology, 55*, 654–659.

Strober, M., & Katz, J. L. (1988). Depression in the eating disorders: A review and analysis of descriptive, family and biological findings. In D. M. Garner & P. E. Garfinkel (Eds.), *Diagnostic issues in anorexia nervosa and bulimia nervosa* (pp. 80–111). New York: Brunner/Mazel.

Sullivan, P. F. (1995). Mortality in anorexia nervosa. *American Journal of Psychiatry, 152*, 1073–1074.

Theander, S. (1996). Anorexia nervosa with an early onset: selection, gender, outcome, and results of a long-term follow-up study. *Journal of Youth and Adolescence, 25*, 419–429.

Thode, N. (1990). A family systems perspective on recovery from an eating disorder. In B. P. Kinoy (Ed.), *Eating disorders: New directions in treatment and recovery* (pp. 61–79). New York: Columbia University Press.

VanderHam, T., Meulman, J. J., VanStrien, D. C., VanEngeland, H. (1997). Empirically based subgrouping of eating disorders in adolescents: A longitudinal perspective. *British Journal of Psychiatry, 170*, 363–368.

Vanfurth, E. F., Vanstrien, D. C., Martina, L. M. L., Vanson, M. J. M., Hendrickx, J. J. P., & VanEngeland, H. (1996). Expressed emotion and the prediction of outcome in adolescent eating disorders. *International Journal of Eating Disorder, 20*, 19–31.

Vitousek, K. B. (1995). Cognitive behavioral therapy for anorexia nervosa. In K. D. Brownell & C. G. Fairburn (Eds.), *Eating disorders and obesity–A comprehensive handbook* (pp. 324–329). New York: Guilford.

Vogeltanz-Holm, N. D., Wonderlich, S. A., Lewis, B. A., Wilsnack, S. C., Harris, T. R., Wilsnack, R. W., & Kristjanson, A. F. (2000). Longitudinal predictors of binge eating, intense dieting, and weight concerns in a national sample of women. *Behavior Therapy, 31*, 221–235.

Wakeling, A. (1996). Epidemiology of anorexia nervosa. *Psychiatry Research, 62*, 3–9.

Ward, A., Tiller, J., Treasure, J., & Russell, G. (2000). Eating disorders: Psyche or soma? *International Journal of Eating Disorders, 27*, 279–287.

Wheeler, H. B., Polivy, J., & Herman, C. P. (2002). *The precarious identities of restrained eaters: Effects of a threat.* Unpublished manuscript.

Wilfley, D. E., Friedman, M. A., Dounchis, J. Z., Stein, R. I., Welch, R. R., & Ball, S. A. (2000). Comorbid psychopathology in binge eating disorder: Relation to eating disorder severity at baseline and following treatment. *Journal of Consulting and Clinical Psychology, 68*, 641–649.

Williamson, D. A., Muller, S. L., Reas, D. L., & Thaw, J. M. (1999). Cognitive bias in eating disorders: Implications for theory and treatment. *Behavior Modification, 23*, 556–577.

Wilson, G. T. (1991). The addiction model of eating disorders: A critical analysis. *Advances in Behavior Research and Therapy, 13*, 27–72.

Wilson, G. T. (1996). Treatment of bulimia nervosa: when CBT fails. *Behavior Research and Therapy, 34*, 197–212.

Wilson, G. T. (1999). Cognitive behavior therapy for eating disorders: Progress and problems. *Behavior Research and Therapy, 37*, S79–S95.

Wilson, G. T., & Fairburn, C. G. (2000). The treatment of binge eating disorder. *European Eating Disorders Review, 8*, 351–354.

Wolfe, B. E., Metzger, E. D., & Jimerson, D. C. (1997). Research update on serotonin function in bulimia nervosa and anorexia nervosa. *Psychopharmacology Bulletin, 33*, 345–357.

Wonderlich, S. (1995). Personality and eating disorders. In K. D. Brownell & C. G. Fairburn (Eds.), *Eating disorders and obesity: A comprehensive handbook* (pp. 171–176). New York: Guilford.

Wonderlich, S., & Mitchell, J. E. (2001). The role of personality in the onset of eating disorders and treatment implications. *Psychiatric Clinics of North America, 24*, 249–258.

Woods, S. C., & Brief, D. J. (1988). Physiological factors. In D. M. Donovan & G. A. Marlatt (Eds.), *Assessment of addictive behaviors* (pp. 296–322). New York: Guilford.

Zubieta, J. K., Demitrack, M. A., Fenick, A., & Krahn, D. D. (1995). Obsessionality in eating disorder patients: Relationship to clinical presentation and two year outcome. *Journal of Psychiatric Research, 29*, 333–342.

12

Sexual Dysfunctions and Disorders

Nathaniel McConaghy
University of New South Wales

The majority of men and women have occasional experiences that could be labeled sexual dysfunctions or disorders. The most common are occasional failures to obtain or maintain an erection, or to ejaculate before they wish to do so in men, and in women failure to reach orgasm when they desire to do so. Others include sexual fantasies usually considered deviant, such as in men, having sex with nonconsenting or under-age partners, and in women, being forced to have sex. Many male adolescents carry out illegal sexual behaviors, that is, sexual offenses, such as sexual exhibitionism, voyeurism, and making obscene phone calls, most of which are not reported to authorities. The decision of what is normal sexual behavior is arbitrary, determined by social attitudes. Masturbation and homosexuality, strongly condemned in the past as immoral and unnatural, subsequently became classified as sexual disorders, and are now accepted as normal expressions of sexuality.

DEFINITIONS AND DESCRIPTIONS OF THE DISORDERS

In the absence of nonarbitrary criteria as to what are sexual dysfunctions and disorders, recourse is made to decisions by authorities. The prestige of the *Diagnostic and Statistical Manual of Mental Disorders* (DSM), published and regularly revised by the American Psychiatric Association, has resulted in its classification of disorders in patients with sexual problems being that accepted by the majority of clinicians and researchers. The current version, the DSM–IV–TR (American Psychiatric Association [APA], 2000) introduced some minor revisions to the DSM–IV (American Psychiatric Association [APA], 1994). Both classify sexual disorders as sexual dysfunctions, paraphilias, and gender identity disorders. As most of the behaviors that can be given these diagnoses are dimensionally distributed in the population, to discriminate those considered to justify the label of disorder, both manuals provided additional requirements to the criteria for diagnosis of the disorders, namely that the conditions cause distress or interpersonal problems.

Sexual Dysfunctions

The DSM–IV–TR provided diagnostic criteria for four groups of sexual dysfunctions.

- Sexual desire disorders—hypoactive sexual desire, deficiency or absence of sexual fantasies and desire for sexual activity; and sexual aversion disorder, aversion to and active avoidance of genital sexual contact with a sexual partner. The aversion can be to nongenital sexual activities, such as kissing and general body touching, including touching mutilated areas, such as those due to breast surgery.
- Sexual arousal disorders—in women, inability to attain, or to maintain until completion of the sexual activity, an adequate lubrication-swelling response of sexual excitement; in men, erectile disorder, a similar inability in relation to adequate erection.
- Orgasm disorders—in women and men, delay in, or absence of, orgasm following a normal sexual excitement phase; also in men, premature ejaculation, onset of orgasm and ejaculation with minimal sexual stimulation before, on, or shortly after penetration and before the person wishes.
- Sexual pain disorders—dyspareunia, genital pain in either males or females before, during, or after sexual intercourse; and vaginismus, involuntary spasm of the musculature of the outer third of the vagina that interferes with sexual intercourse. Vaginismus usually prevents penetration of any object above a certain size into the vagina, such as a finger or tampon. If intercourse is attempted, vaginismus is commonly accompanied by spasm of the adductor muscles of the thighs preventing their separation. Vaginismus does not prevent women experiencing sexual arousal and orgasm with activities that do not involve vaginal penetration.

To receive a DSM–IV–TR diagnosis of sexual dysfunction in these four categories, the condition must be recurrent or persistent and cause marked distress or interpersonal difficulty. The latter requirement means that most of the conditions just described would not be diagnosed as dysfunctions in the large number of subjects who report them on questioning but do not consider them problems for themselves or their partners.

DSM–IV–TR Definitions of Sexual Dysfunctions Are Not Operational

To diagnose hypoactive sexual desire, arousal, and orgasmic disorders, DSM–IV–TR states the clinician should take into account factors affecting sexual functioning. These include adequacy of sexual stimulation in focus, intensity, and duration; novelty of the sexual partner; recent frequency of sexual activity; and the subject's age and sexual experience. The DSM was introduced with the expectation that it would increase the reliability of clinical diagnosis, that is, the likelihood that different clinicians would make the same diagnosis with a particular patient. To achieve this goal, the diagnostic definitions it supplied were intended to be operational. Criteria were to be supplied for each step or operation in reaching the diagnosis, and these criteria were to be defined sufficiently precisely that all clinicians would make the same decision concerning them. No such operational criteria were provided in DSM–IV or DSM–IV–TR, however, to enable the clinician to take into account the factors mentioned earlier as affecting sexual functioning, perhaps because it was not considered possible. Hence it is unlikely that the reliability of the diagnoses of sexual dysfunctions made using the DSM–IV–TR definitions would be high if clinicians give significant weight to these factors in making their diagnoses, rather than to the patient's decision that the condition causes marked distress or interpersonal difficulty. Unfortunately, as O'Donohue, Regev, and Hagstrom (2000) pointed out, there is no empirical information of the reliability or validity of DSM–IV diagnoses of sexual disorders, because of their being ignored in DSM field trials.

High reliability is necessary in research to ensure that patients given a particular diagnosis in one study have the same condition as those given the diagnosis in other studies. This approach requires not only the use of operationally defined diagnoses, but of standardized interviews to obtain the information on which the diagnoses are made. Such interviews ensure that interviewers in different studies base their diagnoses on information obtained in the same way. Unlike most psychiatric conditions, no standardized structured interviews have been developed to make such diagnoses for the dysfunctions or the other sexual disorders (Raymond, Coleman, Ohlerking, Christenson, & Miner, 1999). Hence, though the DSM classification of sexual disorders is generally accepted, its diagnostic criteria are rarely used in research studies. Some researchers created their own operationally defined criteria. These included, for orgasmic dysfunction in women, that orgasm resulted from 5% or less of all sexual activities with their partners (Kelly, Strassberg, & Kircher, 1990). However few clinicians would consider making a diagnosis on the basis of a single variable. Rowland, Cooper, and Schneider (2001) reported a flowchart designed to produce an operationally defined diagnosis of premature ejaculation based on DSM–IV criteria. Its complexity and ideal requirement that subjects time their latency to ejaculation with a stopwatch over a 6-month period makes its use in clinical practice unlikely. Use of arbitrary criteria for diagnosis of hypoactive or inhibited sexual desire has allowed the diagnosis to be made for women and men who show evidence of significant sexual interest (McConaghy, 1993). If subjects who report acceptable frequencies of sexual activity complain of reduced desire, it is necessary to establish that they are having intercourse from obligation to their partner rather than from desire. Subjects who report low frequencies may be avoiding sexual activity because of dissatisfaction with their sexual relationship rather than reduced desire.

Sexual Difficulties

Reflecting its development from a medical rather than a social model, the DSM–IV–TR classification of sexual dysfunction does not include what have been termed sexual difficulties. A study of White middle-class happily married couples found 77% of the women and 50% of the men reported difficulties related to the emotional tone of their sexual relations (Frank, Anderson, & Rubinstein, 1978). Those in women included inability to relax, too little foreplay before intercourse, disinterest, their partner choosing an inconvenient time, and/or being "turned off." The men reported attraction to persons other than the spouse, too little foreplay before intercourse, too little tenderness after intercourse, disinterest, and their partner choosing an inconvenient time. Dysfunctions were reported by 63% percent of the women and 40% of the men. The most common dysfunctions in women were difficulty getting excited and difficulty reaching orgasm; and in men, ejaculating too quickly, and difficulty getting and maintaining an erection. However, 85% of both men and women stated their sexual relations were very or moderately satisfying, so that most of these conditions would not receive a DSM–IV–TR diagnosis of sexual dysfunction, in view of the requirement that the disturbance causes marked distress or interpersonal difficulty.

Sexual Difficulties Are More Strongly Related to Sexual Satisfaction Than Are Dysfunctions.
Frank et al. (1978) found that the presence of the sexual difficulties in both the women and men correlated more highly with the subjects' lack of sexual satisfaction than did the presence of dysfunctions. Other studies of nonpatients found no relationship between the presence of sexual dysfunctions and sexual satisfaction (McConaghy, 1993).

Nettelbladt and Uddenberg (1979) concluded that couples' sexual satisfaction was related to their emotional relationship rather than their sexual function. Hallstrom and Samuelsson (1990) at 6-year follow-up of middle-aged women found that decrease in self-reported desire was predicted by lack of a confiding relationship and insufficient support from their spouses. Phelps, Albo, Dunn, and Joseph (2001) found partner satisfaction, relationship quality, and sexual desire were significantly related to the sexual satisfaction and behavior of fifty married or partnered men with spinal cord injury. Erectile function, level of genital sensation, and orgasmic capacity, all of which varied widely, were not. Snyder and Berg (1983) showed that the conclusions of Frank et al. (1978) and Nettelbladt and Uddenberg (1979) also applied to patients. In couples presenting with lack of sexual satisfaction to a sexual dysfunctions clinic, though dysfunctions were common complaints of both the men and women, their prevalence was lower than more general interpersonal difficulties. No dysfunctions reported by the women correlated with their sexual dissatisfaction, and only failure to ejaculate during intercourse correlated with that of men. Among both sexes, dissatisfaction correlated strongly with the partner's lack of response to sexual requests and with the frequency of intercourse being too low. Though sexual difficulties and the related sexual dissatisfaction are not classified as sexual disorders by the DSM–IV–TR, clearly they require assessment, as does the couple's emotional relationship, if their problems with their sexual lives are to be appropriately diagnosed and treated.

Paraphilias

DSM–IV–TR Definition of Paraphilias

The DSM–IV–TR states the essential features of paraphilias are recurrent, intense sexually arousing fantasies, sexual urges, or behaviors generally involving (a) nonhuman objects, (b) the suffering or humiliation of oneself or one's partner, or (c) children or other nonconsenting persons that occur over a period of at least 6 months. DSM–IV–TR gives descriptive criteria for commoner paraphilic behaviors, including exhibitionism, voyeurism, sexual masochism, sexual sadism, frotteurism (sexual arousal by touching and rubbing against a nonconsenting person), fetishism (sexual arousal to nonliving objects), and transvestic fetishism (sexual arousal involving cross-dressing). Despite the reference to nonconsenting persons, rape or sexual assault is not classified as a paraphilia. Pedophilia is, and is defined as recurrent, intense sexually arousing fantasies, sexual urges, or behaviors, occurring over a period of at least 6 months, that involve sexual activity with a prepubescent child or children (generally age 13 years or younger) by a person aged at least 16 years and 5 years older. Hebephilia, sexual activity of an adult with pubertal or immediately postpubertal subjects, is not classified as a paraphilia, though male hebephiles and male pedophiles with male victims share common features. Compared to male hebephiles and male pedophiles with female victims, male hebephiles and male pedophiles with male victims are more likely to commence their offenses in adolescence, and they usually have many more victims against whom they offend less frequently. Their victims are more likely to be unknown to them. Also they are less likely to form close friendships with or be sexually attracted to adults of either sex (McConaghy, 1993).

DSM–IV–TR retained as a diagnostic criterion for a paraphilia that the condition should cause clinically significant distress or impairment in social, occupational, or other important areas of functioning. Many clinicians criticized the criterion as inappropriate for those paraphilic behaviors that are indisputably unacceptable and illegal, yet appear to have caused no distress or impairment to the offender until they were detected (McConaghy, 1997). This was in fact recognized in DSM–IV, when it stated that many individuals with such paraphilias as pedophilia or sexual sadism assert that the behavior causes them no distress and that their only problem is social dysfunction as a result of the reaction of others to their behavior.

As discussed subsequently, the behavior of most pedophiles and sexual sadists is never detected, and so is not reacted to by others. The DSM–IV–TR took the clinicians' criticism into account by changing the specific criteria for pedophilia, voyeurism, exhibitionism, and frotteurism to enable the diagnosis to be made if the person has acted on the urges, and for sexual sadism, if the person has acted on the urges with a nonconsenting person. However, it retained the criterion that the condition should cause clinically significant distress or impairment for the remaining paraphilias. The common offensive behavior of obscene telephoning, which is seldom detected, would therefore not be diagnosed as a paraphilia except in the unusual event that it caused the offender clinically significant distress or impairment in social, occupational, or other important areas of functioning.

The requirement that the paraphilic urges or behaviors must be present over at least 6 months also has generated some controversy. Marshall and Eccles (1991) pointed out that many rapists, incest offenders, exhibitionists, and a substantial number of nonfamilial child molesters do not display or report deviant sexual urges, yet they persistently engage in sexually offensive behaviors. If all their offensive behaviors occurred in a period of less than 6 months, they would not qualify for a DSM–IV–TR diagnosis of paraphilia. Marshall and Eccles (1991) considered that most clinicians tend to ignore DSM diagnoses of paraphilias, a conclusion agreed with by O'Donohue et al. (2000). The subjects who carry out illegal paraphilias are commonly called sex offenders, a term requiring legal definition, not a psychiatric definition.

Social Attitudes and the Exclusion of Homosexuality From Classification of Paraphilias

As pointed out earlier, changes in social values resulted in homosexuality being no longer classified as a sexual disorder in the DSM classification. Acceptance of the term homosexuality for same-sex activities and regarding it as a medical condition rather than a chosen socially and morally unacceptable behavior occurred earlier in the context of the development of sexology as a scientific discipline in late nineteenth century Europe. Foucault in *The History of Sexuality* (1990) claimed that before this "medicalization" of homosexuality,

> *sodomy was a category of forbidden acts; their perpetrator was nothing more than the juridical subject of them. The nineteenth-century homosexual became a personage, a past, a case history, and a childhood . . . Nothing that went into his total composition was unaffected by his sexuality . . . The sodomite had been a temporary aberration; in addition to being a type of life the homosexual was now a species. (p. 43).*

Homosexuality was largely a taboo subject to write about in Europe from the late Roman empire until its medicalization. Nevertheless, there is sufficient evidence that throughout this period both men and women who carried out homosexual acts were regarded as personages (to use Foucault's term). They were considered to show characteristic behavioral features, in particular feminine characteristics in the men and masculine characteristics in the women (McConaghy, 1999a, in press). In eighteenth century England, the men were termed "mollies" and the women "sapphists or tommies" (Trumbach, 1994). Van der Meer (1994) reported evidence from records of the legal persecution of sodomites in the Netherlands that the concept that men and women who carried out same-sex activity had characteristic behavioral features was accepted there from the late seventeenth to the second half of the nineteenth centuries. That is to say, before the medicalization of the nineteenth century, men labeled sodomites were not, as claimed by Foucault, regarded as men who carried out an aberrant act. Rather, they were considered to have behavioral features different from those of other men. Nevertheless, to cite

Jagose (2002), the distinction made by Foucault between the sodomite and the homosexual "has had a massive influence on gay history, everywhere evidenced in the frequent quotation or paraphrase of this passage" (that is, the passage by Foucault cited earlier; p. 11).

Once homosexuality was regarded as a medical disorder, many homosexual subjects, mainly men, sought treatment with the aim of becoming heterosexual. As part of the ideology of liberation movements that developed in the 1960s, gay activists demanded that homosexuality not be seen as a medical disorder, and that such treatment not be attempted. They disrupted a session of the annual conference of the American Psychiatric Association held in San Francisco in 1971 following the presentation of a paper by the author evaluating the effect of aversive therapy in homosexuality. Their demand was probably an important reason for the acceptance of a background report on homosexuality by the Board of Trustees of the American Psychiatric Association in 1973. This report stated that homosexuality, per se, does not meet the requirements for a psychiatric disorder because many homosexual men and women are not distressed by, but are quite satisfied with, their sexual orientation and demonstrate no generalized impairment in social effectiveness or functioning. In its 1973 December meeting, the Board approved the removal of homosexuality from the diagnostic nomenclature. There was opposition by some psychiatrists to its removal, and it was replaced with the diagnosis of "sexual orientation disturbance" in the DSM–II. This diagnosis was criticized as implying that homosexuality was a disorder, and in the 1980 publication of the DSM–III (American Psychiatric Association [APA], 1980), this term was replaced with the diagnosis "ego dystonic homosexuality," which also proved controversial. The DSM–III–R introduced instead a diagnosis of "persistent and marked distress about sexual orientation," a diagnosis retained in the DSM–IV–TR.

Effect of Declassification of Homosexuality as a Paraphilia on Therapist Training.

Once homosexuality ceased to be classified in the DSM, articles about it ceased appearing in journals of clinical psychology (Rothblum, 1994). Consequently, there was comparatively little focus on mental health and treatment issues concerning lesbians and gay men. These issues were dealt with in detail in the *Textbook of Homosexuality and Mental Health* (Cabaj & Stein, 1996). Several contributors noted that although homosexuality was not a disorder, the negative treatment of gays and lesbians and aspects of their lifestyle put them at high risk for mental health problems, particularly in adolescence and early adulthood. A 1989 U.S. Department of Health and Human Services task force report was cited (Hartstein, 1996), which concluded that studies indicated a high rate of suicide attempts among lesbians and gay males, particularly during their youth. It suggested that suicides among lesbians and gay males comprise up to 30% of youth suicides annually. It did not cite research to support this estimate. The report also stated that approximately 30% of lesbians and gay men suffered from substance abuse, particularly alcohol abuse, compared with 10% to 12% of the general population. A greater percentage than members of the general population sought counseling and received mental health services. However, lesbians and gays who received treatment reported that some mental health workers had marked negative reactions to homosexuality, so that many did not reveal their sexual orientation to their therapists.

The authors of one chapter commented that despite the growing body of research that documented the existence of negative attitudes to homosexuality among health care providers, little effort is made to educate them about homosexuality as a normal variant of human sexuality. When education about homosexuality was removed from courses in sexual disorders, previously part of the training of health care providers, it was not replaced with education concerning homosexuality in sexual behavior courses. In a 1992 survey in which 65% of 126 U.S. medical schools responded, only one reported that gay and lesbian issues were integral to its curriculum. The authors suggested that students were not likely to supplement the absence of exposure in their coursework with up-to-date resources. While retaining the emphasis that homosexuality is not a disorder, the education and training of mental health professionals should include more information about the problems and the lifestyles of gays and lesbians. This education should encourage trainees to examine their own attitudes to sexually diverse behaviors and their suitability for working with people with these behaviors.

Coleman and Rosser (1996) suggested that some DSM–IV diagnoses reflect a heterosexist bias. Although terms such as "vaginismus" and "dyspareunia" were used to describe problems in peno-vaginal functioning, there was no equivalent term for problems in anal intercourse. If its absence was due to heterosexism, it indicated a lack of awareness of the prevalence of anal intercourse among heterosexual men and women. Most couples who practice anal intercourse do so in heterosexual activities (McConaghy, 1993). Coleman and Rosser also pointed out that the only example of compulsive sexual behavior in the DSM–IV was that of a heterosexual man who had repeated sexual conquests and saw women as objects to be used. Compulsive sexual behavior is a common problem among gay men, and its recognition and effective treatment is crucial in decreasing the likelihood of their exposure to HIV infection and other sexually transmitted diseases.

Should Sadism, Masochism, and Fetishism Continue to Be Considered Sexual Disorders?

Men and women who perform sexual sadistic and masochistic acts have not actively campaigned for their removal from classification as paraphilias in the DSM. This removal could by justified for the same reasons that homosexuality was removed—that performance of the acts does not meet the requirements for a psychiatric disorder because many who engage in them are not distressed by their behavior and do not demonstrate generalized impairment in social effectiveness or functioning. Men and women with sadistic and masochistic behaviors rarely seek treatment for them, so that information concerning sadomasochists has been mainly obtained by investigating members of "S and M" clubs. About 20% to 30% of the members of such clubs were women, who were more likely to be bisexual than the men, most of whom were predominantly heterosexual. Beating, bondage, and fetishistic practices were common, and more extreme and dangerous practices were rare. The members were of above-average intelligence and social status and most wished to continue sadomasochistic activities (McConaghy, 1993).

The few reports of practicing sadomasochists seeking medical treatment indicate that significant physical damage as a result of their sexual behavior is uncommon. That which is reported usually is the result of fisting, the insertion of the hand and arm into the rectum or the vagina, or of self-insertion of implements. Twenty percent or more men and women report nondistressing sadistic or masochistic sexual fantasies (McConaghy, 1993). The majority of subjects who identify as sadomasochists by joining clubs would not meet the DSM–IV–TR diagnostic criteria for a paraphilia. Diagnosis of sexual masochism requires that the fantasies, urges, or behaviors cause clinically significant distress or impairment in social, occupational, or other important areas of functioning. Diagnosis of sexual sadism requires that the person has acted on the sexual urges with a nonconsenting person or the urges or fantasies cause marked distress or interpersonal difficulty. Acting on heterosexual or homosexual urges with a nonconsenting postpubertal women or man is not diagnosed as a sexual disorder. Homosexual urges or fantasies can cause distress or impairment in some persons, yet homosexuality is not classified as a sexual disorder. It would seem justifiable that sexual sadism and masochism also should not be considered sexual disorders.

A sexual act with a nonconsenting person, whether the act is heterosexual, homosexual, or sadistic, is best viewed as an illegal act rather than a symptom of a psychological disorder (Marshall and Kennedy, 2003). Green (2002) suggested that pedophilia be treated similarly, not as a disorder but an illegal act with a child, who, of course, is a nonconsenting person. He pointed out that sexual arousal patterns to children are reported by and physiologically demonstrable in a substantial minority of people. In the male population, this minority is about 20% (McConaghy, 1993). Green further pointed out that sexual activity of adults with children has been common historically and accepted by various cultures at various times, though this past acceptance did not justify its moral and legal acceptance today. He argued that if arousal to children and sexual activity constituted a mental illness, a lot of people in many cultures and in much of the past must be considered to have been mentally ill. Giving violent sex offenders any kind of diagnosis carries the risk that it absolves them of responsibility for their behavior. Treating their behavior as illegal strengthens the acceptance of the rights of victims of such violence, who are usually women and children.

DSM–IV–TR defined fetishistic behaviors as recurrent, intense sexually arousing fantasies, sexual urges, or behaviors involving the use of nonliving objects (e.g., female undergarments). The behaviors are almost exclusively shown by men, many of whom appear to experience no distress with their fantasies, urges or behaviors and demonstrate no generalized impairment in social effectiveness or functioning. The fetishism of these men is not a sexual disorder, as it does meet the DSM–IV–TR requirement for the diagnosis that distress or impairment is present. When a person with a fetish does seek treatment, it is usually the result of impairment of their emotional relationship due to their partner objecting to such requests as that they wear shoes during sexual activity. Similar impairment can occur with subjects with partialism, when the partner objects to their preoccupation with a bodily part, such as feet or hair.

Compulsive or Addictive Sexuality

Black, Kehrberg, Flumerfelt, and Schlosser (1997) commented that DSM–IV was mute concerning the condition labeled by some therapists as compulsive sexuality and by others as addictive sexuality. Their statement could be contested on the grounds that the DSM–IV diagnosis of "sexual disorder not otherwise specified" (retained in the DSM–IV–TR) included "distress about a pattern of repeated sexual relationships involving a succession of lovers who are experienced by the individual only as things to be used" (p. 582). This diagnosis could be given to many of the people diagnosed as having compulsive sexuality. The fact that this diagnosis does not state that the pattern of repeated relationships is driven by a compulsive or addictive urge was what Black et al. (1997) considered in need of correction. They pointed out the existence of such driven sexual behaviors have recently been the subject of growing interest in professional and lay literature, though they were described by Krafft-Ebbing in the nineteenth century. There is no accepted definition of compulsive sexuality, though inclusion of inability to control repeated sexual acts or thoughts that are experienced as distressing or harmful should be central in any definition. Black et al. (1997) quoted Goodman's (1992) definition that sexual addiction was a form of behavior that could function both to produce pleasure and to provide escape from internal discomfort, and could not be controlled but was continued despite significant harmful consequences.

Black et al. (1992) investigated thirty-six subjects who responded to advertisements for persons who have problems with compulsive sexual behavior. The main compulsive non-paraphilic sexual behaviors they reported were compulsive "cruising," compulsive "fixation," multiple lovers, compulsive sex within relationships, and compulsive masturbation. The typical subject was a 27-year-old man who reported experiencing the compulsive behavior for over

8 years. Compulsive paraphilias were less common and included exhibitionism, sexual sadism, and transvestic fetishism. The respondents showed considerable psychiatric comorbidity, with nearly two-thirds meeting DSM–III–R criteria for a current (past 6 months) major mental disorder, most commonly a substance abuse disorder, anxiety disorder, or a mood disorder. The reader should keep in mind that 30% of a random sample of adult Americans were found to have a DSM–III–R psychiatric or substance abuse disorder in the preceding 12 months (Kessler et al., 1994). Psychoanalyst Bloland (2000) recently diagnosed John F. Kennedy and Bill Clinton as sexual addicts. Bloland pointed out that they were both charismatic figures who achieved enormous popularity as presidents, and that both were revealed as compulsive womanizers who risked their political careers, if not the welfare of the country, in the addictive pursuit of sexual gratification.

DSM–IV–TR Diagnosis of Transvestic Fetishism

The DSM–IV–TR diagnostic criteria for transvestic fetishism are the presence in a hetero-sexual male over a period of at least 6 months, of recurrent, intense sexually arousing fantasies, sexual urges, or behaviors involving cross-dressing. Person, Terestman, Myers, Goldberg, and Salvadori (1989) found that 4% of female university students reported experiencing these fantasies, urges, or behaviors. However, the condition in women rarely comes to the attention of clinicians. In its typical form it is shown by adolescent males who have cross-dressed before puberty, with variable degrees of sexual arousal. The arousal becomes markedly greater at puberty, when the urge to obtain female clothes secretly may lead them to steal from clothes-lines or from neighboring houses, resulting at times in criminal charges. Probably the behavior remains undetected in many of these adolescents.

Cross-Dressing in Adults

An unknown percentage of the male adolescent transvestic fetishists continue to cross-dress periodically into adulthood, when most report the associated sexual arousal diminishes or dis-appears. It is replaced by feelings of being a woman, which they experience as relaxation, relief from responsibility, and/or of sensuality, elegance, and beauty. Initially, many of these men are disturbed by their continuing urges to cross-dress. Croughan, Saghir, Cohen, and Robins (1981) studied seventy men with the condition, 85% of whom belonged to cross-dressing clubs. Half the men had sought help from a mental health professional in relation to their cross-dressing, about half of whom self-referred and half responded to pressure from courts, wives, parents, or friends. In this author's experience, most adult cross-dressers who persist with treatment aimed at eliminating the behavior do so to please their female partners. Because treatment can often reduce, but only rarely eliminate, their urges to cross-dress, most do not persist with treatment and come to accept their feelings. When they do, they may commence to attend in cross-dress a group of other cross-dressed men, commonly adopting a female name in their company. When cross-dressing alone, they may spend an hour or more grooming themselves to appear more like women, applying makeup while examining themselves in a mirror. They are predominantly sexually attracted to members of the opposite sex and most marry. They often work in male-dominated professions, such as engineering, and many are involved in sports regarded as masculine, such as car racing. As these men no longer experi-ence recurrent, intense sexually arousing fantasies, sexual urges, or behaviors involving cross-dressing, the diagnosis of transvestic fetishism that was appropriate when they did experience sexual arousal in adolescence seems inappropriate for their adult condition. Their periodic ex-periences of feeling like women would justify their being considered to have an atypical gender identity. They prefer to refer to themselves by the previously accepted term, transvestites, or as TVs. Nevertheless their condition remains classified in the DSM–IV–TR as transvestic fetishism, a paraphilia, not a gender identity disorder.

Gender Identity Disorder

Adolescents and Adults With Gender Identity Disorder

The term transsexualism was previously used for the condition of adolescents and adults classified in DSM–IV–TR as gender identity disorder. The diagnostic criteria include that the person must have a strong and persistent cross-gender identification and persistent discomfort with his or her sex or sense of inappropriateness in the gender role of that sex. Like adult men diagnosed as transvestic fetishists, they give a history of cross-dressing in childhood and adolescence, but typically do not report having experienced sexual arousal with the activity. As they age they cross-dress for longer periods, but do not devote a marked amount of time to self-grooming when doing so. In late adolescence or early adulthood, an unknown percentage seek physical sex-conversion by hormones and surgery and hence come to professional attention. Both men and women who seek sex-conversion commonly express negative feelings about their genitals and in women, breast development. The women commonly reduce the appearance of breast development by binding, and more rarely men attempt to surgically remove their genitals. Typically both the women and the men are predominantly or exclusively attracted to members of the same biological sex and adopt occupations and have interests more typical of members of the opposite sex. A similar relationship between degree of homosexual feelings, opposite sex interests, and feelings of being of the opposite sex was found in men and women in the total population (Dunne, Bailey, Kirk, & Martin, 2000; McConaghy, 1993). Men with gender identity disorder have a lower mean socioeconomic status and are less stable in their relationships and occupation compared to adult transvestic fetishists.

Transvestic Fetishists Who Seek Sex-Conversion

A series of studies by Buhrich and McConaghy (1977, 1978) compared men who sought physical sex-conversion with men who had joined a club for men who identified as transvestites. They found that some men showed features of both the conditions classified in DSM–IV–TR as transvestic fetishism and gender identity disorder. In the studies these men were termed fetishistic transsexuals as they experienced sexual arousal with cross-dressing at puberty but sought sex-conversion at the time of the study. Many had identified in early adulthood as transvestites. When they sought physical sex-conversion it was at a significantly older age than the age of the men studied who sought the procedure, but had not experienced sex arousal with cross-dressing at puberty. In the studies the latter group of men were termed classical trans-sexuals. When the men termed fetishistic transsexuals sought sex-conversion, they resembled the men who identified as transvestites but did not seek sex-conversion (termed typical transvestites) rather than the classical transsexuals, in having higher socioeconomic status and commonly being married. Their penile volume responses to films of men and women, a valid measure of sexual orientation discussed subsequently, indicated they had approximately equal sexual interest in men and women. The penile volume responses of the typical transvestites indicated predominant heterosexual interest, and the responses of the classical transsexuals in-dicated predominant or exclusive homosexual interest. In regard to their gender identity, typical transvestites and fetishistic and classical transsexuals all said that they felt like women when they were cross-dressed. All typical transvestites and about half the fetishistic transsexuals said they felt like men when nude, and all classical transsexuals said they felt like women when nude. The findings of these studies indicated the condition termed fetishistic transsexualism was intermediate between the conditions termed typical transvestism and classical transsexualism.

The views of sex researchers remain conflicted concerning the conditions until recently termed transvestism and transsexualism in the research literature. Some argued that a history of sexual arousal to cross-dressing in men who seek sex-conversion should preclude a diagnosis of transsexualism and that their requests for surgery should be rejected (Stoller, 1971). Carroll (2000) commented that in the past men with this history were usually labeled transvestites or secondary transsexuals and were not considered appropriate for surgery. Now professionals understand they may benefit from gender reassignment, and they make up the majority of men seeking it. He termed their condition a form of gender dysphoria. It was not clear whether he included DSM–IV–TR diagnosed transvestic fetishists who had not sought sex conversion in this diagnosis. Zucker (1997) defended the DSM–IV statement (retained in DSM–IV–TR) that transvestic fetishism has been described only in heterosexual men and rejected the substantial evidence reviewed by Bullough and Bullough (1997) that sexual arousal with cross-dressing occurs in some men who identify as homosexual.

Is Gender Identity Categorical or Dimensional?

DSM–TR–IV diagnostic criteria were developed by committees that attempted to accommodate the various views of sex researchers as to the nature of transvestism and transsexualism and their association with gender identity. The concept of gender identity was introduced in the middle of the last century when the existence of men and women who reported feelings of belonging to the opposite gender was recognized. Benjamin (1954) named their condition transsexualism and considered the conviction of male transsexuals that they were really females with faulty sex organs to be profound and passionate. Worden and Marsh suggested (1955) that "the existence of persons who have this distorted subjective perception of their sexual identity offers an opportunity to study the whole problem of how human beings normally get their sense of being a male or a female" (p. 1292).

This suggestion was generally accepted. It required the assumption that the sense of gender identity in normal women and men developed similarly to that of transsexuals as a powerful and unified sense that they were either male or female. Their same sex identity was considered to be held with the same persistence and intensity as was the opposite sexual identity that drove transsexuals to undergo the emotional and physical demands of sex-conversion. Research was not considered necessary to establish this categorical concept that the sex identity of people without a gender identity disorder was totally female in women and totally male in men. Spence and Buckner (1995), in agreeing with the concept, claimed that sex identity was what they termed an existential sense and therefore could not be measured. The belief that the gender identity of people without gender identity disorder is categorical is not consistent with the evidence that gender identity is dimensional in normal men and women. In response to anonymous questionnaires, normal men and women reported degrees of feeling like members of the same versus the opposite sex that correlated with the ratios of their heterosexual to homosexual feelings and behaviors (Dunne et al., 2000; McConaghy, 1993).

The issue of whether gender identity is dimensional rather than categorical was by-passed in DSM–IV–TR. The compromise it adopted was to ignore the fluctuating gender identity in the men referred to as typical transvestites in the studies discussed by diagnosing their condition as a paraphilia, transvestic fetishism. It did accept that in some of the men so diagnosed, sexual arousal to cross-dressing diminished or disappeared while they continued to cross-dress. The fact that this change made the diagnosis of fetishism inappropriate was ignored. The intermediate group of men who in early adulthood identify as transvestites but later seek sex-conversion were labeled as a subtype of the paraphilia, transvestic fetishism, with gender dysphoria. These DSM categories fail to capture the complex nature of the relationship between age, cross-dressing, and gender identity.

The compromises made in the DSM–IV–TR reclassification of transvestism and transsexualism have been unsuccessful in accommodating the views of all researchers. Like Carroll (2000), many clinicians prefer the term gender dysphoria instead of gender identity disorder as being a broader category. Carroll pointed out that many men and women experience an identity they do not wish to change, which is outside the simple categories of male or female and which they refer to as transgender. Not wishing sex-conversion, many do not come to the attention of clinicians. Carroll commented of those who do that "The clinician is now confronted with an often bewildering array of individuals with transgendered experiences, including transsexuals, transvestites, she-males, third sex, two spirit, drag queens and kings, and cross-dressers" (p. 369). It is likely that recognition of existence of these women and men will lead to further changes in the DSM classification of transvestic fetishism and gender identity disorder. These changes will need to take into account the "new ferment concerning transsexualism" (Swartz, 1998) discussed subsequently.

Most Children With Gender Identity Disorder Become Normal Adults

The DSM–IV–TR category of gender identity disorder includes children who cross-dressed, showed behaviors typical of the opposite sex, and expressed wishes to belong to the opposite sex. Its onset was usually between the ages of 2 and 4 years. DSM–IV–TR states that only a very small number of children with gender identity disorder continue to have symptoms that meet the criteria for the diagnosis in adolescence or adulthood. Most show less overt cross-gender behaviors with time, parental intervention, or response from peers. By late adolescence or adulthood about three-quarters of the boys with a childhood history of gender identity disorder report a homosexual or bisexual orientation without concurrent gender disorder, and most of the remainder report a heterosexual orientation without concurrent gender disorder. DSM–IV–TR further states that the corresponding percentages of outcomes for girls with gender identity disorder are not known. Homosexual activists have criticized the provision in the DSM–IV of diagnostic criteria for gender identity disorder in children as pathologizing a condition when most subjects who conform to the criteria do not show subsequent pathology.

CULTURAL AND GENDER ISSUES

Transgender Activism

Swartz (1998) argued that the transgender liberation movement has discredited the medical model of transsexualism, and that deference to medical authority should be substantially diminished. He pointed out some transgender activists are demanding that access to sex reassignment surgery should be available based solely on self-diagnosis and request. They consider psychological screening and diagnosis for the surgery and related procedures to be invalid and corrupt, expensive, and demeaning, and believe they encourage the client to lie. Swartz predicted that gender identity disorder and transsexualism will eventually disappear as categories of medical pathology.

Internet Sexuality

As pointed out by McGrath and Casey (2002), the growth of the internet has not only revolutionized how society conducts business; the sexual predator and the obsessional harasser use it to meet their needs in contacting victims, avoiding apprehension, and communicating with other offenders. Black et al. (1997) did not mention its use in subjects with compulsive sexual behavior. Schneider (2000) found forty-five men and ten women, aged 18 to 64 years, in response to an online request, who self-identified as experiencing adverse consequences from online sexual activities. The consequences included worsening of their sexual relationship with spouse or partner, harm to their marriage or primary relationship, exposure of children to on-line pornography, decreased job performance, career loss, other financial difficulties, and legal charges. In a 2001 study of 5,925 men who reported online sexual activity, Cooper, Griffin-Shelley, Delmonico, and Mathy found 6.5% self-identified as having sexual problems resulting from their online activity. In the author's clinical practice a number of men have reported these problems, which were treated as compulsive sexual behaviors.

Gender Differences in Sexual Disorders

Possibly the most striking gender difference in sexual behavior is difference in motivation. Markedly more adolescent and adult women than men report an emotional involvement is a prerequisite for participating in sexual intercourse (McConaghy, 1993). In an English random sample population, sexual problems were associated with physical problems such as hyper-tension, diabetes, and prostate disease in men, but with marital difficulties and emotional problems in women (Dunn, Croft, & Hackett, 1999). It has been suggested that the importance of the emotional relationship to women's sexual life reflects evolutionary pressures for survival. Men's genes, are more likely to be passed on if they impregnate as many women as possible. For women to pass on their genes, they must successfully rear their children. Hence, men should be most sexually attracted to women who are young and healthy, and hence likely to be fertile. Women should be sexually attracted to men who are likely to set up a committed relationship with them, so they can provide better child care. Both these and other predictions concerning evolutionary pressures on attraction to, selection of, and jealousy of mates have been supported (Buss, 1996). This evolutionary theory also suggests that as men are more motivated to initi-ate intercourse at the earliest opportunity, their sexual interest, and pleasure and orgasm with intercourse would be greater than that of women. Laumann, Gagnon, Michael, and Michaels (1994) asked a representative U.S. population sample whether they had experienced a number of sexual dysfunctions for several months or more in the preceding 12 months. In the subjects aged 18 to 59 years, about 15% of men and 32% of women lacked interest in sex, 9% compared to 24% found sex not pleasurable, and 8% compared to 26% were unable to reach orgasm. Climaxing too quickly was reported by 28% of men and 12% of women. Provided the majority of the men ejaculated in the vagina, premature ejaculation could increase the likelihood of impregnating a partner in the earlier societies in which human sexual behavior developed. Another major difference in men and women that may reflect the reduced influence of sexual desire as compared to emotional involvement on women's behavior is the virtual absence of many paraphilias among women, including exhibitionism, voyeurism, fetishism, frotteurism, transvestism, and telephone scatologia.

THEORY AND RESEARCH ON ETIOLOGY

Etiology of Sexual Dysfunctions

There is little rigorous research on the etiology of sexual disorders. It is generally accepted that heterosexual attraction is largely biologically determined in view of its widespread presence in the animal world and its necessity for survival of the species. The nature of the factors that influence sexual attraction and its expression to produce modifications and disorders, including the extent to which such factors are biological or social, remains controversial. The evolutionary theory discussed earlier predicts that women's sexual behavior is more likely that that of men to be determined by social and emotional factors than by identifiable biological factors. Evidence supporting this conclusion includes the failure of numerous studies to find consistent relationships between women's sexual interest or behavior and the wide fluctuations in level of the sex hormones (i.e., estrodial, progesterone, and testosterone) that occur throughout the menstrual cycle. In contrast, men's sexual interest is strongly influenced by changes in their normal level of testosterone, falling when the level is reduced by antiandrogen medication, and erectile dysfunction occurring when it falls below about 20% (McConaghy, 1993).

Laumann et al. (1994) found that most sexual dysfunctions in women, including inability to be sexually aroused or to reach orgasm, decreased with age. The decrease has been attributed to learning (McConaghy, 1993). Adolescence social expectations, at least in the past, required that girls but not boys controlled their sexual arousal to remain virgin until marriage. They then needed to learn to relinquish this control to fully experience sexual arousal. In Hunt's survey (1974) of sexual behavior in the United States in the 1970s, women emphasized the role of men in helping them to learn to become aroused. This finding could seem inconsistent with the lack of evidence for the widely held belief that there is a relationship between the sexual technique of men and their women partners' ability to reach orgasm (Morokoff, 1978). However it may be that having learned to reach orgasm, women are no longer dependent on the technique of the partner. Also the type of learning suggested by the statements of the women in Hunt's survey did not appear to involve physical techniques so much as encouragement to relinquish emotional control. The available evidence also does not support the other common belief that inadequate genital stimulation in sexual relationships is an important determinant of women's inability to reach orgasm. Duration of intercourse did not differ between married women who usually and who rarely experienced orgasm (Gebhard, 1966; Terman, 1938). Huey, Kline-Graber, and Graber (1981) found no difference in duration of foreplay or intromission reported by 153 women who did not experience orgasm with coitus or other sexual activities, 114 women who reached orgasm with other sexual activities apart from coitus, and 24 women who experienced orgasm with coitus and usually with other sexual activities. Irrespective of the importance of sexual technique, throughout life women's sexual interest and activity is more dependent than is that of men on the existence and nature of a relationship with a partner (McConaghy, 1993). The role of learning in women's becoming able to experience orgasm in sexual relationships was supported by studies that found that this ability was common in societies in which women were expected to possess it, and rare or absent in those in which they were not (Morokoff, 1978). These data suggest that in treating female orgasmic dysfunction, emphasis should be put on encouraging women to accept and express rather than control their feelings of sexual arousal. Their partners should be instructed to reinforce this expression of the women's arousal, rather than focusing only on sexual techniques.

Learned Anxiety as a Cause of Sexual Dysfunctions

The most accepted theory of the cause of sexual dysfunctions in individual men and women is that of Wolpe (1958), who pioneered the application of behavior therapy to psychological disorders. Before Wolpe, the most commonly held theory of the cause of sexual dysfunctions was the psychodynamic view that sexual dysfunctions resulted from unconscious castration anxiety established in the first 5 years of the child's life. Wolpe believed that anxiety could be conditioned to sexual activity by experiences that occurred at any stage of life. These experiences included exposure to beliefs that masturbation weakened the body and the mind, that sexual activity was sinful and would be punished by hellfire, or that sexual behaviors were painful or aggressive. The last beliefs could result from experiences in childhood of overhearing or observing the sexual activities of parents or others. A single episode of impotence or of premature ejaculation due to fatigue, illness, or indulgence in alcohol could lead to anxiety about future sexual performance, particularly in men whose ability to perform well sexually was important to them. When anxiety occurred in association with sexual activity, the two would be linked by conditioning. The anxiety would then recur when sexual activity was subsequently considered or initiated, even though the experiences may have been forgotten or the beliefs abandoned that originally produced the anxiety.

The conditioned anxiety could result in sexual dysfunctions. By partially or totally inhibiting the person's sexual responsiveness, it would result in sexual activities not being enjoyed and therefore not desired. If people who did not desire sexual activities felt under pressure from themselves or partners to carry them out, they could develop sexual aversion. Fear of loss of control could cause the person to inhibit the increase of sexual arousal necessary for orgasm. Fear that sexual activity would be painful or would result in an undesired pregnancy or an agonizing labor could lead the subject to become physically tense, resulting in inability of the muscles of the vagina and thighs to relax and allow penile penetration. Attempts at intercourse would therefore be painful, producing vaginismus. Anxiety is associated with heightened activity of the sympathetic nervous system, which is involved in ejaculation in the male. Anxiety could therefore lead to premature ejaculation, which would then be maintained by a fear of its recurrence. Though unacknowledged by them, Wolpe's theory was popularized in the United States by Masters and Johnson (1970) whose term for the anxiety involved, performance anxiety, remains widely used. Clinicians considered other negative emotional responses, such as anger at the partner, could also lead to sexual dysfunctions.

Despite the logical appeal of Wolpe's theory, experimental studies investigating whether anxiety could impair sexual arousal have produced inconsistent findings. Hale and Strassberg (1990) pointed out that the anxiety commonly studied was to stimuli such as threat of electric shock, rather than those producing sexual anxiety. They investigated the effect of both types of stimuli in men with no history of sexual dysfunctions. Sexual anxiety was produced by showing the men false graphs of their penile responses recorded before the experiment and informing them that the graphs indicated they could be likely to develop a sexual problem. Both threat of shock and sexual anxiety reduced sexual arousal, as assessed by penile circumference responses to videotapes of couples involved in heterosexual intercourse. Hale and Strassberg concluded that their study provided empirical support for the concept that anxiety about sexual performance was a factor in erectile dysfunctions in men. They commented that if the sexually functional men in their study were sufficiently concerned by the possibility that their sexual performance was subnormal, the effect of such cognitions could be expected to be much greater in men with reasons for concern, such as an episode of erectile failure following heavy alcohol intake. A related study in women by Elliott and O'Donohue (1997) failed to produce meaningful results. Their attempt to produce sexual anxiety in their subjects by videotaping them while they watched erotic material was unsuccessful. The degree of the women's sexual arousal was assessed by their self-reports and their vaginal vasocongestion. The correlation between the two measures was not reported. It is commonly low or negative. Palace (1996) suggested that in women generalized sympathetic arousal associated with anxiety, laughter, or exercise could facilitate genital vascular changes, reducing their validity in assessing sexual arousal. Nevertheless, these changes are regularly used for this purpose.

Sexual abuse of children and sexual assault of adults are commonly believed to result in sexual disorders in the victims. However, studies reporting the relationship usually investigate patients with psychiatric illness and therefore could overestimate the significance of sexual abuse in producing sexual disorders. Rind, Bauserman, and Tromovitch (2000) reported a meta-analysis of fifty-nine studies of the effect of childhood sexual abuse on college students. In regard to seventeen behaviors, including sexual adjustment, the abused students were slightly less well adjusted than the nonabused students. The authors considered the poorer adjustment could not be attributed to the abuse because family environment was consistently confounded with it and explained much more variance in adjustment. Clinical studies of women victims of sexual assault found that their satisfaction with sexual behaviors with their partner was significantly reduced following the assault, particularly their satisfaction with behaviors that had been forced on them during the assault. Not all studies reported that the frequency of the behaviors was reduced (Foley, 1985). Dysfunctions reported by the assaulted women included vaginismus, dyspareunia, and difficulties with arousal and orgasm, which could persist for years following the assault. Sexual disorders were also reported to follow the sexual assault of men by women and men (Sarrel & Masters, 1982). In a community study, Koss (1985) questioned female university students concerning whether they had experienced intercourse with dates against their will by force or threat of force. Of the students who reported the experience, those who at the time of the study accepted it was rape, compared to those who did not, reported more liberal sexual values and a larger number of sexual partners. Koss considered this finding was consistent with the hypothesis that sexual victimization altered sexual standards and behavior. The students who did not consider the experience was rape showed no difference in sexual behavior from the women who reported they had not had the experience.

Organic Causes of Sexual Dysfunctions

In contrast to the decrease in sexual dysfunctions with age in women being attributed to learning, the marked increase in men of erectile dysfunction with age is due to organic causes. The most common is reduction in blood flow in the arteries supplying the penis, which can be demonstrated by Doppler ultrasound probe. This investigation is not necessary in the usually young men whose erectile dysfunction results from performance anxiety in relation to intercourse. They attain adequate erections in nonthreatening situations such as masturbation or during sleep and early morning waking. Impairment of sexual desire, arousal, and orgasm in both sexes can result from use of drugs of abuse as well as a wide range of medications, including antihypertensive agents, diuretics, vasodilators, medications used to treat psychiatric disorders, and anticonvulsant drugs (Schiavi & Segraves, 1995). Depression and physical illnesses also are significant etiological factors.

Etiology of Paraphilias

Paraphilias and sexual offenses are generally attributed to the presence in the perpetrator, usually a man, of related sexual urges that are regarded as deviant from those socially accepted. It is possible that a number of such deviant urges are biologically determined to some extent. Those that are reported predominantly by males include wishing to observe naked persons, wishing to be observed by them when in a state of sexual arousal, attempting to sexually arouse persons by touching, acting in a dominant fashion, and inflicting some degree of pain on sexual partners. Acting submissively appears to be more predominant in females. Sixty-five percent of fifty-seven undergraduate men reported having engaged in some form of sexual misconduct, including voyeurism (42%), frotteurism (35%), and making obscene phone calls (8%; Templeman & Stinnett, 1991). Fifty percent of normal men expressed some likelihood that if they could not be reported they would engage in bondage, and 35% some likelihood they would engage in whipping and spanking a women (Malamuth, 1989). During heterosexual activity, 40% percent of normal men had erotic fantasies of tying up a woman, 30% of raping a woman, 26% of behaving aggressively, and 10% of beating a woman up (Crepault & Couture, 1980). Person et al. (1989) investigated university students' sexual experiences in the previous 3 months. Sexual fantasies of men included forcing a partner to submit (reported by 31%), being forced to submit (15%), being tied or bound (15%), torturing a partner (6%), and whipping or beating a partner (5%). Sexual fantasies of women included being forced to submit and being tied or bound during sex activity (20%), being sexually degraded (12%), being a prostitute (10%), being tortured by a sex partner (9%), being whipped or beaten by a partner (8%), forcing a partner to submit (5%), whipping or beating a partner (1%), and degrading a partner (1%). Half of 141 married upper-class New York women (median age 32) reported their second most popular coital fantasy was of being overpowered or forced to surrender; 14% reported using this fantasy on almost every occasion of intercourse (Hariton & Singer, 1974). About 15% of male and 2% of female university students in the United States and Australia reported some likelihood of having sexual activity with a prepubertal child if they could do so without risk (Malamuth, 1989; McConaghy, Zamir, & Manicavasagar, 1993). Freund and Watson (1991) assessed the penile volume responses of normal male volunteers to color film clips of males and females, aged from 5 to adulthood. Twenty percent of the men showed responses indicating a greater sexual preference for prepubertal children than for adults. The percentage of men who sexually assault children and adults during wartime, when the risk of punishment is reduced, has not been investigated.

A widely accepted theory of why sex-offending men act on their deviant urges is that they have cognitions supportive of the offenses. These include what have been termed rape myths, such as that women say No when they mean Yes, and that children enjoy sexual activity with adults. Ageton (1983) investigated this hypothesis in a study of sexually assaultive offenders identified from the United States national sample of adolescents. Though the offenders differed markedly from nonoffenders in showing increased evidence of delinquency, they did not differ in their beliefs concerning sex roles or their attitudes toward sexual assault. The cognitive theory has also been tested in a number of studies of college men but has received only weak support (McConaghy, 1993). The theory that male pedophiles become abusers because they were sexually abused themselves in childhood, the so-called "cycle of child sexual abuse theory advanced by Russell (1986), has become widely accepted. It is supported by the fact that more pedophiles than nonoffenders report that they were sexually abused in childhood. Some therapists have argued that the reports were not reliable, but were attempts to gain attention and sympathy (Marshall, 1996a). Hindman (1988) found the number of child molesters making the claim fell from 67% to 29% when on the second occasion they were interviewed using a polygraph, which they were told would detect lying.

Marshall (1996b) considered there was evidence that the parents of sex offenders were either physically, sexually, or emotionally abusive and many offenders were also abused by other people, and emphasized the role of low self-esteem as an important factor in sex offending. He suggested that deviant sexual preferences and activities were adopted by men in part because they were unable to meet their needs for intimacy, sexual gratification, need for power and control, and search for self-confirmation with consenting adult partners. In accounting for the correlation between the childhood parental relationships and later deviant behaviors, the possibility it could be due to genetic factors (DiLalla & Gottesman, 1991) was rarely considered.

Etiology of Gender Identity Disorders

There is no convincing evidence for any particular explanation for gender identity disorders. Biologically oriented researchers believe they are determined genetically or by sex hormone fluctuations in intrauterine development. It is argued that there is a critical period in the development of the brain of the fetus when gender identity is established. If at this period the balance of male to female sex hormones is above the mean, the female fetus will show greater male gender identity in childhood and adulthood. If the balance is below the mean, the male fetus will subsequently show greater female gender identity. Social learning theorists believe that social factors are responsible for gender identity. The theory that gender identity is largely determined by the sex in which a person was reared rather than by biological forces was considered discredited by the account of the boy called John/Joan, which received widespread media attention. The claim was advanced repeatedly over several years that he was successfully reared as a girl following hormonal and surgical sex-conversion after his penis was accidentally severely damaged during circumcision. The claim was eventually found to be false. In fact, he had been severely distressed by having to live as a girl. He subsequently demanded hormonal and surgical sex-reconversion so he could live as a man, which he successfully did (Kipnis & Diamond, 1999). His situation was one stimulus for the appeal of the Intersex Society of North America that the accepted procedure of immediate surgical "correction" of the sexually anomalous external genitalia of children born with intersex conditions should be ceased. They argued that assignment to a male or female gender should be delayed or not done at all and that intersex should be accepted as an alternative gender.

RESEARCH ON EMPIRICALLY VALIDATED TREATMENTS

There are few methodologically adequate studies evaluating treatments of sexual disorders, as reflected by the limited number in the Cochrane Library's database of systematic reviews, a regularly updated collection of evidence-based health care databases. The reviews are full text articles reviewing the effects of health care and are currently the most rigorous, and hence considered the most authoritative, in establishing which treatments are empirically based. They include only evaluative studies that are randomized and controlled by comparison with another treatment, a placebo treatment, treatment as usual, or, in some reviews, waiting list controls. Unfortunately, until the present, most studies evaluating sexual disorders have used waiting list or untreated controls. By not using controls treated with placebo, they do not control for the effect of suggestibility.

Treatment of Sexual Dysfunctions

The only Cochrane review of interventions for sexual dysfunctions evaluated studies treating vaginismus (McGuire & Hawton, 2002). They found three studies eligible for inclusion, but only one that could be analysed statistically, that by Schnyder, Schnyder-Luthi, Ballinari, and Blaser (1998). Forty-four patients with vaginismus were randomly allocated to in vivo or in vitro systematic desensitization. The in vivo desensitization consisted of provision of information, relaxation exercises, and introduction of appropriately sized vaginal dilators by the physician. The in vitro procedure differed in that, although the information provision and relaxation exercises were the same, the physician provided the patient with verbal instructions as to how she was to insert the dilators. Following treatment, forty-three of the forty-four women reported being able to engage in intercourse, and the two interventions did not differ in effectiveness. The review pointed out the high success rate was comparable to that of uncontrolled trials and case studies.

Baucom, Shoham, Mueser, Daiuto, and Stickle (1998) identified four possibly efficacious psychological treatments of sexual dysfunctions for women, which met their criteria of adequate sample size and inclusion of controls, including waiting list controls. All four treatments involved training in sexual skills and/or reduction in sexual anxiety by desensitization procedures. Two that compared the treatments administered in groups, one of women only and one of women with their partners, found the latter to be more effective. Baucom et al. (1998) concluded that women with sexual dysfunctions should be treated with rather than without their partners, and that a direct focus on sexual interactions was important. These features, together with improvement of partners' communication about their sexual interactions, characterize the procedures most widely used to treat sexual dysfunctions in both men and women. They are modifications of the treatment introduced by Wolpe (1958) and developed by Masters and Johnson (1970), who described their form of treatment as sensate focusing. The program developed by Masters and Johnson involved the subjects and their partners being seen both individually and jointly by a male and a female therapist, at times working individually and at times jointly. The majority of subjects treated came from elsewhere in the United States to St. Louis to receive the treatment, which was carried out in daily sessions for 2 or 3 weeks. In addition, the couples were given nightly homework assignments. Most therapists do not follow the format of the Masters and Johnson approach precisely, as the majority of patients are unwilling or unable to give up 2 or 3 weeks for treatment and can do homework assignments of an hour's duration a few times weekly at most. Also many sex therapists, finding their results satisfactory, continue to work individually rather than involve a cotherapist of the opposite sex. They see the couple weekly or less frequently.

Treatment is initiated with the cognitive phase of Wolpe's (1958) approach, so that the couple is provided with appropriate information and their faulty cognitions corrected. They are then given instructions concerning their homework activities, and their performance of these is monitored in the following interview. They are asked to organize their activities so that they can put aside weekly, two or more periods of an hour's duration, when they are relaxed and will not be disturbed. This often takes a good deal of negotiation, dealing with issues of how interruptions from children and house and external work demands are to be managed. In the initial phase of the homework sessions, the patients are instructed that one is to be passive and the other active for half the session, and then change roles. While both are naked, the active partner sensuously stimulates the passive partner by massaging, stroking, or kissing, how and where he or she is told by the passive partner. Touching of genitals and women's breasts is prohibited. The goal of this prohibition is to allow the gradual extinction of anxieties conditioned from past experiences of unpleasant or painful coitus or failures to meet self-imposed performance standards. The partner in the passive role learns to inform her/his partner about what she/he enjoys in foreplay. The partner in the active role learns how to carry out the activities his or her partner enjoys.

When the couple report that they are communicating effectively during the homework sessions and are enjoying the sensuous stimulation from their partner without anxiety, they are instructed to proceed to stimulation of the genitals and breasts of the partner in the passive role. Intercourse is still prohibited. If they feel it is appropriate and it will not involve subjecting either partner to any pressure, one or both can reach orgasm by manual or oral stimulation at the end of the session. Men who are unable to ejaculate or, as is more common, women who are unable to reach orgasm in sexual activities with their partner, are instructed to attempt to do so during these later sessions. They are told that it may take an hour or more of masturbatory stimulation (commonly termed directed masturbation) for them to reach orgasm initially and that they will need to experiment to find the type of stimulation that most arouses them.

The partners of men with premature ejaculation are instructed at this stage to sit between the men's legs facing them, and to masturbate them. The men are told to monitor their arousal and to tell their partners when they feel they are about to ejaculate; the partners then cease stimulation until told the sensation has disappeared. They then recommence masturbation. The man's erection may subside temporarily. As the man learns to prolong his erection and postpone ejaculation, his anxiety that he will ejaculate prematurely begins to diminish. This stop–start procedure was first recommended as a treatment for premature ejaculation by Semans in 1956. Masters and Johnson (1970) modified the procedure, so that when ejaculation was imminent, the partner squeezed the glans of the penis (a penile squeeze) rather than ceasing stimulation. This inhibited ejaculation and usually resulted in some loss of erection. Masturbation was then recommenced as with the stop–start procedure. The good initial response to these treatments does not appear to persist at long-term follow-up. This may also be true of the response of premature ejaculation to clomipramine taken before intercourse, as no long-term reports of its use are available.

Baucom et al. (1998) pointed out the paucity of studies evaluating psychological treatment of male dysfunctions. They considered the resulting lack of evidence of the effectiveness of psychological treatments could account for the increasing tendency to treat male dysfunctions, particularly erectile dysfunctions, with physical rather than psychological treatments. Previous physical means of creating erections (e.g., vacuum constriction and injection of vasodilators) have largely been replaced as initial treatments by the recently introduced oral medication, sildenafil citrate (Viagra), shown to be effective in producing erections in patients with erectile dysfunction in double-blind placebo-controlled trials. Since its approval by the U.S. Food and Drug Administration in March 1998, Viagra has been used by millions of men (Boyce & Umland, 2001). Its effectiveness had been demonstrated for erectile dysfunction associated with prostatectomy, radiation therapy, diabetes mellitus, some neurological disorders, and drug therapies, such as the antidepressant serotonin reuptake inhibitors (SSRIs; Boyce & Umland, 2001). It is less effective in women with sexual dysfunctions, with the exception of those associated with use of SSRIs. Rosen and Ashton (1993) had earlier criticized the dearth of studies of the effects of prosexual drugs in women.

There is insufficient evidence to support the administration of sexual hormones in the treatment of sexual dysfunctions in women or men, except for the use of testosterone in men with hypogonadism and local estrogen for postmenopausal women with vaginal atrophy.

Treatment of Paraphilias

The Cochrane Library provided two reviews of treatment for paraphilias and sex offenses. One reviewed studies in which only men with learning disabilities were treated (Ashman & Duggan, 2002), and one reviewed studies of the treatment of adult males (White, Bradley, Ferriter, & Hatzipetrou, 2000). The former found no studies and the latter, three studies that met criteria of randomized controlled trials suitable for inclusion. The most important was a large controlled trial carried out by Marques and colleagues in which jailed offenders were offered treatment. Of those who accepted the offer, half were assigned to receive the treatment, relapse prevention, and the other half were assigned to a notreatment condition. Relapse prevention concepts provide the framework of cognitive-behavioral programs for sex offenders in North America (Marshall, 1999). They incorporate skills training designed to help the offender recognize high-risk situations in which he is likely to reoffend, assertiveness training, stress management, relaxation training, anger management, enhancement of empathy for victims, communication skills, and general social and/or dating skills.

In their review, White et al. (2000) ignored the report circulated by Marques in 1995 and published by her in 1999, in favor of an earlier report. In the later report Marques (1999) followed up the treated and untreated sex offenders at an average time of 4 years after release. Of the 172 who commenced treatment, 13% of the 138 who completed treatment and 17.7% of the 34 who dropped out had sexually reoffended. Of the 184 offenders denied treatment, 12.5% had sexually reoffended. In a post hoc analysis in the 1999 report, Marques found that treated married subjects showed a better outcome than untreated married subjects. Post hoc findings, of course, have a higher probability of being due to chance than findings predicted before the study, and the procedure of seeking them has been criticized (McConaghy, 1999b). If the post hoc finding was valid, it meant that though married subjects did better with treatment, the larger group of unmarried subjects did worse. Of the unmarried men, 17.6% of 91 who completed treatment, 24% of 25 who dropped out, and 14.3% of 105 who were denied treatment reoffended sexually. Leading sex researchers accepted that the study showed a modest treatment effect (McConaghy, 1999a).

Penile Volume Assessment More Valid Than Penile Circumference Assessment of Sexual Deviance

Penile circumference assessment is much more widely used than penile volume assessment of sexual arousal as it is considered more convenient. To accurately assess arousal, penile circumference responses to sexual stimuli require 2 minutes or more to develop (McConaghy, 1974). This time allows men so motivated to modify their responses to the stimuli presented by fantasying alternative stimuli, for example, fantasying aversive stimuli when shown pictures of children. The more rarely used penile volume assessment accurately assesses arousal to sexual stimuli within about 10 seconds. With these brief presentations, few pedophiles requested to produce penile volume responses indicating a preference for adult women were able to do so (Freund, 1971). With fifty-four second presentations, seventeen of twenty university students on request were able to produce responses indicating either a preference or equal interest in female children as adults (Wilson, 1998).

Should Control Rather Than Modification of Deviant Urges Be the Aim of Treatment?

Using penile volume assessment, it was found that men's ratio of homosexual to heterosexual interest was not changed by various behavioral techniques (McConaghy, 2003). Though this finding, of course, cannot be generalized to other forms of sexual interest, so far no evidence has been advanced that behavioral techniques can modify urges to rape adults or molest children, using the valid penile volume response assessment (McConaghy, 2002). In view of the lack of valid evidence that sexual interest can be modified, treatment should be aimed not at attempting to modify offenders' deviant interests but at encouraging them to learn to control their behavior. Treatments that encourage development of control include imaginal desensitization and antiandrogen medication. Imaginal desensitization aims to decrease or eliminate compulsions to act on deviant urges by teaching control directly. It was shown to be more effective in doing so than the still commonly employed aversive therapy, covert sensitization (McConaghy & Armstrong, 1985). Imaginal desensitization was developed on the basis of a theory that compulsive behaviors, sexual and nonsexual, were driven by behavior completion mechanisms established in the brain when behaviors were carried out regularly. If the behavior was not carried out in the presence of cues for it, the mechanisms produced increased arousal, experienced as anxiety or tension, which was sufficiently aversive as to cause the subject to complete the behavior against his or her will. With imaginal desensitization, the subjects were trained to relax and while relaxed to visualize being exposed to the cues for the compulsive behavior. They then visualized not completing the behavior, but carrying out an alternative behavior while remaining relaxed. Antiandrogen medication lowers the offender's testosterone level and therefore his deviant sexual urges. He is then able not to act on the urges while in the community where he is exposed to the stimuli that activated the urges on which he previously acted compulsively. He is able to learn to control the urges to these stimuli, so that the urges are reduced by lack of reinforcement. After several months, the medication can be gradually withdrawn.

The second study in the Cochrane review of White et al. (2000) reported the response of thirty male sex offenders who were randomly allocated, ten to imaginal desensitization, ten to a low dose of intramuscular medroxyprogesterone given for 6 months, and ten to the combination of these two treatments (McConaghy, Blaszczynski, & Kidson, 1988). The reduction in deviant compulsions at 1 month and 1 year reported by the men who received medroxyprogesterone alone correlated .82, and .74 respectively with the degree of reduction in their testosterone levels at those times. They were unaware of their testosterone levels, so that the correlation of their self-reported degree of reduction in urge with the objective measure of testosterone level reduction provided evidence for the validity of their self-reports. No sexual offenses in the year following commencement of treatment were reported by seven subjects who received imaginal desensitization, eight who received medroxyprogesterone alone, and nine who received the combination. Four of the six patients who did not respond adequately to the original treatment did so when given an alternative, medroxyprogesterone in three and electrical aversive therapy in one.

In the third study reviewed by White et al. (2000), 231 convicted sex offenders undergoing intensive probation were randomized to group therapy or standard care (Romero & Williams, 1983). There was no significant difference in rearrest rate at 10 years. White et al. (2000) pointed out this finding was disturbing given the widespread use of group therapy in treatment of sex offenders. White et al. (2000) concluded that relapse prevention seems to have the most promise and that it was difficult to justify the use of antilibidinal drugs (such as medroxyprogesterone) outside a well-conducted trial. The opposite conclusions seem more reasonable, in view of (a) the finding of the lack of response to relapse prevention in the 1999 report of Marques and (b) the marginal superiority of medroxyprogesterone to the cognitive behavioral approach reported by McConaghy et al. (1988). Pointing out the need for more randomized controls of different therapies for sexual offending, White et al. (2000) were justifiably dismissive of the arguments of researchers that studies of less methodological rigor were sufficient in this area.

Understandably, there are strong economic reasons for believing that the cognitive-behavioral therapy widely used in treating sex offenders is effective. Reviews and meta-analyses have concluded that it is, by accepting the results of studies that compared it with no treatment in subjects who were not randomly allocated to the two procedures. In these studies, control groups compared with the treated groups consisted of subjects who could be at greater risk of reoffending, as they had refused treatment, left treatment without approval, or decided they lived too far away (McConaghy, 1999b). Marshall (1996a), in his review of treatments of sex offenders, gave no attention to the issue of random assignment. Only random allocation controls for all differences between the two groups that could affect outcome.

Evaluation of treatment of paraphilias that are not sex offenses has received little attention. In the author's experience, they have responded similarly to imaginal desensitization, or if this approach proved inadequate, to use of medroxyprogesterone, if the subject finds them sufficiently distressing to justify this treatment.

Treatment of Gender Identity Disorders

Initially for men and women to obtain sex-conversion surgery it was necessary that they provide a classical history that they felt they belonged to the opposite sex since childhood. However, it was apparent in the discussion in an Open Forum that concluded the Fourth International Conference on Gender Identity (1978) that many clinicians no longer required this history. Rather, the transgendered person needed to have lived without problems in the role of the opposite sex for an acceptable period. Fisk commented in the Open Forum discussion that "In our follow-up there are people who came with a transvestite, or effeminate homosexual, or virile lesbian history, and seem to do as well as those who had a classical transsexual history" (p. 402).

The *Standards of Care for Gender Identity Disorders*, now in its sixth version (2001) and available on the internet, provides authoritative guidelines for management, including the recommended minimal credentials for the treating professional. It gives as an eligibility requirement for surgical treatment that the patient has lived full time in the preferred gender for 12 months. The treating professional also needs to judge that the patient meets readiness criteria of further consolidation of evolving gender identity or improved mental health in the new or confirmed gender role. Indicative of the more liberal requirements for surgical intervention, wishes to be neutered rather than sexually converted are accepted by some clinicians as acceptable requirements. Others prescribe female hormones for breast development of sex-workers who dress as women but use their penis in sexual activity. However, it is likely that most, like many other transgendered men, obtain their hormones illegally. It does not seem possible to evaluate the sex-conversion of transgendered persons, other than by the finding that following the procedure almost all subjects report greatly increased satisfaction (McConaghy, 1993).

DSM–IV–TR definitions of the sexual dysfunctions and disorders are discussed, with attention to their limitations. They ignore sexual difficulties, which are more strongly related to sexual satisfaction than sexual dysfunctions. Problems remain with the DSM–IV–TR exclusion from classification as paraphilias, sex-offending behaviors that are not experienced by the subjects as distressing, do not cause impairment of their social functioning, and have not been recurrent over at least 6 months. Exclusion of homosexuality as a disorder has resulted in limited training of clinicians in health issues related to it. Sadism, masochism, and fetishism could be excluded as disorders on the same grounds as homosexuality was excluded. DSM–IV–TR does not give adequate attention to compulsive sexuality, and its classification of adult cross-dressers as transvestic fetishists is inappropriate. Most are not sexually aroused by cross-dressing, and it ignores their periodic feelings of opposite-sex identity. Theories of etiology of sexual disorders are reviewed, as is research on empirically validated treatments. Treatments of sexual dysfunction in women are more effective if their partners are involved and there is a direct focus on sexual interactions. Dysfunctions in men are more commonly treated by physical therapies, with sildenafil citrate (Viagra) for erectile dysfunction being very widely used. The only randomly controlled trial of the commonly used relapse prevention therapy for sex offenders found at 4-year follow-up that more treated than untreated offenders had reoffended. It is suggested that treatment should aim at giving offenders control of deviant urges, rather than attempting to modify them by behavioral methods. Clinicians' requirements to approve of sex-conversion for transgendered men and women who seek the procedure have become more liberal, though some activists demand that access to sex-reassignment surgery should be available based solely on self-diagnosis and request.

REFERENCES

Ageton, S. S. (1983). *Sexual assault among adolescents*. Lexington, MA: Lexington Books.

American Psychiatric Association. (1980). *Diagnostic and statistical manual of mental disorders* (3rd ed.). Washington, DC: Author.

American Psychiatric Association. (1994). *Diagnostic and statistical manual of mental disorders* (4th. ed.). Washington, DC: Author.

American Psychiatric Association. (2000). *Diagnostic and statistical manual of mental disorders* (4th. ed., text rev.). Washington, DC: Author.

Ashman, L., & Duggan, L. (2002). Interventions for learning disabled sex offenders. In *The Cochrane Library, 2*. Oxford: Update Software.

Baucom, D. H., Shoham, V., Mueser, K. T., Daiuto, A. D., & Stickle, T. R. (1998). Empirically supported couple and family interventions for marital distress and adult mental health problems. *Journal of Consulting and Clinical Psychology, 66*, 53–88.

Benjamin, H. (1954). Transsexualism and transvestism as psychosomatic and somatopsychic syndromes. *American Journal of Psychotherapy, 8*, 219–230.

Black, D. W., Kehrberg, L. L. D., Flumerfelt, D. L., & Schlosser, S. S. (1997). Characteristics of 36 subjects reporting compulsive sexual behavior. *American Journal of Psychiatry, 154*, 243–249.

Bloland, S. E. (2000). Bill Clinton and John F. Kennedy: The dark side of charisma. *Psychoanalytic Dialogues, 10*, 285–289.

Boyce, E. G., & Umland, E. M. (2001). Sildenafil citrate: A therapeutic update. *Clinical Therapeutics, 23*, 2–23.

Buhrich, N., & McConaghy, N. (1977). The discrete syndromes of transvestism and transsexualism. *Archives of Sexual Behavior, 6*, 483–495.

Buhrich, N., & McConaghy, N. (1978). Two clinically discrete syndromes of transsexualism. *British Journal of Psychiatry, 133*, 73–76.

Bullough, B., and Bullough, V. (1997). Are transvestites necessarily heterosexual? *Archives of Sexual Behavior, 26*, 1–12.

Buss, D. M. (1996). The evolutionary psychology of human social strategies. In E. T. Higgins & A. W. Kruglanski (Eds.), *Social psychology: Handbook of basic principles* (pp. 3–38). New York: Guilford.

Cabaj, R. P., & Stein, T. S. (1996). *Textbook of homosexuality and mental health* (pp. 267–288). Washington, DC: American Psychiatric Press.

Carroll, R. A. (2000). Assessment and treatment of gender dysphoria. In S. R. Leiblum & R. C. Rosen (Eds.), *Principles and practice of sex therapy* (3rd ed., pp. 368–397). New York: Guilford.

Coleman, E., & Rosser, B. R. (1996). Gay and bisexual male sexuality. In R. P. Cabaj & T. S. Stein (Eds.), *Textbook of homosexuality and mental health* (pp. 707–721). Washington, DC: American Psychiatric Press.

Cooper, A., Griffin-Shelley, E., Delmonico, D. L., & Mathy, R. M. (2001). Online sexual problems: Assessment and predictive variables. *Sexual addiction and compulsivity, 8*, 267–285.

Crepault, C., & Couture, M. (1980). Men's erotic fantasies. *Archives of Sexual Behavior, 9*, 565–581.

Croughan, J. L., Saghir, M., Cohen, R., & Robins, E. (1981). A comparison of treated and untreated male cross-dressers. *Archives of Sexual Behavior, 10*, 515–528.

DiLalla, L. F., & Gottesman, I. I. (1991). Biological and genetic contributions to violence: Widom's untold tale. *Psychological Bulletin, 109*, 125–129.

Dunn, K. M., Croft, P. R., & Hackett, G. I. (1999). Association of sexual problems with social, psychological, and physical problems in men and women: A cross sectional population survey. *Journal of Epidemiology & Community Health, 53*, 144–148.

Dunne, M. P., Bailey, J. M., Kirk, K. M., & Martin, N. G. (2000). The subtlety of sex-atypicality. *Archives of Sexual Behavior, 29*, 549–565.

Elliott, A. N., & O'Donohue, W. T. (1997). The effects of anxiety and distraction on sexual arousal in a nonclinical sample of heterosexual women. *Archives of Sexual Behavior, 26*, 607–624.

Foley, T. S. (1985). Family response to rape and sexual assault. In A. W. Burgess (Ed.), *Rape and sexual assault.* (pp. 159–188). New York: Garland.

Foucault, M. (1990). *The history of sexuality*: Vol. 1. An introduction. Robert Hurley, Trans. London: Penguin.

Frank, E., Anderson, B., & Rubinstein, D. (1978). Frequency of sexual dysfunction in "normal" couples. *New England Journal of Medicine, 299*, 111–115.

Freund, K. (1971). A note on the use of the phallometric method of measuring mild sexual arousal in the male. *Behavior Therapy, 2*, 223–228.

Freund, K., & Watson, R. J. (1991). Assessment of the sensitivity and specificity of a phallometric test: An update of phallometric diagnosis of pedophilia. *Psychological Assessment: A Journal of Consulting and Clinical Psychology, 3*, 254–260.

Gebhard, P. H. (1966). Factors in marital orgasm. *Journal of Social Issues, 22*, 88–95.

Goodman, A. (1992). Diagnosis and treatment of sexual addiction. *Journal of Sex and Marital Therapy, 18*, 303–314.

Green, R. (2002). Is pedophilia a mental disorder? *Archives of Sexual Behavior, 31*, 467–471.

Hale, V. E., & Strassberg, D. S. (1990). The role of anxiety on sexual arousal. *Archives of Sexual Behavior, 19*, 569–581.

Hallstrom, T., & Samuelsson, S. (1990). Changes in women's sexual desire in middle life: The longitudinal study of women in Gothenburg. *Archives of Sexual Behavior, 19*, 259–268.

Hariton, E. B., & Singer, J. L. (1974). Women's fantasies during sexual intercourse. *Journal of Consulting and Clinical Psychology, 42*, 313–322.

Hartstein, N. B. (1996). Suicide risk in lesbian, gay, and bisexual youth. In R. P. Cabaj & T. S. Stein (Eds.) *Textbook of homosexuality and mental health* (pp. 819–837). Washington, DC: American Psychiatric Press.

Hindman, J. (1988). New insights into adult and juvenile sex offenders. *Community Safety Quarterly*, *1*, 1.

Huey, C. J., Kline-Graber, G., & Graber, B. (1981). Time factors and orgasmic response. *Archives of Sexual Behavior*, *10*, 111–118.

Hunt, M. (1974). *Sexual behavior in the 1970's*. Dell: New York.

Jagose, A. (2002). *Inconsequence. Lesbian representation and the logic of sexual sequence*. Ithaca: Cornell University Press.

Kelly, M. P., Strassberg, D. S., & Kircher, J. R. (1990). Attitudinal and experiential correlates of anorgasmia. *Archives of Sexual Behavior*, *19*, 165–177.

Kessler, R. C., McGonagle, K. A., Zhao, S., Nelson, C. B., Hughes, M., Eshleman, S., Wittchen, H. U., & Kendler, K. S. (1994). Lifetime and 12-month prevalence of DSM-III-R psychiatric disorders in the United States: Results from the National Comorbidity Survey. *Archives of General Psychiatry*, *51*, 8–19.

Kipnis, K., & Diamond, M. (1999). Pediatric ethics and the surgical assignment of sex. In A. D. Dreger (Ed.), *Intersex in the age of ethics* (pp. 173–193). Hagerstown, MD: University Publishing Group.

Koss, M. P. (1985). The hidden rape victim: Personality, attitudinal, and situational characteristics. *Psychology of Women Quarterly*, *9*, 193–212.

Laumann, E. O., Gagnon, J. H., Michael, R. T., & Michaels, S. (1994). *The social organization of sexuality*. Chicago: University of Chicago Press.

Malamuth, N. M. (1989). The attraction to sexual aggression scale: Part two. *Journal of Sex Research*, *26*, 324–354.

Marques, J. (1999). How to answer the question "Does sex offender treatment work?" *Journal of Interpersonal Violence*, *14*, 437–451.

Marshall, W. L. (1996a). Assessment, treatment, and theorizing about sex offenders. *Criminal Justice and Behavior*, *23*, 162–199.

Marshall, W. L. (1996b). The sexual offender: Monster, victim, or everyman? *Sexual Abuse: A Journal of Research and Treatment*, *8*, 317–335.

Marshall, W. L. (1999). Current status of North American assessment and treatment programs for sex offenders. *Journal of Interpersonal Violence*, *14*, 221–239.

Marshall, W. L., & Eccles, A. (1991). Issues in clinical practice with sex offenders. *Journal of Interpersonal Violence*, *6*, 68–93.

Marshall, W. L., & Kennedy, P. (2003). Sexual sadism in sexual offenders: An elusive diagnosis. *Aggression and Violent Behavior*, *8*, 1–22.

Masters, W. H., & Johnson, V. E. (1970). *Human sexual inadequacy*. Boston: Little, Brown.

McConaghy, N. (1974). Measurements of change in penile dimensions. *Archives of Sexual Behavior*, *3*, 381–388.

McConaghy, N. (1993). *Sexual behavior: Problems and management*. New York: Plenum.

McConaghy, N. (1997). Sexual and gender identity disorders. In S. M. Turner & M. Hersen (Eds.), *Adult psychopathology and diagnosis* (3rd ed., pp. 409–464). New York: Wiley.

McConaghy, N. (1999a). Unresolved issues in scientific sexology. *Archives of Sexual Behavior*, *28*, 285–318.

McConaghy, N. (1999b). Methodological issues concerning evaluation of treatment for sexual offenders: Randomization, treatment dropouts, no-treatment controls, and within-treatment studies. *Sexual Abuse: A Journal of Research and Treatment*, *11*, 183–193.

McConaghy, N. (2002). Orgasmic reconditioning. In M. Hersen & W. Sledge (Eds.), *Encyclopedia of psychotherapy*, (Vol. 2, pp. 299–305). New York: Elsevier Science.

McConaghy, N. (2003). *So you say you're straight: The one in five hidden homosexual heterosexuals*, in press.

McConaghy, N. (2003). Penile plethysmography and change in sexual orientation. *Archives of Sexual Behavior*, *32*, 444–445.

McConaghy, N., & Armstrong, M. S. (1985). Expectancy, covert sensitization, and imaginal desensitization. *Acta Psychiatrica Scandanavica*, *72*, 176–187.

McConaghy, N., Blaszczynski, A., & Kidson, W. (1988). Treatment of sex offenders with imaginal desensitization. and/or medroxyprogesterone. *Acta Psychiatrica Scandinavica*, *77*, 199–206.

McConaghy, N., Zamir, R., & Manicavasagar (1993). Non-sexist sexual experiences survey and scale of attraction to sexual aggression. *Australian and New Zealand Journal of Psychiatry*, *27*, 686–693.

McGrath, M. G., & Casey, E. (2002). Forensic psychiatry and the internet: Practical perspectives on sexual predators and obsessional harassers in cyberspace. *Journal of the American Academy of Psychiatry and the Law*, *30*, 81–94. Oxford: Update Software.

McGuire, H. & Hawton, K. (2002). Interventions for vaginismus. In *The Cochrane Library*, 2.

Morokoff, P. (1978). Determinants of female orgasm. In J. LoPiccolo & L. LoPiccolo (Eds.), *Handbook of sex therapy* (pp. 147–165). New York: Plenum.

Nettelbladt, P., & Uddenberg, N. (1979). Sexual dysfunction and sexual satisfaction in 58 married Swedish men. *Journal of Psychosomatic Research*, *23*, 141–147.

O'Donohue, W., Regev, L. G., & Hagstrom, A. (2000). Problems with the DSM-IV diagnosis of pedophilia. *Sexual Abuse: A Journal of Research and Treatment, 12*, 95–105.

Open Forum. (1978). *Archives of Sexual Behavior, 7*, 387–415.

Palace, E. M. (1996). Modification of dysfunctional patterns of sexual response through autonomic arousal and false physiological feedback. *Journal of Consulting and Clinical Psychology, 63*, 604–615.

Person, E. S., Terestman, N., Myers, W. A., Goldberg, E. L., & Salvadori, C. (1989). Gender differences in sexual behaviors and fantasies in a college population. *Journal of Sex and Marital Therapy, 15*, 187–198.

Phelps, J., Albo, M., Dunn, K., & Joseph, A. (2001). Spinal cord injury and sexuality in married or partnered men: Activities, function, needs, and predictors of sexual adjustment. *Archives of Sexual Behavior, 30*, 591–602.

Raymond, N. C., Coleman, E., Ohlerking, F., Christenson, G. A., & Miner, M. (1999). Psychiatric comorbidity in pedophile sex offenders. *American Joural of Psychiatry, 156*, 786–788.

Rind, B., Bauserman, R., & Tromovitch, P. (2000). Science versus orthodoxy: Anatomy of the congressional condemnation of a scientific article and reflections on remedies for future ideological attacks. *Applied and Preventative Psychology, 9*, 211–225.

Romero, J. J., & Williams, L. M. (1983). Group psychotherapy and intensive probation supervision with sex offenders: A comparative study. *Federal Probation, 47*, 36–42.

Rosen, R. C., & Ashton, A. K. (1993). Prosexual drugs: Empirical status of the "new aphrodisiacs." *Archives of Sexual Behavior, 22*, 521–543.

Rothblum, E. D. (1994). Introduction to the special section: Mental health of lesbians and gay men. *Journal of Consulting and Clinical Psychology, 62*, 211–212.

Rowland, D. L., Cooper, S. E., & Schneider, M. (2001). Defining premature ejaculation for experimental and clinical investigation. *Archives of Sexual Behavior, 30*, 235–253.

Russell, D. E. H. (1986). *The secret trauma. Incest in the lives of girls and women.* New York: Basic Books.

Sarrel, P., & Masters, W. (1982). Sexual molestation of men by women. *Archives of Sexual Behavior, 11*, 117–133.

Schiavi, R. C., & Segraves, R. T. (1995). The biology of sexual function. *Psychiatric Clinics of North America, 18*, 7–23.

Schneider, J. P. (2000). A qualitative study of cybersex participants: Gender differences, recovery issues, and implications for therapists. *Sexual Addiction and Compulsivity, 7*, 249–278.

Schnyder, U., Schnyder-Luthi, C., Ballinari, P., & Blaser, A. (1998). Therapy for vaginismus: In vivo versus in vitro desensitization. *Canadian Journal of Psychiatry, 43*, 941–944.

Semans, J. H. (1956). Premature ejaculation: A new approach. *Southern Medical Journal, 49*, 373–377.

Snyder, D. K., & Berg, P. (1983). Determinants of sexual dissatisfaction in sexually distressed couples. *Archives of Sexual Behavior, 12*, 237–246.

Spence, J. T., & Buckner, C. (1995). Masculinity and femininity: Defining the indefinable. In P. J. Kalbfleish & M. J. Cody (Eds.), *Gender, power, and communication in human relationships* (pp. 105–138). Hillsdale, NJ: Lawrence Erlbaum Associates.

Standards of Care for Gender Identity Disorders. (2001; Version 6). http://www.hbigda.org/socv6.html

Stoller, R. J. (1971). The term "transvestism." *Archives of General Psychiatry, 24*, 230–237.

Swartz, L. H. (1998). Legal implications of the new ferment concerning transsexualism. http://www.symposium.com/ijt/ijtc0604.htm

Templeman, T. L., & Stinnett, R. D. (1991). Patterns of sexual arousal and history in a "normal" sample of young men. *Archives of Sexual Behavior, 20*, 137–150.

Terman, L. M. (1938). *Psychological factors in marital happiness.* New York: McGraw-Hill.

Trumbach, R. (1994). London's sapphists: From three sexes to four genders in the making of modern culture. In G. Herdt (Ed.). *Third Sex, Third Gender* (pp. 111–136). New York: Zone Books.

van der Meer, T. (1994). Sodomy and the pursuit of a third sex in the early modern period. In G. Herdt (Ed.). *Third Sex, Third Gender* (pp. 137–212). New York: Zone Books.

White, P., Bradley, C., Ferriter, M., & Hatzipetrou, L. (2000). Management for people with disorders of sexual preference and for convicted sex offenders. In *The Cochrane Library, 3*. Oxford: Update Software.

Wilson, R. J. (1998). Psychophysiological signs of faking in the phallometric test. *Sexual Abuse: A Journal of Research and Treatment, 10*, 113–126.

Wolpe, J. (1958). *Psychotherapy by reciprocal inhibition.* Stanford, CA: Stanford University Press.

Worden, F. G., & Marsh, J. T. (1955). Psychological factors in men seeking sex transformation. *Journal of the American Medical Association, 157*, 1292–1298.

Zucker K. J. (1997). Letter to the Editor. *Archives of Sexual Behavior, 26*, 671–672.

13

Somatoform Disorders

Georg H. Eifert
Chapman University

Michael J. Zvolensky
The University of Vermont

Individuals exhibiting multiple somatic symptoms often present to medical practitioners believing that they are physically sick, yet upon evaluation, are informed that there are no known physiological mechanisms underlying their reports of distress. Although many of these patients will be satisfied with negative medical examination results and some reassurance to that effect, a significant subgroup will anxiously continue to ruminate about the possibility of suffering from a yet undiagnosed physical disease, a phenomenon known as *somatization*. Specifically, somatization denotes the presence of physical symptoms (e.g., chest pain, gastrointestinal distress) for which no demonstrable disease process or bodily oriented pathology can be identified at the current time. These individuals are likely to continue to seek help for their physical symptoms, demand more physical examinations and specialist referrals, undergo costly laboratory tests, and in rare cases, even end up on an operating table (Warwick & Salkovskis, 1990). At the extreme, such somatization behavior can interfere with life activities and goals, resulting in clinically significant impairment, a phenomenon typically classified as *somatization disorder*. Yet, somatization processes frequently occur in other somatic disorders, including hypochondriasis, pain disorder, conversion disorder, and body dysmorphic disorder, as well as many other psychiatric conditions (e.g., panic disorder, major depressive disorder).

Somatization is a relatively common occurrence in the general medical system. For instance, a study by van Hemert, Hengeveld, Bolk, Rooijmans, and Vandenbroucke (1993) found that among 191 new referrals to a general medical outpatient clinic, 52% of patients had symptoms that ultimately remained unexplained. An earlier study reported that of ninety-five patients visiting a general practitioner and presenting with somatic complaints, 41% had no demonstrable somatic pathology (Pilowsky, Smith, & Katsikitis, 1987). Comparable percentages have been reported in different countries (Eifert, 1992; Harvey, Salih, & Read, 1983; Mayou, Bryant, Forbar, & Clark, 1994), highlighting the cross-cultural relevance of this problem. Somatization can cause a high degree of personal suffering measured in both financial and human terms. For example, somatization is a common cause of absenteeism, and many physicians spend large amounts of time working with individuals who exhibit multiple somatic symptoms (Kellner, 1990). The best estimates indicate that the per capita expenditure for the health care service for individuals demonstrating somatization behavior are approximately nine times the average per capita amount for other individuals. It is important to note from the onset that somatization does not necessarily rule out the possibility of a true physical illness. In fact, many physical health care problems, typically quite mild, can be found among this group (e.g., hypertension). Thus, somatization denotes an excess degree of worry about physical health and overuse of medical services, relative to the severity of *identifiable* illness. Perhaps not surprisingly, these same individuals report a higher degree of physical, social, and occupational impairment compared to individuals who are seriously ill (Kellner, 1990). Typically, these impairment concerns are long-standing (occur across most phases of life) and tend to be exacerbated by concurrent stressors in everyday life. Although somatization is indeed a vexing health care problem, this domain represents an exciting opportunity for researchers from diverse disciplines to work together in a collaborative manner to better understand the relations between body and mind and health and disease.

The main aim of this chapter is to provide a contemporary overview of the process of somatization as it applies to somatoform disorders. To some extent, our discussion is necessarily organized around the categories and classification of somatoform disorders in the *Diagnostic and Statistical Manual of Mental Disorders* (4th Ed., DSM–IV; American Psychiatric Association, 1994). However, we attempt to move beyond DSM categories toward a more function-based dimensional perspective of somatization problems. We believe such an approach is potentially useful because it analyzes fundamental biobehavioral processes and thereby provides information that is likely to be directly useful for the design of clinical interventions. The first section of the chapter briefly reviews somatoform disorders from a traditional DSM–IV perspective, highlighting their prevalence, nature, and the diagnostic validity of such diagnoses. We then outline how a dimensional perspective that focuses on key biobehavioral processes may be a more useful approach for understanding somatoform disorders. We then address some key vulnerability processes for somatoform disorders. Finally, we address how a dimensional perspective and focus on dysfunctional processes related to illness behavior can be translated into treatments for somatoform disorders.

CLASSIFICATION, PREVALENCE, AND COURSE OF SOMATOFORM DISORDERS

According to DSM–IV (APA, 1994), the common feature of the somatoform disorders is the presence of physical symptoms that suggest a general medical condition (hence the term somatoform) but are not fully (currently) explained by a general medical condition, the direct effects of substance, or by another mental disorder. Physical symptoms result in substantial personal, social, and occupational impairment and are not feigned or voluntarily produced, as in malingering or factitious disorder. Although symptoms are not feigned, the fact that no medical explanation can be found for patient complaints makes it hard at times to differentiate somatoform disorders from malingering.

Although the exact prevalence of specific somatoform disorders is not exactly known, most estimates place these problems collectively at under 1% of the general population. DSM–IV distinguishes between five somatoform disorders: somatization disorder, hypochondriasis, pain disorder, conversion disorder, and body dysmorphic disorder. By way of background, we begin our discussion with a brief overview of these conditions from a traditional DSM–IV perspective.

Somatization Disorder.   Somatization disorder is characterized by many physical complaints without clear or known physical causes. The condition may last for many years and, in some cases, extend over the entire adult life span. To meet the DSM–IV diagnostic criteria, an individual needs to present with a history of pain related to at least four different sites or functions (e.g., head, back, abdomen, joints), two gastrointestinal symptoms (e.g., diarrhea, food intolerance), one sexual symptom (e.g., irregular menses, indifference to sex), and one pseudoneurological symptom (e.g., poor balance, numbness, paralysis). These symptoms lead to frequent and multiple medical consultations, complex medical history, and to alterations of the person's lifestyle. Physical and laboratory findings cannot detect a plausible medical condition as the cause of the symptoms. Somatization disorder is a relatively rare phenomenon with recent community and epidemiological studies citing prevalence rates between 0.4% and 0.7% (4–7 per 1,000; Bass & Murphy, 1990). Its onset is in early adulthood, its course is often chronic, and the prognosis is generally regarded as poor.

Hypochondriasis. Perhaps the most well-known somatoform disorder is hypochondriasis, defined as fears, suspicions, or convictions that one has a serious and often fatal illness such as heart disease, cancer, or AIDS. Patients frequently seek reassurance, check their bodies, and avoid illness-related situations. Merely informing patients of the absence of a disease process, or explaining the benign nature of the symptoms, results in only temporary reassurance that is followed by renewed worry over symptoms and continuing overuse of medical services (Salkovskis & Warwick, 2001). The onset of hypochondriasis is frequently in early adulthood. The course of hypochondriasis is typically chronic, and the condition frequently takes on a dominant role in the person's life and relationships.

Pain Disorder. Pain Disorder is characterized by acute or chronic pain in one or more body parts that is not easily understood or cannot be fully accounted for by a known medical condition. Pain is considered acute when it exists for less than 6 months and chronic when it persists beyond 6 months. Chronic pain, in particular, is often associated with major changes in behavior such as decreased activity and somatic preoccupation (Pilowsky, Chapman, & Bonica, 1977). Pain disorder is relatively common, may occur in adults of all ages, and is the most common complaint of individuals presenting to a physician. The proliferation of special pain clinics could be seen as another indication of the high number of pain patients seeking professional help. A study of internal medicine private practice patients found that 13% of patients suffered from chronic pain (Margolis, Zimny, & Miller, 1984).

Conversion Disorder. Conversion Disorder is characterized by symptoms suggesting a neurological disorder with medical investigations failing to identify a neurological or general medical disorder. At times, the particular symptoms may even be inconsistent with general neurological knowledge. Patients may present with any one or a combination of motor symptoms (e.g., paralysis), seizures or convulsions, and sensory deficits (e.g., blindness, anesthesia, and aphonia). An important requirement for the diagnosis is the temporal relation between conversion symptoms and a psychological stressor such as acute grief or victimization. Patients are typically unaware of any psychological basis for their symptoms and report being unable to control them. The diagnosis of conversion disorder is rare and difficult to establish with estimates ranging between 0.001% and 0.3% (1–300 per 100,000; APA, 1994). One reason is that symptoms seemingly indicative of conversion disorder are later discovered to be linked to a gradually developing physical (neurological) disease such as a brain tumor or multiple sclerosis (Fishbain & Goldberg, 1991). Although this condition may occur at any age, onset is typically in late childhood or early adulthood. Onset is often sudden and in response to conflicts or stressful situations such as unresolved grief and sexual trauma (Sharma & Chaturvedi, 1995).

Body Dysmorphic Disorder. Body dysmorphic disorder (BDD) is characterized by a preoccupation with an imagined or exaggerated body disfigurement or an excessive concern that there is something wrong with the shape or appearance of body parts. The perceived defect or abnormality is generally not or hardly noticeable to others. Objects of concern typically refer to the face (e.g., shape or size of nose), head (e.g., hair thinning), sexual characteristics (size of penis, breasts), or general body appearance (tallness/shortness). Other concerns may involve scars, wrinkles, or body odor. Cognitive features are excessive preoccupation, intrusive thoughts, and sometimes ideas of reference. For instance, an individual may persist in the belief that he or she is physically ill because of blemishes on the skin or somewhat atypical marks on the skin. On a behavioral level, features include avoidance (e.g., of body exposure, direct social contact, talking about the problem, looking in the mirror), camouflaging or concealing imagined deformities (wearing a hat or glasses), excessive grooming and checking, and reassurance seeking. BDD is not very common. Rosen (1995), in a representative study, found that only about 1% of a community sample met criteria for BDD with virtually no gender differences in prevalence. Onset of BDD may be gradual or sudden, and its course is generally continuous and chronic, though fluctuating in intensity. BDD is thought to start in adolescence when preoccupation with physical appearance is very common. Sociocultural factors influencing people's attitudes toward and dissatisfaction with their bodies seem to play a role in determining the extent to which a real or imagined physical abnormality becomes a cause for concern and preoccupation.

It should be noted that a preoccupation with physical appearance and distorted body image can also be found in persons with eating disorders. The difference is that individuals with eating disorders also exhibit abnormal patterns of eating (binging, purging, extreme dieting), whereas such abnormal eating patterns are not typical for persons with BDD.

Is the Diagnostic Validity of DSM-Defined Somatoform Disorders Questionable?

The diagnostic validity of somatoform disorders in relation to each other as well as to other clinical syndromes is problematic. First, most scholars have observed that these conditions do not necessarily represent distinct conditions. Second, they are highly influenced by contextual factors (social-verbal communities). Third, difficulties distinguishing between symptoms of somatoform disorders and physical health problems abound.

In terms of diagnostic validity, the distinct status of the somatoform disorders has been questioned repeatedly. Even the authors of the DSM–IV concede that the grouping of these disorders in a single section is based on clinical utility rather than on assumptions regarding shared etiology (APA, 1994). Murphy (1990) indicated that the disorders are often not qualitatively distinct, but rather, merge into each other making distinctions between individual somatoform disorders challenging. For example, pain may occur in any of the somatoform disorders. Ambiguous criteria such as "the person's concern is markedly excessive," "grossly in excess of what would be expected," and "slight physical abnormality" further hamper clear differentiation of these problems. The distinction between BDD and normal concerns about appearance is as difficult to make as the distinction between BDD and delusional disorder (somatic subtype). The relation and distinction between somatoform disorders and personality disorders also has been questioned for similar reasons (Bass & Murphy, 1995). Based on these limitations, Fava (1992) suggested that the somatoform disorders should be replaced by the concept of abnormal illness behavior because it is easier to operationalize. Fink (1996) made a similar point, arguing that researchers have been overly preoccupied with physical symptoms in their search for reliable and valid diagnostic criteria for somatization, but have neglected the behavioral emotional factors. Moreover, symptom-focused diagnoses may be artifacts biased by patient suggestibility, a clinician's preoccupation with some disease, and the social-verbal community (culture) in which such persons live.

The cross-cultural influences of somatization processes, in particular, are well documented (Escobar, Allen, Nervi, & Gara, 2001). In a review, Escobar et al. (2001), conclude that data from cross-cultural studies have documented "considerable cultural variation in the expression of somatizing syndromes. The available evidence further elaborates the well-accepted tenet that the presentation of personal/social distress in the form of somatic complaints appears to be the norm for most cultures" (p. 226). Thus, the specific symptoms of certain disorders often appear to be more a function of the individual's culture than of some underlying (distinct) biologically based disease process. Even DSM–IV suggests that the types and frequency of somatic symptoms differ across cultures and that symptom lists should be adjusted to the culture. For example, people in Africa and Southern Asia report burning hands and feet or the nondelusional experience of worms in the hands or ants in the head, whereas such reports are virtually unheard of among persons in Europe and North America. By comparison, people living in Europe and North America tend to be preoccupied with heart disease and cancer.

From Differential Diagnosis to a Dimensional Framework for Understanding Pathogenic Processes

Although diagnostic distinctions often cannot be made to a satisfactory degree, the origin of somatic complaints plays an important role in the present diagnostic criteria, particularly for differential diagnosis purposes. Specifically, DSM–IV distinguishes symptoms as part of a real disease (general medical condition) from symptoms for which medical reasons cannot be found. Health professionals are very much aware of the danger of misdiagnosing a somatoform disorder and of missing the presence of actual physical problems, particularly life-threatening diseases with a slow and diffuse onset such as multiple sclerosis, brain tumors, or systemic lupus (Fishbain & Goldberg, 1991). Additionally, there is frequently a reciprocal relation between health anxiety and somatic symptoms. For instance, Salkovskis (1996) describes how safety-seeking behavior designed to reduce anxiety frequently increases the symptoms that are the focus of anxiety. He cites the example of patients who palpate or rub lumps until they swell and cause pain. Several authors also point to potential pathophysiological mechanisms that may underlie unexplained physical symptoms (Sharpe & Bass, 1992). Thus, both in fairness to the patient and to design the most appropriate intervention, terms such as unexplained physical symptoms, functional defects, and nonorganic should be avoided when talking to patients.

We have previously argued (Eifert, Lejuez, & Bouman, 1998; Eifert, Zvolensky, & Lejuez, 2000) that overlap between related categories is not necessarily a problem of comorbidity or inaccurate definitions but a result of similar psychological processes involved in these conditions. Accordingly, we suggest adopting a dimensional approach to understanding illness-related concerns that can identify key biobehavioral processes. To illustrate this approach, we discuss focal dimensions of health anxiety, a psychological process that characterizes, in part, many somatoform disorders as well as related conditions (e.g., panic disorder). We view health anxiety as a psychological process where persons present with problems that fall on a continuum along four dimensions (Eifert et al., 2000):

1. Preoccupation with the body and its functioning—such bodily preoccupation, especially when coupled with somatic complaints, may produce a state of somatic uncertainty and form the basis for the other three dimensions of the disorder.

2. Disease suspicion or conviction—the person has the suspicion or is convinced of having a serious physical disease; suspicion and conviction are on a continuum of strength, and in rare cases the conviction may reach delusional intensity.
3. Disease fear—the person fears having a serious physical disease.
4. Safety-seeking behavior—the function of behavior such as repeated requests for medical examinations and tests, bodily checking, verbal complaints, and seeking reassurance is to reduce worry and anxiety over physical illness.

A person could obtain a high score on any one or all four dimensions of health anxiety. For example, disease suspicion/conviction may or may not be accompanied by a strong fear of the suspected disease. Clinically, this feature is most apparent in patients' resistance to medical reassurance. For instance, patients may remain extremely worried about their health even though their fear of suffering from a specific disease may have been eliminated by a medical examination (Fava & Grandi, 1991). Accordingly, a dimensional classification system could help overcome some challenges inherent to a traditional diagnostic perspective of somatoform disorders. Moreover, identifying dimensions that allow a classification of illness behavior based on the function that such behavior serves, rather than just its topography, might lead to a better understanding and improved treatments of persons with somatoform problems (Eifert & Lau, 2001). Apart from the number and type of physical complaints, some of these dimensions include the presence and extent of preoccupation with body and health, symptom misinterpretation, disease suspicion or conviction, disease fear, and safety-seeking behavior.

GENERAL VULNERABILITY PROCESSES FOR ABNORMAL ILLNESS BEHAVIOR

Given our previous discussion as to prototypical characteristics of health anxiety, the next logical question pertains to the types of processes that increase or decrease the risk for developing abnormal illness behavior. As discussed at the onset of this chapter, many, if not all, people experience distressing physical sensations at some point in their lives. Moreover, a substantial percentage will even experience robust internal physical (interoceptive) reactions in the form of panic attacks, limited symptom panic attacks, gastrointestinal distress, respiratory infections, strained muscles, and so on. In fact, such bodily distress is so common to the human experience that it seems almost inconceivable to imagine a person going through life without experiencing at least some significant somatic disturbance.

Although systematic knowledge about causes is lacking, factors such as parental modeling, stressful life events, high negative affect, and aspects of the relationship and communication between patients and doctors appear to be related to the development of somatoform disorders (e.g., Bass & Murphy, 1990). In addition, there are a number of biopsychosocial processes that increase vulnerability for the development of somatoform pathology or abnormal illness behavior generally. The processes that we discuss in this section include (a) an inherited risk for emotional responsivity to physical sensations, (b) deficits in emotion regulatory skills, and (c) language-based and observational learning. Before this discussion, however, we need to briefly define what we mean by the term abnormal illness behavior.

Pilowsky (1993, p. 62) defined *abnormal illness behavior* as the "persistence of a maladaptive mode of experiencing, perceiving, evaluating, and responding to one's own health status, despite the fact that a doctor has provided a lucid and accurate appraisal of the situation and management to be followed (if any), with opportunities for discussion, negotiation and clarification, based on adequate assessment of all relevant biological, psychological, social and cultural factors." Thus abnormal illness behavior refers to the disagreement between the doctor and patient about the sick role to which the patient feels entitled. Sharpe, Mayou and Bass (1995) argued that the concept of abnormal illness behavior is valuable not only for understanding patients with functional somatic symptoms but also for understanding the behavioral aspects of all illness. We now turn to a discussion of variables that may increase the risk of developing abnormal illness behavior.

Inherited Risk for Emotional Responsivity to Physical Sensations

There is convincing evidence that there is an inherited component or substrate for negative emotionality. Researchers have referred to this inherited disposition by a number of different terms, including negative affectivity, trait anxiety, and neuroticism (Barlow, 2001). These synonymous labels are intended to capture a general predisposition to experience negative affect (e.g., anxiety) and perhaps abrupt emotional reactivity (e.g., panic) to challenging or stressful life events.

Although the characteristics of negative affectivity vary across specific negative emotional experiences (e.g., panic versus anger), they all posit that high degrees of negative emotionality are associated with a lower threshold of initial affective response, slower recovery to baseline, and greater reactivation of arousal with repeated exposure to stressful events. High reactivity is generally associated with inhibited temperament, whereas low reactivity is associated with uninhibited temperament (Kagan, 1989). Thus, individual differences in temperament are often related to the experience and regulation of affect because they constrain or facilitate certain types of responding. For example, the temperamental characteristics of behavioral inhibition are believed to relate to tendencies to experience high levels of autonomic arousal in evocative contexts as well as the propensity to react in a defensive manner in response to threat (e.g., avoidance-oriented coping strategies; Kagan, Snidman, & Arcus, 1992).

As behavioral genetic research continues to make important strides in our understanding of emotional functioning, we may eventually have specific models articulating the extent to which a specific gene or combination of genes contributes to a specific anxiety disorder or health disorder. At this stage, however, it appears that a general disposition for negative affectivity is inherited. The contribution of this inherited component is estimated to be at approximately 30% in the development of somatoform-related disorders (Kendler, Walters, Truett, & Heath, 1995). No research has documented the exact proportion of explained variance for the development of a specific disorder, although there is some evidence that there are both shared and specific genetic vulnerabilities across anxiety-related disorders (Kendler et al., 1995). It is likely that a genetic predisposition creates the biological conditions that make people prone to respond with anxiety and panic reactions to certain bodily changes and processes. One research challenge in this domain will be to specify how genetic vulnerabilities (once they are identified) might influence the pathogenesis of a specific disorder.

Development of Emotion Self-Regulatory Skills

Research has shown that early in life humans develop a repertoire of regulatory-oriented skills to deal with elevated levels of bodily arousal and concomitant emotional distress. For example, crying as an infant is a signal to caregivers that the infant is in need of something (e.g., food), and ceasing to cry and related behavioral responses (e.g., smiling) reinforce caregiver behavior (Rothbart, Ziaie, & O'Boyle, 1992). Thus, the effective management of bodily states, particularly negative emotional experiences, is a critical (primary) early step in psychological development. As children mature, they learn to approach and avoid salient environmental stimuli, and the various segments of society increasingly expect them to gain better emotion regulatory skills (e.g., suppression of crying in school). By adulthood, the individual is expected to have sophisticated emotional control skills and the ability to learn new regulatory skills for a variety of changing sociocultural contexts. As one illustrative example, adults are not supposed to demonstrate signs of emotional distress in social, performance, or work settings. Research indicates that individuals with low levels of emotional regulation skills, or an inability to readily alter regulation strategies, evidence less capacity to function flexibly and successfully in social environments relative to those who have such emotion regulation skills (Rothbart, 1989).

The preceding discussion highlights that emotion regulation skills are expected to increase consistently across the life span and are an integral component of mental health. When individuals lack the ability to effectively alter their emotional experiences, they are more susceptible to physical discomfort, negative affect, and anxiety (Rothbart et al., 1992). A major source of learning for emotion regulation skills is the degree to which children exercise the capacity to explore their world, both literally and metaphorically. Developmental researchers have referred to these experiences as mastery learning opportunities (Rothbart, 1989). Impoverished environments where parents or caregivers (e.g., teachers) respond to children in a noncontingent manner produce more emotional distress compared to environments associated with contingent outcomes. For example, Chorpita, Brown, and Barlow (1998) found that parents who discourage autonomy (through modeling, vicarious learning, rule-governed behavior, and/or instrumental learning) while simultaneously excessively protecting their children from any potential source of threat are more likely to foster a perceived sense of limited control in their children. Similar findings have been observed in studies of nonhuman animals raised in environments with little control over important outcomes (e.g., availability of food; Mineka, Gunnar, & Champoux, 1986). Such findings are important to understanding somatoform disorders because greater degrees of perceived uncontrollability are predictive of the tendency to view ambiguous internal stimuli as threatening (Zvolensky, Lejuez, & Eifert, 2000).

Coping with emotional distress is, of course, a multidimensional process. Recent work indicates that coping responses are best viewed from a hierarchical model that includes first-order and higher-order dimensions (Compas, Conner-Smith, Saltzman, Thomsen, & Wadsworth, 2001). Indeed, researchers increasingly suggest that coping with emotional distress involves strategic (voluntary) and automatic (involuntary) responses. Additionally, Compas et al. (2001) have categorized these coping responses along the dimensions of engagement and disengagement. Engagement responding includes active, primary control-oriented responding aimed at altering the immediate situation in some sort of direct manner (e.g., leaving a situation that one finds uncomfortable because of cardiac-related distress and tension). Disengagement responding includes secondary control-oriented responding aimed at adapting to an uncontrollable situation by purposively altering one's cognitive-affective response to that situation (indirect responding). For instance, individuals might adapt to pain or other aversive bodily sensations by altering their cognitive response to such events (e.g., acceptance, distraction, reframing). Overall, it is likely that individuals will develop varying degrees of emotion regulatory skills across the life span, and these skills are likely to be a product of early learning experiences. How such regulatory skills moderate clinical outcome for the development, maintenance, and remediation of specific somatoform disorders promises to be an exciting area of future research.

Deficits in Emotion Processing (Alexithymia)

Alexithymia literally means no words for feelings. Its key features are a relative constriction of emotional functioning, poverty of fantasy life, and inability to find appropriate words to describe one's emotions. Bach and Bach (1995) found high alexithymia scores to be predictive of persistent somatization. The concept of alexithymia implies that somatic symptoms have a communicative function, that is, individuals are perhaps trying to tell us something with their symptoms. For example, in a sample of normal volunteers, Vingerhoets, Van Heck, Grim, and Bermond (1995) found strong negative correlations between alexithymia and the expression of emotions, daydreams and fantasies, and planful and rational actions. Individuals with high alexithymia scores seem to be vulnerable to mounting tension from undifferentiated states of unpleasant emotional arousal. This vulnerability probably is caused by a disturbance in the processing of emotional awareness that interferes with the subject's ability to experience and express emotions. There is evidence that alexithymic coping strategies (emotional constriction or lack of emotional expression) are moderated by anxiety sensitivity, or the fear of anxiety-related sensations (Devine, Stewart, & Watt, 1999; Stewart, Zvolensky, & Eifert, 2002).

Language-Based Learning

Aside from direct forms of learning, individuals also experience affective responses to body-related events and sensations through the use of language. Language serves important symbolic functions by providing humans with emotional experiences without exposure to the actual physical stimuli or events that ordinarily elicit those responses (Staats & Eifert, 1990). For instance, both knowing what to do and knowing what to feel involve verbal understanding of the relation between them. Thus, the meaning of health-related anxiety in a psychological sense represents a complex act of relating largely arbitrary verbal-symbolic events with other events and psychological functions within a particular context (Forsyth & Eifert, 1996). For instance, words such as anxiety and fear either implicitly or explicitly establish relations with other events such as "I am anxious or afraid of . . . something, some event, or someone."

The relational quality of terms denoting emotions, in turn, must be tied to descriptions of behavior and events with a variety of stimulus functions (e.g., eliciting, evoking, reinforcing, and punishing) and meanings (e.g., good, bad, pleasant, unpleasant, painful). In turn, people often describe their emotional experiences metaphorically in ways that others can understand (e.g., "When I feel anxious, it's like a knife going through my chest"). These metaphorical extensions have no real counterpart inside the person. Instead, they function to communicate the meaning of emotional experience (feeling threatened to the point of fearing death) by identifying and relating events with known stimulus functions (a sharp knife can cut into a chest and cause death).

The social-verbal community determines what kind of stimuli and events are placed in a relation and the nature of that relation (Hayes & Wilson, 1994), and these arbitrary relations are learned and function in a variety of ways (Sidman, 1994; Staats & Eifert, 1990). Individuals become health anxious about particular experiences or "symptoms" because they read and hear about them in the specific cultural context they live in. This may be one of the main reasons why cultural variations in somatoform disorders are widespread and can be observed with such great regularity (Escobar et al., 2001). For instance, people in Western societies become anxious when they notice a fast or irregular heart beat because they have seen or heard about that event being related to heart attack many times.

The most important point is that persons with somatoform disorders have likely developed complex repertoires of verbal and other symbolic responses that elicit negative affect and serve as discriminative stimuli for escape/avoidance behavior (Staats & Eifert, 1990). Thus, for otherwise healthy people, the sensations of a beating heart or chest pain may lead to a sequence of verbal and autonomic events that result in the belief that they are having a heart attack (Eifert, 1992). In this instance, a fast or irregular heartbeat is not just a felt beating heart. Instead, it is an acquired and verbally mediated formulation of what it means to have a fast or irregular heartbeat or chest pain (e.g., "I have heart disease" or "I am suffering from a heart attack"). Not only may the person respond to such sensations by rushing to an emergency room, but also any other public or private stimulus events associated with this response may now acquire similar negative functions (e.g., physical exercise, smoking, working hard). In this way, a variety of behaviors and events can come to elicit the physiological event that the person then misconstrues as dangerous (Forsyth & Eifert, 1996).

Observational Learning

Aside from the general vulnerability dimensions already discussed, it is likely that persons who develop somatoform disorders have been exposed to negative health-related events to a greater degree than persons who do not develop this disorder. For example, some studies indicate that a significant number of persons with cardiophobia have observed heart disease and its potentially lethal effects (e.g., death) in relatives and close friends (Eifert & Forsyth, 1996). These persons had been exposed directly to the physical and emotionally painful consequences of heart disease. As a result, they may also have had more exposure to heart-focused perceptions and interpretations of physical symptoms and physiological processes.

Observational learning is strongly involved in learning pain tolerance, pain ratings, and nonverbal expressions of pain (Flor, Birbaumer, & Turk, 1990). Such observational learning may increase the likelihood of expressing and interpreting arousal and pain in later life as a heart problem, because socially acquired perceptions and interpretations of symptoms largely determine how people deal with illness. For instance, if one or both parents have heart disease, children might observe their parent's response to a heart problem. If that modeling is inappropriate (e.g., excessive illness behavior), these children will not only be more likely to respond to stress with increased cardiovascular activity, but they will have also learned inappropriate labeling and interpretation of such symptoms and have fewer appropriate coping skills.

Taken together, research suggests a variety of general factors that may promote the development of the type of abnormal illness behavior found in somatoform disorders. These processes are likely nonspecific in the sense that they increase the chance of negative emotional responding and poor affect regulatory strategies. Exposure to specific illnesses or to persons who model the potential dangers of certain physical disorders may increase an individual's general vulnerability. Continued research in each of these general domains will improve our ability to predict who will develop a specific type of somatoform disorder.

TREATMENT OF SOMATOFORM DISORDERS

Cognitive-behavioral theories and research have been helpful in providing a fledgling basis for a better understanding and treatment of persons with somatization problems. Important progress has been made in particular for persons with health anxiety (Eifert & Lau, 2001; Salkovskis & Warwick, 2001) and chronic pain (e.g., Flor et al., 1990; Schermelleh-Engel, Eifert, Moosbrugger, & Frank, 1997). We now overview these treatment strategies at a general level and how they can be applied to specific types of somatoform disorders.

General Strategies

Psychologically distressed patients who present with unexplained somatic symptoms are high users of medical care, and their doctors regard them as frustrating and difficult to treat (Mayou & Sharpe, 1995). There is often a mismatch between the expectations of these patients and their doctors' abilities and communication skills. For instance, terms such as *functional heart problem, nervous heart, atypical chest pain*, and *pseudoangina*, when used to "diagnose" unexplained chest pain, can easily be misinterpreted by a patient who is determined to believe that some significant cardiac disease is being described (Eifert et al., 2000). Health care providers often feel frustrated and emotionally drained because these patients obviously need psychological support but resent being referred to a psychologist or psychiatrist.

Patients often perceive the use of diagnostic labels such as hypochondriasis as an insult because these labels seem to imply that the patients' problems are not real and "just in their head." Accepting and understanding, rather than refuting or arguing with the patient's symptoms, is therefore the most important condition for engaging the patient in a therapeutic working relationship (cf. Bass & Benjamin, 1993). In the engagement stage of treatment, patients are helped to see that there may be an alternative explanation for the difficulties they are experiencing (Salkovskis, 1996). For instance, although chest pain can be due to coronary artery disease, it can also be caused by hyperventilation-induced chest wall muscle tension (Eifert et al., 2000). The general treatment strategy is to test such alternative or benign medical explanations for symptoms and to conduct therapy in the context of an experiment that provides an opportunity for testing alternative hypotheses (Eifert & Lau, 2001; Salkovskis, 1996).

Rather than merely telling patients there is no organic reason for their chest pain, an explanation of symptoms that overcomes the nonorganic–organic dualism provides the patient with a more acceptable rationale and reassurance (Eifert, Hodson, Tracey, Seville, & Gunawardane, 1996). For instance, to provide a patient with a credible explanation of how anxiety and chest wall muscle tension can result in chest pain, patients may be given a chest-focused relaxation with electromyogram (EMG) feedback that literally shows them how they can change their chest tension levels. Salkovskis and Warwick (2001) found that reassurance that only informs the patients that there is nothing organically wrong with their body will actually increase future reassurance seeking rather than decrease it. On the other hand, appropriate reassurance and feedback that provides the patient with new and alternative explanations is the key to successful treatment, and in some cases, may help prevent the development of chronic somatization problems in the first place. In a controlled case study, Eifert and Lau (2001) found that behavioral experiments were not only useful in developing alternative symptom explanations but also in teaching the patients to reassure themselves rather than seeking therapist reassurance. The treatment strategies and techniques targeting the dimensions of abnormal illness behavior related to heart-focused anxiety are summarized in Table 13.1.

Medical professionals need to be trained to provide alternative explanation rather than vague pseudomedical labels and to acknowledge rather than dismiss patients' concerns. At the same time, withholding unnecessary medication and medical examinations (response prevention for safety-seeking behavior) is a crucial part of treatment. For example, Goldberg, Gask, and O'Dowd (1989) developed a training program for primary care physicians that included empathic listening to complaints and symptoms, thus changing the agenda of the actions to be undertaken from a somatomedical focus on bodily symptoms to a psychological perspective focusing on emotional distress. Physicians were also taught how to help patients reattribute bodily symptoms to psychological factors. Two other studies (Rost, Kashner, & Smith, 1994; Smith, Rost, & Kashner, 1995) also focused on changing physician behavior in primary care settings. Physicians were taught to use empathic listening techniques with their patients without reinforcing patients' abnormal illness behavior by denying expensive diagnostic procedures, surgeries, and hospitalizations. Such denials also prevent iatrogenic diseases and counteract patients' disease convictions. The results of these studies suggest that this balanced approach to patient care can reduce health care costs and at the same time increase the psychological adjustment of patients.

TABLE 13.1

Key Treatment Components Targeting Dimensions and Symptoms of Heart-Focused Anxiety

Dimensions	Treatment Strategies and Techniques
Preoccupation with heart	Demonstrate that chest pain/heart sensations are not dangerous *Reduce avoidance; expose to cardiac-related stimuli*
Disease fear	Extinction of fear and exposure to avoided activities *Expose to interoceptive (particularly cardioceptive) cues* *Reinforce "dangerous" behavior (e.g., strenuous exercise)*
Disease conviction	Testing alternative symptom explanations *Explain impact of anxiety & tension on body (chest pain)* *Conduct behavioral experiments to test hypotheses* *Review evidence for/against heart disease* *Review evidence for cardiac vs. tension chest pain*
Safety/reassurance seeking	Extinction of help and reassurance seeking *Review results of previous tests* *Withhold reassurance* *Refuse further tests* *Do physical exercise while preventing pulse checking*
Physical (panic) symptoms	Reduce chronic tension and overbreathing *Relax chest muscles* *Teach slow diaphragmatic vs. thoracic breathing*

Note: Although this example deals with heart-focused anxiety, the process dimensions are adaptable and applicable to other somatization problems. Adapted from "Using Behavioral Experiments in the Treatment of Cardiophobia. A case study," by G. H. Eifert and A. Lau, 2001, *Cognitive and Behavioral Practice, 8,* 305–317.

Finally, it is essential that we move patients from an almost exclusive focus on symptoms, which may or may not be changeable and/or controllable, to goals and behavior that are controllable and changeable. For instance, Rief, Hiller, Geissner, and Fichter (1995) suggest that after an initial empathic discussion of symptoms, treatment needs to shift toward more changeable behavioral targets, such as occupational problem solving, social skills training, and quality of life enhancement. Behavioral activation treatment programs (Hopko, Lejuez, Ruggiero, & Eifert, 2003) appear to be valuable therapist tools to help move patients in their "valued direction" (Hayes, Strosahl, & Wilson, 1999) and at the same time reduce negative affect.

SPECIFIC TREATMENT RECOMMENDATIONS

Somatization Disorder

Most articles seem to imply that it is best to think of somatic problems as requiring management rather than treatment (e.g., Bass & Benjamin, 1993). Early diagnosis and the prevention of unnecessary medical and surgical investigation are of primary importance. Most somatization patients have distinct expectations regarding treatment goals and procedures and try to persuade their doctors to follow their wishes for further medical investigations and treatments. Bass and Murphy (1990) state that treatment often involves long-term supportive psychotherapy and must be directed toward controlling the demands on medical care as well as the treatment of symptoms and social disability. They recommend the following five steps: (a) encourage a long-term supportive relationship with only one understanding primary care physician to prevent doctor shopping and to coordinate all actions; (b) see patients on regular appointments rather than on demand to prevent reinforcement of illness behavior; (c) view patients' physical complaints as a form of communication rather than as evidence of disease; and (d) minimize the use of psychotropic drugs and/or analgesic medication. In general, adaptive behavior is encouraged and promoted, whereas sick role behavior is ignored as much as possible. A study by Kashner, Rost, Cohen, Anderson, and Smith (1995) focused on coping with the nature and consequences of the physical symptoms, general problem solving, and helping patients take more control of their lives. These authors found that eight sessions of brief group therapy improved physical and mental health at 1-year follow-up.

A randomized controlled trial examining a comprehensive cognitive-behavioral approach for dealing with medically unexplained physical symptoms was conducted by Speckens and associates (1996). A cognitive-behavioral intervention group of thirty-nine general medical outpatients was compared with a control group of forty patients receiving optimized medical care. Treatment included imaginary exposure and distraction techniques to break the vicious circles of cognitive avoidance and preoccupation; activity scheduling, exposure in vivo, and response prevention to decrease avoidance behavior; relaxation training, breathing exercises, and physical exercises; and problem-solving or social skills training to overcome any problems in interpersonal relationships. At both 6- and 12-months follow-up, the intervention group reported lower intensity and frequency of symptoms, reduced illness behavior, less sleep impairment, and fewer limitations in social and leisure activities than did the control group.

Hypochondriasis

Traditionally, individuals with hypochondriasis were considered difficult to treat and their prognosis was regarded as poor. For instance, early studies assessing the effectiveness of a variety of psychological interventions available at that time (e.g., Kenyon, 1964) found 40% of patients with primary hypochondriasis to be unchanged or worse following treatment. Although patients with unexplained physical symptoms and/or health anxiety still pose a considerable challenge for therapists, cognitive-behavioral interventions have yielded encouraging results.

The first comprehensive cognitive-behavioral treatment formulations were provided by Warwick and Salkovskis (1990). Patients are instructed to self-monitor during hypochondriacal episodes, paying careful attention to environmental events, physical symptoms, associated cognitions, and their resulting hypochondriacal behavior. As indicated, their treatment is directed at evaluating alternative, nonthreatening explanations of body-related observations that they misinterpret as signs of serious disease. Two possible explanations for the patient's problem are considered alongside each other rather than as mutually exclusive alternatives (Salkovskis, 1996). Patients are then asked to engage in a variety of behavioral experiments to test these new explanations, and therapy proceeds as an evaluation of the relative merits of the alternative views. Salkovskis (1996) emphasizes that inappropriate safety seeking prevents individuals from discovering that their fears are groundless. Hence, the key function of exposure exercises and response prevention is to bring patients into contact with the actual rather than expected consequences of their behavior (Eifert & Lau, 2001). By allowing patients to repeatedly experience feared bodily sensations without the dreaded consequences, they learn that what they are afraid of does not actually happen.

A system of differential reinforcement may need to be added for individuals who gain sympathy or interest for physical complaints but may receive little attention otherwise. In those cases, family members and other individuals the patient has contact with (including the therapist) should reinforce patient initiation of conversation on any topic other than symptoms (healthy conversation). This reinforcement could consist of praise or increased attention. As the patient engages in more healthy conversation, the natural contingencies (e.g., reduced medical bills, more pleasant interactions with others) should begin to maintain behavior and the frequency and magnitude of artificial reinforcement can be slowly reduced.

Salkovskis and Warwick (1986) reported two successfully treated single cases of primary hypochondriasis using cognitive-behavioral methods. In another study, Visser and Bouman (1992) found that four of six hypochondriacal patients improved significantly following in vivo exposure, response suppression, and cognitive therapy. In this study exposure and response suppression (behavioral components) appeared to have accounted for more of the improvement than the cognitive component (i.e., attempting to change directly the patient's misconceptions about symptoms). The positive results of these series of single case studies were supported in a first controlled trial that showed cognitive-behavioral therapy to be superior to a wait-list control condition (Warwick, Clark, Cobb, & Salkovskis, 1996).

For patients whose main concern is fear of a specific disease, without significant conviction of having the disease, a more focused program of tension reduction (e.g., through relaxation), exposure to the feared stimuli, and prevention of checking and safety seeking can be sufficient (Eifert, 1992). For instance, Warwick and Marks (1988) used exposure to feared stimuli, paradox (deliberate attempts to induce a panic attack), and response prevention such as banning reassurance seeking and physician visits. There was a significant decrease in illness fear and an increase in work and social adjustment for the group of seventeen patients who were treated.

Overall, cognitive-behavioral treatments are promising and prognosis for patients who are treated with such interventions seems more favorable than previously thought. More extensive and controlled studies are needed to determine the most crucial treatment components and the mechanisms that explain their success.

Pain Disorder

Earlier approaches for pain management were based on psychodynamic principles and used hypnotic suggestions to help people deal with pain. A review by Turk, Meichenbaum, and Genest (1983) found that these techniques are ineffective when used alone and that treatment effects are due to the unwitting inclusion of behavioral and cognitive treatment components.

Pain behavior is not an expression or side effect of a pain problem, instead it is the problem (Rachlin, 1985). Therefore, the goal of treatment is to extinguish maladaptive pain behavior and teach and reinforce the use of more adaptive pain coping strategies (Nicholas, Wilson, & Goyen, 1991). Treatment begins with a thorough functional analysis of current pain behavior and the environmental contingencies associated with that behavior. Once the consequences maintaining the maladaptive pain behavior are determined, attempts are made to reduce reinforcement for that behavior and increase reinforcement for adaptive pain coping behavior (cf. Fordyce, Roberts, & Sternbach, 1985; Nicholas et al., 1991). In addition to changing a patient's maladaptive pain behavior, cognitive-behavioral therapy also attempts to alter associated thought patterns and the patient's perceived competence in dealing with pain (Schermelleh-Engel et al., 1997). Pain management programs typically require active patient participation and include fostering a patient's real and perceived competence to deal with pain, teaching skills and adaptive responses to problems (including self-attribution for change and success), and planning maintenance.

Based on the assumption that pain is mediated by thoughts and images, cognitive methods involving imagery and distraction have often been added to pain management programs (Turk et al., 1983). Patients are encouraged to create and focus on those thoughts and images that alleviate pain while ignoring those that exacerbate pain. Particularly for patients who engage in few activities, a behavioral activation program is beneficial in more than one way

(Lejuez et al., 2001). Such programs encourage and reinforce patients engaging in a host of activities. As patients continue with these activities, they frequently recognize the intrinsically reinforcing value of the activities and their mood enhancement effects.

The cognitive-behavioral approach to pain management has been identified as an empirically validated treatment by the Task Force on Promotion and Dissemination of Psychological Procedures (Chambless, 1995). Which specific components are most effective, however, remains unclear. In a review of the experimental research, Turk et al. (1983) concluded that cognitive strategies are effective but that the data "do not convincingly establish the efficacy of any cognitive coping strategy relative to the strategies that subjects bring to experiments" (p. 96). They also conclude that there is not sufficient evidence "to support the use of any one strategy compared to any one other" (p. 96). Others have raised more fundamental criticisms and argued that the effects attributed to direct cognitive manipulations could be due to associated environmental manipulations (Rachlin, 1985).

Conversion Disorder

An important first step in the treatment of conversion symptoms is their early recognition in which a physical examination plays a crucial role. In many cases, a positive diagnosis can be made on the basis of the rather untypical or bizarre symptoms. Because conversion symptoms vary widely across patients, treatment needs to be individualized. Identifying precipitating stressors is crucial so that patients can be taught more adaptive ways of coping with these stressors. Occasionally, manipulation of the patient's social environmental is necessary to reduce the influence of secondary gain, such as attention from family and friends. Partners and significant others may have to learn how to reinforce the patients nonsymptomatic behavior.

Body Dysmorphic Disorder

Behavioral interventions for BDD aim at changing avoidance behavior, reassurance seeking, checking, and excessive grooming. Exposure in vivo is used to counter avoidance of social situations (meeting people, having a conversation, being in the spotlight) and prevent individuals from attempting to cover their ostensible blemishes (e.g., by wearing camouflaging clothing such as baggy pants, long hair, sunglasses). Patients are encouraged to expose themselves to social situations rather than avoid them and to observe the reactions of other people to their imagined deformity. Rosen (1995) suggests exposure assignments such as wearing trendy clothes, using makeup to accentuate features, standing closer to people, undressing in front of one's spouse. Response prevention may involve refraining from looking in the mirror for excessive periods of time, the use of makeup, and inspecting skin blemishes.

There are few controlled treatment outcome studies for BDD, but several case studies and uncontrolled trials using exposure and response prevention (Neziroglu & Yaryura-Tobias, 1993) and social skills training (Braddock, 1982) have been reported. Schmidt and Harrington (1995) describe a successful cognitive-behavioral therapy in a 24-year-old male who was preoccupied with having small hands. Nine 1-hour sessions with behavioral experiments aimed at challenging beliefs about size of his hands and other people's attention to his hands. Treatment resulted in a decrease in BDD–related cognitions, distress and avoidance behavior, and Beck Depression and Beck Anxiety Inventory scores.

The first controlled outcome study of the treatment of BDD (Rosen, Reiter, & Orosan, 1995) compared the effectiveness of cognitive-behavioral therapy with a wait-list control condition in fifty-four females. Treatment involved eight 2-hour small group sessions and was aimed at modifying dysfunctional thoughts about the patients' body image, reducing checking of their appearance, and increasing exposure to avoided situations. Results at posttest and 4-months follow-up showed improvement in the active treatment condition on several measures of body image, whereas no such changes occurred in the control condition. The results of this study are promising, but more controlled studies are needed to corroborate existing data and to examine the role of the various treatment components.

Unexplained and unexplainable somatic symptoms are very common in the general population. These problems are costly to the individuals concerned in terms of distress and financial expense as well as to society in terms of lost productivity and health care costs. Compared to other common psychological dysfunctions (e.g., anxiety and depression), our present conceptual understanding of somatoform disorders is poor and comprehensive integrative models are still lacking.

One factor that has impeded a better understanding of the somatoform disorders is the unsatisfactory and somewhat arbitrary way of their current DSM classification. In view of the existing conceptual and diagnostic confusion, vagueness, and imprecision, we question the utility of the current criteria for and distinctions among somatoform disorders and the wisdom of keeping hypochondriasis in particular separate from the anxiety disorders. Comorbidity of somatoform disorders with anxiety disorders and depression is not a diagnostic problem, but an indication that there are similarities in the underlying psychopathological processes (Aikens, Zvolensky, & Eifert, 2001). We have outlined some commonalities in emotional dysregulation processes, particularly in relation to anxiety. A practical consequence for researchers and clinicians is to give up their focus on the individual disorders and increase their efforts at identifying the common functions of symptoms in persons with different somatoform problems (Eifert, 1996).

The complex relationships between the physical and psychological aspects of somatoform disorders has led to much confusion. We caution against an overreliance on medical diagnostic procedures and medical theory. At the same time, research and service delivery would benefit from a more balanced approach. This approach should focus not just on finding or excluding somatic abnormalities but also combine current medical knowledge and diagnostic techniques with the psychological assessments of a patient's behavior, cognitive processes, and social relationships (cf. Fink, 1996). In our work with cardiac patients, we observed how a simple reliance on one source of information (medical or psychological) was inadequate for many patients. Instead, it was the combination of sophisticated medical tests and psychological information that yielded the type of knowledge that was most useful for recommending and designing the most appropriate treatment for the individual patient.

Hence, one of the most compelling conclusions arising from this chapter is that somatoform disorders cannot be adequately understood, assessed, and treated from a single perspective. Both the classification and research could be improved by adopting a multidisciplinary approach and an integrated biopsychosocial perspective. For example, Mayou, Bass and Sharpe (1995) propose a multidimensional classification of patients with functional somatic symptoms along five dimensions: (a) number and type of somatic symptoms; (b) mental state (mood and psychiatric disorder); (c) cognitions (e.g., symptom misinterpretations, disease conviction); (d) behavioral and functional impairment (illness behavior, avoidance, use of health services); and (e) pathophysiological disturbance (organic diseases, physiological mechanisms such as hyperventilation). As indicated in the section on health anxiety, individuals may be assigned different positions on all of these dimensions across the various types of somatoform disorders. Rather than attempting to find the correct diagnosis, we recommend assessment along the crucial dimensions involved in the regulation of maladaptive illness behavior and devising treatment programs based on such assessments. Beyond the number and type of physical complaints, some of these dimensions include the presence and extent of preoccupation with body and health, symptom misinterpretation, disease suspicion or conviction, disease fear, safety-seeking behavior, focus and modulation of worry and fear, and pathophysiological processes.

A multicausal perspective suggests several potentially fruitful lines for future psychological research into somatoform disorders, such as an increased focus on information processing behavior (attribution, attention, and memory) and environmental contingencies for illness behavior (e.g., social, occupational, medical). Psychoneuroimmunological studies may help clarify particular aspects of the nature of the interface between pathophysiological changes and individual responses to such changes as exemplified in some chronic pain research (cf. Flor et al., 1990). Although the past emphasis on the problems of patients with no demonstrable physical pathology was worthwhile and deserves continued attention, the gray area of persons with some organic pathology, bodily symptoms, and psychological distress deserves greater recognition and needs to be investigated more carefully.

Treatment programs and outcomes are likely to be enhanced by an improved conceptual understanding of these problems. The need for better theories and treatments is even more pressing for those somatoform problems that have been particularly neglected in the past such as BDD and conversion problems. The relative success of recent cognitive-behavioral treatment programs for persons with unexplained physical symptoms, health anxiety, or chronic pain is promising. These treatment successes may help change the common perception of health care providers that people with such problems are just a "pain in the neck" and invariably difficult, or even impossible, to treat.

REFERENCES

Aikens, J. E., Zvolensky, M. J., & Eifert, G. H. (2001). Fear of cardiopulmonary sensations in emergency room noncardiac chest pain patients. *Journal of Behavioral Medicine, 24*, 155–167.

American Psychiatric Association. (1994). *Diagnostic and statistical manual of mental disorders* (4th ed.). Washington, DC: Author.

Barlow, D. H. (2001). *Anxiety and its disorders: The nature and treatment of anxiety and panic* (2nd ed.). New York: Guilford.

Bass, C. M., & Benjamin, S. (1993). The management of the chronic somatizer. *British Journal of Psychiatry, 162*, 472–480.

Bass, C. M., & Murphy, M. R. (1990). Somatization disorder: Critique of the concept and suggestions for future research. In C. M. Bass (Ed.), *Somatization. Physical symptoms and psychological illness* (pp. 301–332). Oxford: Blackwell.

Bass, C. M., & Murphy, M. R. (1995). Somatoform and personality disorders: Syndromal comorbidity and overlapping developmental pathways. *Journal of Psychosomatic Research, 39*, 403–427.

Braddock, L. E. (1982). Dysmorphophobia in adolescence: A case report. *British Journal of Psychiatry, 140*, 199–201.

Chambless, D. L. (1995). Training in and dissemination of empirically validated psychological treatments: Report and recommendations by the Task Force on Psychological Procedures. *The Clinical Psychologist, 48*, 3–23.

Chorpita, B. F., Brown, T. A., & Barlow, D. H. (1998). Perceived control as a mediator of family environment in etiological models of childhood anxiety. *Behavior Therapy, 29*, 457–476.

Compas, B. E., Conner-Smith, J. K., Saltzman, H., Thomsen, A. H., & Wadsworth, M. E. (2001). Coping with stress during childhood and adolescent: Problems, progress, and potential in theory and research. *Psychological Bulletin, 127*, 87–127.

Devine, H., Stewart, S. H., & Watt, M. C. (1999). Relations between anxiety sensitivity and dimensions of alexithymia. *Journal of Psychosomatic Research, 47*, 145–158.

Eifert, G. H. (1992). Cardiophobia: A paradigmatic behavioral model of heart-focused anxiety and non-anginal chest pain. *Behaviour Research and Therapy, 30*, 329–345.

Eifert, G. H. (1996). More theory-driven and less diagnosis-based behavior therapy. *Journal of Behavior Therapy and Experimental Psychiatry, 27*, 75–86.

Eifert, G. H., & Forsyth, J. F. (1996). Heart-focused and general illness fears in relation to parental medical history and separation experiences. *Behaviour Research and Therapy, 34*, 735–739.

Eifert, G. H., Hodson, S. E., Tracey, D. R., Seville, J. L., & Gunawardane, K. (1996). Heart-focused anxiety, illness beliefs, and behavioral impairment: Comparing healthy heart-anxious patients with cardiac and surgical inpatients. *Journal of Behavioral Medicine, 19*, 385–399.

Eifert, G. H., & Lau, A. (2001). Using behavioral experiments in the treatment of cardiophobia: A case study. *Cognitive and Behavioral Practice, 8*, 305–317.

Eifert, G. H., Lejuez, C. W., & Bouman, T. K. (1998). Somatoform disorders. In A. S. Bellack & M. Hersen (Series Eds.). *Comprehensive Clinical Psychology* (Vol. 6, pp. 543–565). Oxford: Pergamon.

Eifert, G. H., Zvolensky, M. J., & Lejuez, C. W. (2000). Heart-focused anxiety and chest pain: A conceptual and clinical review. *Clinical Psychology: Science and Practice, 7*, 403–417.

Escobar, J. I., Allen, L. A., Nervi, C. H., & Gara, M. A. (2001). General and cross-cultural considerations in a medical setting for patients presenting with medically unexplained symptoms. In G. J. G. Asmundson, S. Taylor, & B. Cox (Eds.), *Health anxiety: Clinical research perspectives on hypochondriasis and related disorders* (pp. 220–245). New York: Wiley.

Fava, G. A. (1992). The concept of psychosomatic disorder. *Psychotherapy and Psychosomatics, 58*, 1–12.

Fava, G., & Grandi, S. (1991). Differential diagnosis of hypochondriacal fears and beliefs. *Psychotherapy and Psychosomatics, 55*, 114–119.

Fink, P. (1996). Somatization–Beyond symptom count. *Journal of Psychosomatic Research, 40*, 7–10.

Fishbain, D. A., & Goldberg, M. (1991). The misdiagnosis of conversion disorder in a psychiatric emergency service. *General Hospital Psychiatry, 13*, 177–181.

Flor, F., Birbaumer, N., & Turk, D. C. (1990). The psychobiology of chronic pain. *Advances in Behaviour Research and Therapy, 12*, 47–84.

Fordyce, W. E., Roberts, A. H., & Sternbach, R. A. (1985). The behavioural management of chronic pain: A response to critics. *Pain, 22*, 113–125.

Forsyth, J. P., & Eifert, G. H. (1996). The language of feeling and the feeling of anxiety: Contributions of the behaviorisms toward understanding the function-altering effects of language. *The Psychological Record, 46*, 607–649.

Goldberg, D., Gask, L., & O'Dowd, T. (1989). The treatment of somatization: Teaching techniques of reattribution. *Journal of Psychosomatic Research, 33*, 689–695.

Harvey, R. F., Salih, W. Y., & Read, A. E. (1983). Organic and functional disorders in 2000 gastroenterology outpatients. *Lancet, i*, 632–634.

Hayes, S. C., Strosahl, K., & Wilson, K. (1999). *Acceptance and commitment therapy: Understanding and treating human suffering.* New York: Guilford.

Hayes, S. C., & Wilson, K. G. (1994). Acceptance and commitment therapy: Altering the verbal support for experiential avoidance. *The Behavior Analyst, 17*, 289–303.

Hopko, D. R., Lejuez, C. W., Ruggiero, K. J., & Eifert, G. H. (2003). Behavioral activation as a treatment for depression: Procedures, principles, and progress. *Clinical Psychology Review, 23*, 699–717.

Kagan, J. (1989). Temperamental contributions to social behavior. *American Psychologist, 44*, 668–674.

Kagan, J., Snidman, N., & Arcus, D. M. (1992). Initial reactions to unfamiliarity. *Current Directions in Psychological Science, 1*, 171–174.

Kashner, T. M., Rost, K., Cohen, B., Anderson, M., & Smith. G. R. (1995). Enhancing the health of somatization disorder patients. Effectiveness of short-term group therapy. *Psychosomatics, 36*, 462–470.

Kellner, R. (1990). Somatization: Theories and research. *The Journal of Nervous and Mental Disease, 178*, 150–160.

Kendler, K. S., Walters, E. E., Truett, K. R., & Heath, A. C. (1995). A twin-family study of self-report symptoms of panic, phobia, and somatization. *Behavior Genetics, 25*, 499–515.

Kenyon, F. E. (1964). Hypochondriasis: A clinical study. *British Journal of Psychiatry, 110*, 478–488.

Lejuez, C. W., Hopko, D. R., & Hopko, S. D. (2001). A brief behavioral activation treatment for depression. *Behavior Modification, 25*, 255–286.

Margolis, R. B., Zimny, G. H., & Miller, D. (1984). Internists and the chronic pain patient. *Pain, 20*, 151–156.

Mayou, R., Bass, C. M., & Sharpe, M. (Eds.) (1995). *Treatment of functional somatic symptoms.* Oxford: Oxford University Press.

Mayou, R., Bryant, B., Forbar, C., & Clark, D. (1994). Non-cardiac chest pain and benign palpitations in the cardiac clinic. *British Heart Journal, 72*, 548–553.

Mayou, R., & Sharpe, M. (1995). Patients whom doctors find difficult to help. *Psychosomatics, 36*, 323–325.

Mineka, S., Gunnar, M., & Champoux, M. (1986). Control and early socioemotional development: Infant rhesus monkeys reared in controllable versus uncontrollable environments. *Child Development, 57*, 1241–1256.

Murphy, M. R. (1990). Classification of the somatoform disorders. In C. M. Bass (Ed.), *Somatization. Physical symptoms and psychological illness* (pp. 10–39). Oxford: Blackwell.

Neziroglu, F. A., & Yaryura-Tobias, J. A. (1993). Exposure, response prevention, and cognitive therapy in the treatment of body dysmorphic disorder. *Behavior Therapy, 24*, 431–438.

Nicholas, M. K., Wilson, P. H., & Goyen, J. (1991). Operant-behavioural and cognitive-behavioural treatment of chronic low back pain. *Behaviour Research and Therapy, 29,* 225–238.

Pilowsky, I. (1993). Aspects of abnormal illness behaviour. *Psychotherapy and Psychosomatics, 60,* 62–74.

Pilowsky, I., Chapman, C. R., & Bonica, J. J. (1977). Pain, depression, and illness behavior in a pain clinic population. *Pain, 4,* 183–192.

Pilowsky, I., Smith, Q. P., & Katsikitis, M. (1987). Illness behavior and general practice utilisation: A prospective study. *Psychosomatic Research, 31,* 177–183.

Rachlin, H. C. (1985). Pain and behavior. *Behavioral and Brain Sciences, 8,* 43–83.

Rief, W., Hiller, W., Geissner, E., & Fichter, M. M. (1995). A two-year follow-up study of patients with somatoform disorders. *Psychosomatics, 36,* 376–386.

Rosen, J. C. (1995). The nature of body dysmorphic disorder and treatment with cognitive behavior therapy. *Cognitive and Behavioral Practice, 2,* 143–166.

Rosen, J. C., Reiter, J., & Orosan, P. (1995). Cognitive behavioral body image therapy for body dysmorphic disorder. *Journal of Consulting and Clinical Psychology, 63,* 263–269.

Rost, K., & Kashner, T. M., & Smith, G. R. (1994). Effectiveness of psychiatric intervention with somatization disorder patients. *General Hospital Psychiatry, 16,* 381–387.

Rothbart, M. K. (1989). Temperament and development. In G. Kohnstamm, J. Bates, & M. Rothbart, M. K. (Eds.), *Temperament in childhood* (pp. 187–248). Chichester: Wiley.

Rothbart, M. K., Ziaie, H., & O'Boyle, C. G. (1992). Self-regulation and emotion in infancy. In N. Eisenberg & R. A. Fabes (Eds.), *Emotion and its regulation in early development: New directions for child development* (pp. 7–24). New York: Jossey-Bass.

Salkovskis, P. M. (1996). The cognitive approach to anxiety: Threat beliefs, safety seeking behavior, and the special case of health anxiety and obsessions. In P. M. Salkovskis (Ed.), *Frontiers of cognitive therapy* (pp. 49–74). New York: Guilford.

Salkovskis, P. M., & Warwick, H. M. C. (1986). Morbid preoccupations, health anxiety and reassurance: A cognitive-behavioural approach to hypochondriasis. *Behaviour Research and Therapy, 24,* 597–602.

Salkovskis, P. M., & Warwick, H. M. C. (2001). Making sense of hypochondriasis: A cognitive model of health anxiety. In G. J. G. Asmundson, S. Taylor, & B. Cox (Eds.), *Health anxiety: Clinical research perspectives on hypochondriasis and related disorders* (pp. 46–64). New York: Wiley.

Schermelleh-Engel, K., Eifert, G. H., Moosbrugger, H., & Frank, D. (1997). Perceived competence and anxiety as determinants of maladaptive and adaptive coping strategies of chronic pain patients. *Personality and Individual Differences, 22,* 1–10.

Schmidt, N. B., & Harrington, P. (1995). Cognitive behavioral treatment of body dysmorphic disorder: A case report. *Journal Behaviour Therapy and Experimental Psychiatry, 26,* 161–167.

Sharma, P., & Chaturvedi, S. K. (1995). Conversion disorder revisited. *Acta Psychiatria Scandinavica, 92,* 301–304.

Sharpe, M., & Bass, C. M. (1992). Pathophysiological mechanisms in somatization. *International Review of Psychiatry, 4,* 81–97.

Sharpe, M., Mayou, R., & Bass, C. M. (1995). Concepts, theories, and terminology. In R. Mayou, C. M. Bass, & M. Sharpe (Eds.), *Treatment of functional somatic symptoms* (pp. 3–16). Oxford: Oxford University Press.

Sidman, M. (1994). *Equivalence relations and behavior: A research story.* Boston, MA: Authors Cooperative.

Smith, G. R., Rost, K., & Kashner, T. M. (1995). A trial of the effect of a standardized psychiatric consultation of health outcomes and cost in somatizing patients. *Archives of General Psychiatry, 52,* 238–243.

Speckens, A. E. M., van Hemert, A. M., Spinhoven, P., Hawton, K. E., Bolk, J. H., & Rooijmans, H. G. M. (1996). Cognitive behavioral therapy for medically unexplained physical symptoms: A randomised controlled trial. *British Medical Journal, 311,* 1328–1332.

Staats, A. W., & Eifert, G. H. (1990). A paradigmatic behaviorism theory of emotion: Basis for unification. *Clinical Psychology Review, 10,* 539–566.

Stewart, S. H., Zvolensky, M. J., & Eifert, G. H. (2002). The relations of anxiety sensitivity, experiential avoidance, and alexithymic coping to young adults' motivations for drinking. *Behavior Modification, 26,* 274–296.

Taylor, G. J., Bagby, R. M., & Parker, J. D. A. (1991). The alexithymia construct. A potential paradigm for psychosomatic medicine. *Psychosomatics, 32,* 153–164.

Turk, D. C., Meichenbaum, D., & Genest, M. (1983). *Pain and behavioral medicine: A cognitive-behavioral perspective.* New York: Guilford.

van Hemert, A. M., Hengeveld, M. W., Bolk, J. H., Rooijmans, H. G. M., & Vandenbroucke, J. P. (1993). Psychiatric disorders in relation to medical illness among patients of a general outpatient clinic. *Psychological Medicine, 23,* 167–173.

Vingerhoets, A. J. J. M., Van Heck, G. L., Grim, R., & Bermond, B. (1995). Alexithymia: A further exploration of its nomological network. *Psychotherapy and Psychosomatics, 64,* 32–42.

Visser, S., & Bouman, T. (1992). Cognitive-behavioural approaches in the treatment of hypochondriasis: Six single case cross-over studies. *Behaviour Research and Therapy, 30*, 301–306.

Warwick, H. M. C., Clark, D. M., Cobb, A. M., & Salkovskis, P. M. (1996). A controlled trial of cognitive-behavioural treatment of hypochondriasis. *British Journal of Psychiatry, 169*, 189–195.

Warwick, H. M. C., & Marks, I. M. (1988). Behavioural treatment of illness phobia. *British Journal of Psychiatry, 152*, 239–241.

Warwick, H. M. C., & Salkovskis, P. M. (1990). Hypochondriasis. *Behaviour Research and Therapy, 28*, 105–117.

Zvolensky, M. J., Lejuez, C. W., & Eifert, G. H. (2000). Prediction and control: Operational definitions for the experimental analysis of anxiety. *Behaviour Research and Therapy, 38*, 653–663.

14

Substance Use Disorders

William Fals-Stewart
University at Buffalo
The State University of New York

Of the major public health concerns of the 20th century, alcoholism and drug addiction certainly are among the most insidious and devastating. However defined, excessive use of alcohol and other drugs is an all-too-common problem, not only in the United States, but across the globe. A large national survey sponsored by the National Institute on Alcohol Abuse and Alcoholism found the lifetime prevalence of alcoholism in the U.S. population to be 13.4%; thus, one in seven people have had a problem with alcohol use in their lifetimes (Grant, 1997). Although the prevalences of other drug use disorders are much lower than for alcohol, they are sizable by nearly any standard. For illicit psychoactive substances, the lifetime prevalence of drug abuse or dependence is roughly 6% in the United States, with lifetime cannabis abuse (i.e., 4.6%) being the most common after alcohol (Grant, Peterson, Dawson, & Chou, 1994). The World Health Organization (1997) estimates that 28 million people worldwide incur significant health risks by using psychoactive substances other than alcohol. Annually, substance use in the United States claims 600,000 lives, including 440,000 attributable to nicotine use, 125,000 from alcohol use, and 10,000 from heroin and cocaine (exclusive of deaths from HIV; McCrady & Epstein, 1999).

The pernicious effects of excessive alcohol or drug use—for the individuals who use them, their immediate and extended families, and society in general—are legion. Moreover, they are interwoven into many of the most pressing of our societal ills, including illness, crime, violence, and homelessness. For instance, alcoholism is the third major cause of death in the United States (behind coronary heart disease and cancer), with the life span of individuals with alcoholism being about 12 years shorter than their nonalcoholic counterparts. Abuse of alcohol and other drugs has significant deleterious effects on the body, including cirrhosis of the liver, malnutrition, and stomach problems (Maher, 1997). Substance use also has significant long-term effects on brain functioning, including significant reductions in cognitive abilities such as abstract reasoning and problem solving. At its most severe, extensive alcohol use can lead to Korsakoff's syndrome, which is marked by extensive, debilitating memory loss (for a review, see Fals-Stewart et al., 1994).

In addition to the serious problems individuals with alcohol or drug problems create for themselves, victims of family violence, accidents, and violent crime add to the numbers of those adversely affected. In the home, drug and alcohol use by husbands is associated with a ten- to fifteen-fold increase in physical violence against their partners (e.g., Fals-Stewart, 2003). Parental substance use is associated with a host of emotional, behavioral, and social problems for children who live in the environments these caregivers provide (e.g., Fals-Stewart, Kelley, Cooke, & Golden, 2002) that often evolve into problems with alcohol and drugs as these children enter adolescence and adulthood. Thus, the effects of alcoholism and substance abuse can be accurately described as being part of an intransigent multigenerational vicious cycle.

When viewed from a broader social perspective, the negative impact of substance abuse is immense. Alcohol abuse is associated with half of the deaths and major injuries suffered in automobile accidents each year (e.g., Brewer et. al., 1994), 50% of all murders (Bennett & Lehman, 1996), and over 50% of all rapes (Seto & Barbaree, 1995). Aside from the toll in human suffering, estimates of yearly direct and indirect economic social costs arising from substance abuse (i.e., the sum of private costs incurred by individuals abusing drugs and external costs imposed on nonparticipating individuals as a result of drug abuse) have ranged from 58 to 300 billion dollars in the United States alone (e.g., Kozel & Adams, 1986; Lowinger, 1992). Individuals who abuse alcohol and other drugs consume a disproportionately large share of social resources from a variety of sources, some of which include specialized drug abuse treatment (Institute of Medicine, 1990), treatment of secondary health effects (Langenbucher, 1994), use of social welfare programs (Plotnick, 1994), and criminal justice system use (e.g., arrests, incarceration, parole, and probation) (Deschenes, Anglin, & Speckart, 1991; Harwood, Hubbard, Collins, & Rachal, 1988).

Thus, the size and scope of substance abuse and dependence in our society has drawn significant and increasing scientific and public attention. Although our present understanding of addiction to alcohol and drugs is far from complete, there has been great progress in the understanding of the etiology, course, and treatment of alcoholism and drug abuse. However, progress is not to be confused with consensus. There remains much heated controversy, not only about the etiology and treatment of substance misuse, but also, on a far more fundamental level, about how to conceptualize and operationalize substance use disorders.

DEFINITION AND DESCRIPTION OF SUBSTANCE USE DISORDERS

For most of U.S. history, chronic and excessive substance use has been viewed either as immoral conduct or as a disease. More recently, with the rising influence of the behavioral sciences in this dialogue, addictive behavior has also been viewed as maladaptive behavior subject to reinforcement contingencies that govern all learned human behavior. In turn, the definition and description of addictive behavior can vary considerably, based on which view (i.e., moral, disease, or behavioral) is emphasized.

Defining Addictive Behavior

Over the last two decades, the research community has gradually moved toward an encompassing view of what constitutes addictive behavior. The evolution in thinking about what defines addictive behavior is based in large part on the observation that a number of processes are common to excessive behaviors that have been characterized as addictive. Individuals who have problems with eating, drinking alcohol, consuming drugs, gambling, smoking, sexuality, and so forth present very similar descriptions and somewhat converging views of the phenomenology of their problems (e.g., Cummings, Gordon, & Marlatt, 1980). To capture the essence of addiction that spans across these behaviors, a broad definition has evolved that can be generally applied to all addiction, including addiction to psychoactive substances. From this vantage point, addiction is viewed as a complex, progressive behavior pattern having biological, psychological, and sociological components. What distinguishes this pattern of behavior from others is the individual's overwhelming pathological involvement in or attachment to it, subjective compulsion to continue it, and reduced ability to exert control over it. The behavior pattern continues despite its negative impact on the physical, psychological, and social functioning of the individual.

Although this depiction provides an overarching description of addictive behavior, it provides little insight into how to discern when use of drugs or alcohol crosses over from normal to problematic use, and from problematic use to disorder. More specifically, because of widely divergent social attitudes toward and prejudices about alcohol and drug use, there have been few generally accepted and agreed-on operational criteria for what level of use constitutes social use, abuse, and dependence. Substance use can follow one of several patterns; addiction "is not an all-or-nothing" phenomenon, but a continuum from recreational use to severe compulsion (Peele, Brodsky, & Arnold, 1991, p. 133).

Diagnostic Systems

Although use, abuse, and addiction are best viewed as a continuum of behavior, much effort has been put forth to delineate boundaries between different critical points on this continuum. There are several different definitional frameworks used to categorize various levels of addictive behavior that are widely referenced in the scientific and lay press. The most widely used framework is the psychiatric diagnostic approach, exemplified in the *Diagnostic and Statistical Manual of Mental Disorders* (DSM–IV; American Psychiatric Association, 1994) and the *International Classification of Diseases* (ICD–10, World Health Organization, 1992). Using the DSM–IV system as an example, the diagnosis of alcohol or psychoactive substance use disorders includes two general subcategories: abuse and dependence. *Substance dependence* is marked by a cluster of cognitive, behavioral, and physiological symptoms indicating that the individual continues to use a given psychoactive substance despite significant substance-related problems. To meet diagnostic criteria for dependence on a psychoactive substance, an individual must display at least three of the following seven symptoms:

- Physical tolerance.
- Withdrawal.
- Unsuccessful attempts to stop or control substance use.
- Use of larger amounts of the substance than intended.
- Loss or reduction in important recreational, social, or occupational activities.
- Continued use of the substance despite knowledge of physical or psychological problems that are likely to have been caused or exacerbated by the substance.
- Excessive time spent using the substance or recovering from its effects.

In contrast, the essential feature of *substance abuse* is a maladaptive pattern of problem use leading to significant adverse consequences. This includes one or more of the following:

- Failure to fulfill major social obligations in the context of work, school, or home.
- Recurrent substance use in situations that create the potential for harm (e.g., drinking and driving).

- Recurrent substance-related legal problems.
- Continued substance use despite having persistent social or interpersonal problems caused or exacerbated by the effects of the substance.

Although the developers of the ICD–10 and DSM–IV claim the definitions of alcohol and drug use disorders are largely atheoretical, some have persuasively argued that the classifications arise from a traditional medical model conceptualization of disease states and are inherently flawed by their reductionist view of illness (e.g., Pattison, Sobell, & Sobell, 1977). Given the complexity of addictive behavior, it appears that a binary, either-or view implicit in the psychiatric diagnostic approach is too simplistic and provides little understanding of the complexities of the addictive process and how to change it. As noted by Shaffer and Neuhaus (1985), addictive behavior is not easily categorized and, as such, is not easily defined by a set of consensually agreed-on criteria. Indeed, different diagnostic systems often place greater emphases on different aspects of behavioral and physiological functioning in their definitions. In turn, these differences lead to fairly divergent estimates about the prevalence of alcohol and drug use disorders in the general population (for a review of this issue, see Grant & Dawson, 1999).

A Biopsychosocial Perspective

Behavioral scientists have proposed an alternative biopsychosocial approach to defining alcoholism and drug abuse. In this framework, alcohol and drug use disorders are not defined as a unitary disease, nor is it implicitly assumed that the observed substance use symptoms are the manifestation of a disease state. Symptoms are viewed as acquired habits that emerge from a combination of genetic, social, pharmacological, and behavioral factors. Both biological and nonbiological processes are seen as essential to the development of addiction (Peele, 1985). Addiction is viewed as involving physiological changes in individuals (many of whom may be genetically and/or psychologically predisposed) and the complex interaction of environmental stressors and individual aspects of the person (including his or her experiential history) that produce addictive behavior.

A comprehensive understanding of the synergistic relationship among these factors is essential not only to understanding the degree and severity of substance use, but also for understanding treatment when use becomes abuse. Labeling and diagnosis are largely de-emphasized, and greater emphasis is placed on understanding the interplay between multiple factors that have led to and maintain the observed behavior.

CULTURAL AND SOCIAL ISSUES

Definitions of substance abuse do not develop in isolation; the point at which substance use moves from recreational to disordered is determined by the social and cultural context in which the behavior occurs (e.g., Thombs, 1998). Thus, societal norms and definitions of substance use and abuse are inextricably intertwined. How we determine what qualifies as an alcohol or drug problem is drawn largely from the boundaries implicitly (e.g., social stigma associated with being labeled an alcoholic or drug addict) or explicitly (e.g., laws prohibiting use of certain substances) drawn by the society in which the behavior occurs. In many respects, the norms for acceptable drinking and other drug use are delineated and implicitly or explicitly communicated to members of the society by the way the culture defines addiction.

A Sociocultural View of Alcoholism and Drug Abuse

From a sociological perspective, clinical diagnostic criteria for alcoholism and other drug abuse are derived from societal norms and thus vary depending on when and where the diagnosis is made. More specifically, those drinking or drug-taking behaviors that are considered disordered are those that deviate from what are considered socially acceptable standards. Perhaps the cultural foundations of alcoholism, which can also be applied to other addictive behaviors, are best captured by Vaillant (1990), who stated: "Normal drinking merges imperceptibly with pathological drinking. Culture and idiosyncratic viewpoints will always determine where the line is drawn" (p. 6).

Clearly, the sociocultural foundations of substance use diagnoses have certain important implications, even calling into question the veneer of objectivity in our official definitions of substance use disorder. Diagnosing a person as being alcohol dependent may not be very different from offering a personal opinion about his or her alcohol or drug use. The application of the label may be based not so much on scientific evidence as on the values, beliefs, and experiences of the person making the diagnosis. From a sociological perspective, alcoholism and other drug addiction are forms of social deviance, and the deviance is a function of the perceptions and biases of the person observing. Treatment then becomes an effort to force the alcoholic or drug abuser to conform to a socially acceptable standard of conduct.

Moreover, problems with alcoholism and drug abuse have become medicalized, and certain factions appear to have an agenda in viewing these behaviors as symptoms of a disease state and convincing others to view them that way. If addictive behavior is defined as disease, the label itself gives credibility to physicians' efforts to control, manage, and supervise the care provided to individuals seeking treatment. Thus, the medical community may have a strong, vested interest in defining addictive behavior as a disease (Schwartz & Kart, 1978). The label serves to make legitimate such financially lucrative efforts as hospital admissions, insurance billing, expansion of the pool of patients available for hospital admission, consulting fees, and so forth. In addition, the disease label may serve to restrict the number of nonmedical treatment providers (e.g., counselors, psychologists, social workers) who can independently provide care for substance-abusing clients.

However, it would be myopic to assume that societal norms alone shape the parameters for defining alcoholism and drug addiction. In some respects, the process of labeling what constitutes substance abuse or dependence restricts drinking and drug use behavior by members of a given culture. In essence, the definition of alcoholism and substance abuse provides guidelines for drinking and drug use practices for members of a given society. In our culture, obvious drunkenness, drinking early in the morning, drinking while at work, and drinking and driving are considered signs of problem drinking and such indicators of alcoholism appear in many of our widely used diagnostic instruments, such as the Michigan Alcoholism Screening Test (Selzer, 1971). Clearly, these "symptoms" are culturally derived and are based on a commonly held set of beliefs about acceptable substance use; the nature of the symptoms would likely be different in another culture that had a different set of social norms.

The Disease–Moral Model of Addictive Behavior

The disease model of alcoholism and abuse of other drugs is not the only theoretical conceptualization of these disorders and, in some contexts, not the predominant one. From a social policy perspective, the idea that addictive behavior is deviant and immoral is on at least an equal footing with the disease model. This disease–moral model is summed up by a passage from a turn-of-the-century temperance lecturer, John B. Gough (1881), who wrote that he considered "drunkenness as a sin, but I consider it also a disease. It is a physical as well as moral evil" (p. 443). The disease and moral models of substance abuse are, in many respects, strange bedfellows. These models hold divergent and, at times, inconsistent views about the etiology and maintenance of addictive behavior. In essence, the moral view holds that drinking and drug use are freely chosen acts for which individuals are responsible; the disease model, in many respects, espouses the opposite position. In turn, the conclusions and outcomes of the disease–moral model are, at times, rife with contradiction. For example, it is difficult to reconcile the inherent contradiction in treating the "illness" of psychoactive substance abuse with punishment (e.g., incarceration). How many other illnesses are routinely punished?

At a social policy level, much energy and effort is expended in veering between these two models. Yet, it is the disease–moral model that is the guiding hand that drives alcohol and drug policies today, with neither perspective completely supplanting the other. For instance, judges sentence offenders to treatment, those convicted of driving while intoxicated (DWI) are sentenced to attend Alcoholics Anonymous (AA) meetings or face jail, and so forth. Peele (1996) describes this as the "disease law enforcement model," which perhaps manifests itself most clearly in the debate between those who believe drug abusers should be treated and those who believe they should be incarcerated.

GENDER ISSUES

Although social norms provide a context in which to understand addictive behavior, it is also important to understand that science does not stand above or outside of its social context, but is immersed in and highly influenced by it (Kuhn, 1962). As with all areas of inquiry, social and cultural factors influence the way scientists study alcoholism and drug abuse. The relationship between addictive behavior and gender is an important case in point. Alcoholism and other addictions have traditionally been considered problems of men; as such, it has been the study of addictive behavior among men that has shaped our understanding of the nature and course of these disorders. Perhaps the two most widely known and influential investigations of alcoholism, Jellinek's (1952) on the phases of alcoholism and Vaillant's (1995) 45-year prospective longitudinal study of alcohol abuse in an inner-city and college cohorts, were limited to male participants. Other studies that did include information about women often failed to analyze or report these data (Blume, 1980). Treatment methods and programs were also initially designed to treat male substance abuse; it was not unusual for women who needed treatment for addictive disorders to be placed on psychiatric wards whereas men were treated in specialized alcoholism or drug abuse treatment programs (Blume, 1998).

Because the majority of research conducted in the area of substance abuse has been based largely on studies with male participants, a significant concern is that conclusions drawn from these studies may not generalize to women with substance use disorders. More recently, women have become the focus of increased attention by the research and treatment communities. Comparisons of substance use by men and women have revealed several important differences in the epidemiology, development, and treatment of substance abuse.

Epidemiological and Etiological Comparisons

Data from the Center on Addiction and Substance Abuse (1996) reveal that men are more likely than women to use psychoactive substances, including alcohol and nicotine. However, changes in use patterns over time appear to be different based on gender. For example, over the last three decades, the proportion of U.S. men who smoke tobacco products has fallen at a much greater rate (52% to 28%) than the corresponding decrease among women (34% to 22%). Although the National Comorbidity Study (Warner, Kessler, Hughes, Anthony, & Nelson, 1995) revealed the prevalences of substance use disorders in the general population are higher for men than women, other important gender differences did emerge. Women between the ages of 45 and 54 years reported a higher lifetime prevalence of drug dependence (other than alcohol or nicotine) than did men (3.8% compared to 2.1% for men). This finding reflects the higher prevalence of prescription drug dependence in women, whereas men have higher rates of dependence on illicit drugs.

Several important risk factors for the development of problems with alcohol or other drugs have also been identified in women. For example, Winfield, George, Swartz, and Blazer (1990) found the lifetime prevalence of alcohol abuse or dependence was three times higher and that of other drugs abuse was four times higher among women who reported a history of sexual assault. It also appears that male significant others who use drugs have a significant influence on women's patterns of substance use. In comparison to women, men are more likely to introduce women to the use of drugs and to supply drugs to their female partners (e.g., Amaro & Hardy-Fosta, 1995).

Another area of difference between men's and women's substance use are the reasons they give for drinking and drug use. Women misuse psychoactive substances in response to current psychosocial stressors more often than do men; this may be particularly problematic for middle-aged women because several stressful life events often occur during midlife (e.g., children leaving the home, death of parents, divorce; Allan & Cooke, 1985). In both the general population (e.g., Helzer & Pryzbeck, 1988) and clinic populations (e.g., Hesselbrock, Meyer, & Keener, 1985; Rounsaville et al., 1991), female alcoholics and substance abusers have higher rates of comorbid (i.e., co-occurring) psychiatric disorders, especially depressive and anxiety disorders, than do men. In addition, these disorders typically predate the onset of the substance use problems (Brady & Randall, 1999). Moreover, Annis and Graham (1995) found women were more likely to drink in response to negative emotional states and interpersonal conflict than men. Taken together, these findings suggest that women rely on substance use as a form of self-medication for mood disturbances more than do men.

The Stigma of Addiction for Women

Sociocultural factors also play important roles in the substance use patterns of men and women. In nearly all societies in which alcohol or other drugs are consumed, the cultural norms, attitudes, stereotypes, and legal sanctions often differ for males and females. Most cultures expect that women will drink less alcohol than men. These expectations may serve as a protective factor, reducing the incidence of alcohol use disorders among women (e.g., Klee & Ames, 1987; Kubicka, Csemy, & Kozeny, 1995).

However, the intense stigma associated with drinking and drug use by women can also create serious social problems. Society tolerates some behaviors exhibited by intoxicated men but views the same behavior as scandalous if exhibited by intoxicated women. For example, women who use alcohol or other drugs are seen as promiscuous. As Blume (1991) argues, women who are intoxicated are often the object of unwanted sexual overtures, and men believe that intoxicated women who say No to these advances really mean Yes. In a study of beliefs about rape, participants viewed rapists who were intoxicated as less responsible for their crimes than nonintoxicated rapists and viewed rape victims who had been drinking as more to blame for the rape than victims who had not been drinking (Richardson & Campbell, 1982). Thus, it is not surprising that alcoholic women are much more likely to be victims of violent crime, including rape, than matched nonalcoholic controls (Miller & Downs, 1986). Some contend that society at large views women who abuse alcohol or other drugs as partially or fully responsible for sexual advances made by men, thus making these women acceptable targets for physical and sexual aggression (e.g., Blume, 1991).

An important result of the stigma associated with women's alcohol and drug use is denial by the person, the family, and society. These stigmas, in turn, are important barriers that often prevent women from seeking treatment. As noted by Schober and Annis (1996), women often are reluctant to acknowledge a substance use problem publicly by seeking treatment because of intense fear of being stigmatized as a substance abuser. In comparison to their male counterparts, fears about the stigma associated with the label of *alcoholic* or *substance abuser* may be more powerful disincentives for women to seek treatment than denial of having a problem or accessibility and cost of treatment (Marlatt, Tucker, Donovan, & Vuchinich, 1997).

Along with personal denial, family denial is also a significant barrier to women entering treatment for substance abuse. In fact, the response by family members of women entering treatment appears to be more negative than it is for men. For example, Beckman and Amaro (1986) found that nearly 25% of women in a treatment sample reported opposition from family or friends, compared to only 2% of men. In addition, child-care and child custody issues influence the decision to seek treatment. Women often fear that entering treatment will lead to the perception that they are unfit as mothers and may be deprived of custody of their children.

These fears are not unfounded. Recently, women who use alcohol and other drugs during pregnancy have been prosecuted on charges of prenatal child abuse or delivery of a controlled substance to a minor (via the umbilical cord). Such practices have not prevented substance use during pregnancy, but have discouraged pregnant substance users from seeking prenatal or addiction treatment (Blume, 1997).

In addition to these personal and familial barriers, several factors related to the types and process of treatment have increased women's reluctance to seek help. Less than 14% of all women who need treatment for substance abuse receive it; less than 12% of pregnant women receive help (Center on Addiction and Substance Abuse, 1996). These findings, although disturbing, are not surprising; most treatments for addictive behaviors have been developed largely to meet the needs of men and thus may not be as effective for women (e.g., Jordan & Oei, 1989; Ramlow, White, Watson, Leukfield, 1997). A major reason women do not enter treatment is that most programs do not provide services (e.g., child care, obstetrician services) that make it easier for women to enter treatment (Nelson-Zlupko, Dore, Kaufmann, & Kaltenbach, 1996). Some studies do, in fact, suggest that treatment programs designed specifically to meet the treatment needs of substance-abusing women have higher retention and better outcome than standard outpatient or residential treatment programs (e.g., Dahlgren & Willander, 1989; Roberts & Nishimoto, 1996).

ETIOLOGY OF ALCOHOL AND OTHER DRUG USE DISORDERS

Research on the etiology of substance use disorders is a multidimensional, multidisciplinary effort, and the findings that have appeared in the literature are truly voluminous. This diversity and volume are a consequence of the multiple theoretical conceptualizations of the development and maintenance of these disorders. For instance, investigators who view alcoholism and drug abuse as diseases are often most interested in examining genetic and biological contributions to these disorders. Behavior-oriented researchers are more apt to explore antecedent and consequent events that may serve to initiate and reinforce substance use. Sociologists are likely to look at more macrolevel variables, such as peer and societal influences, that contribute to the development and maintenance of addictive behavior. The development of an addiction to alcohol or other drugs is a complex process involving many factors; however, the exact role of each of these ingredients has not been fully determined, and they may operate differently for each individual. However, genetics, biology, environment, sociocultural factors and the biochemical properties of the psychoactive substances themselves appear to contribute substantially to the process (e.g., Kalint, 1989; Sandbak, Murison, Sarviharju, & Hyytiae, 1998).

Neurobiology of Addiction

Psychoactive substances vary widely in terms of their biochemical properties, how they enter the body, and how they ultimately enter the brain. Central to the neurochemical process underlying addiction is the process by which alcohol or other drugs activate what is often referred to as the pleasure pathway. Although several regions of the central nervous system are responsive to psychoactive substances, the neuroanatomical system that is most often implicated is the mesocorticolimbic dopamine pathway (MCLP; Stine & Kosten, 1992).

The MCLP consists of dopaminergic neurons in the middle portion of the brain known as the ventral tegmental region and connects to other brain centers such as the nucleus accumbens and then to the frontal cortex. The MCLP appears to be involved in memory, gratification, and the regulation of emotions. Ingestion of opiates, alcohol, and other drugs is reinforcing because they stimulate this part of the brain. Several studies suggest that direct electrical stimulation of the MCLP produces great pleasure and has strong reinforcing properties (e.g., Liebman & Cooper, 1989). Thus, use of drugs that activate the brain's reward system is reinforced and, thereby, furthers use. With continued use of the drug, tolerance develops and more of the drug is needed to obtain the same pleasurable effect.

Genetic Propensity

Many studies have examined the genetic predisposition to alcohol and drug abuse and addiction, and a substantial literature suggests that addiction problems and disorders have a genetic component. The familial nature of alcoholism has long been recognized and is well documented (Dawson, Harford, & Grant, 1992). Cotton's (1979) review of thirty-nine family history studies estimated a four- to five-fold increase in developing alcoholism among first-degree relatives of alcoholics compared to the general population. More recently, Merikangas (1990) found that risk of developing alcoholism among first-degree relatives of alcoholics is seven times higher than among first-degree relatives of nonalcoholics.

While alcoholism appears to run in families, it is difficult to separate genetic factors from environmental influences because members of nuclear families typically share both genetic and environmental factors. Adoption studies enable the separation of genetic and environmental factors and usually reveal a strong link between paternal alcoholism and the development of alcoholism, particularly among male offspring (e.g., Bohman, Sigvardsson, & Cloninger, 1981; Goodwin et al., 1974). Studies of twins also support the role of genetic factors in the development of alcoholism, with the majority of twin studies reporting a greater concordance rate of alcoholism among monozygotic twins than among dizygotic twins (e.g., Kendler, Heath, Neale, Kessler, & Eaves, 1992; McGue, Pickens, & Svikis, 1992). In general, heritability is much stronger for alcohol dependence than for abuse and has been shown to be stronger for men than for women (National Institute on Alcohol Abuse and Alcoholism, 1993).

Much support for a genetic link in alcoholism has been derived from animal studies. For example, in a recent study, investigators demonstrated that rats bred to lack a particular gene stayed intoxicated longer than normal rats (Miyakawa et al., 1997). Mice can also be bred for alcohol preference and tolerance. Consistent with what we have inferred from data on humans, highly tolerant mice show the greatest preference for alcohol when given a choice (Le & Kiianma, 1988). In short, evidence from animal studies indicates that alcohol preference has some genetic determination and that higher tolerance is associated with more drinking.

Research on the genetic risk factors for abuse of drugs other than alcohol is far less evolved to date; only a few studies have sought to determine a familial influence in the development of substance use disorders other than alcohol. Croughan (1985) reviewed several family history studies and found antisocial personality disorder and criminal behavior tend to cluster in families in which there is drug dependence. Others have found a significantly greater prevalence of drug dependence among the biological relatives of inpatients with nonalcoholic chemical dependence than matched non-substance-abusing controls. In addition, a preference for specific types of drugs may occur among family members of drug abusers; monozygotic twins appear to display a greater similarity than dizygotic twin pairs in their preference for, and response to, certain types of drugs (Schuckit, 1987).

Examining the genetic link for other drug abuse, compared to alcoholism, is often far more difficult because individuals must be exposed to the psychoactive substance for the behavioral manifestation of the genetic propensity toward a certain behavior to appear. Most individuals in the world have extensive exposure to alcohol; this is not the case for many other drugs of abuse (e.g., heroin, cocaine).

Although the evidence supports the role of genetics in the etiology of addictive behavior, particularly for alcoholism, the size and extent of this role continues to be the subject of heated debate. For example, many children who have alcoholic parents do not themselves become alcoholic. In a study by Schulsinger, Knop, Goodwin, Teasdale, and Mikkelsen (1986) of high-risk children of alcoholics, young men (ages 19 to 20 years) who were presumably at high risk for developing alcoholism were carefully evaluated for signs of psychopathology and alcohol abuse. No differences were found on these factors compared to a control sample. Others have failed to find differences in drinking behavior or alcohol-related symptoms between a group of supposedly high-risk participants (i.e., those who had alcoholic fathers) and a group of non-high-risk participants (Alterman, Searles, & Hall, 1989). At present, few would argue that genetics alone account for the full range of observed addictive behaviors. Psychosocial and sociocultural factors are still considered powerful influences on both the availability of and motivation to use alcohol and other drugs.

Family Environment Influences

Not only do individuals who abuse alcohol and other drugs often develop physiological dependence, they can also develop a strong psychological dependence. Essentially, they become dependent on the drug to help them cope with negative emotional states and stressful social situations. Because substance use so often leads to significant problems for people across multiple domains of functioning, we must ask, "How is psychological dependence on alcohol or other drugs learned?"

As has been argued by many investigators, the family is an extremely important molding influence for children. Although the misuse of alcohol and other psychoactive substances by adults often has serious physical, emotional, behavioral, and economic consequences, the ancillary short- and long-term negative effects on those who live with these adults are often no less destructive. In particular, children who live with parents who abuse alcohol and other drugs often are victimized by the deleterious environments these caregivers frequently create. Findings from several studies suggest that children who live in homes with substance-abusing parents are at an increased risk for developing substance abuse problems and other emotional and behavioral problems in adolescence and early adulthood (e.g., Hops, Duncan, Duncan, & Stoolmiller, 1996). It appears that alcoholic parents are less likely than are nonalcoholic parents to monitor what their children are doing, which can lead to affiliation of their adolescent children with drug-using peers (Chassin, Pillow, Curran, Molina, & Barrera, 1993). Stress and negative affect, which are comparatively high in families with an alcoholic family member, are associated with alcohol use in adolescents (Chassin, Curran, Hussong, & Colder, 1996).

Personality and Psychiatric Factors

A number of psychoanalytic explanations for the development and maintenance of alcoholism and drug abuse have been proposed. For example, Wurmser (1984) viewed substance abusers as having overly harsh superegos and proposed that these individuals use alcohol and other drugs to escape intense feelings of anger and fear. Khantzian, Halliday, and McAuliffe (1990) theorized that inadequacies of the ego underlie substance misuse. In addition, these authors argue that a person's drug of choice has particular self-medicating properties for his or her particular type of ego deficit. Other psychoanalytic formulations also have been put forth (for a review, see Leeds and Morgenstern, 1995); however, because they are difficult to test scientifically, these models have not been widely accepted in the research community.

A related theory that is often used to explain substance abuse (most often in the popular press) is the idea of an alcoholic personality—a type of character organization that predisposes a person to use alcohol rather than some other strategy for coping with emotional and social stress. Some investigators have found that persons at high risk for developing alcoholism are significantly more impulsive and aggressive than those at low risk for abusing alcohol (e.g., Morey, Skinner, & Blashfield, 1984). However, results of studies regarding a predisposition to drinking or other drug use have been mixed, and most alcoholism and drug abuse investigators have largely dismissed the traditional notion of the existence of an alcoholic personality. However, there is strong evidence that certain disorders and substance abuse are linked. For example, roughly half of those individuals diagnosed with schizophrenia have either alcohol or drug dependency as well (Kosten, 1997). The relationship between antisocial personality and substance use is also strong (Harford & Parker, 1994; Kwapil, 1996), although the direction of the causal link (if there is one at all) is unclear (Carroll, Ball, & Rounsaville, 1993). Some investigators have also suggested that there is a strong relationship between depressive disorders and alcoholism (Kranzler, Del Boca, & Rounsaville, 1997); this relationship may be stronger among women than among men (Moscato et al., 1997).

Although the nature of the relationship between substance abuse and other mental disorders is unclear, this relationship is certainly a very important consideration for treatment. Providing the best possible treatment for substance-abusing clients who have co-occurring psychiatric disorders requires (a) more cross-disciplinary collaboration, (b) greater integration of substance abuse and mental health treatments, and (c) more comprehensive training to treatment providers in the assessment of and intervention with common co-occurring conditions.

Behavior-Oriented Explanations

Early learning explanations for substance abuse were based on two fundamental assumptions: (a) Substance use is a learned behavior, and (b) substance use is reinforced because it reduces anxiety and tension. Perhaps in the most widely known investigation, Masserman, Yum, Nicholson, and Lee (1944) induced an experimental neurosis in cats. After the cats were trained to eat food at a food box, they were given an aversive stimulus (e.g., an air blast to the face or an electric shock) whenever they approached the food. In turn, the cats stopped eating and displayed various symptoms, including anxiety, psychophysiological disturbances, and peculiar behaviors. When the cats were given alcohol, however, their symptoms were alleviated and they were able to eat again. It was concluded that the anxiety-reducing properties of the alcohol are reinforcing and are thus largely responsible for maintaining drinking behavior.

In general, however, the tension reduction model of substance use is difficult to test, and research with alcoholic participants has produced conflicting findings. Paradoxically, in some individuals, prolonged drinking is associated with increased anxiety and depression (e.g., McNamee, Mello, & Mendelson, 1968). In addition, if tension reduction alone explained the development of substance use disorders, anyone who finds drugs or alcohol tension reducing would be in danger of becoming a substance abuser. We would expect alcoholism and drug abuse to be far more common than it is, because psychoactive substances such as alcohol do tend to reduce tension for most people who use them.

Recently, several investigators have concluded that expectancies play a central role in the initiation and maintenance of alcohol and drug use disorders (Connors, Maisto, & Derman, 1994; Marlatt et al., 1998). Expectancies of the positive effects of substance use develop from repeated pairings of alcohol or other drugs with their reinforcing effects. Thus, expectancies can be conceptualized as conditioned cognitions, which can themselves be associated with positive experiences, or positive subjective responses, to alcohol or other drugs. Positive expectancies can facilitate more frequent alcohol or drug use and thus contribute to the development of dependence (Rotgers, 1996). Expectancy theory has been supported by research. For example, expectancies of social benefit can influence adolescents' decisions to start drinking and predict their consumption of alcohol (Christiansen, Smith, Roehling, & Goldman, 1989).

Sociocultural Factors in the Etiology of Substance Abuse

What is ultimately labeled alcoholism or drug addiction varies based on the temporal, geographic, and religious context. In the mid 1800s, the average American consumed roughly three times more alcohol than he or she consumes today. Thus, what would be considered alcoholic drinking then would differ substantially from our present-day definition. During the 1600s and much of the 1700s, alcohol was not even seen as an addictive substance and habitual drunkenness was not, by and large, seen as problematic (Levine, 1978).

Additionally, the effect of cultural attitudes toward drinking is well illustrated by Mormons and Muslims, whose religious values prohibit the use of alcohol. As such, the prevalence of alcoholism using standard diagnostic systems is rare in these groups. Any use of alcohol is considered problem use by members of these religious groups. This is not dissimilar from many cultures that consider any use of "hard drugs" (e.g., heroin, cocaine) to be problematic use.

Although alcohol plays a significant role in Jewish family rituals (Lawson & Lawson, 1998), excessive consumption is viewed as inexcusable behavior. Thus, within the Jewish culture, norms are for frequent drinking of alcohol, but in small amounts. These cultural norms serve to protect Jewish people from developing problems with alcohol (Glassner & Berg, 1980). In general, among cultures where drinking is integrated into religious rites and social customs and where self-control, sociability, and "knowing how to hold one's liquor" are important, alcoholism is rare (e.g., Blum & Blum, 1969).

In comparison, the prevalence of alcoholism is high in Europe and those countries that have been highly influenced by European culture (i.e., Argentina, Canada, Chile, Japan, the United States, and New Zealand). Although these countries make up less than 20% of the world's population, they consume 80% of the alcohol (Barry, 1982). In particular, the French have the highest rate of alcoholism in the world (i.e., roughly 15% of the population); France is also marked by the highest per capita alcohol consumption and the highest death rate from cirrhosis of the liver (Noble, 1979).

It is also generally accepted that Irish Catholics have a comparatively high rate of alcoholism (Lawson & Lawson, 1998). Vaillant (1983) found Irish subjects in his prospective study on the longitudinal course of alcoholism were more likely to develop alcohol problems than were those from other ethnic groups. Interestingly, Irish subjects were also more likely to abstain as a way of controlling drinking. As noted by Vaillant (1983), "It is consistent with Irish culture to view alcohol in terms of black or white, good or evil, drunkenness or complete abstinence ... " (p. 226). Viewing drinking behavior dichotomously, as either good or sinful, may serve to effectively eliminate models of social drinking. In the Irish culture, there appears to be a shared norm that drinking is an effective and acceptable method to deal with personal distress (Bales, 1980).

When comparing cultures that generally engage in moderate drinking and those where a disproportionately large percentage of its members appear to have drinking problems, certain differences consistently emerge (Maloff, Becker, Fonaroff, & Rodin, 1982; Peele & Brodsky, 1996). Cultural groups with comparatively low rates of alcoholism share four characteristics regarding alchohol use. First, drinking alcohol is accepted and is governed by social custom; thus, individuals in these cultures learn constructive norms for drinking. Second, differences between "good" and "bad" patterns of drinking are explicitly taught. Third, skills for drinking responsibly are taught. Fourth, drunkenness and misbehavior under the influence of alcohol are disapproved. In cultures where alcohol consumption is more problematic, agreed-on social standards for alcohol use have not been established, so drinkers must rely on an internal standard or their peer group's standards. Drinking is largely disapproved by members of the culture and, moreover, and abstinence is encouraged by members of the culture; thus, norms of social drinking are not available. Finally, people in these cultures expect that alcohol will overpower the individual's capacity for self-management.

Thus, social customs and cultural norms have an enormous influence on substance use. In addition, the behavior that is displayed while under the influence of psychoactive substances also appears to be influenced by cultural factors. For example, Lindman and Lang (1994) studied alcohol-related behavior in eight countries and found that participants generally believed that aggression frequently would follow many alcoholic drinks. However, the authors found significant national differences in the expectancy that excessive alcohol consumption leads to aggression. These differences were unrelated to self-reported alcoholic beverage preference, frequency of drinking to intoxication, or rates of personal involvement in episodes of alcohol-related aggression. The authors concluded that the expectation that drinking leads to aggression is determined to a significant extent by contextual factors and cultural traditions related to alcohol use. Importantly, it is the expectancy that alcohol will lead to aggressive behavior. For example, studies using real and mock alcoholic beverages have shown that individuals who believe they have consumed alcohol begin to act more aggressively, regardless of the beverage they actually consumed (Bushman, 1997).

Thus, how we learn to drink alcohol and consume other drugs is determined largely by the drinking and drug use we observe and by the people with whom we engage in these behaviors. There is a strong interdependence between the drinking and substance use patterns of those who associate with each other regularly in the same social circle. Indeed, in the broadest sense, each individual is linked, to a greater or lesser extent, to all other members of his or her culture. It is within this social fabric that patterns of belief and behaviors about alcohol and other drug use are modeled through a combination of example, reinforcements, punishments, encouragement, and the many other means that societies use to communicate norms, attitudes, and values (Heath, 1982).

TREATMENT

The conceptualizations of addiction have varied throughout history and, in turn, different treatment approaches have predominated based largely on the theoretical model holding sway. At present, the range of treatment possibilities is fairly extensive, varying greatly in terms of philosophy and general treatment goals. Thus, those seeking help now have a broad range of choices in their attempts to resolve substance abuse problems.

Pharmacotherapy

Intuitively, a reasonable solution to drug or alcohol addiction is to identify molecules that oppose the actions of these substances (i.e., antidotes to the substances of abuse). Much scientific effort has been put forth, based largely on this idea, and is manifested in the large variety of pharmacotherapies now available to treat addictive behavior. Medications are now used widely as primary or adjunctive interventions to treat alcoholism and other drug abuse. These include medications to reduce cravings to use drugs, to reduce the reinforcing effects of the psychoactive substances, to make taking drugs aversive, and to treat co-occurring mental disorders that may potentially underlie the drinking or drug use (Romach & Sellers, 1998).

Several pharmacotherapy options have been developed for the treatment of alcoholism. Disulfiram (Antabuse) is a drug that causes intense vomiting when followed by alcohol consumption; this reaction is a deterrent for further drinking by alcoholic clients. However, the effectiveness of disulfiram has been mixed, particularly if used as the sole intervention (Gorlick, 1993). Because it is generally self-administered, the alcoholic client can simply cease taking the disulfiram, wait for the drug to leave his or her system (roughly 2 weeks), and resume drinking. Disulfiram has been shown to be effective when another party is enlisted to observe the partner consume the disulfiram (Chic, Gough, Falkowski, & Kershaw, 1992). In addition, some studies have shown that clients with concurrent alcohol and cocaine problems reduce their intake of both drugs when taking disulfiram (e.g., Carroll, Ziedonis, et al., 1993; Higgins, Budney, Bickel, Hughes, & Foerg, 1993).

Another type of medication that has been used to treat alcoholism is naltrexone, an opiate agonist that helps to reduce craving for alcohol by blocking the pleasure-producing effects of ethanol. O'Malley and colleagues (1996) have shown that use of naltrexone reduced alcohol intake and lowered the incentive to drink for alcoholics compared to those given a placebo. Volpicelli and colleagues (1992) have shown that, in general, use of naltrexone has a moderate effect in reducing drinking and, in particular, reducing relapse to heavy drinking by alcohol-dependent patients. However, as with most medications, compliance with the naltrexone regimen plays an important role in the effectiveness of naltrexone (Volpicelli et al., 1997).

Acamprosate has also demonstrated effectiveness in treating alcoholics. In one large-scale study, clients treated with it were twice as likely to remain abstinent than were those treated with placebo (Mann, Chabac, Lehert, Potgieter, & Henning, 1995). A review of studies conducted in several countries reveals an increase in complete abstinence for acamprosate-treated clients. Although acamprosate appears to reduce craving for alcohol, the mechanism underlying acamprosate's action remains unknown, although some evidence suggests that it blocks the glutamate receptor (Spanagel & Zieglgansberger, 1997).

Finally, antidepressant medications have been used to treat alcoholics with co-occurring depression. Mason, Kocsis, Ritivo, and Cutler (1996) reported that tricyclic antidepressants reduced depressive symptoms, and, to a certain extent, drinking behavior. Others have found that selective serotonin reuptake inhibitors, such as Prozac, reduce the frequency of drinking among alcoholic patients with major depression (e.g., Cornelius et al., 1997).

Significant progress also has been made in the pharmacotherapy of opiate addiction. Methadone, L-alpha-acetylmethadol (LAAM), and naltrexone have all been approved in the United States to treat opiate dependence. Methadone and LAAM reduce the subjective effects of heroin and other opiates through cross-tolerance. Its usefulness in treatment lies in the fact that it satisfies the craving for heroin or other opiate-based illicit drugs, yet it is equally addictive physiologically. Thus, the advantage of methadone and LAAM over heroin is that methadone and LAAM are administered in a controlled environment as part of treatment. Methadone and LAAM are often combined with other psychosocial treatments to be fully effective (e.g., McLellan, Arndt, Metzger, Woody, & O'Brien, 1993; Fals-Stewart, O'Farrell, & Birchler, 2001). LAAM is similar to methadone but is administered every 3 days rather than daily. The main difficulty with LAAM is that it takes time to achieve initial stabilization, thus increasing relapse risk (Jaffe, 1995).

Both LAAM and methadone also reduce such concomitant negative behaviors as crime and needle sharing. They also enable those dependent on opiates to function well enough to maintain employment and other social obligations. Many who are involved in LAAM or methadone maintenance programs are also able to function in their communities and their families. The quality and dosing of LAAM and methadone is strictly controlled via well-monitored government standards compared to that of street heroin and other illegal opiate-based substances. However, the practice of weaning drug abusers from heroin only to addict them to a government-controlled substance is considered by many to be morally and ethically questionable. Moreover, LAAM and methadone maintenance treatments are often difficult for participants because they often require secrecy from employers, friends, and family members due to concerns about the stigma associated with being maintained on these drugs. It also is difficult for participants to develop a drug-free social network—a task that many see as a crucial part of successful recovery.

Naltrexone operates by blocking opioid receptor sites, thus preventing activation by heroin and other illicit opiates. However, unlike with alcohol treatment, naltrexone has not been very successful in treating opiate dependence, largely because of poor patient compliance (O'Brien & McLellan, 1996). Naltrexone appears to be effective with individuals highly motivated to quit, particularly those in high-level professional positions, such as physicians, lawyers, and executives (Meandzija & Kosten, 1994), and as part of other psychosocial treatments (e.g., Fals-Stewart & O'Farrell, 2003).

Buprenorphine, an experimental drug that is awaiting approval by the Food and Drug Administration for the treatment of opiate addiction, blocks the subjective effects of heroin and other opiates and has been shown to reduce heroin use and increase compliance with psychosocial treatment (Strain, Stitzer, Liebson, & Bigelow, 1994). An advantage of buprenorphine is that it has less abuse potential than methadone and it can be withdrawn or tapered with ease (e.g., Litten, Allen, Gorelick, & Preston, 1997).

No medication has been demonstrated to treat cocaine dependence effectively. Several medications have been investigated, including stimulants, antidepressants, cocaine antagonists, opioid agents, and anticonvulsants (e.g., Mendelson & Mello, 1996). In addition, no medications are yet available to treat clients suffering from abuse of other drugs, such as cannabis, steroids, phencyclidine, and inhalants (Wilkins & Gorelick, 1994).

Psychosocial Interventions

Although medications are an important part of the treatment armamentarium of clinicians working with clients suffering from psychoactive substance use disorders, most experts agree that the mainstay of treatment for addiction is some form of peer support or psychosocial therapy. Alcoholics Anonymous (AA) and other twelve-step peer support groups (e.g., Narcotics

Anonymous, Cocaine Anonymous) are the largest and most widely known self-help support groups for treating persons with alcohol and other drug problems. These programs operate primarily as self-help counseling programs in which both person-to-person and group relationships are emphasized. Meetings consist mainly of discussions of participants' problems with alcohol and other drugs, with testimonials from those who have recovered. Participants are encouraged to work the twelve steps of AA, which include admitting powerlessness over alcohol, believing that a higher power can restore sanity, making a searching and fearless moral inventory of oneself, and so forth (Alcoholics Anonymous, 1976). The program promotes total abstinence from psychoactive substances. Although widely used, evidence for the effectiveness of AA and the related peer support groups is mostly anecdotal rather than based on well-controlled studies of outcome, largely because AA does not endorse participation in external research. However, Morganstern, Labouvie, McCrady, Kahler, and Frey (1997) reported that affiliation with AA after outpatient treatment was associated with better outcome than non–AA involvement.

A commonly used formal treatment approach derived from AA and the disease model is twelve-step facilitation (TSF). In TSF, substance dependence is viewed not as symptomatic of another illness but as a primary problem with biological, emotional, and spiritual underpinnings and presenting features. Alcoholism and drug abuse are seen as progressive illnesses, marked largely by denial. The primary goals of treatment are to encourage clients to work through their denial and work the twelve steps of AA. This is typically done in the context of individual and group therapy and involves strong encouragement to attend twelve-step self-help groups on a regular basis. Along with individual and group counseling, medical services and religious services are also considered important parts of treatment because the disease of alcoholism and other drug use is viewed as effecting the biological and spiritual realms as well as psychosocial functioning. Although there has been little research on the efficacy of treatments derived from the disease model, it is the most common form of treatment in the United States.

One of the strongest predictors of success of treatment for alcoholism has been motivation to change. A treatment intervention that has grown out of this observation is motivational enhancement therapy (MET), which attempts to get clients to assume responsibility for helping themselves and increasing their desire to change through a technique referred to as motivational interviewing (Yahne & Miller, 1999). Motivational interviewing is defined as a directive, client-centered therapy style designed to elicit change by assisting clients with exploring and resolving ambivalence. Exploring ambivalence about change is the central goal of motivational interviewing; therapists are directive in pursuing this objective (Rollnick & Miller, 1995). Several studies have now demonstrated that MET is an effective treatment for alcoholism and other drug abuse (e.g., Miller et al., 1995).

Behavioral and cognitive behavioral treatments have been among the most widely used and investigated psychosocial treatments for substance abuse and dependence. Cognitive-behavioral therapy (CBT) teaches clients coping skills to reduce or eliminate drinking or substance use. Techniques that characterize this approach include identifying high-risk situations for relapse, instruction and rehearsal strategies for coping with those situations, self-monitoring and behavioral analysis of substance use, strategies for recognizing and coping with cravings, coping with lapses, and instruction on problem-solving (Carroll, 1998).

It has long been maintained that treatment for substance use disorders would be more effective if important patient characteristics were taken into account in selecting treatments (e.g., Mattson et al., 1994). This hypothesis was tested in the most comprehensive study of patient–treatment matching for alcoholism, Project MATCH. In this investigation, the efficacy of TSF, MET, and CBT were compared. Overall, the study involved 1,726 participants who were treated in twenty-six alcohol treatment programs in the United States by eighty different therapists.

The investigators evaluated patients on ten characteristics shown to predict treatment outcome (Project MATCH Group, 1997): diagnosis, cognitive impairment, conceptual ability level, gender, desire to seek meaning in life, motivation, psychiatric severity, severity of alcohol involvement, social support for drinking versus abstinence, and the presence of antisocial personality disorder.

The results of the study were somewhat surprising to many in the treatment and research communities—matching the patients to particular treatments did not appear to influence treatment effectiveness. TSF, MET, and CBT were equally effective across multiple domains of functioning. One conclusion drawn from these findings was that clients receiving interventions in competently run programs will do equally well with any of the three treatments (Gordis, 1997).

Relapse Prevention

Without question, one of the most vexing problems facing substance abuse treatment providers is relapse. For example, Polich, Armor, and Braiker (1981) found that, over a 4-year posttreatment period, only 7% of their total sample (i.e., 922 males) abstained from alcohol during the entire follow-up interval; 54% continued to show alcohol-related problems. Thus, increasing the durability of gains made during any primary intervention has become a major part of overall treatment planning.

A cognitive-behavioral approach to preventing relapse that has been widely used is that described in the classic work by Marlatt and Gordon (1985), in which relapse is viewed as a key behavior in substance abuse treatment. The behaviors underlying relapse are seen as indulgent behaviors based on an individual's learning history. When a person is abstinent, he or she gains a greater sense of personal control over the indulgent behaviors. The longer the person stays abstinent, the greater his or her sense of self-efficacy. In this model, relapse is a process that begins with a series of small, seemingly irrelevant decisions, even while maintaining abstinence. These decisions make relapse inevitable. For example, an alcoholic who buys beer to keep in his house to be prepared for visits by friends who drink has made a decision that may ultimately lead to relapse.

Another relapse behavior that is also often observed involves the abstinence violation effect, in which any use of drugs or alcohol is viewed by the substance abuser as complete failure. In many respects, this notion is advocated by many treatment programs and grows from an axiom often heard at AA meetings: "One drink, one drunk." Thus, when a substance user who has been abstinent for an extended period drinks or uses drugs, he or she may lose a certain degree of self-efficacy over the ability to control the addictive behavior. Because the goal of complete abstinence has been violated, the individual's self-efficacy for abstinence plummets, and he or she may therefore assume that a return to regular use of the drug is inevitable and then behave in a way that fulfills this prophecy.

As part of the relapse prevention program, clients are taught to recognize the apparently irrelevant decisions that serve as warning signals of the possibility of relapse. High-risk situations are identified and targeted, and the individuals learn to assess their own vulnerability to relapse. To counter the abstinence violation effect, clients are also taught not to become excessively discouraged if they do relapse. Clients are taught that relapse is part of the recovery process and are encouraged **to** develop plans to address relapse when it does happen.

Controlled Drinking: A Controversial Outcome

Although the goal of the treatments described thus far is abstinence from alcohol and other drugs, other interventions are based on the hypothesis that some individuals need not give up drinking or drug use but can learn to use moderately (Lang & Kidorf, 1990; Sobell & Sobell, 1995). Several approaches have been used to teach controlled drinking, and some research has suggested that certain alcoholics can control their drinking. For example, self-control training techniques, in which the goal of treatment is to have alcoholic clients reduce their drinking without necessarily abstaining from alcohol, has much appeal for some clients (Miller, Leckman, Tinkcom, & Rubenstein, 1986). A computer program is now available that provides instruction on self-control training and has been shown in a well-controlled study to reduce problem drinking (Hester & Delaney, 1997). Miller and colleagues (1986) have concluded that controlled drinking was most likely to be successful with persons who have less severe drinking problems.

In the United States, the vast majority of treatment professionals have rejected the idea that substance users can control their drinking or drug use and thus insist on a total abstinence approach. However, controlled drinking interventions are less controversial in other parts of the world (e.g., The Netherlands, Australia), and have been used effectively in other countries (e.g., Dawe & Richmond, 1997). The debate regarding controlled drinking as an acceptable treatment goal has raged for over 25 years. Some investigators have noted that controlled drinking can be efficacious (Heather, 1995; Kahler, 1995), whereas others have argued that alcoholics cannot maintain control over drinking and, as such, controlled drinking is not an acceptable treatment objective (Glatt, 1995).

Substance use disorders are among the most pressing and intransigent mental health problems facing society today. Concerns about abuse of alcohol, tobacco, and other psychoactive substances date as far back as Biblical times: "He shall separate himself from wine and strong drink, and shall drink no vinegar of wine, or vinegar of strong drink, neither shall he drink any liquor of grapes, nor eat moist grapes, or dried" (Num. 6:3). Despite such a long history, scientific scrutiny of these problems is fairly recent. For example, the National Institute on Alcohol Abuse and Alcoholism and the National Institute on Drug Abuse were formed in the early 1970s. However, an impressive body of knowledge about the epidemiology, etiology, neurobiology, and treatment of addictive behavior has accumulated. These and other aspects of addictive behavior continue to be the focus of extensive clinical and experimental research.

The study of addictive behavior has been marked by extensive controversy and heated debate. The conflicts have been fueled by a fundamental disagreement among scientists, clinicians, social policy makers, and the public about whether to view addiction as a disease in need of medical treatment, as sin in need of punishment and containment, or as learned behaviors that can be modified by contingencies. The debate is not simply over semantics but has implications for research, treatment, and social policy. For example, treatments that are shown to be effective in research settings are often ignored in the treatment community because the interventions are viewed as philosophically opposed to a conventional wisdom about what works best. Unfortunately, the conventional wisdom about what constitutes effective treatment is often not supported by the empirical research. Those who view alcoholism and other drug use as diseases are ethically and, in some instances, morally opposed to the use of controlled use treatments, which they view as irresponsible, perhaps akin to using cigarette smoking as a treatment for lung cancer. Drug users fill our criminal justice system, while treatment providers lament the criminalization of these "diseases." Yet, proponents of legalization of drugs, who are in the minority, note that legalization will help contain many of the social ills associated with substance use. Others see such a stance as irresponsible and immoral because it would increase the exposure of those with a genetic propensity for addiction to the substances that would activate the addictive process. In turn, they believe that such policies would contribute to greater social decay. Because the emotional, legal, and economic stakes in the debate are so high, no end to the debate is in sight.

QUESTIONS

1. What are the advantages and limitations of viewing addictive behavior as diseases? As learned behaviors? As immoral and sinful?

2. Should harm reduction approaches to treatment (e.g., controlled drinking, methadone maintenance) be made more widely available in treatment programs?

3. What would be the advantages and disadvantages of legalizing certain illicit substances, such as cannabis?

ACKNOWLEDGMENT

This project was supported, in part, from grants from the National Institute on Drug Abuse (R01DA12189 and R01DA14402) and the Alpha Foundation.

REFERENCES

Alcoholics Anonymous. (1976). *Living sober: Some methods A.A. members have used for not drinking.* New York: Alcoholics Anonymous World Services.

Allan, C. A., & Cooke, D. J. (1985). Stressful life events and alcohol misuse in women: A critical review. *Journal of Studies on Alcohol, 46,* 147–152.

Alterman, A. I., Searles, J. S., & Hall, J. G. (1989). Failure to find differences in drinking behavior as a function of familial risk for alcoholism: A replication. *Journal of Consulting and Clinical Psychology, 98,* 50–53.

Amaro, H., & Hardy-Fosta, C. (1995). Gender relations in addiction and recovery. *Journal of Psychoactive Drugs, 27,* 325–333.

American Psychiatric Association. (1994). *Diagnostic and statistical manual of mental disorders* (4th ed.). Washington, DC: Author.

Annis, H. M., & Graham, J. M. (1995). Profile types on the Inventory of Drinking Situations: Implications for relapse prevention counseling. *Psychology of Addictive Behaviors, 9,* 176–182.

Bales, F. (1980). Cultural differences in roles of alcoholism. In D. Ward (Ed.), *Alcoholism: Introduction to theory and treatment.* Dubuque, IA: Kendall/Hunt.

Barry, H., III. (1982). Cultural variations in alcohol abuse. In I. Al-Issa (Ed.), *Culture and psychopathology.* Baltimore: University Park Press.

Beckman, L. J., & Amaro, H. (1986). Personal and social difficulties faced by women and men entering alcoholism treatment. *Journal of Studies on Alcohol, 47,* 135–145.

Bennett, J. B., & Lehman, W. E. K. (1996). Alcohol, antagonism, and witnessing violence in the workplace: Drinking climates and social alienation-integration. In G. R. Vandenbox & E. Q. Bulatao (Eds.), *Violence in the workplace* (pp. 105–152). Washington: American Psychological Association.

Blum, R. H., & Blum, E. M. (1969). A cultural case study. In R. H. Blum (Ed.), *Drugs I: Society and drugs* (pp. 226–227). San Francisco: Jossey-Bass.

Blume, S. B. (1980). Researches on women and alcohol. In *Alcohol and women* (Research Monograph No. 1, DHEW Publication No. ADM 80-834, pp. 121–151). Washington, DC: U.S. Department of Health, Education and Welfare.

Blume, S. B. (1991). Sexuality and stigma: The alcoholic woman. *Alcohol Health and Research World, 15*(2), 139–146.

Blume, S. B. (1997). Women and alcohol: Issues in social policy. In R. Wilsnack & S. Wilsnack (Eds.), *Gender and alcohol: Individual and social perspectives.* New Brunswick, NJ: Rutgers Center of Alcohol Studies.

Blume, S. B. (1998). Addictive disorders in women. In R. J. Frances & S. I. Miller (Eds.), *Clinical textbook of addictive disorders* (2nd ed.). New York: Guilford.

Bohman, M., Sigvardsson, S., & Cloninger, C. (1981). Maternal inheritance of alcohol abuse: Cross-fostering analysis of adopted women. *Archives of General Psychiatry, 38,* 965–969.

Brady, K. T., & Randall, C. L. (1999). Gender differences in substance use disorders. *Psychiatric Clinics of North America, 22,* 241–252.

Brewer, R. D., Morris, P. D., Cole, T. B., Watkins, S., Patetta, M. J., & Popkin, C. (1994). The risk of dying in alcohol-related automobile crashes among habitual drunk drivers. *New England Journal of Medicine, 331,* 523–527.

Bushman, B. J. (1997). Effects of alcohol on human aggression: Validity of proposed explanations. In M. Galanter (Ed.), *Recent Developments in Alcoholism* (pp. 27–243). New York: Plenum.

Carroll, K. M. (1998). *Treating cocaine dependence: A cognitive behavioral approach*. Rockville, MD: National Institute on Drug Abuse.

Carroll, K. M., Ball, S. A., & Rounsaville, B. J. (1993). A comparison of alternate systems for diagnosing antisocial personality disorder in cocaine abusers. *Journal of Nervous and Mental Diseases, 181*, 436–443.

Carroll, K., Ziedonis, D., O'Malley, S., McCance-Katz, E., Gordon, L., & Rounsaville, B. (1993). Pharmacologic interventions for alcohol- and cocaine-abusing individuals. *American Journal on Addictions, 2*, 77–79.

Center on Addiction and Substance Abuse. (1996). *Substance abuse and American women*. New York: Author.

Chassin, L., Curran, P. J., Hussong, A. M., & Colder, C. R. (1996). The relation of parent alcoholism to adolescent substance use: A longitudinal follow-up. *Journal of Abnormal Psychology, 105*(1), 70–80.

Chassin, L., Pillow, D. R., Curran, P. J., Molina, B. S., & Barrera, M. (1993). Relation of parental alcoholism in early adolescent substance use: A test of three mediating mechanisms. *Journal of Abnormal Psychology, 102*, 3–19.

Chic, J., Gough, K., Falkowski, W., & Kershaw, P. (1992). Disulfiram treatment of alcoholism. *British Journal of Psychiatry, 161*, 84–89.

Christiansen, B. A., Smith, G. T., Roehling, P. V., & Goldman, M. S. (1989). Using alcohol expectancies to predict adolescent drinking behavior after one year. *Journal of Consulting and Clinical Psychology, 57*, 93–99.

Connors, G. J., Maisto, S. A., & Derman, K. H. (1994). Alcohol-related expectancies and their applications to treatment. In R. R. Watson (Ed.), *Drug and alcohol abuse reviews: Vol. 3. Alcohol abuse treatment* (pp. 203–231). Totowa, NJ: Humana.

Cornelius, J. R., Salloum, I. M., Ehler, J. G., Jarrett, P. J., Cornelius, M. D., Perel, J. M., Thase, M. E., & Black, A. (1997). Fluoxetine in depressed alcoholics: A double-blind placebo-controlled trial. *Archives of General Psychiatry, 54*, 700–705.

Cotton, N. S. (1979). The familial incidence of alcoholism. *Journal of Studies on Alcohol, 40*, 89–116.

Croughan, J. L. (1985). Contribution of family studies to understanding drug abuse. In L. N. Robins (Ed.), *Studying drug abuse* (series in psychosomatic epidemiology, Vol. 6, pp. 93–116). New Brunswick, NJ: Rutgers University Press.

Cummings, C., Gordon, J. R., & Marlatt, G. A. (1980). Relapse: Prevention and prediction. In W. R. Miller (Ed.), *The addictive behaviors* (pp. 291–321). New York: Pergamon.

Dahlgren, L., & Willander, A. (1989). Are special treatment facilities for female alcoholics needed? A controlled 2-year follow-up study from a specialized female unit (EWA) versus a mixed male/female treatment facility. *Alcoholism: Clinical and Experimental Research, 13*, 499–504.

Dawe, S., & Richmond, R. (1997). Controlled drinking as a treatment goal in Australian alcohol treatment agencies. *Journal of Substance Abuse, 14*(1), 81–86.

Dawson, D. A., Harford, T. C., & Grant, B. F. (1992). Family history as a predictor of alcohol dependence. *Alcoholism: Clinical and Experimental Research, 16*, 572–575.

Deschenes, E. P., Anglin, M. D., & Speckart, G. (1991). Narcotics addiction: Related criminal careers, social and economic costs. *Journal of Drug Issues, 21*, 383–411.

Fals-Stewart, W. (2003). The occurrence of interpartner violence on days of alcohol consumption: A longitudinal diary study. *Journal of Consulting and Clinical Psychology, 71*, 41–52.

Fals-Stewart, W., Kelley, M. L., Cooke, C. G., & Golden, J. (2002). Predictors of the psychosocial adjustment of children living in households in which fathers abuse drugs: The effects of postnatal social exposure. *Addictive Behaviors, 27*, 1–19.

Fals-Stewart, W., & O'Farrell, T. J. (2003). Behavioral family counseling and naltrexone for male opioid-dependent patients. *Journal of Consulting and Clinical Psychology, 71*, 432–442.

Fals-Stewart, W., O'Farrell, T. J., & Birchler, G. R. (2001). Behavioral couples therapy for male methadone maintenance patients: Effects on drug-using behavior and relationship adjustment. *Behavior Therapy, 32*, 391–411.

Fals-Stewart, W., Schafer, J., Lucente, S., Rustine, T., & Brown, L. (1994). Neurobehavioral consequences of prolonged alcohol and substance abuse: A review of findings and treatment implications. *Clinical Psychology Review, 14*, 775–778.

Glassner, B., & Berg, B. (1980). How Jews avoid drinking problems. *American Sociological Review, 45*, 647–664.

Glatt, M. M. (1995). Controlled drinking after a third of a century. *Addiction, 90*, 1157–1160.

Goodwin, D. W., Schulsinger, F., Moller, N., Hermansen, L., Winokur, G., & Guze, S. (1974). Drinking problems in adopted and nonadopted sons of alcoholics. *Archives of General Psychiatry, 31*, 164–169.

Gordis, E. (1997). Patient-treatment matching. *Alcohol Alert, 36*, 1–4.

Gorlick, D. A. (1993). Overview of pharmacologic treatment approaches for alcohol and other drug addiction. *Psychiatric Clinics of North America, 16*, 141–156.

Gough, J. B. (1881). *Sunlight and shadow*. Hartford, CT: Worthington.

Grant, B. F. (1997). Prevalence and correlates of alcohol use and DSM-IV alcohol dependence in the United States: Results of the National Longitudinal Alcohol Epidemiologic Survey. *Journal of Studies on Alcohol, 58*, 464–473.

Grant, B. F., & Dawson, D. A. (1999). Alcohol and drug use, abuse, and dependence: Classification, prevalence, and comorbidity. In B. S. McCrady & E. E. Epstein (Eds.), *Addiction: A comprehensive textbook* (pp. 9–29). New York: Oxford University Press.

Grant, B. F., Peterson, L. A., Dawson, D. S., & Chou, S. P. (1994). *Source and accuracy statement for the National Longitudinal Alcohol Epidemiologic Survey*. Rockville, MD: National Institute on Alcohol Abuse and Alcoholism.

Harford, T. C., & Parker, D. A. (1994). Antisocial behavior, family history, and alcohol dependence symptoms. *Alcoholism, 18*, 265–268.

Harwood, H. J., Hubbard, R. L., Collins, J. J., & Rachal, J. V. (1988). The costs of crime and the benefits of drug abuse treatment: A cost-benefit analysis using TOPS data. In C. G. Luekefeld & F. M. Tims (Eds.), *Compulsory treatment of drug abuse: Research and clinical practice*. (Research Monograph Series 86, pp. 209–235). Rockville, MD: National Institute on Drug Abuse.

Heath, D. B. (1982). Sociocultural variants in alcoholism. In E. M. Pattison & E. Kaufman (Eds.), *Encyclopedic Handbook of Alcoholism* (pp. 426–440). New York: Gardner.

Heather, J. (1995). The great controlled drinking consensus. Is it premature? *Addiction, 90*, 1160–1163.

Helzer, J. F., & Pryzbeck, T. R. (1988). The co-occurrence of alcoholism with other psychiatric disorders in the general population and its impact on treatment. *Journal of Studies on Alcohol, 49*, 219–224.

Hesselbrock, M. N., Meyer, R. E., & Keener, J. J. (1985). Psychopathology in hospitalized alcoholics. *Archives of General Psychiatry, 42*, 1050–1055.

Hester, R. K., & Delaney, H. D. (1997). Behavioral self-control program for Windows: Results of a controlled clinical trial. *Journal of Consulting and Clinical Psychology, 65*, 686–693.

Higgins, S. T., Budney, A. J., Bickel, W. K., Hughes, J. R., & Foerg, F. (1993). Disulfiram therapy in patients abusing cocaine and alcohol. *American Journal of Psychiatry, 150*, 675–676.

Hops, H., Duncan, T. E., Duncan, S. C., & Stoolmiller, M. (1996). Parent substance use as a predictor of adolescent use: A six-year lagged analysis. *Annals of Behavioral Medicine, 18*, 157–164.

Institute of Medicine. (1990). *Treating drug problems*. Washington, DC: National Academy Press.

Jaffe, J. H. (1995). Pharmacological treatment of opioid dependence: Current techniques and new findings. *Psychiatric Annals, 25*, 369–375.

Jellinek, E. M. (1952). Phases of alcohol addiction. *Quarterly Journal of Studies on Alcohol, 13*, 673–684.

Jordan, C. M., & Oei, T. P. S. (1989). Help-seeking behaviour in problem drinkers: A review. *British Journal of Addiction, 84*, 979–988.

Kahler, C. W. (1995). Current challenges and an old debate. *Addiction, 90*, 1169–1171.

Kalint, H. (1989). The nature of addiction: An analysis of the problem. In A. Goldstein (Ed.), *Molecular and cellular aspects of the drug addictions* (pp. 1–28). New York: Springer-Verlag.

Kendler, K., Heath, A. C., Neale, M. C., Kessler, R. C., & Eaves, L. J. (1992). A population-based twin study of alcoholism in women. *Journal of the American Medical Association, 268*, 1877–1882.

Khantzian, E. J., Halliday, K. S., & McAuliffe, W. E. (1990). *Addiction and the vulnerable self: Modified dynamic group therapy for substance abusers*. New York: Guilford.

Klee, L., & Ames, G. (1987). Reevaluating risk factors for women's drinking: A study of blue collar wives. *American Journal of Preventive Medicine, 3*, 31–41.

Kosten, T. R. (1997). Substance abuse and schizophrenia. *Schizophrenia Bulletin, 23*, 181–186.

Kozel, N. J., & Adams, E. H. (1986). Epidemiology of drug abuse: An overview. *Science, 234*, 970–974.

Kranzler, H. R., Del Boca, F. K., & Rounsaville, B. (1997). Comorbid psychiatric diagnosis predicts three-year outcomes in alcoholics: A posttreatment natural history study. *Journal of Studies on Alcohol, 57*, 619–626.

Kubicka, L., Csemy, L., & Kozeny, J. (1995). Prague women's drinking before and after the "velvet revolution" of 1989: A longitudinal study. *Addiction, 90*, 1471–1478.

Kuhn, T. (1962). *The structure of scientific revolutions*. Chicago: University of Chicago Press.

Kwapil, T. R. (1996). A longitudinal study of drug and alcohol use by psychosis-prone and impulsive-non-conforming individuals. *Journal of Abnormal Psychology, 105*(1), 114–123.

Lang, A. R., & Kidorf, M. (1990). Problem drinking: Cognitive behavioral strategies for self control. In M. E. Thase, B. A. Edelstein, & M. Hersen (Eds.), *Handbook of outpatient treatment of adults* (pp. 413–442). New York: Plenum.

Langenbucher, J. (1994). Offsets are not add-ons: The place of addictions treatment in American health care reform. *Journal of Substance Abuse, 6*, 117–122.

Lawson, A., & Lawson, G. (1998). *Alcoholism and the family: A guide to treatment and prevention* (2nd ed.). Gaithersburg, MD: Aspen.

Le, A. D., & Kiianma, K. (1988). Characteristic of ethanol tolerance in alcohol drinking (AA) and alcohol avoiding (ANA) rats. *Psychopharmacology, 94*, 479–483.

Leeds, J., & Morgenstern, J. (1995). Psychoanalytic theories of substance abuse. In F. Rotgers, D. S. Keller, & J. Morgenstern (Eds.), *Treating substance abuse: Theory and technique* (pp. 68–83). New York: Guilford.

Levine, H. G. (1978). The discovery of addiction: Changing conceptions of habitual drunkenness in America. *Journal of Studies on Alcohol, 39,* 143–174.

Liebman, J. M., & Cooper, S. J. (1989). *The neuropharmacological basis of reward.* New York: Clarendon.

Lindman, R. E., & Lang, A. R. (1994). The alcohol-aggression stereotype: A cross-cultural comparison of beliefs. *International Journal of Addictions, 29,* 1–13.

Litten, R. Z., Allen, J. P., Gorelick, D. A., & Preston, K. (1997). Experimental pharmacological agents to reduce alcohol, cocaine, and opiate use. In N. S. Miller (Ed.), *The principles and practice of addictions in psychiatry* (pp. 532–567). Philadelphia: Saunders.

Lowinger, P. (1992). Drug abuse: Economic and political basis. In J. H. Lowinson, P. Ruiz, R. B. Millman, & J. G. Langrod (Eds.), *Substance abuse: A comprehensive textbook* (pp. 138–143). Baltimore: Williams & Williams.

Maher, J. J. (1997). Exploring effects on liver function. *Alcohol, Health, & Research, 2,* 5–12.

Maloff, D., Becker, H. S., Fonaroff, A., & Rodin, J. (1982). Informal social controls and their influence on substance use. In N. E. Zinberg & W. M. Harding (Eds.), *Control over intoxicant use* (pp. 53–76). New York: Human Sciences Press.

Mann, K., Chabac, S., Lehert, P., Potgieter, A., & Henning, S. (1995, December). *Acamprosate improves treatment outcome in alcoholics: A polled analysis of 11 randomized placebo controlled trials in 3338 patients.* Poster presented at the annual conference of the American College of Neuropsychopharmacology, Puerto Rico.

Marlatt, G. A., Baer, J. S., Kivahan, D. R., Dimeoff, L. A., Larimer, M. E., Quigley, L. A., Somers, J. M., & Williams, E. (1998). Screening and brief intervention for high-risk college student drinkers: Results from a 2-year follow up assessment. *Journal of Consulting and Clinical Psychology, 66,* 604–615.

Marlatt, G. A., & Gordon, J. R. (Eds.). (1985). *Relapse prevention: Maintenance strategies in the treatment of addictive behaviors.* New York: Guilford.

Marlatt, G. A., Tucker, J. A., Donovan, D. M., & Vuchinich, R. E. (1997). Help-seeking by substance abusers: The role of harm reduction and behavioral-economic approaches to facilitate treatment entry and retention. In L. S. Onken, J. D. Blaine, & J. J. Boren (Eds.), *Beyond the therapeutic alliance: Keeping the drug-dependent individual in treatment* (pp. 44–84). Rockville, MD: National Institute on Drug Abuse.

Mason, B. J., Kocsis, J. H., Ritvo, E. C., & Cutler, R. B. (1996). A double-blind placebo-controlled trial of desipramine in primary alcoholics stratified on the presence or absence of major depression. *Journal of the American Medical Association, 275,* 1–7.

Masserman, J., Yum, K., Nicholson, J., & Lee, S. (1944). Neurosis and alcohol: An experimental study. *American Journal of Psychiatry, 101,* 389–395.

Mattson, M. E., Allen, J. P., Longabaugh, R., Nickless, C. J., Connors, G. J., & Kadden, R. M. (1994). A chronological review of empirical studies matching alcoholic clients to treatment. *Journal of Studies on Alcohol, 12,* 16–29.

McCrady, B. S., & Epstein, E. E. (1999). Introduction. In B. S. McCrady & E. E. Epstein (Eds.), *Addiction: A comprehensive textbook* (pp. 3–8). New York: Oxford University Press.

McGue, M., Pickens, R. W., & Svikis, D. S. (1992). Sex and age effects on the inheritance of alcohol problems: A twin study. *Journal of Abnormal Psychology, 101,* 3–17.

McLellan, A. T., Arndt, I. O., Metzger, D. S., Woody, G. E., & O'Brien, C. P. (1993). The effects of psycho-social services in substance abuse treatment. *Journal of the American Medical Association, 260,* 1953–1959.

McNamee, H. B., Mello, N. K., & Mendelson, J. H. (1968). Experimental analysis of drinking patterns of alcoholics: Concurrent psychiatric observations. *American Journal of Psychiatry, 124,* 1063–1069.

Meandzija, B., & Kosten, T. R. (1994). Pharmacologic therapies for opioid addiction. In N.S. Miller (Ed.), *Principles of addiction medicine* (sect. XII, chap. 4, pp. 1–5). Chevy Chase, MD: American Society of Addiction Medicine.

Mendelson, J. H., & Mello, N. K. (1996). Management of cocaine abuse and dependence. *New England Journal of Medicine, 334,* 965–972.

Merikangas, K. R. (1990). Comorbidity for anxiety and depression: Review of family and genetic studies. In J. D. Maser & C. R. Cloninger (Eds.), *Comorbidity of mood and anxiety disorders.* Washington, DC: American Psychiatric Press.

Miller, B. A., & Downs, W. R. (1986, July). *Conflict and violence among alcoholic women as compared to a random household sample.* Paper presented at the 38th annual meeting of the American Society of Criminology, Atlanta, GA.

Miller, W. R., Brown, J. M., Simpson, T. L., Handmaker, N. S., Bien, T. H., Luckie, L. F., Montgomery, H. A., Hester, R. K., & Tonigan, J. S. (1995). What works? A methodological analysis of the alcohol treatment outcome literature. In R. K. Hester & W. R. Miller (Eds.), *Handbook of alcoholism treatment approaches: Effective alternatives* (pp. 12–44). Needham, MA: Allyn & Bacon.

Miller, W. R., Leckman, A. L., Tinkcom, M., & Rubenstein, J. (1986, August). *Longterm follow-up of controlled drinking therapies*. Paper presented at the ninety-fourth annual meeting of the American Psychological Association, Washington, DC.

Miyakawa, T., Yagi, T., Kitazawa, H., Yasuda, M., Kawai, N., Tsuboi, K., & Niki, H. (1997). Fyn-Kinase as a determinant of ethanol sensitivity: Relation to NMDA receptor function. *Science, 278,* 698.

Morey, L. C., Skinner, H. A., & Blashfield, R. K. (1984). A typology of alcohol abusers: Correlates and implications. *Journal of Abnormal Psychology, 93,* 403–417.

Morganstern, J., Labouvie, E., McCrady, B. S., Kahler, C. W., & Frey, R. M. (1997). Affiliation with Alcoholics Anonymous after treatment: A study of its therapeutic effects and mechanisms of action. *Journal of Consulting and Clinical Psychology, 65,* 768–777.

Moscato, B. S., Russell, M., Zielezny, M., Bromet, E., Egri, G., Mudar, P., & Marshall, J. R. (1997). Gender differences in the relation between depressive symptoms and alcohol problems: A longitudinal perspective. *American Journal of Epidemiology, 146,* 966–974.

National Institute on Alcohol Abuse and Alcoholism. (1993). Genetic and other risk factors for alcoholism. In *Alcohol and Health: Eighth Special Report to the U.S. Congress* (NIH Publication No. 94-3699, pp. 61–83). Washington, DC: National Institute of Health.

Nelson-Zlupko, L., Dore, M. M., Kauffman, E., & Kaltenbach, K. (1996). Women in recovery: Their perceptions of treatment effectiveness. *Journal of Substance Abuse Treatment, 13,* 51–59.

Noble, E. P. (Ed.). (1979). *Alcohol and health: Technical support document*. Third special report to the U.S. Congress (DHEW Publication No. ADM 79-832). Washington, DC: U.S. Government Printing Office.

O'Brien, C. P., & McLellan, A. T. (1996). Myths about the treatment of addiction. *Lancet, 347,* 237–240.

O'Malley, S. S., Jaffe, A. J., Chang, G., Rode, S., Schottenfeld, R., Meyer, R. E., & Rounsaville, B. (1996). Six month follow-up of naltrexone and psychotherapy for alcohol dependence. *Archives of General Psychiatry, 53,* 217–224.

Pattison, E. M., Sobell, M. B., & Sobell, L. C. (1977). *Emerging concepts of alcohol dependence*. New York: Springer.

Peele, S. (Ed.). (1985). *The meaning of addiction: A compulsive experience and its interpretation*. Lexington, MA: Lexington Books.

Peele, S. (1996). Assumptions about drugs and the marketing of drug policies. In W. K. Bickel & R. J. DeGrandpre (Eds.), *Drug policy and human nature: Psychological perspectives on the prevention, management, and treatment of illicit drug abuse*. New York: Plenum.

Peele, S., & Brodsky, A. (1996). The antidote to alcohol abuse: Sensible drinking messages. In S. Peele (Ed.), *Wine in context: Nutrition, physiology, and policy* (pp. 66–70). Davis, CA: American Society for Enology and Viticulture.

Peele, S., Brodsky, A., & Arnold, M. (1991). *The truth about addiction and recovery*. New York: Simon & Schuster.

Plotnick, R. D. (1994). Applying benefit-cost to substance use prevention programs. *International Journal of the Addictions, 29,* 339–359.

Polich, J. M., Armor, D. J., & Braiker, H. B. (1981). *The course of alcoholism: Four years after treatment*. New York: Wiley Interscience.

Project Match Group. (1997). Project MATCH: Rationale and methods for a multisite clinical trial matching patients to alcoholism treatment. *Alcoholism: Clinical and Experimental Research, 17,* 1130–1145.

Ramlow, B. E., White, A. L., Watson, M. A., & Leukefeld, C. G. (1997). The needs of women with substance use problems: An expanded vision for treatment. *Substance Use and Misuse, 32,* 1395–1404.

Richardson, D., & Campbell, J. (1982). The effect of alcohol on attributions of blame for rape. *Personality and Social Psychology Bulletin, 8,* 468–476.

Roberts, A. C., & Nishimoto, R. H. (1996). Predicting treatment retention of women dependent on cocaine. *American Journal of Drug and Alcohol Abuse, 22,* 313–333.

Rollnick, S., & Miller, W. R. (1995). What is motivational interviewing? *Behavioral and Cognitive Psychotherapy, 23,* 325–334.

Romach, M. K., & Sellers, E. M. (1998). Alcohol dependency: Women, biology, and pharmacotherapy. In E. F. McCance-Katz & T. R. Kosten (Eds.), *New treatments for chemical addictions*. Washington, DC: American Psychiatric Press.

Rotgers, F. (1996). Behavioral theory of substance abuse treatment: Bringing science to bear on practice. In F. Rotgers, D. S. Keller, & J. Morgenstern (Eds.), *Treating substance abuse: Theory and technique*. New York: Guilford.

Rounsaville, B. J., Anton, S. F., Carroll, K., Budde, D., Prusoff, B. A., & Gawin, F. (1991). Psychiatric diagnoses of treatment-seeking cocaine abusers. *Archives of General Psychiatry, 48,* 43–51.

Sandbak, T., Murison, R., Sarviharju, M., & Hyytiae, P. (1998). Defensive burying and stress gastric erosions in alcohol-preferring AA and alcohol-avoiding ANA rats. *Alcoholism: Clinical and Experimental Research, 22,* 2050–2054.

Schober, R., & Annis, H. M. (1996). Barriers to help-seeking for change in drinking: A gender-focused review of the literature. *Addictive Behaviors, 21,* 81–92.

Schuckit, M. A. (1987). Biological vulnerability to alcoholism. *Journal of Consulting and Clinical Psychology, 55*, 301–310.

Schulsinger, F., Knop, J., Goodwin, D. W., Teasdale, T. W., & Mikkelsen, U. (1986). A prospective study of young men at high risk for alcoholism. *Archives of General Psychology, 43*, 755–760.

Schwartz, H. D., & Kart, C. S. (1978). *Dominant issues in medical sociology*. Reading, MA: Addison-Wesley.

Selzer, M. L. (1971). The Michigan Alcoholism Screening Test: The quest for a new diagnostic instrument. *American Journal of Psychiatry, 127*, 1653–1658.

Seto, M. C., & Barbaree, H. E. (1995). The role of alcohol in sexual aggression. *Clinical Psychology Review, 15*, 545–566.

Shaffer, H. J., & Neuhaus, C., Jr. (1985). Testing hypotheses: An approach for the assessment of addictive behaviors. In H. B. Milkman & H. J. Shaffer (Eds.), *The addictions: Multidisciplinary perspectives and treatments* (pp. 87–103). Lexington, MA: Lexington Books.

Sobell, M. B., & Sobell, L. C. (1995). Controlled drinking after 25 years: How important was the great debate? *Addiction, 90*, 1149–1153.

Spanagel, R., & Zieglgansberger, W. (1997). Anti-craving compounds for ethanol: New pharmacological tools to study addictive processes. *Trends in Pharmacological Sciences, 18*, 54–59.

Stine, S. M., & Kosten, T. R. (1992). The use of drug combinations in treatment of opioid withdrawal. *Journal of Clinical Psychopharmacology, 12*, 203–209.

Strain, E. C., Stitzer, M. L., Liebson, I. A., & Bigelow, G. E. (1994). Comparison of buprenorphine and methadone in the treatment of opioid dependence. *American Journal of Psychiatry, 151*, 1025–1030.

Thombs, D. L. (1998). *Introduction to addictive behavior* (2nd ed.). New York: Guilford.

Vaillant, G. E. (1983). *The natural history of alcoholism*. Cambridge, MA: Harvard University Press.

Vaillant, G. E. (1990). We should retain the disease concept of alcoholism. *Harvard Medical School Mental Health Letter, 6*, 4–6.

Vaillant, G. E. (1995). *The natural history of alcoholism revisited*. Cambridge, MA: Harvard University Press.

Volpicelli, J. R., Alterman, A. I., Hayashida, M., & O'Brien, C. P. (1992). Naltrexone in the treatment of alcohol dependence. *Archives of General Psychiatry, 49*, 876–80.

Volpicelli, J. R., Rhines, K. C., Rhines, J. S., Volpicilli, L. A., Alterman, A. I., & O'Brien, C. P. (1997). Naltrexone and alcohol dependence: role of subject compliance. *Archives of General Psychiatry, 54*, 737–42.

Warner, L. A., Kessler, R. C., Hughes, M., Anthony, J. C., & Nelson, C. B. (1995). Prevalence and correlates of drug use and dependence in the United States. *Archives of General Psychiatry, 52*, 219–228.

Wilkins, J. N., & Gorelick, D. A. (1994). Pharmacologic therapies for other drugs and multiple drug addiction. In N. S. Miller (Ed.), *Principles of addiction medicine* (sect. XII, chap. 6, pp. 1–6). Chevy Chase, MD: American Society of Addiction Medicine.

Winfield, I., George, L. K., Swartz, M., & Blazer, D. G. (1990). Sexual assault and psychiatric disorders among a community sample of women. *American Journal of Psychiatry, 147*, 335–341.

World Health Organization. (1992). *ICD-10 classification of mental and behavioral disorders: Clinical descriptions and diagnostic guidelines*. Geneva: Author.

World Health Organization. (1997). *World Health Organization Report, 1997: Conquering suffering, furthering humanity*. Geneva: Author.

Wurmser, L. (1984). The role of superego conflicts in substance abuse and their treatment. *International Journal of Psychoanalytic Psychotherapy, 10*, 227–258.

Yahne, C. E., & Miller, W. M. (1999). Enhancing motivation for treatment and change. In B. S. McCrady & E. E. Epstein (Eds.), *Addiction: A comprehensive textbook* (pp. 235–249). New York: Oxford University Press.

15

Externalizing Disorders of Childhood and Adolescence

Paul J. Frick and Eva R. Kimonis

University of New Orleans

It is becoming increasingly clear that a significant number of children and adolescents have severe and impairing emotional or behavioral problems. Prevalence estimates of childhood psychopathology vary greatly depending on the age group studied, the type of disorders included, and the method of assessment used. However, epidemiological studies conducted in the United States, New Zealand, Canada, Puerto Rico, and the Netherlands indicate that from 9% to 22% of children and from 18% to 22% of adolescents have signs of significant problems in adjustment (Frick & Silverthorn, 2001). Furthermore, research has indicated that the form that these problems take can largely be conceptualized along two major dimensions. One dimension, which is the focus of the current chapter, has been labeled as undercontrolled or externalizing and includes various acting out, disruptive, delinquent, hyperactive, and aggressive behaviors. The second broad dimension of childhood psychopathology has been labeled as overcontrolled or internalizing and includes such behaviors as social withdrawal, anxiety, and depression. This basic distinction between internalizing and externalizing problems has been well supported by a number of factor analytic studies. There is even debate as to whether or not more fine grained distinctions within these broad categories provide any additional useful information for understanding children with psychopathological conditions (Achenbach, 1995; Achenbach & Edelbrock, 1978; Quay, 1986).

The distinction within the externalizing dimension that has received the strongest support in research is the distinction between (a) the problems of attention, impulsivity, and hyperactivity associated with the diagnostic category of attention deficit hyperactivity disorder (ADHD) and (b) the conduct problems and aggressive behavior associated with the diagnostic categories of oppositional defiant disorder (ODD) and conduct disorders (CD). Research indicates that these two problem domains can be separated in factor analyses and they have a number of different correlates (Frick, 1994, 1998; Hinshaw, 1987; Lilienfeld & Waldman, 1990). For example, ADHD seems to be more specifically associated with parental problems of attention and impulsivity, poor academic achievement, and problems in executive functioning, whereas conduct problems appear to be more specifically associated with parental criminality/antisocial behavior, socioeconomic disadvantage, and dysfunctional family backgrounds. The importance of these correlates for understanding the two types of externalizing disorders is discussed in later sections of this chapter.

Although research supports distinguishing between these two forms of externalizing disorders, it is also important to note that they overlap considerably. For example, between 40% and 60% of children with ADHD have a co-occurring conduct problem diagnosis (Hinshaw, 1987), and between 65% and 90% of children with either ODD or CD have a co-occurring ADHD diagnosis (Abikoff & Klein, 1992). This overlap is important in understanding research in this area because many studies have failed to control for this comorbidity when studying externalizing disorders. This failure makes it unclear whether the correlates documented in research are due to one or the other or both types of externalizing disorders (Hinshaw, 1987; Lilienfeld & Waldman, 1990). Furthermore, this comorbidity predicts a more chronic course for both ADHD and conduct disorders (Barkley, Fischer, Smallish, & Fletcher, 2002; Frick & Loney, 1999) and can influence the type of treatment that may be most effective for children with these disorders (Abikoff & Klein, 1992; Frick, 1998, 2001). Therefore, although the following sections provide somewhat separate reviews of the two types of externalizing disorders, it is important to recognize that many children show both patterns of behavior. In addition, understanding this overlap can be important for effectively treating children with disruptive behavior problems.

ATTENTION DEFICIT HYPERACTIVITY DISORDER

Definition and Description

Diagnosis.   In the psychiatric literature, there has been a form of childhood psychopathology recognized since the mid-19th century that has, as its primary feature, extreme and impairing levels of motor activity (Barkley, 1996). However, there has been great debate regarding the primary cause of this condition and the best method for diagnosing it in children. This debate is reflected in numerous changes in its name (e.g., minimal brain dysfunction, hyperactive child syndrome, attention deficit disorder) and changes in the diagnostic criteria used to classify children with the disorder over the years (see Frick & Lahey, 1991, for a review).

In the most recent revision of the *Diagnostic and Statistical Manual of Mental Disorders* (DSM–IV–TR; American Psychiatric Association [APA], 2000), ADHD has two core symptom dimensions—an inattention–disorganization cluster (e.g., has difficulty sustaining attention, does not listen when spoken to directly, is easily distracted by extraneous stimuli) and a hyperactivity–impulsivity cluster (e.g., fidgets, runs or climbs excessively, talks excessively, has difficulty awaiting turn, interrupts others). Dividing symptoms into these two dimensions was based on a substantial number of factor analyses conducted in both clinic-referred and community samples (Lahey, Carlson, & Frick, 1997). Like the criteria for all childhood disorders, some level of these symptoms is normative in childhood. Therefore, the DSM–IV–TR specifies

- The severity (i.e., six or more symptoms),
- The duration (i.e., persists for 6 months and evident before age 7),
- The pervasiveness (i.e., impairment present in two or more settings), and
- The degree of impairment (i.e., clear evidence of impaired social, academic, or occupational functioning)

that is necessary for a diagnosis of ADHD (APA, 2000).

Subtypes. An important aspect of most recent definitions of ADHD is the specification of several distinct subtypes of the disorder. The most common subtype is the ADHD–combined type, in which children show significant problems in both inattention–disorganization and impulsivity–hyperactivity (APA, 2000). This subtype accounts for about 55% of all children referred to clinics with ADHD (Lahey et al., 1994), and much of the research on ADHD has focused on this group of children (Lahey et al., 1997).

A second group of children with ADHD have ADHD–predominantly inattentive type (ADHD–PI; APA, 2000). This group of children constitutes approximately 27% of ADHD children referred to clinics for treatment and, as the name implies, this subtype includes children who have problems with inattention–disorganization, but who do not show problems of overactivity (Lahey et al., 1994). In fact, rather than being hyperactive, many of these children are described as being hypoactive, drowsy, and sluggish (McBurnett, Pfiffner, & Frick, 2001). The designation of this subtype was first made in the third edition of the DSM (DSM–III; APA, 1980) under the category of attention deficit disorder without hyperactivity. This diagnostic category has prompted debate for a number of reasons. First, in many past definitions of the disorder, hyperactivity was considered a core and defining feature of the diagnostic category (Stewart, Pitts, Craig, & Dieruf, 1966). Inclusion of this subtype explicitly acknowledges that the presence of increased motor activity is neither necessary nor sufficient for the disorder and supports research on the importance of attentional deficits in defining the disorder (Frick & Lahey, 1991). Second, in addition to the defining difference in the amount of motor activity, children with ADHD–PI exhibit a number of other differences from other children with ADHD. Specifically, they are less likely to show conduct problems and aggression, they are less likely to be rejected by peers, they show higher rates of anxiety and depression, and they tend to respond to lower doses of stimulant medication (Barkley, DuPaul, & McMurray, 1991; Frick & Lahey, 1991; Lahey et al., 1997). Also, their cognitive and attentional difficulties differ from other children with ADHD and appear to be characterized by slower retrieval and information processing (as opposed to fast and impulsive processing of information) and low levels of alertness (Barkley, 1997; McBurnett et al., 2001). These differences have led some authors to suggest that this form of ADHD may be a discrete disorder characterized by a different etiology from other forms of ADHD, rather than a subtype of the same disorder (Barkley, 1997; Milich, Balentine, Lynam, 2001). Third, because problems of inattention typically are manifested later in development, when demands for sustained attention increase (Loeber, Green, Lahey, Christ, & Frick, 1992), the appropriateness of the diagnostic criterion that symptoms must cause impairment before age 7 has been questioned for this subtype. For example, in a sample of clinic-referred youth ages 4 to 17 who were diagnosed with ADHD, 82% who met symptom severity criteria for the ADHD–combined type had an onset of impairment before age 7, whereas only 57% with ADHD–PI met this age-of-onset criterion (Applegate et al., 1997). In comparing children with ADHD–PI who did and did not meet the age-of-onset criterion, but who met all other criteria for the disorder, there were no differences in their current level of impairment as documented by teachers, parents, and clinicians.

The third and least common of the ADHD subtypes recognized by the DSM–IV–TR is the predominantly hyperactive–impulsive type (ADHD–PHI). Children in this category show problems of hyperactivity–impulsivity without problems of inattention–disorganization. This subgroup accounts for about 18% of children diagnosed with ADHD (Lahey et al., 1994). Barkley (1997) has proposed that the predominantly hyperactive subtype of ADHD is best considered a developmental precursor to the ADHD–combined subtype, with children in this category not yet experiencing demands for sustained attention. In support of this hypothesis, a study of 276 children diagnosed with ADHD found that the average age for the ADHD–PHI subgroup was 5.68 years, compared with 8.52 years for the ADHD–combined Type ($n = 152$) and 9.80 years for the ADHD–PI type ($n = 74$; Lahey et al., 1994).

Developmental Course. As noted earlier, by definition ADHD symptoms start early in development. In fact, many studies have documented symptoms of overactivity emerging as early as ages 3 to 4 years (Loeber et al., 1992). Until recently, there was a general view that ADHD was limited to childhood and that children with ADHD outgrew the disorder by adolescence, or at least by adulthood (Lambert, 1988) However, there are now several prospective longitudinal studies that have followed children diagnosed with ADHD into adulthood and have called into question this view of a developmentally limited disorder (Barkley, 1996; Barkley et al., 2002).

Estimates of the stability of ADHD are somewhat dependent on the method and criteria used to assess ADHD in childhood and the method and criteria used to assess later adult adjustment (Barkley et al., 2002). However, there are several general statements that can be made about the developmental course of the disorder. First, there are variations in the manifestation of ADHD symptoms over the life span that need to be considered in estimating the stability of the disorder. For example, the symptoms of inattention–disorganization seem to be much more stable in adolescence than the hyperactive–impulsive symptoms (Hart et al., 1995). However, this difference in stability may be partly due to the fact that the hyperactive–impulsive symptoms show age variations in their manifestations, such as being manifested in driving problems in adolescents (Barkley, Guevremont, Anastopoulos, DuPaul, & Shelton, 1993) or relationship instability in adults (Barkley et al., 2002). Second, when the core symptoms of ADHD are assessed first in childhood and then again in adolescence and young adulthood, between 50% and 70% of children with ADHD have clinically significant levels of symptoms in adolescence and between 30% and 45% have clinically significant levels of symptoms in adulthood (Barkley et al., 2002; Mannuzza, Klein, Bessler, Malloy, & LaPadula, 1998; Rasmussen & Gillberg, 2001; Weiss & Hechtman, 1993). Third, although many children with ADHD do not maintain all of the symptoms of ADHD necessary to meet diagnostic criteria as adults, a large proportion still show significant impairments in their social, occupational, or psychological functioning as adults, even if the core symptoms of the disorder have remitted (Barkley et al., 2002).

Co-occurring Problems. Although the diagnosis of ADHD focuses on the two main symptom domains of inattention–disorganization and hyperactivity–impulsivity, research has consistently documented that children with ADHD often have a number of co-occurring problems in adjustment, in addition to the primary symptoms. These co-occurring or comorbid conditions can have a great impact on the most appropriate treatment for children with ADHD (Abikoff & Klein, 1992), and the presence of co-occurring problems may be a strong predictor of later adjustment (Weiss & Hechtman, 1993).

As noted earlier, many children with ADHD (40% to 60%) have a comorbid conduct disorder (Hinshaw, 1987; Lilienfeld & Waldman, 1990). It is important that the presence of significant conduct problems may be one of the strongest predictors of adult outcome, especially risk for delinquency and substance abuse (Weiss & Hechtman, 1993). Additionally, about 30% to 50% of children with ADHD have significant academic problems, such as learning disabilities or early school dropout (Frick, Kamphaus et al., 1991; Jensen, Martin, & Cantwell, 1997; Weiss & Hechtman, 1993). A similar percentage of children with ADHD (30% to 50%) have comorbid emotional disorders, such as an anxiety or depressive disorder (Jensen, Martin, & Cantwell, 1997; Kitchens, Rosen, & Braaten, 1999). Based on these figures, it is evident that comorbid diagnoses are the rule rather than the exception for children diagnosed with ADHD.

The families of ADHD children differ from the families of non-ADHD children in several ways. In a review of studies examining family functioning, Johnston and Mash (2001) found that the presence of an ADHD child in the home is associated with a number of difficulties, including poorer parenting practices, more parental negative and controlling behaviors, more parental stress, and higher levels of parental psychopathology. It is unclear whether these familial factors precede the child's development of ADHD, or whether the child's ADHD symptoms lead to a change in the family environment. For example, the stress and difficulty involved in parenting a child with ADHD may make it more likely that parents of children with ADHD will engage in less effective parenting strategies (e.g., more negative and controlling parenting) and will be more susceptible to depression (Barkley & Cunningham, 1979; Fisher, 1990). Furthermore, familial factors may play a greater role in maintaining the disorder (Johnston & Mash, 2001) or in predicting the development of some of the co-occurring conditions often found in children with ADHD (e.g., conduct problems; Frick, 1998) than in causing the primary symptoms of the disorder.

Cultural and Gender Issues

A number of studies have compared the prevalence of ADHD in various countries and cultures. These studies have documented some significant variation, especially when compared with the 3% to 5% prevalence rate of ADHD estimated for school-aged children in the United States (Silverthorn & Frick, 1999). For example, in a sample of Spanish children, Gomez-Beneyto, Bonet, Catala, and Puche (1994) found a prevalence of 14.4% in a community sample of 8-year-olds. Researchers in New Zealand determined prevalence rates of 4.8% and 6.7% for 11- and 15-year-olds, respectively (Anderson et al., 1987; Fergusson, Horwood, Lynskey, 1993). Estimates of prevalence in Sweden and the Netherlands were observed at 2% for 6-year-olds (Landgren, Petterson, Kjellman, & Gillberg, 1996) and 2.6% for adolescents (Verhulst et al., 1997). Finally, in a sample of Taiwanese children ages 5 to 13, estimates of prevalence were found at 9.9% (Wang, Chong, Chou, et al., 1993). It is difficult to disentangle the many factors that may account for these differences in prevalence rates across countries, including differences in sample age and differences in diagnostic definitions used across studies. In addition, most estimates were based on reports from parents and teachers and, as a result, different prevalence rates may be a function of differences in cultural expectations for children's behavior by adults rather than true variations in the level and severity of the child's behavior. Within the United States, studies have not found consistent differences in the prevalence of ADHD across cultural groups (Barkley, 1996).

One consistent finding across countries and cultures is that ADHD shows some of the strongest and most consistent evidence for male predominance of any form of childhood psychopathology, with male-to-female ratios ranging from 2:1 to 6:1 in community samples from 6:1 to 9:1 in clinic-referred samples (Barkley, 1996). An important caveat to this overall male predominance is that there is emerging evidence that the male-to-female ratio may not be similar across all types of ADHD. Although boys tend to be more likely to have all forms of ADHD, the male:female ratio seems to be less for the ADHD–PI subtype (Biederman et al., 2002; Lahey et al., 1994). Despite these differences in prevalence rates, when girls do show ADHD, the types and severity of symptoms and the co-occurring problems in adjustment appear to be quite similar between boys and girls with ADHD (Gaub & Carlson, 1997; Gershon, 2002; Silverthorn, Frick, Kuper, & Ott, 1996). The most consistent differences that emerge are that girls tend to show less severe hyperactivity and fewer conduct problems than do boys with ADHD, but greater intellectual impairments, especially deficits in verbal intelligence (e.g., Rucklidge & Tannock, 2001; Silverthorn et al., 1996). In contrast, boys with ADHD tend to show a stronger family history of ADHD, especially a paternal history of ADHD (Silverthorn et al., 1996).

Etiology

Research on the etiology of ADHD has three main foci. The first is defining the core cognitive deficit that can lead to the primary and secondary characteristics of children with ADHD. The second is investigating the neurological substrate of this core deficit. The third is trying to understand the causes of this neurological substrate. This research has made it increasingly clear that the core symptoms of ADHD are related to a neurological deficit and that, as noted previously, the child's psychosocial context (e.g., family environment, quality of educational services) largely influences the severity and level of impairment associated with the child's symptoms and the development of co-occurring problems (e.g., conduct problems). However, there are two important considerations in this general conceptualization of ADHD. First, because the diagnostic criteria of ADHD are based solely on behavioral criteria, documentation of a cognitive and/or neurological deficit is not necessary for the diagnosis. Second, although the child's psychosocial context may not be critical in many etiological theories, intervening in the child's social context (e.g., improving parenting skills, improving the child's educational environment) is nonetheless a critical component of treatment. Limiting the impairment associated with ADHD and preventing the development of secondary problems are both critical to effective intervention for children with ADHD. These goals are often best accomplished through interventions into the child's psychosocial context, a point that is discussed later in this chapter.

Core Deficit. Although there have been many theories as to the core cognitive deficit that can lead to ADHD symptoms, the most extensive and best articulated theory is Barkley's (1997). This theory posits that ADHD results from a core deficit in behavioral inhibition. Behavioral inhibition is defined as the ability to inhibit a prepotent response long enough to consider the consequences of the response; the ability to stop an ongoing response in reaction to environmental feedback; and the ability to suppress stimuli that might interfere with a primary response (i.e., interference control) (see also Nigg, 2000). According to Barkley's (1997) theory, the core deficit in behavioral inhibition leads to secondary impairments in several executive functions (EF). Executive functions are cognitive actions that are self-directed and allow for self-regulation. Four EFs depend on behavioral inhibition for their adequate performance: (a) working memory (e.g., maintaining events in the mind, hindsight, forethought), (b) self-regulation of affect, motivation, and arousal (e.g., self-control of emotions, social perspective taking), (c) internalization of speech (e.g., problem-solving, moral reasoning), and (d) reconstitution (e.g., verbal and behavioral fluency).

Barkley (1997) and Nigg (2000) provide comprehensive reviews of a large number of studies documenting impairments in these four EFs in samples of children with ADHD. Furthermore, these impairments can explain a number of the problems in self-regulation exhibited by children with ADHD. Specifically, the deficit in behavioral inhibition and the resulting impairments in the four domains of EF cause the behavior of ADHD individuals to be controlled by the immediate context rather than internal representations of information (Nigg, 2000). Also, these deficits can explain not only the core symptoms of inattention–disorganization and hyperactivity–impulsivity but also a number of secondary features of the disorder, such as an impaired sense of time and higher levels of emotional reactivity. Furthermore, the importance of the immediate context can explain why the behavior of a person with ADHD can be so strongly influenced by his or her immediate environment, such as the novelty of the task, the intrinsic interest of the child in the activity, the level of fatigue of the child, and the degree of immediate reinforcement present in the task (Barkley, 1996, 1997).

Neurological Substrates. Attempting to tie the deficits associated with ADHD to specific neurological abnormalities has a long and controversial history (see Frick & Lahey, 1991). Early conceptualizations of ADHD assumed a central nervous system dysfunction because of the similarity in symptomatology between persons with ADHD and persons with known brain injury. These similarities led to the use of the term *minimal brain dysfunction* to refer to this syndrome (Strauss & Lehtinen, 1947). However, early research into potential neurological differences between persons with ADHD and controls failed to document clear neurological abnormalities in most persons with the disorder, leading some to question the usefulness of assuming a neurological deficit without clear evidence that such a deficit exists (Rutter, 1977).

With recent advances in neurological imaging techniques, an emerging body of research has begun to document structural differences in the brains of persons with ADHD compared to controls. For example, studies using magnetic resonance imaging (MRI) show reduced size in the corpus callosum, reduced cerebellar volume, and overall reduced total brain volume in ADHD individuals (Giedd et al., 1994; Hynd et al., 1991; Zametkin & Liotta, 1998). In addition, studies using techniques that examine cerebral blood flow, which provides an index of brain function rather than structure, have begun to document diminished brain function in persons with ADHD, specifically in the prefrontal regions of the brain and pathways connecting to this region from the caudate and striatal regions (Lou, Henriksen, & Bruhn, 1984; Lou, Henriksen, Bruhn, Borner, & Nielson, 1989; Zametkin et al., 1990). These imaging studies are informative because the implicated brain areas, the prefrontal and associated regions, have been associated with deficits in inhibition and executive functions and, thus, could explain the core deficits described previously (Barkley, 1997; Nigg, 2000). Furthermore, there is evidence that stimulant medication, which reduces the symptoms of ADHD, increases activity in the prefrontal regions of the brain, thus providing rationale for the method of action of this medication in reducing the symptoms of ADHD (Lou et al., 1989).

Despite these promising findings, this research on the neurological underpinnings of ADHD is limited in several ways. First, as in earlier research, it is still evident that many persons with ADHD do not show clear deficits in brain structure or function. Second, the studies documenting neurological deficits are still few in number and have generally used small samples. Therefore, replications of these results are needed before firm conclusions can be made on their importance. Third, the findings of deficits in persons with ADHD have not always been consistent across studies. For example, some studies have found more defuse abnormalities in cerebral blood flow that is not limited to prefrontal regions of the brain in adults with ADHD (Zametkin et al., 1990). Other studies have found that diminished blood flow is limited to adolescent girls with ADHD and is not found in adolescent boys with ADHD (Ernst et al., 1994; Zametkin et al, 1993). Fourth, these studies do not indicate what causes these neurological deficits.

Causes of the Neurological Abnormalities. There are many different pathways through which a neurological deficit can develop in the brain systems involved in inhibition. One way is through an inherited deficit. This possibility is supported by family studies that have shown evidence for a familial transmission of ADHD symptoms (Frick, Lahey, Christ, Loeber, & Green, 1991). Evidence for genetic involvement in this transmission is provided by twin studies. These studies estimated that between 50% and 90% of the variance in measures of ADHD can be attributable to genetic influences (Edelbrock, Rende, Plomin & Thomson, 1995; Levy, Hay, McStephen, Wood, & Waldman, 1997), thus making it one of the more heritable forms of childhood psychopathology (Stevenson, 1992). However, in addition to potential genetic routes to the neurological deficits, some evidence suggests that biological trauma could be involved in the development of ADHD for some children. For example, children with ADHD are more likely to be born premature than other children because of higher rates of birth complications during pregnancy (James & Taylor, 1990). In addition, exposure to environmental toxins, such prenatal exposure to alcohol and tobacco (Bennett, Wolin, & Reiss, 1988) and high lead blood levels (Stein, Schettler, Wallinga, & Valenti, 2002) have been linked to ADHD symptoms. Taken together, these results suggest that there may be multiple pathways to any neurological deficit involved in the development of ADHD.

Empirically Validated Treatments

There have been many treatment approaches attempted for ADHD, most of which have received only limited support for their effectiveness (Barkley, 1996; Hinshaw, 1994). Only two treatments have demonstrated consistent effectiveness in controlled treatment outcomes studies (Pelham, Wheeler, & Chronis, 1998). These two effective treatments are pharmacological intervention using central nervous system (CNS) stimulants and behavioral therapy that focuses on developing very structured contingency management systems for the child with ADHD in his or her home and school environments. To illustrate the effectiveness of these two treatment approaches, the National Institute of Mental Health's (NIMH) recently funded the Collaborative Multimodal Treatment Study of Children with ADHD (MTA), the largest treatment trial to date to focus on treating a childhood disorder (Richters et al., 1995). The MTA is a 5-year multisite treatment study of 579 children ages 7 to 9 years diagnosed with ADHD. The controlled treatment trial compared four treatment groups: (a) psychosocial treatment only, (b) stimulant medication only, (c) combined psychosocial and pharmacological treatment, and (d) standard community treatment (being whatever treatment was typically delivered in that specific community). All treatments lasted for 14 months of systematic, well-delivered treatment followed by a number of follow-up assessments (Wells et al., 2000).

The choice of stimulant medication as a key component to treatment was based on 30 years of research indicating that it leads to significant improvements in ADHD symptoms in 70% to 80% of children with this diagnosis (see Swanson, McBurnett, Christian, & Wigal, 1995, for a review). Furthermore, research has shown that stimulant medication not only reduces the core symptoms of ADHD but also alleviates many secondary problems, such as conduct problems, aggression, poor peer relations, academic problems, and problematic interactions with parents and teachers (Pelham, 1993; Richters et al., 1995; Swanson et al., 1995). In addition, the side effects encountered with appropriate and carefully monitored trials of stimulant medication have been fairly mild, with the most common side effects being appetite suppression and increased irritability. In fact, in some studies, the side effects encountered with an active dose of stimulant medication have been no more than those encountered when the child was on a placebo (Barkley, McMurray, Edelbrock, & Robbins, 1990). It is important to note that much of this literature has focused on the use of one particular stimulant medication, Ritalin (methylphenidate, MPH), which was also used in the MTA treatment study. Other stimulant medications have been tested in controlled treatment outcome studies, showing similar response profiles and typically varying primarily on how quickly they act and the length of time an active dose shows behavioral effects (Greenhill, Halperin, & Abikoff, 1999).

The initial results of the MTA study support the efficacy of stimulant medication. Children on medication showed substantially greater improvements on most outcome measures than the community treatment control group (some of whom were on medication as well) and even showed better effectiveness rates in most domains than the group receiving only the behavioral treatment (MTA Cooperative Group, 1999). The superior performance by stimulant medication over behavioral interventions is consistent with past studies directly comparing these treatments (Pelham, 1993). This study found, however, that this level of improvement required a much more carefully controlled medical regimen than is typically administered in many community settings. For example, the MTA trial involved monthly phone contacts with the child's teacher, through which medication levels were adjusted to determine the optimal dosage for each child (MTA Cooperative Group, 1999).

While the effects of medication found in the MTA study and in other controlled trials have been impressive (Swanson et al., 1995), pharmacological interventions for children with ADHD are limited in several important ways. First, many parents have negative feelings about medication and may not administer it consistently or may even refuse this form of treatment (Richters et al., 1995). For example, about 6% of otherwise eligible participants in the MTA study declined participation because they did not want medication and another 9% refused medication once the trial began (Wells et al., 2000). Of note, 17% of eligible participants also declined participation in the MTA because they did not want to forego medication; the strong feelings about medication acceptability can be either positive or negative. Second, despite the impressive efficacy found for stimulant medication, its effectiveness is limited. For example, it still leaves 10% to 20% of children without significant levels of improvement and, even for those who do demonstrate significant treatment effectiveness, their behavior is not often brought within what would be considered a normal range (Pelham, 1993; Wells et al., 2000). More important, there is little evidence that stimulants change the long-term course of ADHD, with most of the beneficial effects being demonstrated in short-term treatment outcome studies (Pelham et al., 2000). Third, some evidence suggests that medication is more effective when it is used in conjunction with behavioral treatments. Specifically, more children show a clinical response to medication, more children's adjustments are brought within a normative range, and children can often be maintained on lower doses of stimulant medication (and thus reduce the number and severity of side effects) when medication is combined with behavioral interventions (Klein & Abikoff, 1997; Pelham et al., 2000).

As a result of this research, the MTA study included a behavioral intervention that consisted of several psychosocial interventions that have proven effective in treating children with ADHD in past research (Pelham, Wheeler, & Chronis, 1998; Wells et al., 2000). The first component consisted of twenty-seven sessions of group parent training provided by therapist-consultants over 14 months. In these sessions, parents were taught (a) intensive behavior management skills (e.g., effective commands, token economies in the home, effective discipline), (b) methods to manage their stress, anger, and negative moods to enhance their parenting abilities, and (c) how to effectively work with teachers and advocate with school personnel for their child with ADHD. There was also a school intervention component that involved sixteen consultations with teachers over a 14-month period to establish behavioral management techniques in the classroom (e.g., daily report cards, classroom token economies). In addition, paraprofessionals were trained to be in the child's classroom to help in the implementation of these behavioral management programs. The third component of the MTA behavioral intervention was an 8-week summer treatment program that met daily from 8:00 to 5:00 on weekdays during the summer. During this program, children experienced intensive and individualized behavioral management programs (e.g., point system, daily report cards) designed to promote positive behavioral changes. The summer treatment program also included daily social skills training and sports skills training components.

Consistent with past research, the intensive behavioral intervention of the MTA resulted in gains that were superior to those found for the community treatment control group (MTA Cooperative Group, 1999). However, as noted previously, the group of children receiving medication alone showed outcomes superior to the group receiving behavioral intervention on many outcome measures. Also, on many of the outcome indicators, there was no clear benefit from adding this intensive behavioral intervention to the medication treatment (Pelham, 1999). This finding was qualified, however, by the fact that the combined treatment group showed a greater percentage of children who fell into an age-normative range on many outcome measures and the fact that children could be maintained on lower doses of medication, as found in past research (Pelham, 1999). Furthermore, the combined intervention was more effective for children who had coexisting problems with anxiety (March et al., 2000) and was judged as more acceptable by parents than the medication-alone treatment (MTA Cooperative Group, 1999). Critical information about the long-term outcomes of children treated by the MTA is not yet available. It is possible that the combined treatment will show the clearest evidence for its effectiveness in its effects on the long-term adjustment of children with ADHD.

Summary of Treatment for ADHD. The intervention approach used in the MTA study provides an excellent example of the two methods for treating children with ADHD that have proven effective in past treatment outcome studies (although see Barkley, 2000; Greene & Ablon, 2001 for critiques of the intervention). This large-scale treatment trial supports the effectiveness of both stimulant medication and behavioral approaches to treatment, with somewhat stronger effects noted for the stimulant medication across outcome domains. These findings support previous research in suggesting that these types of intervention are currently the state of the art in treating children with ADHD with some support for combining the interventions to optimize the effects for children. However, much of this work on treatment has been conducted with preadolescent children who have ADHD. As a result, more work is needed to determine how well the effectiveness of these interventions generalizes to adolescents and young adults with ADHD. The effectiveness of the use of stimulant medication and behavioral interventions in older age groups with developmentally appropriate modifications has some support (Barkley, Connor, & Kwasnik, 2000; Nadeau, 1995).

Unfortunately, despite the well-documented efficacy for these two treatment modalities, there continues to be a proliferation of unproven therapies with very limited evidence for their effectiveness. These have ranged from biofeedback programs to specialized diets (Hinshaw, 1994). The popularity of these unproven approaches to intervention is likely due to the strong biases against the two empirically supported treatments. Many parents and professionals have strong negative feelings about the use of medication for controlling children's behavioral problems. Furthermore, most parents report having tried a system of rewards and punishments in an effort to control their children's behavior, albeit not at the level and intensity needed to bring about meaningful changes in the child's behavior. As a result, they are often reluctant to agree to interventions focusing on behavior management strategies. These biases often lead to the unfortunate outcome that many children with ADHD do not receive the optimal treatment approach for this disorder: a combination of a carefully controlled trial of stimulant medication and an intensive behavior management program.

OPPOSITIONAL DEFIANT DISORDER AND CONDUCT DISORDER

Definition and Description

Diagnosis. The study of antisocial and aggressive behavior in children has been a major focus of research in child psychology for a number of reasons. First, conduct problems are one of the most common reasons that children and adolescents are referred to mental health clinics (Frick & Silverthorn, 2001) or referred to residential treatment centers (Lyman & Campbell, 1996). Second, severe conduct problems make up the type of psychopathology that has been most strongly associated with delinquency (Moffitt, 1993). There has been an increase in societal concern over the dramatic rise in juvenile crime, especially violent crime, in recent years (Office of Juvenile Justice and Delinquency Prevention, 1995). As a result of this interest, there has been a great deal of research focused on understanding and treating this form of externalizing psychopathology.

The DSM–IV–TR (APA, 2000) specifies two disorders involving conduct problem behavior, with very explicit diagnostic criteria. Oppositional defiant disorder (ODD) is defined as:

- a recurrent pattern of negativistic, defiant, disobedient, and hostile behavior toward authority figures
- that persists for at least 6 months and
- is characterized by the frequent occurrence of at least four of the following behaviors: losing temper, arguing with adults, actively defying or refusing to comply with requests or rules of adults, deliberately doing things that will annoy other people, blaming others for one's own mistakes or misbehavior, being touchy or easily annoyed by others, being angry and resentful, or being spiteful or vindictive (p. 100; APA, 2000).

Conduct disorder (CD) is defined as:

- a repetitive and persistent pattern of behavior that violates the rights of others or violates major age-appropriate societal norms;
- these behaviors fall into four main groupings: aggressive conduct that threatens physical harm to other people or animals, nonaggressive conduct that causes property loss or damage, deceitfulness and theft, and serious violations of rules; and
- three or more characteristic behaviors must have been present during the past 12 months (pp. 93, 94; APA, 2000).

There has been great debate as to the best way to conceptualize the relationship between these two disorders involving conduct problems. Research seems to suggest that the less severe ODD symptoms are linked to the more severe CD symptoms both hierarchically and developmentally. For example, research has found that preadolescent children rarely begin showing the severe conduct problem behaviors associated with CD without first showing the milder ODD behaviors earlier in development. Instead, the typical developmental progression is that children start to show oppositional and argumentative behaviors early in life (e.g., between the ages of 3 and 8) and then gradually progress into increasingly more severe patterns of conduct problem behavior over the course of childhood (Loeber et al., 1992). However, there are two important aspects to this developmental trajectory. First, while most children who show the more severe conduct problems of CD start by showing the less severe ODD symptoms, a large number of children with ODD do not progress on to show the more severe conduct problems (Lahey & Loeber, 1994). Second, most children who progress on to CD do not *change* the types of behaviors they display but instead *add* the more severe conduct problem behaviors (Lahey & Loeber, 1994).

Also supporting the notion that CD is a developmentally advanced form of ODD is research that has fairly consistently linked ODD and CD to similar correlates. This research has shown that children with ODD and children with CD both differ from other clinic-referred children in three important ways. First, they are more likely to be from families of lower socioeconomic status (Faraone, Biederman, Keenan, & Tsuang, 1991; Frick et al., 1992; Rey et al., 1988). Second, their parents are more likely to have a history of antisocial personality disorder (Faraone et al., 1991; Frick et al., 1992). Third, their parents are more likely to use ineffective discipline practices (Frick et al., 1992). CD children are somewhat more divergent from control children on these variables than children with ODD.

Developmental Course. In addition to this developmental progression in severity of conduct problems, a number of studies have documented the stability of conduct problems across development. Frick and Loney (1999) reviewed twelve prospective longitudinal studies of the stability of conduct problems over short periods of time (from 8 months to 5 years) and found that the correlations between initial and follow-up assessments generally fell between .42 and .64. In studies that estimated the degree of stability of diagnoses of conduct disorders, about 50% of the children diagnosed with CD at an initial assessment were rediagnosed with CD at a follow-up assessment. Frick and Loney (1999) also summarized the results of nine prospective longitudinal studies that investigated the stability of conduct problems over longer periods of time (i.e., more than 6 years). As would be expected, the stability estimates are somewhat lower than those found for shorter follow-up periods, although they still indicate fairly substantial stability. Specifically, the correlation coefficients for the long-term follow-up studies generally fell between .20 and .40. Several studies included in the review provided estimates of the stability within samples of youth with severe patterns of behavior that are likely to have met formal diagnostic criteria for CD. However, the degree of stability was somewhat variable across studies. This variability seemed partly related to the choice of outcome measure. For example, Kratzer and Hodgins (1997) found that about 64% of boys and 17% of girls (ages 12–16) with CD had committed a crime during a 16-year follow-up period. In contrast, Robins (1966) reported that 31% of boys and 17% of girls referred to a mental health clinic for CD symptoms were diagnosed with sociopathic personality disorder as adults. The definition of sociopathic personality disorder is similar to the DSM–IV–TR criteria for antisocial personality disorder (APD; APA, 2000), which requires a severe, varied, and chronic pattern of antisocial behavior rather than the commission of a single criminal offense. In fact, in the Robins sample, 43% of the boys and 12% of the girls who had been referred for CD symptoms were later imprisoned at least once as an adult.

Subtypes of Conduct Disorders. Although conduct disorders are remarkably stable over time, not all children with severe conduct problems continue to show problems through adolescence and into adulthood. In fact, much of this stability can be accounted for by a small group of children with very severe and chronic conduct problems (Moffitt, 1993). This finding has led to many attempts to uncover characteristics that distinguish between more severe and chronic forms of conduct problems and more benign and transient forms (see Frick & Ellis, 1999, for a review).

One of the more consistent predictors of poor outcome for children with CD is the severity of the initial disorder. The frequency and intensity of the behavior exhibited, the variety of different types of symptoms displayed, and the presence of symptoms in more than one setting have all been related to a more severe and persistent form of CD (Loeber, 1982; 1991). Also, children with both conduct problems and ADHD seem to have a worse outcome than those with either type of problem alone (Lynam, 1996; Moffitt, 1990), as do children with conduct problems who have lower intelligence (Farrington, 1991; Moffitt, 1990). In addition, family dysfunction and socioeconomic adversity have been linked to poorer outcome in children with conduct problems (Frick & Loney, 1999; Moffitt, 1990).

Perhaps one of the most consistent predictors of poor outcome is the age at which the child begins to show serious conduct problems (Frick & Loney, 1999). For example, in a prospective study of the adult outcomes of a birth cohort in New Zealand, Moffitt, Caspi, Harrington, and Milne (2002) compared two groups of adults who had severe conduct problems as youth. One group began showing serious problems before puberty and showed a continuous pattern of conduct problems across several age periods and was thus labeled as showing life-course persistent conduct problems. The second group, labeled the adolescent-limited group, did not begin showing serious conduct problems until after the onset of puberty. The life-course persistent group made up only 10% of the birth cohort but accounted for 43% of violent convictions in the sample, 40% of the drug convictions, and 62% of the convictions for violence against women. The adolescent-limited group (26% of the sample) continued to have some problems in adulthood as well, showing greater antisocial behavior than control adults who did not show conduct problems as a youth. However, they were 50% to 60% less likely to be convicted of an offense than the life-course persistent group, and their offenses tended to be less serious (e.g., minor theft, public drunkenness) and less violent (e.g., accounting for 50% of the convictions for property offenses). As a result of findings such as these, the most recent versions of the DSM (APA, 2000) have included in their classification a distinction between childhood-onset type and adolescent-onset type of CD.

More recent research has used the presence of a callous and unemotional interpersonal style (e.g., lacking empathy and guilt, constricted emotions) to designate a distinct group of children with severe and chronic CD (see Frick, Barry, & Bodin, 2000; Frick, Cornell, Bodin, Dane, Barry, & Loney, 2003, for reviews). Although these callous–unemotional (CU) traits seem to be more common in the childhood-onset group (Moffitt et al., 2002), they are characteristic of only about a third of these children (Christian, Frick, Hill, Tyler, & Frazer, 1997). CU traits are similar to characteristics associated with the construct of psychopathy in adults, which has proven important for designating a particularly severe, violent, and chronic antisocial individual in adult forensic samples (Hart & Hare, 1997).

Unfortunately, the predictive utility of the construct of psychopathy and its relation to violence severity and type has not been extensively studied in youth (Edens, Skeem, Cruise, & Cauffman, 2001). There are several notable exceptions using samples of institutionalized adolescents. These studies have documented that the presence of CU traits predicts subsequent delinquency, aggression, number of violence offenses, and a shorter length of time to violent reoffending in antisocial youth (Brandt, Kennedy, Patrick, & Curtin, 1997; Forth, Hart, & Hare, 1990; Toupin, Mercier, Dery, Cote, & Hodgins, 1995). Despite these notable exceptions, much of the research attempting to extend the construct of psychopathy to youth has not been prospective in nature but has been cross-sectional. These cross-sectional studies have generally focused on the usefulness of CU traits for designating a particularly severe subgroup of antisocial youth. For example, nonreferred antisocial youth who show CU traits exhibit a greater variety and severity of crimes than other youth with conduct problems (Lynam, 1997). Furthermore, clinic-referred children with conduct problems who show CU traits show a greater number and variety of conduct problems, more police contacts, and stronger family histories of antisocial personality disorder than other children with conduct problems (Christian et al., 1997). The results of these cross-sectional studies are consistent with longitudinal studies of children with CDs (Frick & Loney, 1999). Also, consistent with the research in adults, there seems to be an especially strong link between CU traits and severity and type of aggression. For example, CU traits have been associated with violent sex offending by institutionalized adolescents (Caputo, Frick & Brodsky, 1999) and with more severe and pervasive violence among juvenile offenders, including instrumental (i.e., violence for monetary or social gains) and sadistic violent acts (Kruh, Frick, & Clements, in press).

Cultural and Gender Issues

There is evidence that aggressive, antisocial, and violent behavior varies in rate across cultures. For example, the United States has one of the highest rates of violence of all industrialized societies, showing four to seventy-three times the rates of violence found in other industrialized nations (Fingerhut & Kleinman, 1990). This high rate of violence in the United States has been linked to various factors. One such factor is the high rate of exposure to violence experienced by children, both in their homes and neighborhoods (Osofsky, Wewers, Hann, & Frick, 1993) and through media portrayals (Heath, Bresdin, & Rinaldi, 1989). In addition, the cultural glorification of violence and the availability of handguns have also been considered as factors related to the high rate of violence in this country (O'Donnell, 1995). Still others have focused on the marginalization of ethnic minorities and the structural inequalities in opportunity afforded to minorities in the United States that can increase the risk of antisocial behavior in those without opportunities for obtaining goods and status through socially sanctioned means (McCloyd, 1990).

This latter possibility would predict higher rates of delinquent and antisocial behavior in ethnic minorities, but these associations have not been consistently found. For example, higher rates of delinquency (Gray-Ray & Ray, 1990) and conduct problems (Fabrega, Ulrich, & Mezzich, 1993; Lahey et al., 1995) have been found for African-American youth in some samples, but not others (McCoy, Frick, Loney, & Ellis, 1999). More important, it is unclear whether this association, when found, could be explained largely by the fact that ethnic minorities are more likely to experience economic hardships and live in urban neighborhoods with higher concentrations of crime than nonminority individuals (Peeples & Loeber, 1994).

In contrast to this somewhat mixed picture of the relation between ethnicity and conduct problems, there are clear sex differences in the rate of conduct problems, with most studies showing that boys are more likely to show conduct problems than girls (see Silverthorn & Frick, 1999, for a review). However, these sex differences vary somewhat across development. For example, in preschool children, this sex difference is small and sometimes nonexistent (Keenan & Shaw, 1997), whereas throughout childhood there is a male: female ratio of about 4:1 (Silverthorn & Frick, 1999). This ratio closes to about 2:1 in adolescence, the period in which girls are most likely to be diagnosed with CD (Silverthorn & Frick, 1999). There is some controversy as to whether these differences in prevalence rates in childhood and adolescence are real differences or an artifact of diagnostic criteria that are not sensitive to sex differences in how conduct problems are expressed. For example, it has been argued that girls are less often diagnosed with severe conduct problems than boys because they manifest more indirect or relational aggression (i.e., spreading rumors, hurting others in the context of a relationship), rather than physical aggression (e.g., Crick & Grotpeter, 1995). Others have argued that girls manifest similar types of behaviors as boys, but that they should be diagnosed using a more lenient criteria that compares girls to other girls rather than to mixed samples of girls and boys (e.g., Zocolillo, 1993). Still others have argued that girls manifest antisocial behaviors that are similar to those of boys but are less likely than boys to experience the necessary pathogenic processes that can lead to the development of antisocial behavior (Moffitt & Caspi, 2001; Silverthorn & Frick, 1999).

One additional source of controversy is whether the distinction between childhood-onset and adolescent-onset is equally valid for girls and boys. Specifically, it is generally accepted that girls are less likely to show a childhood-onset to their severe conduct problems, accounting for the changes in the gender ratio found between childhood and adolescence. However, it is not clear whether girls who show an adolescent-onset of conduct problems show a less severe and less chronic disturbance, as is the case for boys. In fact, there is some preliminary evidence that, despite the adolescent-onset, many antisocial girls show the familial, individual, and interpersonal deficits and the negative outcome in late adolescence and adulthood that make them more similar to boys who show a childhood-onset to their conduct problems (Silverthorn & Frick, 1999).

Etiology: Developmental Pathways to Severe Conduct Problems

There has been a substantial body of research on children and adolescents documenting a large number of factors that can place a child at risk for showing conduct problems. These factors range from individual risk factors (e.g., poor impulse control, poor emotional regulation, low intelligence, lack of social skills), to problems in the child's immediate psychosocial context (e.g., poverty, parental psychopathology, inadequate parental discipline, association with a deviant peer group), to problems in the child's broader psychosocial context (e.g., living in a high crime neighborhood, exposure to violence, lack of educational and vocational opportunities) (see Frick, 1998; Moffitt, 1993, for reviews). However, it has been difficult to weave this broad array of risk factors into a coherent, yet comprehensive, causal model for conduct problems both because of the sheer number of factors and because they involve so many different types of causal processes. Additionally, these risk factors are typically not independent of each other and it is quite likely that they operate in a transactional (e.g., one risk factor having an influence on another risk factor) or multiplicative fashion. For example, an impulsive child may be much more difficult to parent effectively than a child who has better emotional and behavioral regulation, thereby making it more likely that he or she will experience less than adequate parenting (Barkley, 1996; Lytton, 1990). However, the impulsive child probably needs effective parenting even more than the well-regulated child to prevent the development of severe conduct problems (Colder, Lochman, & Wells, 1997). As a result, the development of conduct problems for any child is likely the result of a number of different risk factors that interact to place a child at risk for exhibiting behavior that violates the rights of others or major societal norms.

Another complicating factor is the possibility that the causal mechanisms that lead to conduct problems may differ across subgroups of youth who exhibit antisocial behavior. For example, the distinction between childhood-onset and adolescent-onset patterns of CD not only has important predictive utility, as mentioned previously, but the two groups of youth with CD also show a number of different correlates that could suggest divergent etiologies. Specifically, children in the childhood-onset group show more aggression, more cognitive and neuropsychological disturbances (e.g., EF deficits, autonomic nervous system irregularities), greater impulsivity, greater social alienation, and more dysfunctional family backgrounds than do children in the adolescent-onset group (see Frick, 1998; Moffitt, 1993; Moffitt, Caspi, Dickson, Silva, & Stanton, 1996; Moffitt et al., 2002, for reviews).

These differences in the correlates of the two types of CD suggest that the childhood-onset group results in a more severe and enduring disturbance that is the result of an interaction of a vulnerable temperament in the child and his or her experience of an inadequate rearing environment (Frick, 1998; Moffitt, 1993). In contrast, children in the adolescent-onset group show less temperamental and psychosocial adversity, yet they still show a severe and impairing pattern of antisocial behavior (Moffitt et al., 1996; Moffitt et al., 2002). Additionally, they tend to reject traditional status hierarchies and religious rules, and they associate with deviant peers (Moffitt et al., 1996). As a result, adolescents in this group seem to show an exaggeration of the normal developmental process involving separation and individuation that is crucial to identity formation in adolescence. Because of this developmental task, engaging in forbidden behaviors with peers can engender feelings of independence and maturity, albeit in a misguided manner (Moffitt, 1993). Furthermore, although they may continue to have problems in adulthood, their adult adjustment is less impaired than that of children in the childhood-onset group. This is because the impairments are less related to enduring psychosocial vulnerabilities (e.g., neuropsychological impairments, deficits in social skills) and usually is a direct consequence of their antisocial behavior (e.g., poor educational attainment, criminal record, early marriage) (Moffitt et al., 2002).

As mentioned previously, the presence of CU traits appears to designate a more severe and potentially more chronic group of children with the childhood-onset group. These traits also may be a marker for a group of children who have different causal processes leading to their behavioral problems (Frick et al., 2000; Frick et al., 2003; Frick & Ellis, 1999, for reviews). For example, children with conduct problems who show CU traits tend to be more thrill and adventure seeking (Frick et al., 2003; Frick, Lilienfeld, Ellis, Loney, & Silverthorn, 1999), are less sensitive to cues of punishment when a reward-oriented response set is primed (Fisher & Blair, 1998; Frick et al., 2003; O'Brien & Frick, 1996), and are less reactive to threatening and emotionally distressing stimuli (Blair, 1999; Frick et al., 2003; Loney, Frick, Clements, Ellis, & Kerlin, 2003) than other children with conduct problems.

These characteristics suggest that conduct problem children with CU traits may show a temperamental style associated with low emotional reactivity to aversive stimuli, which can contribute to the development of CU traits in several ways (Blair, 1999; Kochanska, 1993). For example, it can place a child at risk for missing some of the early precursors to empathic concern, which involve emotional arousal evoked by the misfortune and distress of others. Also, it could lead a child to be relatively insensitive to the prohibitions and sanctions of parents and other socializing agents. Finally, it could create an interpersonal style in which the child becomes so focused on the potential rewards and gains of aggression or other antisocial means to solve interpersonal conflicts that he or she ignores the potentially harmful effects of this behavior on him- or herself and others. Some research supports these hypotheses. For example, antisocial and delinquent youth who show CU traits are less distressed by the negative effects of their behavior on others (Blair, Jones, Clark, & Smith, 1997; Frick et al., 1999), are more impaired in their moral reasoning and empathic concern towards others (Blair, 1999), and they expect more instrumental gain (e.g., obtaining goods or social goals) from their aggressive actions and are more predatory in their violence than antisocial youth without these traits (Caputo et al., 1999; Kruh et al., in press).

In contrast, children with childhood-onset conduct problems without CU traits are more highly reactive to emotional and threatening stimuli (Loney et al., 2003), more distressed by the negative effects of their behavior on themselves and others (Frick et al., 1999; Frick et al., 2003), and more likely to attribute hostile intent to the actions of peers (Frick et al., 2003). Also, their aggressive and antisocial behavior is more strongly associated with dysfunctional parenting practices (Wootton, Frick, Shelton, & Silverthorn, 1997) and with deficits in intelligence (Loney, Frick, Ellis, & McCoy, 1998) than for children with conduct problems who are high on CU traits. These findings suggest that antisocial children who do not show high rates of CU traits may have difficulties with behavioral and emotional regulation related to high levels of emotional reactivity. Such poor emotional regulation can result from a number of interacting causal factors, such as inadequate socialization in their rearing environments, deficits in intelligence that make it difficult for them to delay gratification and anticipate consequences, or temperamental problems in response inhibition. The problems in emotional regulation can lead to very impulsive and unplanned aggressive acts for which the child may be remorseful afterwards, but which he or she still has difficulty controlling. They can also lead to a higher susceptibility to anger due to perceived provocations from peers leading to violent and aggressive acts within the context of high emotional arousal (Kruh et al., in press).

Empirically Validated Treatments

Given societal concerns over violence and delinquency, it is not surprising that the treatment of antisocial and aggressive behavior in youth has been the focus of a large number of controlled treatment outcome studies. For example, a recent review of published treatment outcome studies focusing only on psychosocial treatments for children and adolescents with conduct problems documented eighty-two studies involving over 5,272 children (Brestan & Eyberg, 1998). Unfortunately, one of the main conclusions one can reach from this extensive effort to find effective treatments for conduct problem youth is that the vast majority of treatment approaches have proven to be largely ineffective (Kazdin, 1995). Of even greater concern is the evidence that some types of intervention, particularly those that involve extensive antisocial peer group interactions, can have iatrogenic effects on the children being treated by actually increasing the level and severity of their antisocial behavior and increasing their risk for negative life outcomes as adults (Dishion, McCord, & Poulin, 1999). Therefore, uninformed and ill-conceived treatments can do more harm than good.

Although this overview of treatment effectiveness is somewhat pessimistic, four treatments have proven effective in controlled outcome studies (see Frick, 1998, 2001, for a more extended discussion of these empirically supported treatments). The first intervention is the use of contingency management programs. The basic components of contingency management programs are (a) establishing clear behavioral goals that gradually shape a child's behavior in those areas of specific concern for the child, (b) monitoring the child's progress toward these goals, (c) reinforcing appropriate steps toward reaching these goals, and (d) providing consequences for inappropriate behavior. These programs can bring about behavioral changes for children with conduct problems in a number of different settings such as at home (Ross, 1981), at school (Abramowitz & O'Leary, 1991), and in residential treatment centers (Lyman & Campbell, 1996).

The second effective treatment is Parent Management Training (PMT). A critical goal of PMT programs is to teach parents how to develop and implement very structured contingency management programs in the home. However, PMT programs also focus on (a) improving the quality of parent–child interactions (e.g., having parents more involved in their children's activities, improving parent–child communication, increasing parental warmth and responsiveness), (b) changing antecedents to behavior that enhance the likelihood that positive prosocial behaviors will be displayed by children (e.g., how to time and present requests, providing clear and explicit rules and expectations), (c) improving parents' ability to monitor and supervise their children, and (d) using more effective discipline strategies (e.g., being more consistent in discipline, using a variety of approaches to discipline). These specific aspects of parenting have been consistently linked to child conduct problems (Frick, 1994, 1998). The effectiveness of this type of intervention has been the most consistently documented of any technique used to treat children with severe conduct problems (Kazdin, 1995).

The third type of intervention that has proven effective in treating children with conduct problems is a cognitive-behavioral approach designed to overcome deficits in social cognition and social problem solving experienced by many children and adolescents with conduct problems. Research on children who are aggressive or who show other conduct problems has consistently documented deficits in the way they process social information, including the way they encode social cues, interpret these cues, develop social goals, develop appropriate responses, decide on appropriate responses, and enact appropriate responses (Crick & Dodge, 1996). For example, as mentioned previously, some children with conduct problems tend to attribute hostile intent to ambiguous interactions with peers that make them more likely to act aggressively towards peers. Other aggressive children overestimate the likelihood that their aggressive behavior will lead to positive results (e.g., enhanced status, obtaining a desired toy) and this cognitive bias makes them more likely to select aggressive alternatives to solving peer conflict (Dodge, Lochman, Harnish, Bates, & Petit, 1997). Most cognitive-behavioral skills-building programs teach the child to inhibit impulsive or angry responding. This inhibition allows the child to go through a series of problem-solving steps (e.g., how to recognize problems, how to consider alternative responses and select the most adaptive one) and overcome deficits in the way they process social information (Lochman, 1992).

The final intervention that has proven to have some effectiveness in reducing conduct problems in children with ADHD is the use of stimulant medication. As mentioned previously, a large proportion of children with conduct problems also show ADHD, and the impulsivity associated with ADHD may directly lead to some of the aggressive and other poorly regulated behaviors of children with severe conduct problems. In addition, the presence of ADHD may indirectly contribute to the development of conduct problems through its effect on (a) children's interactions with peers and significant others (e.g., parents and teachers), (b) parents' ability to use effective socialization strategies, or (c) a child's ability to perform academically (Frick, 1998). Therefore, for many children and adolescents with conduct problems, reducing ADHD symptoms is an important treatment goal. As mentioned previously, one of the more successful treatments for ADHD is the use of stimulant medication. Most important, the effectiveness of stimulants for reducing conduct problems in children with both ADHD and a CD has been shown in several controlled medication trials (e.g., Hinshaw, 1991; Hinshaw, Heller, & McHale, 1992; Pelham et al., 1993). Furthermore, it is effective in addressing many of the secondary problems often associated with severe conduct problems, such as improving peer relations, in children with both conduct problems and ADHD (Whalen, Henker, Buhrmester, Hinshaw, Huber, & Laski, 1989).

Limitations.   Although each of these four interventions has proven to have some effectiveness in controlled outcome studies, this body of research has also found that each of these interventions also possesses substantial limitations (Brestan & Eyberg, 1998; Kazdin, 1995). First, a significant proportion of children with CD do not show a positive response to these interventions and, for those that do respond positively, their behavior problems are often not reduced to a normal level. Second, treatment is most effective with younger children (before age 8) with less severe behavioral disturbances. Third, the generalizability of treatment effects across settings tends to be poor. That is, treatments that are effective in changing a child's behavior in one setting (e.g., mental health clinics) often do not bring about changes in the child's behavior in other settings (e.g., schools). Fourth, improvements in behavior are often difficult to maintain over time.

Given these limitations, there has been an increasing focus on trying to improve treatments by integrating our knowledge about how antisocial behavior develops with the development of innovative approaches to treatment (Frick, 1998, 2001). Each of the four treatments described previously targets basic processes that research has shown to be important in the development of conduct problems (e.g., family dysfunction, problems in impulse control). However, these treatments have ignored two additional characteristics of children with severe conduct problems. First, research clearly suggests that severe conduct problems are multidetermined. Severe antisocial and aggressive behavior is usually the result of a complex interaction of many different types of causal processes. Second, the causes of severe conduct problems are heterogeneous. As a result, any single intervention, even if it targets multiple causal processes, is not likely to be effective for all children with ODD or CD.

Empirical Supported Principles.   Based on this research, there is not likely to be any single best treatment for severe conduct problems. Instead, interventions must be tailored to the individual needs of children with ODD or CD, and these needs will likely differ depending on the specific mechanisms underlying the child's behavioral disturbance. For example, interventions for children in the adolescent-onset pathways will likely be somewhat different from interventions for children in the childhood-onset pathway. Even within the childhood-onset pathway, the focus of intervention may be different depending on the presence or absence of CU traits (see Frick, 1998, 2001, for examples).

By integrating research on developmental models of conduct problems with empirically supported treatments, several general principles for designing and implementing interventions for children with severe conduct problems appear important. First, one must understand the multiple causal processes that can be involved in the development of conduct problems. For example, by recognizing the developmental progressions that often characterize children and adolescents with CD, interventions can be implemented as early as possible in the developmental sequence. In addition, this knowledge base can help in determining which processes may be involved in the development of CD for a particular child and can guide decisions as to the most important targets of interventions. Second, this flexible approach to treatment requires a clear, comprehensive, and individualized case conceptualization that guides the design of a focused and integrated approach to treatment (Frick & McCoy, 2001). A case conceptualization is a theory about the factors most likely involved in the development, exacerbation, and maintenance of conduct problems for an individual child or adolescent. It uses the research on developmental pathways to conduct problems and attempts to apply it to an individual child with a conduct disorder. Third, successful intervention for children and adolescents with severe conduct problems typically involves multiple professionals and multiple community agencies all working together to provide a comprehensive and integrated intervention.

This comprehensive and individualized approach to intervention outlined here and elsewhere (Frick, 1998, 2001) has not been subjected to controlled outcome evaluations. However, one approach to treatment that incorporates many of the features of a developmental approach to treatment that has been tested in controlled outcome studies is multisystemic therapy (MST). MST was originally developed as a general approach to intervention for psychopathological conditions (Henggeler & Borduin, 1990) but has been applied extensively to the treatment of severe antisocial behavior in children and adolescents (Henggeler, Schoenwald, Borduin, Rowland, & Cunningham, 1998). The orientation of MST is an expansion of a systems orientation to family therapy. In systemic family therapy, problems in children's adjustment are viewed as being embedded within the larger family context. MST expands this notion to include other contexts, such as the child's peer, school, and neighborhood contexts. MST is not explicitly developmental in orientation. For example, it does not emphasize the individual child's characteristics that may contribute to the development of severe conduct problems and that may play a role in shaping his or her psychosocial contexts (e.g., the influence of the child on his or her family environment). Nonetheless, MST does emphasize a comprehensive and individualized approach to intervention that is consistent with the treatment principles outlined previously.

MST involves an initial comprehensive assessment that seeks to understand the level and severity of the child's or adolescent's presenting problems and to understand how these problems may be related to factors in the child's familial, peer, and cultural environment. The information from this assessment is used to outline an individualized treatment plan based on the specific needs of the child and his or her family. Unlike the individual interventions described previously,

MST does not emphasize the use of specific techniques. Instead, it emphasizes several principles that follow from its orientation to intervention. These principles include the following:

- The identified problems in the child are understood within the child's familial, peer, and cultural context.
- Therapeutic contacts emphasize positive (strength-oriented) levers for change.
- Interventions promote responsible behavior among family members.
- Interventions are present focused and action oriented, targeting specific and well defined problems.
- Interventions target sequences of behavior within and between multiple systems.
- Interventions must be developmentally appropriate.
- Interventions are designed to require daily or weekly effort by family members.
- Intervention effectiveness must be evaluated continuously from multiple perspectives.
- Interventions are designed to promote maintenance of therapeutic change by empowering caregivers.

A critical component of MST is a system of intensive supervision for the therapists implementing the treatment to determine how these principles should be implemented to meet the needs of each individual case and to ensure that the principles are followed throughout the intervention (Henggeler et al., 1998).

One of the important contributions of MST to the treatment outcome literature is its demonstration that individualized interventions can be rigorously evaluated through controlled treatment outcome studies. The initial findings from studies on the effectiveness of MST in reducing antisocial and aggressive behavior among even very severely disturbed youth have been quite promising. For example, in a controlled treatment outcome study of MST at a university-based outpatient clinic, eighty-eight adolescent repeat offenders underwent MST. To illustrate the individualized nature of the treatment, the length of treatment with MST ranged from 5 to 54 hours (mean of 23 hours). In addition to this variation in intensity, the way in which these hours were used varied depending on the needs of the clients. Eighty-three percent of the MST group participated in family therapy and 60% participated in some form of school intervention, which included facilitation of parent–teacher communication, academic remediation, or help in classroom behavior management. In 57% of the cases, there was some form of peer intervention, which included coaching and emotional support for integration into prosocial peer groups (e.g., scouts, athletic teams) and/or direct intervention with peers. In 28% of the cases, there was individual therapy with the adolescent, which typically involved some form of cognitive-behavioral skills-building intervention. Finally, in 26% of the cases, the adolescent's parents became involved in marital therapy. The outcomes of this group of offenders receiving MST were compared to a control group of sixty-eight offenders who received traditional outpatient services, typically focusing on individual psychotherapy (Borduin et al., 1995). At a 4-year follow-up, only 26% of the youth who underwent MST were rearrested compared to 71% of the control adolescents.

In a second outcome study of MST, master's level therapists provided intervention at a community mental health center (Henggeler, Melton, & Smith, 1992). The sample included adolescents who had been adjudicated as delinquent and had multiple arrests. These adolescents were randomly assigned to receive either MST or standard services provided by the juvenile justice system. The group receiving MST showed half as many arrests and spent an average of 73 fewer days incarcerated than adolescents who received standard services. These two studies illustrate the promise of MST with a difficult population, namely, adolescent juvenile offenders with multiple arrests. Henggeler et al. (1998) provide examples of several additional outcome studies of MST that are currently underway.

Summary of Treatment for Children With Conduct Problems. In conclusion, there have been many advances in recent years in our understanding of the causes of severe antisocial and aggressive behavior and in our development of effective treatments for youth with such behaviors. However, these interventions require a different model for intervention than the ones in which many mental health professionals were trained (i.e., finding the one treatment that works best and using it for all individuals with the disorder). In addition, the goals of these interventions may be different from the goals of interventions that are based on political ideologies related to how aggressive and antisocial individuals should be treated (e.g., boot camps; Henggeler & Schoenwald, 1994). Given the severity and chronicity of conduct problems and their social costs, it is imperative that mental health professionals promote interventions that reflect these advances and contribute to the development of further advances in both research and service delivery. The available evidence does not support the conclusion that children with CD are untreatable but instead, it seems that the field is only now beginning to understand how best to treat them. Granted, the documented evidence for treatment success is still minimal and this optimism may prove to be unfounded. Research suggests, however, a clear framework for designing intervention programs for children with severe conduct problems (Frick, 1998, 2001). This fact alone provides great cause for optimism.

OVERALL SUMMARY

As mentioned previously, externalizing disorders of children constitute one of the most common reasons that children are referred to mental health clinics for treatment (Frick & Silverthorn, 2001). This fact is not surprising, given the disruptions that children with these disorders often cause to those around them, especially to parents and teachers, who are most likely to refer a child for treatment. Furthermore, given the association between externalizing disorders and many costly and impairing outcomes (e.g., substance abuse, delinquency), understanding and effectively treating children with these disorders is an important endeavor for psychologists and other mental health professionals.

Fortunately, there is a large body of research on children with these disorders. As summarized in this chapter, recent research has led to great advances in our understanding of the causes of these disorders and the development of effective interventions to prevent and treat them in youth. Unfortunately, this research is often not translated well into practice and, as a result, many children with these disorders do not receive state-of-the-art treatment. This gap between research and practice can be the result of a number of factors (Frick, 2000). For example, it can be the result of practitioners not being trained on the most current theories and approaches to treatment or not remaining current on this research. Alternatively, the gap between research and practice can be the result of research not being conducted or presented in a way that is useful to the practicing psychologist. In either case, the quality of services provided to children with disruptive behaviors depends heavily on advances in research and our ability to translate these findings into widely used applications. The focus of this chapter was to summarize research on children with externalizing disorders in a way that promotes such a translation.

REFERENCES

Abikoff, H., & Klein, R. G. (1992). Attention-deficit hyperactivity and conduct disorder: Comorbidity and implications for treatment. *Journal of Consulting and Clinical Psychology, 60*, 881–892.

Abramowitz, A. J., & O'Leary, S. G. (1991). Behavioral interventions for the classroom: Implications for students with ADHD. *School Psychology Review, 20*, 220–234.

Achenbach, T. M. (1995). Diagnosis, assessment, and comorbidity in psychosocial treatment research. *Journal of Abnormal Psychology, 23,* 45–65.

Achenbach, T. M., & Edelbrock, C. S. (1978). The classification of child psychopathology: A review and analysis of empirical efforts. *Psychological Bulletin, 85,* 1275–1301.

American Psychiatric Association. (1980). *Diagnostic and Statistical Manual of Mental Disorders* (3rd ed.). Washington, DC: Author.

American Psychiatric Association. (2000). *Diagnostic and Statistical Manual of Mental Disorders* (4th ed., text rev.). Washington, DC: Author.

Anderson, J. C., Williams, S., McGee, R., & Silva, P. A. (1987). DSM-III disorders in preadolescent children: Prevalence in a large sample from the general population. *Archives of General Psychiatry, 44,* 69–76.

Applegate, B., Lahey, B. B., Hart, E. L., Biederman, J., Hynd, G. W., Barkley, R. A., Ollendick, T., Frick, P. J., Greenhill, L., McBurnett, K., Newcorn, J. H., Kerdyk, L., Garfinkel, B., Waldman, I., & Shaffer, D. (1997). Validity of the age-of-onset criterion for ADHD: A report from the DSM-IV field trials. *Journal of the American Academy of Child and Adolescent Psychiatry, 36,* 1211–1221.

Barkley, R. A. (1996). Attention-deficit/hyperactivity disorder. In E. J. Mash & R. A. Barkley (Eds.), *Child Psychopathology* (pp. 63–112). New York: Guilford.

Barkley, R. A. (1997). Behavioral inhibition, sustained attention, and executive functions: Constructing a unifying theory of ADHD. *Psychological Bulletin, 121,* 65–94.

Barkley, R. A. (2000). Commentary on the multimodal treatment study of children with ADHO. *Journal of Abnormal Child Psychology, 28* (6), 595–600.

Barkley, R. A., Connor, D. F., & Kwasnik, D. (2000). Challenges to determining adolescent medication response in an outpatient clinical setting: Comparing Adderall and methylphenidate for ADHD. *Journal of Attention Disorders, 4,* 102–113.

Barkley, R. A., & Cunningham, C. E. (1979). The effects of Ritalin on the mother-child interactions of hyperactive children. *Archives of General Psychiatry, 36,* 201–208.

Barkley, R. A., DuPaul, G. J., & McMurray, M. B. (1991). Attention deficit disorder with and without hyperactivity: Clinical response to three dose levels of methylphenidate. *Pediatrics, 87,* 519–531.

Barkley, R. A., Fischer, M., Smallish, L., & Fletcher, K. (2002). The persistence of attention-deficit/hyperactivity disorder into young adulthood as a function of reporting source and definition of disorder. *Journal of Abnormal Psychology, 111,* 279–289.

Barkley, R. A., Guevremont, D. G., Anastopoulos, A. D., DuPaul, G. J., & Shelton, T. L. (1993). Driving related risks and outcomes of attention deficit hyperactivity disorder in adolescents and young adults: A 3–5 year follow-up survey. *Pediatrics, 92,* 212–218.

Barkley, R. A., McMurray, M. B., Edelbrock, C. S., & Robbins, K. (1990). Side effects of methylphenidate in children with attention deficit hyperactivity disorder: A systematic, placebo-controlled evaluation. *Pediatrics, 86,* 184–192.

Bennett, L. A., Wolin, S. J., & Reiss, D. (1988). Cognitive, behavioral, and emotional problems among school-age children of alcoholic parents. *American Journal of Psychiatry, 145,* 185–190.

Biederman, J., Mick, E., Faraone, S. V., Braaten, E., Doyle, A., Spencer, T., Wilens, T. E., Frazier, E., & Johnson, M.A. (2002). Influence of gender on attention deficit hyperactivity disorder in children referred to a psychiatric clinic. *American Journal of Psychiatry, 159,* 36–42.

Blair, R. J. R. (1999). Responsiveness to distress cues in the child with psychopathic tendencies. *Personality and Individual Differences, 27,* 135–145.

Blair, R. J. R., Jones, L., Clark, F., & Smith, M. (1997). The psychopathic individual: A lack of responsiveness to distress cues? *Psychophysiology, 34,* 192–198.

Borduin, C. M., Mann, B. J., Cone, L. T., Henggeler, S. W., Fucci, B. R., Blaske, D. M., & Williams, R. A. (1995). Multisystemic treatment of serious juvenile offenders: Long term prevention of criminality and violence. *Journal of Consulting and Clinical Psychology, 63,* 569–578.

Brandt, J. R., Kennedy, W. A., Patrick, C. J., & Curtin, J. J. (1997). Assessment of psychopathy in a population of incarcerated adolescent offenders. *Psychological Assessment, 9,* 429–435.

Brestan, E. V., & Eyberg, S. M. (1998). Effective psychosocial treatments of conduct disordered children and adolescents. *Journal of Clinical Child Psychology, 27,* 180–189.

Caputo, A. A., Frick, P. J., & Brodsky, S. L. (1999). Family violence and juvenile sex offending: Potential mediating roles of psychopathic traits and negative attitudes toward women. *Criminal Justice and Behavior, 26,* 338–356.

Christian, R., Frick, P. J., Hill, N., Tyler, L. A., & Frazer, D. (1997). Psychopathy and conduct problems in children: II. Subtyping children with conduct problems based on their interpersonal and affective style. *Journal of the American Academy of Child and Adolescent Psychiatry, 36,* 233–241.

Colder, C. R., Lochman, J. E., & Wells, K. C. (1997). The moderating effects of children's fear and activity level on relations between parenting practices and childhood symptomatology. *Journal of Abnormal Child Psychology, 25,* 251–263.

Crick, N. R., & Dodge, K. A. (1996). Social information-processing mechanisms in reactive and proactive aggression. *Child Development, 67*, 993–1002.

Crick, N. R., & Grotpeter, J. K. (1995). Relational aggression, gender, and social-psychological adjustment. *Child Development, 66*, 710–722.

Dishion, T. J., McCord J., & Poulin F. (1999). When interventions harm: Peer groups and problem behavior. *American Psychologist, 54*, 755–764.

Dodge, K. A., Lochman, J. E., Harnish, J. D., Bates, J. E., & Pettit, G. S. (1997). Reactive and proactive aggression in school children and psychiatrically impaired chronically assaultive youth. *Journal of Abnormal Psychology, 106*, 37–51.

Edelbrock, C. S., Rende, R., Plomin, R., & Thompson, L. (1995). A twin study of competence and problem behavior in childhood and early adolescence. *Journal of Child Psychology and Psychiatry, 36*, 775–786.

Edens, J., Skeem, J., Cruise, K., & Cauffman, E. (2001). The assessment of juvenile psychopathy and its association with violence: A critical review. *Behavioral Sciences & the Law, 19*, 53–80.

Ernst, M., Liebenauer, L. L., King, A. C., Fitzgerald, G. A., Cohen, R. M., & Zametkin, A. J. (1994). Reduced brain metabolism in hyperactive girls. *Journal of the American Academy of Child and Adolescent Psychiatry, 33*, 858–868.

Fabrega, J. H., Ulrich, R., & Mezzich, J. E. (1993). Do Caucasian and Black adolescents differ at psychiatric intake? *Journal of the American Academy of Child and Adolescent Psychiatry, 32*, 407–413.

Faraone, S. V., Biederman, J., Keenan, K., & Tsuang, M. T. (1991). Separation of DSM-III attention deficit disorder and conduct disorder: Evidence from a family genetic study of American child psychiatry patients. *Psychological Medicine, 21*, 109–121.

Farrington, D. P. (1991). Childhood aggression and adult violence: Early precursors and later-life outcomes. In D. J. Pepler & K. H. Rubin (Eds.), *The development and treatment of childhood aggression* (pp. 5–19). Hillsdale, NJ: Lawrence Erlbaum Associates.

Fergusson, D. M., Horwood, J., & Lynskey, M. T. (1993). Prevalence and comorbidity of DSM-III-R diagnoses in a birth cohort of 15 year olds. *Journal of the American Academy of Child and Adolescent Psychiatry, 32*, 1127–1134.

Fingerhut, L. A., & Kleinman, J. C. (1990). International and interstate comparisons of homicide among young males. *Journal of the American Medical Association, 263*, 3292–3295.

Fischer, M. (1990). Parenting stress and the child with attention deficit hyperactivity disorder. *Journal of Clinical Child Psychology, 19*, 337–346.

Fisher, L., & Blair, R. J. R. (1998). Cognitive impairment and its relationship to psychopathic tendencies in children with emotional and behavioral difficulties. *Journal of Abnormal Child Psychology, 26*, 511–519.

Forth, A. E., Hart, S. D., & Hare, R. D. (1990). Assessment of psychopathy in male young offenders. *Psychological Assessment, 2*, 342–344.

Frick, P. J. (1994). Family dysfunction and the disruptive behavior disorders: A review of recent empirical findings. In T. H. Ollendick & R. J. Prinz (Eds.), *Advances in clinical child psychology* (Vol. 16, pp. 203–226). New York: Plenum.

Frick, P. J. (1998). *Conduct disorders and severe antisocial behavior*. New York: Plenum.

Frick, P. J. (2000). Laboratory and performance-based measures of childhood disorders. *Journal of Clinical Child Psychology, 29*, 475–478.

Frick, P. J. (2001). Effective interventions for children and adolescents with conduct disorder. *The Canadian Journal of Psychiatry, 46*, 26–37.

Frick, P. J., Barry, C. T., & Bodin, S. D. (2000). Applying the concept of psychopathy to children: Implications for the assessment of antisocial youth. In C. B. Gacono (Ed.), *The clinical and forensic assessment of psychopathy* (pp. 3–24). Mahwah, NJ: Lawrence Erlbaum Associates.

Frick, P. J., Cornell, A. H., Bodin, S. D., Dane, H. A., Barry, C. T., & Loney, B. R. (2003). Callous-unemotional traits and developmental pathways to severe conduct problems. *Developmental Psychology, 39*(2), 246–260.

Frick, P. J., & Ellis, M. L. (1999). Callous-unemotional traits and subtypes of conduct disorder. *Clinical Child and Family Psychology Review, 2*, 149–168.

Frick, P. J., Kamphaus, R. W., Lahey, B. B., Loeber, R., Christ, M. A. G., Hart, E. L., & Tannenbaum, L. E. (1991). Academic underachievement and the disruptive behavior disorders. *Journal of Consulting and Clinical Psychology, 59*, 289–294.

Frick, P. J. & Lahey, B. B. (1991). The nature and characteristics of attention-deficit hyperactivity disorder. School Psychology Review, 20, 163–173.

Frick, P. J., Lahey, B., Christ, M. A. G., Loeber, R., & Green, S. (1991). History of childhood behavior problems in biological parents of boys with attention-deficit hyperactivity disorder and conduct disorder. *Journal of Clinical Child Psychology, 20*, 445–451.

Frick, P. J., Lahey, B. B., Loeber, R., Stouthamer-Loeber, M., Christ, M. A. G., & Hanson, K. (1992). Familial risk factors to oppositional defiant disorder and conduct disorder: Parental psychopathology and maternal parenting. *Journal of Consulting and Clinical Psychology, 60*, 49–55.

Frick, P. J., Lilienfeld, S. O., Ellis, M. L, Loney, B. R., & Silverthorn, P. (1999). The association between anxiety and psychopathy dimensions in children. *Journal of Abnormal Child Psychology*, 27, 381–390.

Frick, P. J., & Loney, B. R. (1999). Outcomes of children and adolescents with conduct disorder and oppositional defiant disorder. In H. C. Quay & A. Hogan (Eds.), *Handbook of disruptive behavior disorders* (pp. 507–524). New York: Plenum.

Frick, P. J., & McCoy, M. G. (2001). Conduct disorder. In H. Orvaschel, J. Faust, & M. Hersen (Eds.), *Handbook of conceptualization and treatment of child psychopathology* (pp. 57–76). Oxford, England: Elsevier Science.

Frick, P. J., & Silverthorn, P. (2001). Psychopathology in children. In P. B. Sutker & H. E. Adams (Eds.), *Comprehensive handbook of psychopathology* (3rd ed., pp. 881–920). New York: Kluwer.

Gaub, M., & Carlson, C. L. (1997). Gender differences in ADHD: A meta-analysis and critical review. *Journal of the American Academy of Child and Adolescent Psychiatry*, 36, 1036–1045.

Gershon, J. (2002). A meta-analytic review of gender differences in ADHD. *Journal of Attentional Disorders*, 5, 143–154.

Giedd, J. N., Castellanos, F. X., Casey, B. J., Kozuch, P., King, A. C., Hamburger, S. D., & Rapoport, J. L. (1994). Quantitative morphology of the corpus callosum in attention deficit hyperactivity disorder. *American Journal of Psychiatry*, 151, 665–669.

Gomez-Beneyto, M., Bonet, A., Catala, N. A., & Puche, E. (1994). Prevalence of mental disorders among children in Calencia, Spain. *Acta Psychiatra Scandinavia*, 89, 352–357.

Gray-Ray, P., & Ray, M. C. (1990). Juvenile delinquency in the black community. *Youth & Society*, 22, 67–84.

Greene, R. W., & Ablon, J. S. (2001). What does the MTA study tell us about effective psychosocial treatment for ADHD? *Journal of Clinical Child Psychology*, 30, 114–121.

Greenhill, L. L., Halperin, J. M., & Abikoff, H. (1999). Stimulant medications. *Journal of the American Academy of Child and Adolescent Psychiatry*, 38, 503–512.

Hart, E. L., Lahey, B. B., Loeber, R., Applegate, B., Green, S. M., & Frick, P. J. (1995). Developmental change in attention-deficit hyperactivity disorder in boys: A four-year longitudinal study. *Journal of Abnormal Child Psychology*, 23, 729–749.

Hart, S. D., & Hare, R. D. (1997). Psychopathy: Assessment and association with criminal conduct. In D. M. Stoff, J. Brieling, & J. Maser (Eds.), *Handbook of antisocial behavior* (pp. 22–35). New York: Wiley.

Heath, L., Bresdin, L. B., & Rinaldi, R. C. (1989). Effects of media violence on children: A review of the literature. *Archives of General Psychiatry*, 46, 376–379.

Henggeler, S. W., & Borduin, C. M. (1990). *Family therapy and beyond: A multisystemic approach to treating the behavior problems of children and adolescents*. Pacific Grove, CA: Brooks/Cole.

Henggeler, S. W., Melton, G. B., & Smith, L. A. (1992). Family preservation using multisystemic therapy: An effective alternative to incarcerating juvenile offenders. *Journal of Consulting and Clinical Psychology*, 60, 953–961.

Henggeler, S. W., & Schoenwald, S. K. (1994). Boot camps for juvenile offenders: Just say no. *Journal of Child and Family Studies*, 3, 243–248.

Henggeler, S. W., Schoenwald, S. K., Bordvin, C. M., Rowland, M. D., & Cunningham, P. B. (1998). *Multisystemic treatment of antisocial behavior in children and adolescents*. New York: Guilford Press.

Henggeler, S. W., Schoenwald, S. K, & Pickrel, S. G. (1995). Multisystemic therapy: Bridging the gap between university- and community-based treatment. *Journal of Consulting and Clinical Psychology*, 63, 709–718.

Hinshaw, S. P. (1987). On the distinction between attentional deficits/hyperactivity and conduct problems/aggression in child psychopathology. *Psychological Bulletin*, 101, 443–463.

Hinshaw, S. P. (1991). Stimulant medication and the treatment of aggression in children with attention deficits. *Journal of Clinical Child Psychology*, 20, 301–312.

Hinshaw, S. P. (1994). *Attention deficits and hyperactivity in children*. Thousand Oaks, CA: Sage.

Hinshaw, S. P., Heller, T., & McHale, J. P. (1992). Covert antisocial behavior in boys with attention-deficit hyperactivity disorder: External validation and effects of methylphenidate. *Journal of Consulting and Clinical Psychology*, 60, 274–281.

Hynd, G. W., Semrud-Clikeman, M., Lorys, A. R., Novey, E. S., Eliopulos, D., & Lyytinen, H. (1991). Corpus callosum morphology in attention deficit hyperactivity disorder: Morphometric analysis of MRI. *Journal of Learning Disabilities*, 24, 141–146.

James, A., & Taylor, E. (1990). Sex differences in the hyperkinetic syndrome of childhood. *Journal of Child Psychology and Psychiatry*, 31, 437–446.

Jensen, P. S., Martin, D., & Cantwell, D. P. (1997). Comorbidity in ADHD: Implications for research, practice, and DSM-IV. *Journal of the American Academy of Child and Adolescent Psychiatry*, 36, 1065–1079.

Johnston, C., & Mash, E. J. (2001). Families of children with attention-deficit/hyperactivity disorder: Review and recommendations for future research. *Clinical Child and Family Psychology Review*, 4, 183–207.

Kazdin, A. E. (1995). *Conduct disorders in childhood and adolescence (2nd ed.)*. Thousand Oaks, CA: Sage Publications.

Keenan, K., & Shaw, D. (1997). Development and social influences on young girls' early problem behavior. *Psychological Bulletin, 121*, 95–113.

Kitchens, S. A., Rosen, L. A., & Braaten, E. B. (1999). Differences in anger, aggression, depression, and anxiety between ADHD and non-ADHD children. *Journal of Attention Disorders, 3*, 77–83.

Klein, R. G., & Abikoff, H. (1997). Behavior therapy and methylphenidate in the treatment of children with ADHD. *Journal of Attention Disorders, 2*, 89–114.

Kochanska, G. (1993). Toward a synthesis of parental socialization and child temperament in early development of conscience. *Child Development, 64*, 325–347.

Kratzer, L, & Hodgins, S. (1997). Adult outcomes of child conduct problems: A cohort study. *Journal of Abnormal Child Psychology, 25*, 65–81.

Kruh, I. P., Frick, P. J., & Clements, C. B. (in press). Historical and personality correlates to the violence patterns of juveniles tried as adults. *Criminal Justice and Behavior.*

Lahey, B. B., Applegate, B., Barkley, R. A., Garfinkel, B., McBurnett, K., Kerdyck, L., Greenhill, L., Hynd, G. W., Frick, P. J., Newcorn, J., Biederman, J., Ollendick, T., Hart, E. L., Perez, D., Waldman, I., & Shaffer, D. (1994). DSM-IV field trials for oppositional defiant disorder and conduct disorder in children and adolescents. *American Journal of Psychiatry, 151*, 1163–1171.

Lahey, B. B., Carlson, C. L., & Frick, P. J. (1997). Attention deficit disorder without hyperactivity. In T. A.Widiger, A. J. Frances, H. A. Pincus, R. Ross, M. B. First, & W. Davis (Eds.), *DSM-IV sourcebook*, (Vol. 3, pp. 163–188). Washington, DC: American Psychiatric Association.

Lahey, B. B., & Loeber, R. (1994). Framework for a developmental model of oppositional defiant disorder and conduct disorder. In D. K. Routh (Ed.), *Disruptive behavior disorders in childhood* (pp. 139–180). New York: Plenum.

Lahey, B. B., Loeber, R., Hart, E. L., Frick, P. J., Applegate, B., Qhang, Q, Green, S. M., & Russo, M. F. (1995). Four year longitudinal study of conduct disorder in boys: Patterns and predictors of persistence. *Journal of Abnormal Psychology, 104*, 83–93.

Lambert, N. M. (1988). Adolescent outcomes for hyperactive children. *American Psychologist, 43*, 786–799.

Landgren, M., Pettersson, R., Kjellman, B., & Gillberg, C. (1996). ADHD, DAMP, and other neurodevelopmental/psychiatric disorders in 6-year-old children: Epidemiology and co-morbidity. *Developmental Medical Child Neurology, 38*, 891–906.

Levy, F., Hay, D., McStephen, M., Wood, C., & Waldman, I. (1997). Attention deficit hyperactivity disorder: A category or a continuum? Genetic analysis of a large-scale twin study. *Journal of the American Academy of Child and Adolescent Psychiatry, 36*, 737–744.

Lilienfeld, S. O., & Waldman, I. D. (1990). The relation between childhood attention-deficit hyperactivity disorder and adult antisocial behavior reexamined: The problem of heterogeneity. *Clinical Psychology Review, 10*, 699–725.

Lochman, J. E. (1992). Cognitive-behavior intervention with aggressive boys: Three-year follow-up and preventive effects. *Journal of Consulting and Clinical Psychology, 60*, 426–432.

Loeber, R. (1982). The stability of antisocial and delinquent child behavior: A review. *Child Development, 53*, 1431–1446.

Loeber, R. (1991). Antisocial behavior: More enduring than changeable? *Journal of the American Academy of Child and Adolescent Psychiatry, 30*, 393–397.

Loeber, R., Green, S. M., Lahey, B. B., Christ, M. A. G., & Frick, P. J. (1992). Developmental sequences in the age of onset of disruptive child behaviors. *Journal of Child and Family Studies, 1*, 21–41.

Loney, B. R., Frick, P. J., Clements, C. B., Ellis, M. L., & Kerlin, K. (2003). Callous unemotional traits, impulsivity, and emotional processing in adolescents with antisocial behavior problems. *Journal of Clinical Child and Adolescent Psychology, 32*(1), 66–80.

Loney, B. R., Frick, P. J., Ellis, M., & McCoy, M. G. (1998). Intelligence, psychopathy, and antisocial behavior. *Journal of Psychopathology and Behavioral Assessment, 20*, 231–247.

Lou, H. C., Henriksen, L., & Bruhn, P. (1984). Focal cerebral hypoperfusion in children with dysphasia and/or attention deficit disorder. *Archives of Neurology, 41*, 825–829.

Lou, H. C., Henrikson, L., Bruhn, P., Borner, H., & Nielson, J. B. (1989). Striatal dysfunction in attention deficit and hyperkinetic disorder. *Archives of Neurology, 46*, 48–52.

Lyman, R. D., & Campbell, N. R. (1996). *Treating children and adolescents in residential and inpatient settings.* Thousand Oaks, CA: Sage.

Lynam, D. R. (1996). Early identification of chronic offenders: Who is the fledgling psychopath? *Psychological Bulletin, 120*, 209–234.

Lynam, D. R. (1997). Pursuing the psychopath: Capturing the fledgling psychopath in a nomological net. *Journal of Abnormal Psychology, 106*, 425–438.

Lytton, H. (1990). Child and parent effects in boys' conduct disorder: A reinterpretation. *Developmental Psychology, 26*, 683–697.

Mannuzza, S., Klein, R., Bessler, A., Malloy, P., & LaPadula, M. (1998). Adult psychiatric status of hyperactive boys grown up. *American Journal of Psychiatry*, *155*, 493–498.

March , J. S., Swanson, J. M., Arnold, E., Hoza, B., Conners, K., Hinshaw, S. P., Hechtman, L., Kraemer, H. C., Greenhill, L. L., Abikoff, H. B., Elliott, L. G., Jensen, P. S., Newcorn, J. H., Vitiello, B., Severe, J., Wells, K. C., & Pelham, W. E. (2000). Anxiety as a predictor and outcome variable in the multimodal treatment study of children with ADHD (MTA). *Journal of Abnormal Child Psychology*, *28*, 527–541.

McBurnett, K., Pfiffner, L. T., & Frick, P. J. (2001). Symptom properties as a function of ADHD type: An argument for continued study of sluggish cognitive tempo. *Journal of Abnormal Child Psychology, 29*(3), 207–213.

McCoy, M. G., Frick, P. J., Loney, B. R., & Ellis, M. L. (1999). The potential mediating role of parenting practices in the development of conduct problems in a clinic-referred sample. *Journal of Child and Family Studies*, *8*, 477–494.

McLoyd, V. C. (1990). The impact of economic hardship on black families and children: Psychological distress, parenting, and socioemotional development. *Child Development*, *61*, 311–346.

Milich, R., Balentine, A. C., & Lynam, D. R. (2001). ADHD combined type and ADHD predominantly inattentive type are distinct and unrelated disorders. *Clinical Psychology: Research and Practice*, *8*, 463–488.

Moffitt, T. E. (1990). Juvenile delinquency and attention deficit disorder: Boys' developmental trajectories from age 3 to age 15. *Child Development*, *61*, 893–910.

Moffitt, T. E. (1993). Adolescence-limited and life-course persistent antisocial behavior: A developmental taxonomy. *Psychological Review*, *100*, 674–701.

Moffitt, T. E., & Caspi, A. (2001). Childhood predictors differentiate life-course persistent and adolescent-limited antisocial pathways among males and females. *Development and Psychopathology*, *13*, 355–376.

Moffitt, T. E., Caspi, A., Dickson, N., Silva, P., & Stanton, W. (1996). Childhood-onset versus adolescent-onset antisocial conduct problems in males: Natural history from ages 3 to 18 years. *Development and Psychopathology*, *8*, 399–424.

Moffitt, T. E., Caspi, A., Harrington, H., & Milne, B. J. (2002). Males on the life-course persistent and adolescent-limited antisocial pathways: Follow-up at age 26 years. *Development and Psychopathology*, *14*, 179–207.

MTA Cooperative Group. (1999). A 14-month randomized clinical trial of treatment strategies for attention deficit hyperactivity disorder. *Archives of General Psychology*, *56*, 1073–1086.

Nadeau, K. G. (1995). *Attention deficit disorder in adults: Research, diagnosis, and treatment*. New York: Brunner/ Mazel.

Nigg, J. T. (2000). On inhibition/disinhibition in developmental psychopathology: Views from cognitive and personality psychology and a working inhibition taxonomy. *Psychological Bulletin*, *126*, 220–246.

O'Brien, B. S., & Frick, P. J. (1996). Reward dominance: Associations with anxiety, conduct problems and psychopathy in children. *Journal of Abnormal Child Psychology*, *24*, 223–240.

O'Donnell, C. R. (1995). Firearms deaths among children and youth. *American Psychologist*, *50*, 771–776.

Office of Juvenile Justice and Delinquency Prevention (1995). *Juvenile offenders and victims: A focus on violence*. Pittsburgh, PA: National Center for Juvenile Justice.

Osofsky, J. D., Wewers, S., Hann, D. M., & Fick, A. C. (1993). Chronic community violence: What is happening to our children? *Psychiatry*, *56*, 36–45.

Peeples, F., & Loeber, R. (1994). Do individual factors and neighborhood context explain ethnic differences in juvenile delinquency? *Journal of Quantitative Criminology*, *10*, 141–157.

Pelham, W. E. (1993). Pharmacotherapy for children with attention-deficit hyperactivity disorder. *School Psychology Review*, *22*, 199–227.

Pelham, W. E. (1999). The NIMH multimodal treatment study for attention-deficit hyperactivity disorder: Just say yes to drugs alone? *Canadian Journal of Psychiatry*, *44*, 765–775.

Pelham, W. E., Carlson, C., Sams, S. E., Vallan, G., Dixon, M. J., & Hoza, B. (1993). Separate and combined effects of methylphenidate and behavior modification on boys with attention deficit-hyperactivity disorder in the classroom. *Journal of Consulting and Clinical Psychology*, *61*, 506–515.

Pelham, W. E., Gnagy, E. M., Greiner, A. R., Hoza, B., Hinshaw, S. P., Swanson, J. M., Simpson, S., Shapiro, C., Bukstein, O., & Baron-Myak, C. (2000). Behavioral versus behavioral and pharmacological treatment in ADHD children attending a summer treatment program. *Journal of Abnormal Child Psychology*, *28*, 507–526.

Pelham, W. E., Wheeler, T., & Chronis, A. (1998). Empirically supported psychosocial treatments for attention deficit hyperactivity disorder. *Journal of Clinical Child Psychology*, *27*, 190–205.

Quay, H. C. (1986). Classification. In H. C. Quay & J. S. Weery (Eds.), *Psychopathological disorders of childhood* (pp. 1–34). New York: Wiley.

Rasmussen, P., & Gillberg, C. (2001). Natural outcome of ADHD with developmental coordination disorder at 22 years: A controlled, longitudinal, community-based study. *Journal of the American Academic of Child and Adolescent Psychiatry*, *39*, 1424–1431.

Rey, J. M., Bashir, M. R., Schwarz, M., Richards, I. N., Plapp, J. M., & Stewart, G. W. (1988). Oppositional disorder: Fact or fiction? *Journal of the American Academy of Child and Adolescent Psychiatry*, *27*, 157–162.

Richters, J. E., Arnold, L. E., Jensen, P. S., Abikoff, H., Conners, C. K., Greenhill, L. L, Hechtman, L., Hinshaw, S. P., Pelham, W., & Swanson, J. M. (1995). The National Institute of Mental Health collaborative multisite multimodal treatment study of children with attention deficit hyperactivity disorder (MTA): I. Background and rationale. *Journal of the American Academy of Child and Adolescent Psychiatry, 34,* 987–1000.

Robins, L. N. (1966). *Deviant children grown up.* Baltimore: Williams and Wilkins.

Ross, A. O. (1981). *Child behavior therapy: Principles, procedures, and empirical basis.* New York: Wiley.

Rucklidge, J. J., & Tannock, R. (2001). Psychiatric, psychosocial, and cognitive functioning of female adolescents with ADHD. *Journal of the American Academy of Child and Adolescent Psychiatry, 40,* 530–540.

Rutter, M. (1977). Brain damage syndromes in childhood: Concepts and findings. *Journal of Child Psychology and Psychiatry, 18,* 1–21.

Silverthorn, P. & Frick, P. J. (1999). Developmental pathways to antisocial behavior: The delayed-onset pathway in girls. *Development and Psychopathology, 11,* 101–126.

Silverthorn, P., Frick, P. J., Kuper, K., & Ott, J. (1996). Attention-deficit hyperactivity disorder and sex: A test of two etiological models to explain the male predominance. *Journal of Clinical Child Psychology, 25,* 52–59.

Stein, J., Schettler, T., Wallinga, D., & Valenti, M. (2002). In harm's way: Toxic threats to child development. *Journal of Developmental and Behavioral Pediatrics, 23,* 13–22.

Stevenson, J. (1992). Evidence for genetic etiology in hyperactivity in children. *Behavior Genetics, 22,* 337–343.

Stewart, M. A., Pitts, F. N., Craig, A. G., & Dieruf, W. (1966). The hyperactive child syndrome. *American Journal of Orthopsychiatry, 36,* 403–407.

Strauss, A. A., & Lehtinen, L. E. (1947). *Psychopathology and education of the brain-injured child.* New York: Grune & Stratton.

Swanson, J. M., McBurnett, K., Christian, D. L., & Wigal, T. (1995). Stimulant medication and treatment of children with ADHD. In T. H. Ollendick & R. J. Prinz (Eds.), *Advances in clinical child psychology* (Vol. 17, pp. 265–322). New York: Plenum.

Toupin, J., Mercier, H., Dery, M., Cote, G., & Hodgins, S. (1995). Validity of the PCL-R for adolescents. *Issues in Criminological and Legal Psychology, 24,* 143–145.

Verhulst, F. C., van der Ende, J., Ferdinand, R. F., Kasius, M. C. (1997). The prevalence of DSM-III-R diagnoses in a national sample of Dutch adolescents. *Archives of General Psychiatry, 54,* 329–336.

Wang, Y. C., Chong, M. Y., & Chou, W. J., (1993). Prevalence of ADHD in primary school children in Taiwan. *Journal of the Formosan Medical Association, 92,* 133–138.

Weiss, G., & Hechtman, L. T. (1993). *Hyperactive children grown up: ADHD in children, adolescents, and adults.* New York: Guilford.

Wells, K. C., Pelham, W. E., Kotkin, R. A., Hoza, B., Abikoff, H. B., Abramowitz, A., Arnold, L. E., Cantwell, D. P., Conners, C. K., Del Carmen, R., Elliott, G., Greenhill, L. L., Hechtman, L., Hibbs, Euthymia, Hinshaw, S. P., Jensen, P. S., March, J. S., Swanson, J. M., Schiller, E. (2000). Psychosocial treatment strategies in the MTA study: Rationale, methods, and critical issues in design and implementation. *Journal of Abnormal Child Psychology, 28,* 483–505.

Whalen, C. K., Henker, B., Buhrmester, D., Hinshaw, S. P., Huber, A., & Laski, K. (1989). Does stimulant medication improve the peer status of hyperactive children? *Journal of Consulting and Clinical Psychology, 57*(4), 545–549.

Wootton, J. M., Frick, P. J., Shelton, K. K., & Silverthorn, P. (1997). Ineffective parenting and childhood conduct problems: The moderating role of callous-unemotional traits. *Journal of Consulting and Clinical Psychology, 65,* 301–308.

Zametkin, A. J., Liebenauer, L. L., Fitzgerald, G. A., King, A. C., Minkunas, D. V., Herscovitch, P., Yamada, E. M., & Cohen, R. M. (1993). Brain metabolism in teenagers with attention deficit hyperactivity disorder. *Archives of General Psychiatry, 50,* 333–340.

Zametkin, A. J, & Liotta, W. (1998). The neurobiology of attention deficit hyperactivity disorder. *Journal of Clinical Psychiatry, 59,* 17–23.

Zametkin, A. J., Nordahl, T. E., Gross, M., King, A. C., Semple, W. E., Rumsey, J., Hamburger, S., & Cohen, R. M. (1990). Cerebral glucose metabolism in adults with hyperactivity of childhood onset. *New England Journal of Medicine, 323,* 1361–1366.

Zoccolillo, M. (1993). Gender and the development of conduct disorder. *Development and Psychopathology, 5,* 65–78.

16

Internalizing Disorders of Childhood and Adolescence

Thomas H. Ollendick
Alison L. Shortt
Janay B. Sander
Virginia Polytechnic Institute and State University

Internalizing disorders in childhood and adolescence include the anxiety and affective disorders. As such, they consist of problems related to worry, fear, shyness, low self-esteem, sadness, and depression. These emotional problems have frequently been found to be interrelated in clinical settings and to be associated statistically with one another in factor analytic studies. Internalizing problems can be contrasted with externalizing problems—problems frequently associated with inattention, bad conduct, and opposition and defiance (see chapter 15). It is of historic interest to note that these two broad dimensions of childhood and adolescent problems have been recognized for some time. Karen Horney (1945), for example, spoke of children who "move against the world" (i.e., externalizing disorder children) and those who "move away from the world" (i.e., internalizing disorder children).

Although there is little question about the existence of internalizing problems in childhood and adolescence and their detrimental effects on the growing child and adolescent (Ollendick & King, 1994), there is considerable controversy about whether they constitute a single broadband internalizing disorder or whether they constitute multiple narrowband disorders. At the heart of this issue is the frequent observation that anxiety disorders and affective disorders frequently co-occur with one another (i.e., are comorbid disorders) and that they are rarely observed in their "pure" forms, at least in childhood and adolescence (Seligman & Ollendick, 1998). For example, in an early study, Last, Strauss, and Francis (1987) found that 73% of separation-anxious children and adolescents and 79% of overanxious disorder children and adolescents presented at their outpatient clinic for anxious children with one or more additional psychiatric disorders, including major depressive disorders. Similarly, Kovacs, Feinberg, Crouse-Novak, Paulauskas, and Finkelstein (1984) demonstrated early on that a majority of children and adolescents who presented at their outpatient clinic for depressed children were diagnosed with concurrent disorders. In fact, 79% of youths with a major depressive disorder and 93% of the cases who presented with dysthymic disorder had a concurrent psychiatric disorder, of which one of the most common was an anxiety disorder. Of importance for the developmental sequence of these disorders, Kovacs et al. (1984) reported that anxiety disorders tended to precede the depressive disorders when these two conditions were present in the same child or adolescent. Last, Perrin, Hersen, and Kazdin (1992) have reaffirmed these rates of comorbidity and developmental sequellae, as have Seligman and Ollendick (1998), in more recent years.

Although the major anxiety and affective disorders in childhood and adolescence overlap, we will present them as separate entities in this chapter, consistent with nosological approaches, such as DSM–IV (*Diagnostic and Statistical Manual*, 4th edition, American Psychiatric Association [APA], 1994) and ICD–10 (International Classification of Diseases, 10th edition, World Health Organization, 1992). In doing so, we will point out areas of overlap and draw distinctions between them. We recognize this decision is not without controversy, but it is consistent with much of clinical practice and research, and it allows us to present information about the disorders in a coherent and organized manner. Before examining specific aspects of these disorders, however, we first examine basic tenets of developmental psychopathology inasmuch as this approach informs our perspective on clinical disorders in children and adolescents.

BASIC PREMISES OF DEVELOPMENTAL PSYCHOPATHOLOGY

Developmental Theory

Within the field of developmental psychology, theorists have long debated which developmental model best explains the many changes that occur in individuals throughout their development and across their life span. Early debates focused on issues of autonomy and organization and were tied to two major worldviews: the mechanistic and organismic models of development. According to the mechanistic view (Baer, 1982; Skinner, 1938), organisms were viewed as similar to machines that were acted on largely by forces from the outside world. That is, with regard to development, organisms were viewed primarily as passive recipients of information and relatively passive respondents to increasingly complex and varied stimulus input (i.e., a tabula rasa). Furthermore, it was believed that changes in behavior over time reflected gradual modifications in antecedent and consequent stimuli with explanations for development derived largely from principles of learning theory (e.g., conditioning, reinforcement). Skinner (1938), for example, suggested "the basic premise of behavioral psychology (was) that all organisms, human and subhuman, young and old, were subject to the same law of effect (principle of reinforcement) and could be studied in the same basic manner" (p. 27). From this perspective, many clinicians and researchers viewed development and developmental processes as possessing relatively little clinical significance (see Gelfand & Peterson, 1985, and Ollendick & Cerny, 1981, for extended discussions of this point).

In contrast to the passive qualities of the organism portrayed in the mechanistic view, proponents of the organismic model of development (Erickson, 1968; Freud, 1949; Piaget, 1950) asserted that organisms were not passive; rather, they were viewed as agents who were actively involved in the construction of their own environments. Furthermore, organismic theorists often described development as if it passed through discrete and oftentimes invariant stages (e.g., Piaget's stages of cognitive development, Freud's psychosexual stages, and Erickson's stages of identity development). These various theories maintained that basic structures and functions changed across age and that they reflected emerging, qualitatively different ways of interacting with the environment. In its simplest form, this model proposed that change resulted largely from maturational processes that were determined by intrinsic organismic factors rather than by extrinsic environmental ones.

Decades of debate among proponents of these two models, as well as recognition of their limitations, led to the advent of a third model of development, namely, the transactional model. Also known as developmental contextualism, the transactional model moved beyond the mechanismic and organismic points of view (Lerner, Hess, & Nitz, 1991; Sameroff, 1995) and was highly consistent with the tenets of social learning/social cognitive theory (cf. Bandura, 1977b, 1989, 2001; Ollendick & Cerny, 1981). According to this model, developmental changes were proposed to occur as a result of continuous reciprocal interactions (i.e., reciprocal determinism, transactions) between an active organism and its active environmental context. Organisms were said to affect their own development by being both producers and products of their environments (Lerner et al., 1991). Although differences in theory and philosophy remain, most developmental theorists agree that development involves systematic, successive, and adaptive changes within and across life periods in the structure, function, and content of the individual's cognitive, emotional, behavioral, social, and interpersonal characteristics (Lease & Ollendick, 2000; Sameroff, 1995; Silverman & Ollendick, 1999). Inasmuch as developmental changes occur in an orderly and sequential fashion (i.e., they are systematic and successive), changes observed at one point in time will influence subsequent events (although not necessarily in a direct linear fashion, see later). Changes that occur at one point in time (whether due to learning, an unfolding of basic predetermined structures, or some complex, interactive/transactional process) have an impact on subsequent development. Thus, the diversity or variety of changes possible at a later point in time are constrained by, but not solely determined by, those that occur at an earlier point in time.

Developmental Psychopathology

Developmental psychopathology is, of course, firmly grounded in developmental theory (Rutter & Garmezy, 1983). Sroufe and Rutter (1984, p. 18) define developmental psychopathology as "the study of the origins and course of individual patterns of behavioral maladaptation, whatever the age of onset, whatever the causes, whatever the transformations in behavioral manifestations, and however complex the course of developmental pattern may be." Implicit in this definition is concern with development and developmental deviations (i.e., clinical psychopathologies) that occur throughout and across the life span and the processes associated with those perturbations. The study of psychopathology, from this perspective, is organized around milestones, transitions, and sequences in physical, cognitive, and social-emotional development. Thus, development is viewed as a series of qualitative reorganizations within and among various systems. The character of these reorganizations is determined by factors at various levels of analysis (e.g., genetic, constitutional, physiological, behavioral, psychological, environmental, and sociological) that are in dynamic transaction with one another (Cicchetti, 1989; Lewis, 1990). Pathological development is understood, then, as a lack of integration among these systems that contributes synergistically to (mal)adaptation at particular developmental levels (i.e., childhood, adolescence).

Although development at any one point in time is assumed to affect later functioning, direct or isomorphic continuity of behavior is not implied nor expected. Rather, multiple pathways through which developmental outcomes may occur are proposed: Both normal and abnormal development results from individually distinct and unique transactions between a changing organism and its ever-changing environmental context. This notion is captured in the developmental principle of equifinality—the principle that any one outcome (i.e., a depressive disorder) may result from multiple and diverse pathways. From a developmental perspective, the expectation that a singular pathway to a given disorder exists would be the exception, not the rule (Kazdin & Kagan, 1994; Lease & Ollendick, 2000; Toth & Cicchetti, 1999). In contradistinction to the principle of equifinality, the principle of multifinality asserts that varied outcomes can eventuate from the same common starting point. Thus, for example, any one risk factor associated with the development of a disorder (e.g., "behavioral inhibition to the unfamiliar," Kagan, 1994) is likely to result in a variety of outcomes, not just anxiety disorders. It is therefore important to identify and understand intra- and extra-individual characteristics that promote or inhibit early deviations or maintain or disrupt early adaptation and development. Toward this end, the field of developmental psychopathology is primarily concerned with the origins and course of a given disorder, its precursors and sequellae, its variations in manifestation with development, and more broadly, its relations to nondisordered behavior patterns (Rutter, 1985; Toth & Cicchetti, 1999).

As may be evident, the developmental psychopathology perspective does not subscribe to a particular theoretical orientation (i.e., medical model, psychodynamic theory, social learning theory) for the understanding of diverse child psychopathologies, nor does it supplant particular theories; rather, it sharpens our awareness about connections among phenomena that may otherwise seem unrelated or disconnected. Achenbach (1990) refers to it as a macroparadigm that serves to bridge a variety of conceptual models (i.e., microparadigms). The utility of this approach has been demonstrated recently in the conceptualization of depression and anxiety in children and adolescents (Cicchetti & Schneider-Rosen, 1986; Lease & Ollendick, 2000; Ollendick, Grills, & King, 2001; Ollendick & Hirshfeld-Becker, 2002; Vasey & Ollendick, 2000).

ANXIETY DISORDERS IN CHILDREN AND ADOLESCENTS

Phenomenology

For children and adults alike, anxiety is a normal and common emotional response to a perceived threat to one's physical or emotional being. Feeling fearful and fleeing from a genuinely dangerous situation is adaptive. However, if the anxiety response is elicited by a situation or object that is not truly dangerous, then the anxiety and the avoidance associated with it are no longer adaptive. A diagnosis of an anxiety disorder may be warranted if the anxiety response is excessive in frequency, intensity and/or duration, and if it results in significant impairment in functioning. Excessive anxiety is distressing to children and adolescents, and the associated avoidance interferes with their ability to engage in developmentally appropriate tasks and activities. Alarmingly, anxiety disorders are one of the most common psychological difficulties experienced by children and adolescents, and these disorders tend to persist into late adolescence and adulthood unless effective treatment is received (Ollendick & March, 2004).

Consistent with Lang's (1979) tripartite model, anxiety is viewed as a multidimensional construct involving *physiological* features such as increased heart rate and respiration, *cognitive* ideation including catastrophic and unhelpful thoughts (e.g. "I can't do it," "What if something terrible happens?"), and *behavioral* responses such as avoidance of the anxiety provoking object or situation. Furthermore, there are developmental differences in the expression of anxiety. For example, young children may avoid objects or situations that scare them; however, they may have difficulty identifying the exact cognitions associated with the feared situation. Young children may also have trouble relating or connecting their physiological symptoms to their anxiety. For example, a child with separation anxiety might insist that the reason she is sick with a headache and a stomachache when she has to go to school is that she has come down with a physical illness such as the flu, not because she is fearful about separation from her caretaker.

Developmental Considerations. For most, if not all, children and adolescents, fears and worries are a normal part of development. Accordingly, clinicians assessing anxiety in children need to be aware of what constitutes "normal" fears at each level of development. For example, young infants and toddlers tend to fear aspects of their immediate environment such as loud noises, unfamiliar people, separation from their caregivers, or heights. Fears of animals, being alone, and of the dark begin to emerge during the preschool years. As cognitive abilities continue to develop during the early school years, children's fears begin to include abstract, imaginary, or anticipatory fears such as fear of failure or evaluation, death, bodily injury, and supernatural phenomena. Finally, concerns about death, danger, social comparison, personal conduct, and physical appearance extend from adolescence to adulthood (Gullone, 2000; Ollendick, King, & Muris, 2002).

Developmentally normal fears are, by definition, age appropriate and transitory in nature. In contrast, a diagnosis of an anxiety disorder is warranted only when a child experiences anxiety that is not typical of a child his or her age, and when a child experiences anxiety that is severe and causes considerable distress and/or that impairs a child's functioning at home, at school, or in peer and family relationships.

Gender Differences.   Research examining the prevalence of anxiety disorders in boys and girls has produced mixed results. Studies using community samples have found that girls are more likely to report anxiety than boys (Essau, Conradt, & Petermann, 2000; McGee et al., 1990). In contrast, gender differences are usually not found in clinic samples (Strauss et al., 1988). There are at least two plausible explanations for this discrepancy. First, societal expectations of gender-appropriate behavior for boys and girls may mean that girls are more open in reporting anxiety symptoms than boys. Alternatively, anxiety symptoms may be more common in girls, and the equal ratio of males to females in clinic samples may indicate that boys experiencing anxiety are more likely to be referred for treatment than girls with similar symptoms.

The direction and size of the gender difference is also dependent on the diagnostic category being considered. Generalized anxiety disorder (GAD) appears to be similarly prevalent in boys and girls during childhood, although in adolescence it is more common among females than males (Cohen et al., 1993; Werry, 1991). Research concerning gender differences for separation anxiety disorder (SAD) has been mixed. Although some studies find no gender differences for SAD (Cohen et al., 1993; Last et al., 1992), most studies find that girls outnumber boys (e.g., Anderson Williams, McGee, & Silva, 1987; Kashani, Orvaschel, Rosenberg, & Reid, 1989). The research on social phobia is less clear, although few gender differences have been noted (Beidel & Morris, 1995; Ollendick & Ingman, 2001).

Epidemiology

Estimated prevalence rates for the childhood anxiety disorders using DSM criteria have been found to vary dramatically, but typically range between 7% and 12% (Anderson et al., 1987; Kashani et al., 1987; Kashani, Orvaschel, Rosenberg, & Reid, 1989). For example, Anderson et al. (1987) showed that 7.4% of 792 children in the Dundedin, New Zealand, longitudinal study met criteria for an anxiety disorder when they were 11 years of age. At 15 years of age, McGee et al. (1990) reported that 10.7% of the adolescents in this same sample met criteria for an anxiety disorder. A 3.3% increase in the anxiety disorders was evident over the 4-year period. Similar prevalence rates for the anxiety disorders have been found by a host of other researchers, with many indicating that the prevalence of some anxiety disorders increase with age (e.g., GAD, social phobia, panic disorder), whereas others tend to decrease with age (e.g., SAD, specific phobia). Thus, overall prevalence rates vary by gender and age. They also vary by the diagnostic category being considered, as we shall see next.

DSM–IV Diagnostic Categories and Associated Prevalence

The APA describes *separation anxiety disorder* (SAD) as developmentally inappropriate and excessive anxiety associated with separation from home or from those to whom the individual is attached. Often children with SAD worry about danger or harm coming to themselves (e.g., being kidnapped) or their loved one (e.g., becoming ill) when they are separated. Children with SAD exhibit distress when they are separated from their attachment figure and will undertake steps to avoid being apart from them. This may result in children refusing to attend school or sleep away from home. The evidence indicates that as children become older, the prevalence of SAD declines. For example, in the Dunedin study, it was shown that the 12-month prevalence rate for SAD was 3.5% for the 11-year-old children but 2.0% for the 15-year-old adolescents. In adolescence, this disorder seems to become less common compared to other disorders such as GAD, social phobia, and panic disorder (Mattis & Ollendick, 2002).

Generalized anxiety disorder (GAD) is characterized as excessive anxiety and worry, which occurs more days than not for at least 6 months. These children find it difficult to control their worries about a number of events or activities. To meet criteria for GAD, children need to experience at least one associated physiological symptom, although typically these children report multiple physical symptoms. Physical symptoms include stomachaches or nausea, headaches, muscle tension, restlessness, irritability, fatigue, and sleep disturbance. The DSM–IV category of GAD in children replaced overanxious disorder (OAD; DSM–III–R; American Psychiatric Association, 1980). As noted earlier, there is some evidence to suggest that the prevalence of OAD/GAD increases with age (Kashani et al., 1989).

Specific phobia (SP) is defined as persistent fear of a specific object or situation that is excessive or unreasonable. Phobias of certain animals or insects, the dark, heights, storms, and medical procedures are among the most common in children. A recent study conducted in Germany reported a prevalence rate of 2.5% in 12 to 17-year-olds (Essau et al., 2000). Studies in the United States have reported prevalence rates ranging from 3.6% to 9% (Costello et al., 1988; Kashani et al., 1987; Kessler et al., 1994). Taken together, studies suggest a prevalence rate of about 5% for specific phobia in children and adolescents (Ollendick, Hagopian, & King, 1997).

Social phobia (SOP) in children, as in adults, is characterized by a marked or persistent fear of social situations or performance situations. Typically, in these situations, the child is exposed to unfamiliar people and/or is scrutinized by others. SOP is a disorder with a later age of onset (usually around 11 years of age), being rarely diagnosed in children younger than 10 years old (Ollendick & Hirshfeld-Becker, 2002). Of the changes in diagnostic criteria from the DSM–III–R to DSM–IV, the difference between the previous category of avoidant disorder and the new category of social phobia has been found to be the most significant (Kendall & Warman, 1996). This disparity has made comparison of prevalence rates across studies using these two systems more difficult. Using the DSM–III–R, Anderson et al. (1987) found that less than 1% of children aged 11 years and that none of the 15-year-olds in the Dunedin study were diagnosed with avoidant disorder. A later study using DSM–IV criteria reported that 6.3% of adolescents were diagnosed with social phobia. Although these results may suggest an increase in prevalence with age, it is more likely that these results reflect changes in diagnostic criteria from DSM–III–R to DSM–IV (Schniering, Hudson, & Rapee, 2000).

Obsessive-compulsive disorder (OCD) is characterized by obsessions, which are recurrent thoughts, images, and/or impulses that are intrusive and result in an increase in anxiety. These obsessions are most often, though not always, accompanied by compulsions, which are repetitive behaviors that reduce anxiety (e.g., washing hands, or checking). Epidemiological data on the prevalence of OCD in prepubertal children has been reported to be less than 1% (Heyman et al., 2001). The prevalence rates for adolescents, however, range from 1.9% to 3.6% (Cook et al., 2001). The results of the Heyman et al. (2001) study suggest that prevalence may increase with age.

Differential Diagnosis and Comorbidity

Although recent research using the DSM classification system has facilitated the communication of knowledge between researchers and clinicians, the overlap in diagnostic criteria between some of these nosological categories has generated controversy. Briefly, the major problem, as we noted earlier, is the co-occurrence of multiple disorders (i.e., comorbidity) in the same child or adolescent. Several authors (e.g., Caron & Rutter, 1991) have argued that the categorical system of diagnosis does not accurately reflect the true nature of childhood anxiety, and they suggest that a dimensional approach may be preferred in dealing with the overarching issue of comorbidity. Others, however, maintain that the current diagnostic system is sufficiently precise and that we need more refined research to clarify the boundaries among the various anxiety disorders (cf. Ollendick & March, 2004). Undoubtedly, there are positive aspects to both dimensional and categorical systems, depending on the intended use of the information obtained from these somewhat disparate approaches.

In clinical populations, the most common comorbidity with any specific anxiety disorder is another type of anxiety disorder (Kendall, Brady, & Verduin, 2001). Across epidemiological and clinical studies using varied methodologies, disorders have been found to co-occur with one another at rates higher than chance (Caron & Rutter, 1991). Evidence of significant comorbidity is troubling because children with comorbid disorders tend to have a greater severity and persistence of symptoms, more interpersonal problems, and may be more refractory to change and clinically challenging for therapists (Manassis & Monga, 2001).

In addition to comorbidity with other anxiety disorders, anxious children may also exhibit high rates of depression (Brady & Kendall, 1992), as noted previously. Using a large cohort of 1,710 adolescents, the Oregon Adolescent Depression project found that 49% of the adolescents with an anxiety disorder also had comorbid depressive disorders using DSM criteria (Lewinsohn, Hops, Roberts, Seeley, & Andrews, 1993). Similarly high rates of comorbidity were found in the Dunedin, New Zealand, sample of youths (Anderson et al., 1987; McGee et al., 1990; McGee, Feehan, Williams, & Anderson, 1992). This series of studies also found that the rates of comorbid mood disorders increased as the children became older. Rates of comorbidity of anxiety and depressive disorders were higher among adolescents than among children.

Rates of comorbidity between anxiety and externalizing problems such as attention-deficit hyperactivity disorder (ADHD) are also high (Caron & Rutter, 1991). Studies examining this relationship have found that between 13% and 24% of children with an anxiety disorder also have ADHD, oppositional defiant disorder, or conduct disorder (Keller et al., 1992; Last et al., 1987). Consistent with these findings, Kendall, Brady, and Verduin (2001) reported that 25% of their clinical sample of anxious children also met DSM criteria for one of these three disruptive behavior disorders.

Developmental Course and Prognosis

A common misconception is that children and adolescents will outgrow their worries and fears. Although this belief may be true of developmentally normal fears and everyday concerns, research suggests that anxiety disorders tend to persist unless treated. For example, Pfeffer, Lipkins, Plutchik, and Mizruchi (1988) found that for children aged 6 to 12 years who were diagnosed with OAD, 70.6% still met this diagnosis 2 years later. Similarly, in the Dunedin study, longitudinal results showed that girls diagnosed with an anxiety or depressive disorder at one age were more likely to continue to meet diagnostic criteria in subsequent years (McGee et al., 1990; McGee et al., 1992).

Anxiety disorders have been shown to persist not only over time but also to be associated with the development of more severe symptomatology (Albano, Chorpita, & Barlow, 1996). Older children tend to report more severe anxiety and comorbid symptomatology than do younger children with the same diagnosis (Strauss, Lease, Last, & Francis, 1988). Similarly, many adults with anxiety disorders report a lifelong history of anxiety symptoms beginning in childhood (Ollendick, Lease, & Cooper, 1993). For example, a longitudinal study conducted in the United States found that children with an anxiety disorder were at greater risk for future anxiety disorders, and they were at increased risk of developing dysthymic disorders as well (Lewinsohn et al., 1993; Orvaschel, Lewinsohn, & Seeley, 1995).

Etiological Theories of Childhood Anxiety

Understanding the development of anxiety and its disorders requires us to consider the potential for complex, reciprocal interactions and transactions between many etiological factors over the course of a child's development. Empirical efforts to explain the development and maintenance of anxiety have focused on the interaction between personal characteristics of the child (e.g., genetic vulnerability, behavioral inhibition, cognitive processes) and interpersonal factors such as attachment to caregivers and learning processes that occur within the family. Some of these etiological factors will now be addressed briefly.

Biological and Familial Factors. Family studies using both referred and nonreferred samples show that the parents of anxious children, and the children of anxious parents, are more likely to experience anxiety problems than nonclinic controls (McClure, Brennan, Hammen, & Le Brocque, 2001). Although family studies have demonstrated that anxiety disorders tend to run in families, the question about the mechanism of transmission remains unanswered. Twin studies help to distinguish whether this mechanism is genetic, environmental, or a combination of the two. Although specific heritability estimates vary across studies, almost all twin studies support the conclusion that there is a heritable genetic risk for anxiety disorders (see Thapar & McGuffin, 1995, for a review). However, rather than a risk toward developing a specific anxiety disorder, the research is strongest for a genetic vulnerability toward either an anxiety or a depressive disorder (Eley & Stevenson, 1999; Kendler et al., 1995).

One of the proposed mechanisms by which a predisposition for anxiety is transmitted genetically is via inherited temperamental characteristics such as behavioral inhibition. Behavioral inhibition, as described earlier, is a category suggested by Kagan and his colleagues to describe the 15% to 20% of children who react with withdrawal, avoidance, or distress when confronted with unfamiliar people, situations, or objects (Kagan, Reznick, & Snidman, 1987; Kagan, Snidman, Zentner, & Peterson, 1999). Behavioral inhibition has been shown to be a risk factor for later childhood anxiety problems (Biederman et al., 2001). However, it is important to remember that not all behaviorally inhibited children develop anxiety disorders, and it is best conceptualized as one possible predisposing factor that may lead to anxiety given the "right" set of other contextual conditions (Ollendick & Hirshfeld-Becker, 2002).

Learning Theories. The theory of classical conditioning can be used to explain the development of certain fears and phobias, as well as anxiety disorders. For example, a child might develop a dog phobia after the previously neutral stimulus (a dog) was associated with the pain of being bitten (UCS), unconditioned stimulus resulting in a conditioned fear response. However, classical conditioning theory alone cannot explain why some individuals who experience a pairing of trauma or pain with a particular object or situation do not develop a phobia. In more recent years, theorists have integrated information processing theories with classical conditioning theory, suggesting that an individual's internal representation and subsequent evaluation of the unconditioned stimulus mediates the strength of the conditioned response (Davey, 1992). For example, Reiss (1980) suggested that a person's anticipation of social or physical danger, or his or her expectation of anxiety, might make a person more susceptibility to traumatic conditioning.

Operant conditioning theory suggests that behaviors that are reinforced are more likely to occur again and behaviors that are followed by punishment are less likely to occur again (Skinner, 1938). The concept of negative reinforcement is frequently used to explain how avoidant behavior maintains anxiety symptoms over time. Specifically, when an anxious child avoids a feared situation, the child is reinforced by the resultant reduction in anxiety symptoms. The child therefore learns that to prevent experiencing the unpleasantness of anxiety, he needs to avoid the feared situation or object (Ollendick, Vasey, & King, 2001).

Operant conditioning principles can also be used to explain the process by which a child's nonanxious behavior gradually decreases in frequency while the anxious behavior increases. Barrett, Rapee, Dadds, and Ryan (1996) found that parents of clinically anxious children attended more to the anxious and avoidant behaviors of their children than to their brave coping behaviors. Although this study was unable to clarify whether this pattern of parenting behavior existed before or after the development of their child's anxiety, it does indicate that positive reinforcement from parents may serve to maintain the problem.

Childhood anxiety has also been shown to develop as a result of vicarious learning and modeling. Bandura (1977a, 1977b, 1986) suggested that behaviors might be acquired, facilitated, reduced, or eliminated by observing the behavior of others. Accordingly, fears may appear after children have observed their parents or peers reacting fearfully to certain objects or situations. Silverman, Cerny, Nelles, and Burke (1988) studied a group of anxious parents and their children and found that children's anxious behaviors were associated with heightened levels of avoidance evidenced by their parents. Interestingly, these researchers noted that anxiety disorders showing the most pronounced avoidance behaviors (social and simple phobia and agoraphobia) seem to have the highest rates of familial risk.

Cognitive and Information Processing Biases. Cognitive theorists suggest that when processing information, anxious people tend to overestimate the threat of danger and underestimate their abilities to cope with that threat (Beck, 1976, 1991). Using a variety of methodologies, attentional biases toward threat-related stimuli have been demonstrated for clinically and nonclinically anxious adults (e.g., Pury & Mineka, 2001; Wood, Mathews, & Dalgleish, 2001). Similar research has found evidence of attentional bias toward threat-related cues in both clinically anxious (Taghavi, Neshat-Doost, Moradi, Yule, & Dalgleish, 1999) and nonclinically anxious children (Kindt, Brosschot, & Everaerd, 1997).

Findings of biased attention in anxious children have been complemented by research examining the process of threat interpretation. A series of studies by Barrett and colleagues (Barrett et al., 1996; Dadds & Barrett, 1996; Dadds, Barrett, Rapee, & Ryan, 1996) demonstrated that clinically anxious children tended to interpret ambiguous vignettes of social and physical situations as threatening compared to nonclinic controls.

The Role of The Parent–Child Relationship in Child Anxiety Disorders. An increasing number of studies have examined the relations between parenting behavior and anxiety in children. Parents of clinic-referred anxious children have been found to be more controlling (Dumas, LaFreniere, & Serketich, 1995), more restrictive (Krohne & Hock, 1991), more overinvolved emotionally (Hirshfeld, Biederman, Brody, Faraone, & Rosenbaum, 1997), less accepting, and less granting of psychological autonomy (Siqueland, Kendall, & Steinberg, 1996) than are parents of nonreferred children. Because these studies are cross-sectional, however, it is impossible to draw firm conclusions about whether relations between parent behavior and anxiety represent cause or effect, or, for that matter, whether it is more reciprocal in nature. This latter possibility is more consistent with a developmental psychopathology perspective (for extended discussion of these issues, see Rapee, 1997, and Dadds and Roth (2001).

Assessment

Only a brief overview of assessment practices is provided herein (for a more complete review of assessment practices with anxious youths, see Ollendick and Ollendick, 1997, and Silverman and Treffers, 2001). As discussed earlier, anxiety is recognized as a multidimensional construct and as such, a multiinformant and multimethod approach to the assessment of childhood anxiety is recommended. Diagnostic interviews with the child and the child's parents are one of the best ways to distinguish normal, developmentally appropriate fears and anxieties from problematic anxiety disorders. The most commonly used diagnostic interview to assess youth with anxiety disorders is the Anxiety Disorders Interview Schedule for Children (ADIS–C/P) (Silverman & Albano, 1996). This interview can be used to solicit detailed information about a range of individual anxiety symptoms, interference in daily functioning, school refusal behavior, interpersonal functioning, and avoided situations. In addition to the interviews, the child and her or his parents are usually asked to complete self-report questionnaires, and responses on these questionnaires can be compared to available normative data. The Multidimensional Anxiety Scale for Children (MASC; March, Parker, Sullivan, Stallings, & Connor, 1997), the Revised Children's Manifest Anxiety Scale (Reynolds & Richmond, 1985), and the Fear Survey Schedule for Children–Revised (Ollendick, 1983) are examples of questionnaires that are frequently used in this regard. Parents and teachers can complete ratings scales such as the Child Behavior Checklist (CBCL) and Teacher Report Form (TRF; Achenbach, 1991). These scales have the advantage of measuring anxiety/depression symptoms as well as externalizing and other related problems. In addition to these measures, it is recommended that behavioral observation, cognitive assessment, and physiological assessment be considered.

Interventions

Pharmacological Interventions.   There are a limited number of controlled pharmacological treatment trials for anxiety in children and adolescents. Labellarte, Ginsburg, Walkup, and Riddle (1999) conducted an extensive review of psychopharmacological treatments for anxiety disorders in children and concluded that SSRIs (selective serotonin reuptake inhibitors) represent the first-line medical treatment for childhood anxiety disorders (as well as affective disorders). Serotonegic and tricyclic antidepressants are second-line anxiety agents, and buspirone may be used as a second or third-line anxiety treatment. Medication alone is rarely the treatment of choice for children with anxiety disorders, and typically medication is used in combination with psychological treatment (see Ollendick & March, 2004).

Psychosocial Interventions.   Cognitive-behavioral therapy (CBT) for childhood anxiety has the strongest empirical support (Ollendick & King, 1998). CBT consists of four main strategies. First, *exposure* requires the child to approach the object or situation she or he fears or worries about, either directly (in vivo) or imaginally. Exposure is typically conducted in a graduated and progressive manner. Exposure may also take the form of systematic desensitization in which the child receives relaxation training and then practices relaxation while facing his or her feared situations in vivo or imaginally. In vivo and imaginal desensitization are both effective treatments for childhood anxiety disorders.

The second strategy implemented to treat childhood anxiety is *modeling*. Modeling involves a person demonstrating approach behavior in situations that the child finds anxiety provoking. Variants of modeling include filmed modeling where the child watches a videotape, live modeling where the person modeling is in the presence of the anxious child, and participant modeling where a model interacts with the child and guides him or her to approach the feared situation. In their review of nine controlled studies that examined the efficacy of modeling as a treatment for childhood fears and phobias, Ollendick and King (1998) concluded that filmed modeling and live modeling are moderately effective procedures and that participant modeling is a highly effective treatment for childhood fears and phobias.

Progressive exposure and modeling assume that fear must be reduced before approach behavior will occur. In contrast, the third CBT strategy—*contingency management*—based on the principles of operant conditioning, encourages increases in approach behavior by altering the consequences of a child's behavior in the anxiety-provoking situations. Contingency management involves modifying the antecedents of anxiety or the consequences of anxious behavior through positive reinforcement, punishment, extinction, and shaping. For example, positive reinforcement for courageous or approach behaviors to the feared or dreaded stimulus are frequently used in such programs. These procedures are implemented by the therapist during the therapy session and are often taught to parents and teachers for use in the home, school, and other community settings. Treatments involving reinforced practice have been shown to be superior to no-treatment or wait list control conditions and other treatments (verbal coping skills, modeling) in reducing phobic symptoms. As such, reinforced practice is considered to be a well-established treatment for childhood fears and phobias (see Ollendick & King, 1998).

The fourth strategy used in cognitive-behavioral therapy is primarily a cognitive or information-processing one. Cognitive interventions include techniques such as identifying self-talk, cognitive restructuring, and problem solving and they are usually taught in combination with one or more of the behavioral strategies reviewed earlier. Consequently, most published studies have examined treatments combining cognitive and behavioral interventions, and very few have examined the effectiveness of cognitive strategies in isolation. These integrated CBT programs are the most widely used treatments for children suffering from the most common anxiety disorders.

Kendall and his colleagues, for example, pioneered an integrated cognitive-behavioral treatment program for anxiety in children called "Coping Cat" (Kendall et al., 1992). The four coping strategies taught to anxious children were summarized in an acronym (FEAR) that helps children remember the steps to take when they felt anxious: *F*eeling frightened, *E*xpect good things to happen, *A*ctions and attitudes to take, and *R*eward yourself. There have been at least five controlled between-group studies that provide strong evidence that individual CBT programs such as Coping Cat and its variants are more effective than a wait list for reducing anxiety related to SAD, SOP, GAD, and school refusal (Barrett, Dadds, & Rapee, 1996; Heyne et al., 2002; Kendall, 1994; Kendall et al., 1997; King et al., 1998).

Studies have also examined the impact of incorporating parents in the therapeutic process. For example, teaching parents better strategies to manage their own anxiety and informing parents about strategies their children are learning to manage their anxiety may lead to better treatment outcomes than interventions that focus solely on the child (Barrett, Dadds, et al., 1996; Cobham, Dadds, & Spence, 1998). Also, preliminary findings by Cobham et al. (1998) suggest that anxious children who also have an anxious parent benefit the most from combined parent–child interventions.

Although group interventions for anxiety in children have been used for some time (e.g., see Ollendick & King, 1998), it is only recently that group cognitive-behavioral treatment has been investigated in controlled clinical trials. A series of recent studies by different research teams suggests that group format CBT is more effective in reducing anxiety than wait list and placebo conditions (Barrett, 1998; Flannery-Schroeder & Kendall, 2000; Mendlowitz et al., 1999; Shortt, Barrett, & Fox, 2001; Silverman et al., 1999). The question as to whether group CBT is more, less, or equally as effective as individual CBT awaits large-scale studies. Similarly, further research examining whether parent involvement increases the efficacy of child CBT is needed.

Summary of Anxiety Disorders in Children and Adolescents

Anxiety is a common problem in childhood and adolescence. Anxiety problems are frequently comorbid with other anxiety disorders, depression, or externalizing behaviors and have a poor prognosis if not treated. Several etiological theories have been proposed to explain the development and maintenance of anxiety. Although research indicates a familial risk of anxiety, most anxiety problems can be conceptualized as an interaction between temperament and environmental and contextual factors. Anxiety in children and adolescents can be reliably assessed, and promising cognitive-behavioral and pharmacological treatments are available.

DEPRESSIVE DISORDERS IN CHILDREN AND ADOLESCENTS

Phenomenology

Depressive disorders affect a significant number of children and adolescents, and there are important developmental factors to consider when making a diagnosis and in planning effective treatment for youngsters with these disorders (Duggal, Carlson, Sroufe, & Egeland, 2001). A thorough understanding of risk factors, development, family factors, and individual cognitive variables, as well as comorbid disorders, assist in both assessment and treatment of these youngsters (Stark, Sander, Yancy, Bronik, & Hoke, 2000). Although the existence of depressive disorders in children and adolescents is no longer in question as it was in past years, there remain many unanswered questions about etiology, effective treatments, and dealing with depression when it is comorbid with other disorders.

Developmental Considerations. In general, children and adolescents who are depressed do not always report feeling sad or depressed, and developmentally appropriate language is needed to understand and communicate with them about their experiences. In particular, children tend to express their negative emotions as anhedonia (i.e., things that once were fun or reinforcing no longer are), rather than as depressed or sad mood as with adolescents. In addition, both children and adolescents often report greater irritability than sadness, and argumentative behavior may also occur (Hammen & Rudolph, 1996). Although some researchers and clinicians suggest that the observed developmental differences in symptoms warrant different diagnostic categories (not unlike developmental differences between oppositional defiant disorder and conduct disorder), the field appears to have accepted this difference in symptom patterns across development and to embrace them.

Children and adolescents also differ in their perceptions of personal control and resultant depression. A recent model put forth by Weisz, Southam-Gerow, and McCarty (2001) articulated developmental differences in perceived contingency, control, and competence (CCC) related to depression in children and adolescents. Data were collected in several mental health outpatient centers with 360 child and adolescent participants. The CCC model defined perceived control as one's power to influence or engineer a desired outcome. Contingency was determined by how much one's efforts caused the outcome, considering other possible contributing factors. Competence was defined as the degree to which one actually carried out the necessary behaviors to produce the desired outcomes. Both children and adolescents appeared negatively affected by low perceived control and low perceived competence, but adolescents were also sensitive to the contingency or fairness of the circumstances in a more global sense. Such findings may have important implications for current treatments for depression in children versus adolescents.

Differences in prevalence rates for childhood and adolescent depression, regardless of gender, also have implications for our understanding of depression in youth. In a prospective, longitudinal study by Duggal and colleagues (2001), significant differences emerged for factors associated with childhood-onset and adolescent-onset depression. Abuse at an early age, higher maternal stress, and less supportive early care differentiated childhood-onset from adolescent-onset depression. In general, adverse family relationships were associated with childhood-onset depression but not adolescent-onset depression. In the adolescent-onset group, adverse family relationships were less significant; however, greater levels of maternal depression were noted.

Gender Differences. Prevalence rates of depressive disorders are different for boys and girls. The differences change systematically with development, adding an additional factor to consider. Before adolescence, there are approximately equal proportions of depressive disorders among boys and girls. However, beginning in adolescence and continuing into adulthood, depressive disorders occur more frequently among females than males (Kessler, Avenevoli, & Merikangas, 2001), with ratios upward of 2:1 (Axelson & Birmaher, 2001). The exact reasons for these gender differences remain unclear. Biological, cultural, and interpersonal factors have been proposed, with no clear causes emerging (Nolen-Hoeksema, 1995). Still, these gender differences have been found to be robust across cultures. For example, in a large study of Mexican youth, Benjet and Hernandez-Guzman (2001) reported that prevalence of depression was similar for boys and girls prepuberty and increased for females postmenarche but not for males postpuberty.

One theory espoused by Shaw, Kennedy, and Joffe (1995) was that girls are more sensitive to interpersonal rejection and more focused on dissatisfying interpersonal relationship qualities than boys. A modeling theory also proposes that the incidence of depression is greater among women of child-rearing age and that their daughters may learn about depressive symptoms, cognitions, and behaviors, thus placing them at higher risk for depressive symptoms (Goodman & Gotlib, 1999). Benjet and Hernandez-Guzman (2001) also explored family factors, self-esteem, parental education, and attitudes about menstruation as potential modifiers in the puberty-depression relationship among young Mexican females but did not find support for modifying effects.

In a recent review, Beardslee and Gladstone (2001) provided an overview of risk factors for the development of depression in boys and girls. These factors included having a biological relative with a mood disorder, presence of a severe stressor, low self-esteem or hopelessness, being female, and low socioeconomic status (poverty). Males and females were characterized, at least partially, by a unique set of risk factors. For boys, but not girls, neonatal and subsequent health problems posed risk for depression; in girls, but not boys, death of a parent by age 9 years, poor academic performance, and family dysfunction were related to risk for depression. In another review, Duggal and colleagues (2001) indicated that early caregiving patterns, such as household stress and quality of early childhood care, predicted depression for adolescent males but not adolescent females whereas presence of maternal depression predicted depression in adolescent females but not adolescent males. The patterns of gender differences in prevalence and risk are reasonably well established. Yet, the mechanisms contributing to gender differences remain elusive and the field is ripe for new ideas and investigations.

Epidemiology

Prevalence and incidence rates of depressive disorders vary across studies, and large-scale research is sparse in the area of childhood depression. However, on average, narrowly defined DSM major depression is thought to affect 1% to 2% of children (Anderson et al., 1987) and 2% to 4% of adolescents at any given time (Lewinsohn, Clarke, Seeley, & Rohde, 1994), or between 1% and 6% for point prevalence in youths in general (Kessler, Avenevoli, & Merikangas, 2001). Of course, rates increase for subclinical levels of depressive symptoms—depressive symptoms are reported by most children and adolescents at one time or another in their development.

DSM–IV Classification of Depressive Disorders

The *Diagnostic and Statistical Manual*, 4th edition (DSM–IV), lists major depressive disorder, dysthymia, and depressive disorder not otherwise specified within the depressive disorders category (APA, 1994). Some mental health professionals also consider bipolar disorder in the group of depressive disorders because of the depressive features of that disorder. However, given differences in treatment and prognosis for bipolar disorder spectrum illnesses, we do not view them as part of the affective disorders and do not discuss them further in this chapter.

The diagnosis of major depression is warranted if the child is experiencing five of the nine criteria symptoms of depression over a 2-week period. One of those symptoms must be either depressed mood (can be irritable mood in children) or anhedonia (loss of interest or diminished pleasure in what was once reinforcing to the child; APA, 1994). Dysthymia is chronic and less severe than major depression, but symptoms must be present for at least 1 year in children (in contrast to 2 years in adults; APA, 1994). In some cases, a depressed child may appear to have brief moments of enjoyment, such as while playing with friends or winning in a game. When depressed children present for treatment, some clinicians may detect momentary childhood positive moods and mistakenly rule out dysthymia. Children who are dysthymic may have such moments, but they fade quickly and their overall experiences remain affected by chronic depressive symptoms.

Depression is a cyclic, often recurrent, disorder. Emslie and Mayes (2001) reported that 90% of youngsters recovered from a depressive episode within 2 years. Yet, within 6 to 7 years, 25% to 50% of them re-experienced significant symptoms and distress. In addition, within 8 years, 54% to 72% had a recurrent episode of depression.

Differential Diagnosis and Comorbidity

Another important (if not vexing) factor in the diagnosis and treatment of depression is the existence of comorbid disorders. Comorbid disorders include an anxiety disorder, conduct disorder, and substance abuse, with anxiety being most common, as noted earlier in this chapter. Lewinsohn, Zinbarg, Seeley, Lewinsohn, and Sack (1997) reported that depression co-occurs with panic, generalized anxiety, separation anxiety, social phobia, and specific phobia. Although depression may be the first onset with some comorbid disorders (especially with substance abuse disorders), in general, anxiety disorders such as panic disorder and GAD precede its onset (Kessler, Avenevoli, & Merikangas, 2001).

Although anxiety disorders are common comorbid disorders with depression, the two classes of disorders appear to be distinct in children, but related through a common construct of negative affectivity (Axelson & Birmaher, 2001; Seligman & Ollendick, 1998). In depressed youth, up to 75% may have a lifetime prevalence of a comorbid anxiety disorder, and between 45% and 50% may have a disruptive behavior disorder or substance use disorder (Avenevoli, Stolar, Li, Dierker, & Merikangas, 2001). Point prevalence rates for children and adolescents with depression and a comorbid anxiety disorder range from 25% to 50%; in contrast, point prevalence rates for anxious youths with depression range between 15% and 20%. In other words, it is more common for depressed children and adolescents to have a comorbid anxiety disorder than for anxious children and adolescents to have a comorbid depressive disorder. Presence of a comorbid disorder appears to relate to severity of symptoms, such that youngsters with major depression and comorbid anxiety possess more severe depressive symptoms (Axelson & Birmaher, 2001). Comorbidity is particularly relevant in assessment of suicide risk. Youths with substance abuse as either a primary comorbid diagnosis or secondary diagnosis are at increased risk for suicidal behavior. In addition, antisocial behavior, particularly in females, may increase risk for lethal suicidal behaviors (Wannan & Fombonne, 1998).

Etiological Considerations

Biological Factors. Risk of depression in children and adolescents is associated with parental depression, for biological, environmental, and interpersonal reasons. Weissman and colleagues (1987) indicated that childhood-onset depression was more likely in households where the mother was depressed, particularly if the mother's onset of depression was in early adulthood. This finding implies a genetic or heritable component, but environmental factors, of course, cannot be ruled out.

In addition to inherited factors, specific neurotransmitters have been implicated in the onset and course of depression in children and adolescents. One prominent theory suggests that select neurotransmitters such as the monoamines, norepinephrine, serotonin, and dopamine are not available at receptor sites in sufficient supply (Wagner & Ambrosini, 2001). In adults, pharamacological treatment traditionally includes antidepressant medications in the class of monoamine oxidase inhibitors or tricyclic antidepressants, and more recently the selective serotonin reuptake inhibitors (SSRIs) or serotonin-norepinephrine reuptake (SNRIs) inhibitors. Use of such medications is based on this neurotransmitter deficiency theory. Other theories, which have not yet been demonstrated with children, implicate poor growth hormone stimulation, as well as hypothalamic-pituitary-adrenal axis regulation difficulties (Axelson & Birmaher, 2001).

Family and Interpersonal Factors. It is well documented that having a depressed mother makes youth more vulnerable to depression. The mechanisms behind this finding have received increasing attention in recent years. Furthermore, the interpersonal consequences and correlates of depression in children and adolescents have been the subject of much speculation and research. Goodman and Gotlib's (1999) integrative model of risk for transmission of depression from mother to child considers heritability, depressive maternal affect and symptoms, stress within a household with a depressed parent, and neuroregulatory consequences from that environmental circumstance. In addition, they propose that the timing, severity, and duration of depressive symptoms interact with the developmental tasks and challenges for children (Goodman & Gotlib, 1999). Furthermore, the Oregon Adolescent Depression project (Allen, Lewinsohn, & Seeley, 1998) examined prenatal, neonatal, developmental, and family relationship factors in psychopathology. They found several factors increased the risk of adolescent depression, including maternal depression and absence of breastfeeding.

The effect of early relationship quality on later depression in children and adolescents is unclear, as is the contribution made by youngsters with a predisposition for depression to the negative quality of their interpersonal interactions. However, depressed youth do appear to have poorer social competence, perceive less support from peers, and spend less time with peers than do nondepressed youth (Hammen & Rudolph, 1996). Professionals need to acknowledge and integrate interpersonal deficits or struggles, including peer and parental relationships, when conceptualizing and implementing treatment programs for depressed youngsters (Mufson, Weissman, Moreau, & Garfinkel, 1999; Stark et al., 2000). In addition, depression and its associated cognitive distortions appear to be related to interpersonal factors and, therefore, can or should be treated within an interpersonal context (Joiner, Coyne, & Blalock, 1999).

Consistent with research on the role of interpersonal and cognitive variables in depression in youth, a cognitive-interpersonal theory of depression proposes that cognitive style and interpersonal relationship patterns combine to result in depression (see Stark et al., 2000). From this perspective, Bowlby's attachment theory (1980) plays an important role. In brief, the early or primary interpersonal relationships are proposed to either buffer or increase risk for cognitive style associated with depression (Stark et al., 2000). According to this theory, early relationship patterns and caregivers' responsiveness to children shape the children's expectations of how they will be treated by others and how responsive others will be to their needs. An unresponsive caregiver, such as a depressed parent, could inadvertently communicate the message that the child's needs are unimportant, thus predisposing the child to adopt a negative self-schema (Duggal et al., 2001; Stark et al., 2000). Others suggest similar cognitive-interpersonal pathways and theoretical integration (Gotlib & Hammen, 1992).

Individual and Cognitive Variables.   Among individual variables, cognitive style, including attributional style, has received the most attention. In brief, the cognitive model of depression includes the concepts of negative thought patterns, depressive self-schema, and pessimistic attributional style about events (Clark, Beck, & Alford, 1999; Stark, Schmidt, & Joiner, 1996). According to cognitive theory, the self-schema guides information processing and may produce errors in perception that are consistent with a depressive self-schema—typically that the self is unlovable or incompetent (Clark et al., 1999). Attributional style refers to the patterns of causality assigned to events, such as how stable, global, and internal those events are perceived to be (Nolen-Hoeksema, Girgus, & Seligman, 1992). Depressed children and adolescents, in contrast to nondepressed children and adolescents, may often distort events and make information-processing errors that confirm negatively biased assumptions about the self (Stark et al., 1996) and the internal, stable, and global nature of negative events (Nolen-Hoeksema et al., 1992).

Assessment

The scope of this chapter does not allow for thorough review of the assessment process. However, brief recommendations are put forth (see Kendall, Cantwell, & Kazdin, 1989, for a thorough discussion of this topic). Within the field of depression, a common diagnostic interview used for assessing clinical depression is the Kiddie Schedule for Affective Disorders and Schizophrenia (K–SADS) (Orvaschel & Puig-Antich, 1987). Various researchers have adopted versions of the K–SADS, including present episode, epidemiologic version, and combined versions. The K–SADS is a semistructured diagnostic interview designed to be used by clinically trained interviewers and can be administered to the youth and parent separately. The complete interview is cumbersome and was designed for research. However, the specific prompts and questions can be incorporated into an interview for clinical practice (Stark et al., 2000). A common self-report tool for assessing depression is the Children's Depression Inventory (CDI) (Kovacs, 1981). Other tools can be used in community samples, such as the internalizing items on the Child Behavior Checklist or Youth Self Report (Achenbach, 1991), but these are not considered best practice in assessing youth with clinical levels of depression (Stark et al., 2000).

Assessment of suicide risk and behavior is important. In adolescents, there may be a precipitating stressor that has compromised developmental tasks such as establishing autonomy, acceptance by desired peer groups, or conflict with important peers or with family members. The clinician must remain attuned to these potential events in relation to increased risk for suicide in youths (Rudd & Joiner, 1998), as well as assess for substance use and antisocial behavior, as discussed previously (Wannan & Fombonne, 1998).

Interventions

Pharmacological Interventions. As with the anxiety disorders, there have been a limited number of controlled, randomized clinical trials of treatment of depression in children and adolescents, either pharmacological or psychosocial. Pharmacologically, the most promising results have been obtained with use of SSRIs (e.g., fluoxetine, marketed as Prozac) to reduce depressive symptoms. However, rates of improvement have been less than 40% (Wagner & Ambrosini, 2001). Importantly, however, the SSRIs are most likely to reduce depressive symptoms and have fewer and less detrimental side effects than other antidepressants (Emslie & Mayes, 2001). However, major clinical trials are still underway evaluating the efficacy of these other pharmacologic agents.

Psychosocial Interventions. In a review of psychosocial interventions for depressed children and adolescents, Asarnow, Jaycox, and Tompson (2001) acknowledged the merits of efficacious interventions across a range of modalities, including cognitive-behavioral therapy (CBT) and interpersonal psychotherapy for adolescents (IPT–A), both of which are relatively short-term interventions. However, the relapse rates (40%–50%) of clinically depressed youth when these psychosocial treatments are the sole treatment modality are relatively high (Asarnow et al., 2001).

CBT has received the most empirical support of the psychosocial treatments (Curry, 2001). Components of CBT include affective education, planning positive activities, proactive problem solving, social skills training, coping strategies, and cognitive restructuring. Family and interpersonal components may also be included. CBT has been implemented with children as young as 8 to 9 years of age and up to 18 years of age. Among fifteen CBT studies reviewed by Curry (2001), treatment duration ranged from 5 to 16 weeks. Some therapy protocols involved twice-weekly sessions, with an average of eleven sessions total. New treatment investigations include an emphasis on family components, combined with cognitive-behavioral approaches (Asarnow et al., 2001; Curry, 2001).

IPT–A has also received promising empirical support. In IPT–A, focus is on resolving conflicts in current, important, interpersonal relationships and improving communication and relationship skills (Mufson, Moreau, Weissman, & Klerman, 1993). To date, empirical support for this intervention has been limited to one major clinical trial (Mufson et al., 1999).

Managing suicidal risk is a necessary skill when working with depressed youngsters, particularly as outpatients. Managing this risk involves several straightforward strategies (Rudd & Joiner, 1998). The first is to have a proactive stance and a plan for potential hospitalization, to be revised or revisited frequently during suicide risk periods. In addition, treatment progress and goals should be revisited and updated often, particularly noting the changes that co-occur with decreased suicidal ideation. Sessions may need to occur more frequently, and the family's involvement and a phone contact list, as well as availability of emergency 24-hour support, is necessary. Furthermore, medication assessment and monitoring, as well as consultation, is recommended.

In summary, although the available treatments for depressed and suicidal children and adolescents show promise, several important caveats should be kept in mind. Overall, recovery rates across interventions are generally at or below 50% (Asarnow et al., 2001; Curry, 2001). Moreover, relapse rates are high. Also, comorbidity is rarely addressed in treatment efficacy studies, and it remains an important factor to consider in day-to-day clinical practice as well as in major clinical outcome trials (Curry, 2001). Psychosocial interventions, particularly the traditional CBT approaches, are moving in new directions to reflect a more integrative treatment, incorporating individual, cognitive, relational, and interpersonal factors (Seligman, Goza, & Ollendick, 2004).

Summary of Depressive Disorders in Children and Adolescents

The research on child and adolescent depression offers a number of exciting and promising findings. Treatment research is ongoing, including new directions involving biological and interpersonal factors. Although efficacious treatments exist, both pharmacological and psychosocial (primarily CBT and IPT–A), not all youth are being helped by these interventions. Furthermore, the issue of comorbidity has not been adequately addressed nor has the role of culture and ethnicity. The protective factors and risk factors associated with different cultural and ethnic practices have yet to be examined in standard research and clinical practice. These could be pivotal factors in understanding and treating childhood depression in our increasingly diverse society.

FUTURE DIRECTIONS

The internalizing disorders of children and adolescents represent a major challenge to practicing clinicians and researchers alike. As we have seen, the anxiety and affective disorders are highly prevalent in childhood and adolescence. Their effects are distressing in the short run and can be long lasting.

Although we have attempted to articulate a developmental psychopathology perspective on these disorders, it is evident that the field has not yet fully embraced this way of thinking about these problems. As a result, many studies continue to look at single causal pathways and direct, linear outcomes. As we have suggested, it may be more productive to posit that several very different pathways can lead to any one outcome such as depression or anxiety (i.e., the developmental principle of equifinality) and that any one pathway can lead to diverse outcomes (i.e., the principle of multifinality). Thus, a risk factor such as child sexual abuse can and frequently does lead to multiple outcomes, whether they are an internalizing disorder or one of the externalizing disorders reviewed in Chapter 15. Tracking this developmental process is undoubtedly a complex and challenging undertaking, but a necessary one. This effort will benefit greatly from carefully planned, multisite, longitudinal studies (Ollendick & King, 1994).

Moreover, the effects of these risk factors may not be direct and we need to consider conditions that moderate these relations. Direct effects are oftentimes captured by what are referred to as main effect models that imply that a risk factor is directly related to the outcome in a linear fashion. Yet, any one risk factor does not invariably result in any one pathological outcome. For example, it is well known that not all sexually abused children have negative outcomes such as the development of internalizing or externalizing disorders—or at least not the same negative outcomes. Often, a significant minority of abused children do not develop any disorders at all, implying a profound interaction between the experience of abuse and some other internal or external moderating conditions (Kazdin & Kagan, 1994). What does seem most important is the context in which the abuse occurs and the inter-related risk factors that are present. As noted by Kazdin and Kagan, "when one begins with the multiplicity of variables that operate, one might better consider nonlinearity to be the better point of departure in our work" (p. 38).

These same issues have important implications for the treatment and prevention of internalizing disorders. Our treatment and prevention programs must move away from a "one size fits all" mentality. Children and adolescents become depressed or anxious through a variety of pathways, and they express these disorders in a variety of ways. We need to take this complexity into consideration in designing, implementing, and evaluating our interventions. Although current empirically supported or evidence-based interventions work with most (i.e., 50% to 70%) of the children and adolescents and families who come into our practices and research clinics, we must do better. An approach that is individualized and prescriptive, and one that is based in developmental theory and grounded in established principles of behavior change (e.g., exposure, cognitive change, interpersonal relationships), is likely to be most effective, although such remains to be carefully documented.

REFERENCES

Achenbach, T. M. (1990). What is "developmental" about developmental psychopathology? In J. Rolf, A. Matsen, D. Cicchetti, K. Nuuechterlein, & S. Weintraub (Eds.), *Risk and protective factors in the development of psychopathology* (pp. 29–48). New York: Cambridge University Press.

Achenbach, T. M. (1991). *Manual for the Child Behavior Checklist/4–18 and 1991 profile*. Burlington, VT: University of Vermont, Department of Psychiatry.

Albano, A. M., Chorpita, B., & Barlow, D. H. (1996). Anxiety disorders in children and adolescents. In E. J. Mash and R. A. Barkley (Eds.), *Child psychopathology* (pp. 196–241). New York: Guilford.

Allen, N. B., Lewinsohn, P. M., & Seeley, J. R. (1998). Prenatal and perinatal influences on risk for psychopathology in childhood and adolescence. *Development and Psychopathology, 10*, 513–529.

American Psychiatric Association. (1980). *Diagnostic and statistical manual of mental disorders* (3rd ed.). Washington, DC: Author.

American Psychiatric Association. (1994). *Diagnostic and statistical manual of mental disorders* (4th ed.). Washington, DC: Author.

Anderson, J. C., Williams, S., McGee, R., & Silva, A. (1987). DSM-III disorders in pre-adolescent children: Prevalence in a large sample from the general population. *Archives of General Psychiatry, 44*, 69–76.

Asarnow, R., Jaycox, L. H., & Tompson, M. C. (2001). Depression in youth: Psychosocial interventions. *Journal of Clinical Child Psychology, 30*, 33–47.

Avenevoli, S., Stolar, M., Li, J., Dierker, L., & Merikangas, K. R. (2001). Comorbidity of depression in children and adolescents: Models and evidence from a prospective hi-risk family study. *Biological Psychiatry, 49*, 1071–1081.

Axelson, D. A., & Birmaher, B. (2001). Relation between anxiety and depressive disorders in childhood and adolescence. *Depression and Anxiety, 14*, 67–78.

Baer, D. M. (1982). Behavior analysis and development. *Human Development, 25*, 357–361.

Bandura, A. (1977a). Self-efficacy: Toward a unifying theory of behavioral change. *Psychological Review, 84*, 191–215.

Bandura, A. (1977b). *Social learning theory*. Englewood Cliffs, NJ: Prentice-Hall.

Bandura, A. (1986). *Social foundations of thought and action: A social cognitive theory*. Englewood Cliffs, NJ: Prentice Hall.

Bandura, A. (2001). Social cognitive theory: An agentic perspective. *Annual Review of Psychology, 52*, 1–26.

Barrett, P. M. (1998). Evaluation of cognitive-behavioral group treatments for childhood anxiety disorders. *Journal of Clinical Child Psychology, 27*, 459–468.

Barrett, P. M., Dadds, M. R., & Rapee, R. M. (1996). Family treatment of childhood anxiety: A controlled trial. *Journal of Consulting and Clinical Psychology, 64*, 333–342.

Barrett, P. M., Rapee, R. M., Dadds, M. M., & Ryan, S. M. (1996): Family enhancement of cognitive style in anxious and aggressive children. *Journal of Abnormal Child Psychology, 24*, 187–203.

Beardslee, W. R., & Gladstone, T. R. G. (2001). Prevention of childhood depression: Recent findings and future prospects. *Biological Psychiatry, 49*, 1101–1110.

Beck, A. T. (1976). *Cognitive therapy and the emotional disorders*. New York: International Universities Press.

Beck, A. T. (1991). Cognitive therapy: A 30-year retrospective. *American Psychologist, 46*, 368–375.

Beidel, D. C., & Morris, T. L. (1995). Social phobia. In E. J. Mash and R. A. Barkley (Eds.), *Child psychopathology* (pp. 181–211). New York: Guilford.

Benjet, C., & Hernandez-Guzman, L. (2001). Gender differences in psychological well-being of Mexican early adolescents. *Adolescence, 36*, 47–65.

Biederman, J., Hirshfeld-Becker, D. R, Rosenbaum, J. F., Herot, C., Friedman, D., Snidman, N., Kagan, J., & Faraone, S. V. (2001). Further evidence of association between behavioral inhibition and social anxiety in children. *American Journal of Psychiatry, 158*, 1673–1679.

Bowlby, J. (1980). *Attachment and loss: Vol III. Loss, sadness, and depression*. New York: Basic Books.

Brady, E. U., & Kendall, P. C. (1992). Comorbidity of anxiety and depression in children and adolescents. *Psychological Bulletin, 111*, 244–255.

Caron, C., & Rutter, M. (1991). Comorbidity in child psychopathology: Concepts, issues and research strategies. *Journal of Child Psychology and Psychiatry, 32*, 1063–1080.

Cicchetti, D. (1989). Developmental psychopathology: Past, present, and future. In D. Cicchetti (Ed.), *The emergence of a discipline: The Rochester symposium on developmental psychopathology* (Vol. 1, pp. 1–12). Hillsdale, NJ: Lawrence Erlbaum Associates.

Cicchetti, D., & Schneider-Rosen, K. (1986). An organizational approach to childhood depression. In M. Rutter, C. E. Izard, & P. B. Read (Eds.), *Depression in young people: Developmental and clinical perspectives* (pp. 71–134). New York: Guilford.

Clark, D. A., Beck, A. T. & Alford, B. A. (1999). *Scientific foundations of cognitive theory and therapy of depression*. New York: Wiley.

Cobham, V. E, Dadds, R., & Spence, S. H. (1998). The role of parental anxiety in the treatment of childhood anxiety. *Journal of Consulting and Clinical Psychology, 66*, 893–905.

Cohen, P., Cohen, J., Kaasen, S., Noemi Velez, C., Hartmark, C., Johnson, J., Rojas, M., Brookk, J., & Streuning, E. L. (1993). An epidemiological study of disorders in late childhood and adolescence—1. Age and gender specific prevalence. *Journal of Child Psychology and Psychiatry, 34*, 851–867.

Cook, E. H, Wagner, K. D., March, J. S, Biederman, J., Landau, P., Wolkow, R., & Messig, M. (2001). Long-term sertraline treatment of children and adolescents with obsessive-compulsive disorder. *Journal of the American Academy of Child and Adolescent Psychiatry, 40*, 1175–1189.

Costello, E. J., Costello, A. J., Edelbrock, C., Burns, B. J., Dulcan, M. K., Brent, D., & Janiszewski, S. (1988). Psychiatric disorders in pediatric primary care. *Archives of General Psychiatry, 45*, 1107–1116.

Curry, J. F. (2001). Specific psychotherapies for childhood and adolescent depression. *Biological Psychiatry, 49*, 1091–1100.

Dadds, M. R., & Barrett, P. M. (1996). Family processes in child and adolescent anxiety and depression. *Behaviour Change, 13*, 231–239.

Dadds, M. R., Barrett, P. M., Rapee, R. M., & Ryan, S. (1996). Family processes and child psychopathology: An observational analysis of the FEAR effect. *Journal of Abnormal Child Psychology, 24*, 715–735.

Dadds, M. R., & Roth, J. H. (2001). Family processes in the development of anxiety problems. In M. W. Vasey and M. R. Dadds (Eds.), *The developmental psychopathology of anxiety disorders in children* (pp. 278–303). New York: Oxford University Press.

Davey, G. C. L. (1992). Classical conditioning and the acquisition of human fears and phobias: A review and synthesis of the literature. *Advances in Behavior Research and Therapy, 14*, 29–66.

Duggal, S., Carlson, E. A., Sroufe, L. A., & Egeland, B. (2001). Depressive symptomatology in childhood and adolescence. *Development and Psychopathology, 13*, 143–164.

Dumas, J. E., LaFreniere, P. J., & Serketich, W. J. (1995). "Balance of power": A transactional analysis of control in mother-child dyads involving socially competent, aggressive, and anxious children. *Journal of Abnormal Psychology, 104*, 104–113.

Eley, T. C., & Stevenson, J. (1999). Exploring the covariation between anxiety and depression symptoms: A genetic analysis of the effects of age and sex. *Journal of Child Psychology and Psychiatry, 40*, 1273–1282.

Emslie, G. J., & Mayes, T. L. (2001). Mood disorders in children and adolescents: Pharmacological treatment. *Biological Psychiatry, 49*, 1082–1090.

Erickson, E. H. (1968). *Identity, youth, and crisis*. New York: W. W. Norton.

Essau, C. A., Conradt, J., & Petermann, F. (2000). Frequency, comorbidity, and psychosocial impairment of specific phobia in adolescents. *Journal of Clinical Child Psychology, 29*, 221–231.

Flannery-Schroeder, E. C., & Kendall, P. C. (2000). Group and individual cognitive-behavioral treatments for youth with anxiety disorders: A randomized clinical trial. *Cognitive Therapy and Research, 24*, 251–278.

Freud, S. (1949). *Outline of psychoanalysis*. New York: W. W. Norton.

Gelfand, D. M., & Peterson, L. (1985). *Child development and psychopathology*. Beverly Hills, CA: Sage.

Goodman, S. H., & Gotlib, I. H. (1999). Risk for psychopathology in the children of depressed mothers: A developmental model for understanding mechanisms of transmission. *Psychological Review, 106*, 458–490.

Gotlib, I. H., & Hammen, C. (1992). *Psychological aspects of depression: Toward a cognitive-interpersonal integration*. Chichester, England: Wiley.

Gullone, E. (2000). The development of normal fear: A century of research. *Clinical Psychology Review, 20*, 429–458.

Hammen, C., & Rudolph, K. D. (1996). Childhood depression. In E. J. Mash & R. A. Barkley (Eds.), *Child Psychopathology* (pp.153–195). New York: Guilford.

Heyman, I., Fombonne, E., Simmons, H., Ford, T., Meltzer, H., & Goodman, R. (2001). Prevalence of obsessive-compulsive disorder in the British nationwide survey of child mental health. *British Journal of Psychiatry, 179*, 324–329.

Heyne, D., King, N. J., Tonge, B. J., Rollings, S., Young, D., Pritchard, M., & Ollendick, T. H. (2002). Evaluation of child therapy and caregiver training in the treatment of school refusal. *Journal of the American Academy of Child and Adolescent Psychiatry, 41*, 687–695.

Hirshfeld, D. R., Biederman, J., Brody, L., Faraone, S. V., & Rosenbaum, J. F. (1997). Expressed emotion toward children with behavioral inhibition: Associations with maternal anxiety disorder. *Journal of the American Academy of Child and Adolescent Psychiatry, 36*, 910–917.

Horney, K. (1945). *Our inner conflicts*. New York: Norton.

Joiner, T., Coyne, J. C., & Blalock, J. (1999). On the interpersonal nature of depression: Overview and synthesis. In T. Joiner & J. C. Coyne (Eds.), *The interactional nature of depression: Advances in interpersonal approaches*. (pp. 3–20). Washington, DC: American Psychological Association.

Kagan, J. (1994). *Galen's prophecy: Temperament in human nature*. New York: Basic Books.

Kagan, J., Reznick, J. S., & Snidman, N. (1987). The physiology and psychology of behavioral inhibition in children. *Child Development, 58*, 1459–1473.

Kagan, J., Snidman, N., Zentner, M., & Peterson, E. (1999). Infant temperament and anxious symptoms in school age children. *Development and Psychopathology, 11*, 209–224.

Kashani, J. H., Beck, N. C., Hoeper, E. W., Falahi, C., Corcoran, C. M., McAllister, J. A., Rosenberg, T. K., & Reid, J. C. (1987). Psychiatric disorders in a community sample of adolescents. *American Journal of Psychiatry, 144*, 584–589.

Kashani, J. H., Orvaschel, H., Rosenberg, T. K., & Reid, J. C. (1989). Psychopathology in a community sample of children and adolescents: A developmental perspective. *Journal of the American Academy of Child and Adolescent Psychiatry, 28*, 701–706.

Kazdin, A. E., & Kagan, J. (1994). Models of dysfunction in developmental psychopathology. *Clinical Psychology: Science and Practice, 1*, 35–52.

Keller, M. B., Lavori, P., Wunder, J., Beardslee, W. R., Schwarts, C. E., & Roth, J. (1992). Chronic course of anxiety disorders in children and adolescents. *Journal of the American Academy of Child and Adolescent Psychiatry, 312*, 595–599.

Kendall, P. C. (1994). Treating anxiety disorders in children: Results of a randomized clinical trial. *Journal of Consulting and Clinical Psychology, 62*, 100–110.

Kendall, P., Brady, E. U., & Verduin, T. L. (2001). Comorbidity in childhood anxiety disorders and treatment outcome. *Journal of the American Academy of Child & Adolescent Psychiatry, 40*, 787–794.

Kendall, P. C., Cantwell, D. A., & Kazdin, A. E. (1989). Depression in children and adolescents: Assessment issues and recommendations. *Cognitive Therapy and Research, 13*, 109–146.

Kendall, P. C., Chansky, T. E., Kane, M. T., Kim, R., Kortlander, E., Ronan, K., Sessa, F. M., & Siqueland, L. (1992). *Anxiety disorders in youth: Cognitive-behavioral interventions*. New York: MacMillan.

Kendall, P. C., Flannery-Schroeder, E., Panichelli-Mindel, S. M., Southam-Gerow, M., Henin, A., & Warman, M. (1997). Treatment of anxiety disorders in youth: A second randomised clinical trial. *Journal of Consulting and Clinical Psychology, 65*, 366–380.

Kendall, P. C., & Warman, M. J. (1996). Anxiety disorders in youth: Diagnostic consistency across DSM-III-R and DSM-IV. *Journal of Anxiety Disorders, 10*, 453–463.

Kendler, K. S., Karkowski, L. M., & Prescott, C. A. (1999). Fears and phobias: Reliability and heritability. *Psyciatric Medicine, 29*, 539–553.

Kendler, K., Neale, M., Kessler, R., Heath, A., & Eaves, L. (1992). The genetic epidemiology of phobias in women: The interrelationship of agoraphobia, social phobia, situational phobia, and simple phobia. *Archives of General Psychiatry, 49*, 273–281.

Kendler, K. S., Walters, E. E., Neale, M. C., Kessler, R. C., Heath, A. C., & Eaves, L. J. (1995). The structure of genetic and environmental risk factors for six major psychiatric disorders in women: Phobia, generalized anxiety disorder, panic disorder, bulimia, major depression, and alcoholism. *Archives of General Psychiatry, 51*, 8–19.

Kessler, R. C., Avenevoli, S., & Merikangas, K. R. (2001). Mood disorders in children and adolescents: An epidemiologic perspective. *Biological Psychiatry, 49*, 1002–1014.

Kessler, R. C., McGonagle, K. A., Shanyang, Z., Nelson, C. B., Hughes, M., Eshleman, S., Wittchen, H.-U., & Kendler, K. S. (1994). Lifetime and 12-month prevalence of DSM-III-R psychiatric disorders in the United States. *Archives of General Psychiatry, 51*, 8–19.

Kindt, M., Brosschot, J. F., & Everaerd, W. (1997). Cognitive processing bias of children in real life stress situation and a neutral situation. *Journal of Experimental Child Psychology, 64*, 79–97.

King, N. J., Tonge, B. J., Heyne, D., Pritchard, M., Rollings, S., Young, D., Myerson, N., & Ollendick, T. H. (1998). Cognitive-behavioral treatment of school-refusing children: A controlled evaluation. *Journal of the American Academy of Child and Adolescent Psychiatry, 37*, 395–403.

Kovacs, M. (1981). Rating scales to assess depression in school aged children. *Acta Paedopsychiatrica, 46*, 305–315.

Kovacs, M., Feinberg, T. L., Crouse-Novak, M., Paulauskas, S. L., & Finkelstein, R. (1984). Depressive disorders in childhood: I. A longitudinal prospective study of characteristics and recovery. *Archives of General Psychiatry, 41*, 229–237.

Krohne, H. W., & Hock, M. (1991). Relationships between restrictive mother-child interactions and anxiety of the child. *Anxiety Research, 4*, 109–124.

Labellarte, M. J., Ginsburg, G. S., Walkup, J. T., & Riddle, M. A. (1999). The treatment of anxiety disorders in children and adolescents. *Biological Psychiatry, 46*, 1567–1578.

Lang, P. J. (1979). A bio-informational theory of emotional imagery. *Psychophysiology, 6*, 495–511.

Last, C. G., Perrin, S., Hersen, M., & Kazdin, A. E. (1992). DSM-III-R anxiety disorders in children: Sociodemographic and clinical characteristics. *Journal of the American Academy of Child and Adolescent Psychiatry, 31*, 1070–1076.

Last, C. L., Strauss, C. C., & Francis, G. (1987). Comorbidity among childhood anxiety disorders. *Journal of Nervous and Mental Disease, 175*, 726–730.

Lease, C. A., & Ollendick, T. H. (2000). Development and psychopathology. In M. Hersen & A. S. Bellack (Eds.), *Psychopathology in adulthood* (2nd ed., pp. 131–149). Boston: Allyn and Bacon.

Lerner, R. M., Hess, L. E., & Nitz, K. (1991). A developmental perspective on psychopathology. In M. Hersen & C. G. Last (Eds.), *Handbook of child and adult psychopathology: A longitudinal perspective* (pp. 9–32). Elmsford, NY: Pergamon.

Lewinsohn, P. M., Clarke, G. N., Seeley, J. R., & Rohde, P. (1994). Major depression in community adolescents: Age at onset, episode duration, and time to recurrence. *Journal of the American Academy of Child and Adolescent Psychiatry, 33*, 809–818.

Lewinsohn, P. M., Hops, H., Roberts, R. E., Seeley, J. R., & Andrews, J. A. (1993). Adolescent psychopathology: I. Prevalence and incidence of depression and other DSM-III-R disorders in high school students. *Journal of Abnormal Psychology, 102*, 133–144.

Lewinsohn, P. M., Zinbarg, R., Seeley J. R., Lewinsohn, M., & Sack, W. H. (1997). Lifetime comorbidity among anxiety disorders and between anxiety disorders and other mental disorders in adolescents. *Journal of Anxiety Disorders, 11*, 377–394.

Lewis, M. (1990). Models of developmental psychopathology. In M. Lewis & S. M. Miller (Eds.), *Handbook of developmental psychopathology* (pp. 15–27). New York: Plenum.

Manassis, K., & Monga, S. (2001). A therapeutic approach to children and adolescents with anxiety disorders and associated comorbid conditions. *Journal of the American Academy of Child & Adolescent Psychiatry, 40*, 115–117.

March, J., Parker, J., Sullivan, K., Stallings, P., & Conners, C. K. (1997). The Multidimensional Anxiety Scale for Children (MASC): Factor structure, reliability, and validity. *Journal of the American Academy of Child and Adolescent Psychiatry, 36*, 554–565.

Mattis, S. G., & Ollendick, T. H. (2002). Panic disorder and anxiety in adolescence. Oxford, England: Blackwell.

McClure, E. B., Brennan, P. A., Hammen, C., & Le Brocque, R. M. (2001). Parental anxiety disorders, child anxiety disorders, and the perceived parent-child relationship in an Australian high-risk sample. *Journal of Abnormal Child Psychology, 9*, 1–10.

McGee, R., Feehan, M., Williams, S., & Anderson, J. (1992). DSM-III disorders from age 11 to 15 years. *Journal of the American Academy of Child and Adolescent Psychiatry, 31*, 50–59.

McGee, R., Feehan, M., Williams, S., Partridge, F., Silvia, P. A., & Kelly, J. (1990). DSM III disorders in a large sample of adolescents. *Journal of the American Academy of Child and Adolescent Psychiatry, 29*, 611–619.

Mendlowitz, S. L., Manassis, K., Bradley, S., Scapillato, D., Miezitis, S., & Shaw, B. F. (1999). Cognitive-behavioral group treatments in childhood anxiety disorders: The role of parental involvement. *Journal of the American Academy of Child and Adolescent Psychiatry, 38*, 1233–1229.

Mufson, L., Moreau, D., Weissman, M. M., & Klerman, G. L. (1993). *Interpersonal psychotherapy for depressed adolescents*. New York: Guilford.

Mufson, L., Weissman, M. M., Moreau, D., & Garfinkel, R. (1999). Efficacy of interpersonal psychotherapy for depressed adolescents. *Archives of General Psychiatry, 56*, 573–579.

Nolen-Hoeksema, S. (1995). Epidemiology and theories of gender differences in unipolar depression. In M. V. Seeman (Ed.), *Gender and psychopathology* (pp. 63–87). London: American Psychiatric Press.

Nolen-Hoeksema, S., Girgus, J. S., & Seligman, M. E. (1992). Predictors and consequences of childhood depressive symptoms: A 5-year longitudinal study. *Journal of Abnormal Psychology, 101*, 405–422.

Ollendick, T. H. (1983). Reliability and validity of the Fear Survey Schedule for Children-Revised (FSSC-R). *Behaviour Research and Therapy, 21*, 685–692.

Ollendick, T. H., & Cerny, J. A. (1981). *Clinical behavior therapy with children.* New York: Plenum.

Ollendick, T. H., Grills, A. E., & King, N. J. (2001). Applying developmental theory to the assessment and treatment of childhood disorders: Does it make a difference? *Clinical Psychology and Psychotherapy, 8*, 304–314.

Ollendick, T. H., Hagopian, L. P., & King, N. J. (1997). Specific phobias in children. In G. C. L. Davey (Ed.), *Phobias: A handbook of theory, research and treatment* (pp. 201–224). Oxford: Wiley.

Ollendick, T. H., & Hirshfeld-Becker, D. R. (2002). The developmental psychopathology of social anxiety disorder. *Biological Psychiatry, 51*, 41–58.

Ollendick, T. H., & Ingman, K. (2001). Social phobia. In H. Orvaschel, J. Faust, & M. Hersen (Eds.), *Handbook of conceptualization and treatment of child psychopathology* (pp. 191–210). New York: Pergamon.

Ollendick, T. H., & King, N. J. (1994). Assessment and treatment of internalizing problems: The role of longitudinal data. *Journal of Consulting and Clinical Psychology, 62*, 918–927.

Ollendick, T. H., & King, N. J. (1998). Empirically supported treatments for children with phobic and anxiety disorders. *Journal of Clinical Child Psychology, 27*, 156–167.

Ollendick, T. H., King, N. J., & Muris, P. (2002). Fears and phobias in children: Phenomenology, epidemiology, and etiology. *Child Psychology and Psychiatry Review, 7*, 98–106.

Ollendick, T. H., Lease, C. A., & Cooper, C. (1993). Separation anxiety in young adults: A preliminary examination. *Journal of Anxiety Disorders, 7*, 293–305.

Ollendick, T. H., & March, J. S. (Eds.). (2004). *Phobic and anxiety disorders in children and adolescents: A clinician's guide to effective psychosocial and pharmacological interventions.* New York: Oxford University Press.

Ollendick, T. H., & Ollendick, D. G. (1997). General worry and anxiety in children. *In Session: Psychotherapy in Practice, 3*, 89–102.

Ollendick, T. H., Vasey, M. W., & King, N. J. (2001). Operant conditioning influences in child anxiety. In M. W. Vasey & M. R. Dadds (Eds.), *The developmental psychopathology of anxiety* (pp. 231–252). Oxford: Oxford University Press.

Orvaschel, H., Lewinsohn, P. M., & Seeley, R. J. (1995). Continuity of psychopathology in a community sample of adolescents. *Journal of the American Academy of Child and Adolescent Psychiatry, 34*, 1525–1535.

Orvaschel, H., & Puig-Antich, J. H. (1987). *Schedule for affective disorders and schizophrenia for school-age children* (Epidemiologic version, 4th ed.). Pittsburgh, PA: Western Psychiatric Institute and Clinic.

Pfeffer, C. R., Lipkins, R., Plutchik, R., & Mizruchi, M. (1988). Normal children at risk for suicidal behavior: A two-year follow-up study. *Journal of the American Academy of Child and Adolescent Psychiatry, 27*, 34–41.

Piaget, J. (1950). *The psychology of intelligence.* New York: Harcourt Brace Jovanovich.

Pury, C. L., & Mineka, S. (2001). Differential encoding of affective and nonaffective content information in trait anxiety. *Cognition & Emotion, 15*, 659–693.

Rapee, R. M. (1997). Potential role of childrearing practices in the development of anxiety and depression. *Clinical Psychology Review, 17*, 47–68.

Reiss, S. (1980). Pavlovian conditioning and human fear: An expectancy model. *Behavior Therapy, 11*, 380–396.

Reynolds, C. R., & Richmond, B. O. (1985). *Revised children's manifest anxiety scale: Manual.* Los Angeles: Western Psychological Services.

Rudd, D. M., & Joiner, T. E. (1998). An integrative conceptual framework for assessing and treating suicidal behavior in adolescents. *Journal of Adolescence, 21*, 489–498.

Rutter, M. (1985). Resilience in the face of adversity: Protective factors and resistance to psychaitric disorder. *British Journal of Psychiatry, 147*, 498–611.

Rutter, M., & Garmezy, N. (1983). Developmental psychopathology. In E. M. Hetherington (Ed.), *Socialization, personality, and social development: Vol. 4. Mussen's Handbook of Child Psychology* (4th Ed.). New York: Wiley.

Sameroff, A. J. (1995). General systems theories and developmental psychopathology. *Developmental Psychology, 1*, 659–695.

Schniering, C. A., Hudson, J. L., & Rapee, R. M. (2000). Issues in the diagnosis and assessment of anxiety disorders in children and adolescents. *Clinical Psychology Review, 20*, 453–478.

Seligman, L. D., Goza, A. B., & Ollendick, T. H. (2004). Treatment of depression in children and adolescents. In P. M. Barrett & T. H. Ollendick (Eds.), *Handbook of interventions that work with children and adolescents: Prevention and Treatment* (pp. 301–328). Chichester, UK: John Wiley & Sons Ltd.

Seligman, L. D., & Ollendick, T. H. (1998). Comorbidity of anxiety and depression in children and adolescents: An integrative review. *Clinical Child and Family Psychology Review, 1*, 125–144.

Shaw, J., Kennedy, S. H., & Joffe, M. (1995). Gender differences in mood disorders. In M. V. Seeman (Ed.). *Gender and psychopathology*. London: American Psychiatric Press.

Shortt, A. L., Barrett, P. M., & Fox, T. (2001). Evaluating the FRIENDS program: A cognitive behavioral group treatment for anxiety children and their parents. *Journal of Clinical Child Psychology, 30*, 525–535.

Silverman, W. K., & Albano, A. M. (1996). *Anxiety disorders interview schedule for DSM-IV: Child version: Parent interview schedule*. San Antonio, TX: The Psychological Corporation.

Silverman, W. K., Cerny, J. A., Nelles, W. B., & Burke, A. E. (1988). Behavior problems in children of parents with anxiety disorders. *Journal of the American Academy of Child and Adolescent Psychiatry, 27*, 779–784.

Silverman, W. K., Kurtines, W. M., Ginsburg, G. S., Weems, C. G., Lumpkin, P. W., & Carmichael, D. H. (1999). Treating anxiety disorders in children with group cognitive behavioural therapy: A randomised clinical trial. *Journal of Consulting and Clinical Psychology, 67*, 995–1003.

Silverman, W. K., & Ollendick, T. H. (Eds.). (1999). *Developmental issues in the clinical treatment of children*. Boston: Allyn & Bacon.

Silverman, W. K., & Treffers, P. D. A. (2001). *Anxiety disorders in children and adolescents: Research, assessment and intervention*. New York: Cambridge University Press.

Siqueland, L., Kendall, P. C., & Steinberg, L. (1996). Anxiety in children: Perceived family environment and observed family interaction. *Journal of Clinical Child Psychology, 25*, 225–237.

Skinner, B. F. (1938). *The behavior of organisms*. New York: Appelton-Century-Crofts.

Sroufe, L. A., & Rutter, M. (1984). The domain of developmental psychopathology. *Child Development, 55*, 17–29.

Stark, K. D., Sander, J. B., Yancy, M., Bronik, M., & Hoke, J. (2000). Treatment of depression in childhood and adolescence: Cognitive-behavioral procedures for the individual and family. In P. C. Kendall (Ed.). *Child and Adolescent Therapy: Cognitive-Behavioral Procedures* (2nd Ed, pp. 173–234). New York: Guilford.

Stark, K. D., Schmidt, K. L., & Joiner, T. E., Jr. (1996). Cognitive triad: Relationship to depressive symptoms, parents' cognitive triad, and perceived parental messages. *Journal of Abnormal Child Psychology, 24*, 615–631.

Strauss, C., Lease, C., Last, C., & Francis, G. (1988). Overanxious disorder: An examination of developmental differences. *Journal of Abnormal Child Psychology, 11*, 433–443.

Taghavi, M. R., Neshat-Doost, H. T., Moradi, A. R., Yule, W., & Dalgleish, T. (1999). Biases in visual attention in children and adolescents with clinical anxiety and mixed anxiety-depression. *Journal of Abnormal Child Psychology, 27*, 215–223.

Thapar, A., & McGuffin, P. (1995). Are anxiety symptoms in childhood heritable? *Journal of Child Psychology and Psychiatry, 36*, 439–447.

Toth, S. L., & Cicchetti, D. (1999). Developmental psychopathology and child psychotherapy. In S. W. Russ & T. H. Ollendick (Eds.), *Handbook of psychotherapies with children and families* (pp. 15–43). New York: Kluwer Academic/Plenum.

Vasey, M. W., & Ollendick, T. H. (2000). Anxiety. In M. Lewis & A. Sameroff (Eds.), *Handbook of developmental psychopathology* (pp. 511–529). New York: Plenum.

Wagner, K. D., & Ambrosini, P. J. (2001). Childhood depression: Pharmacological therapy/treatment (pharmacology of childhood depression). *Journal of Clinical Child Psychology, 30*, 88–97.

Wannan, G. & Fombonne, E. (1998). Gender differences in rates and correlates of suicidal behavior amongst child psychiatric outpatients. *Journal of Adolescence, 21*, 371–381.

Weissman, M. M., Gammon, G. D., Merikangas, K. R., Warner, V., Prusoff, B. A., & Sholomskas, D. (1987). Children of depressed parents: Increased psychpathology and early onset of major depression. *Archives of General Psychiatry, 44*, 847–853.

Weisz, J. R., Southam-Gerow, M. A., & McCarty, C. A. (2001). Control-related beliefs and depressive symptoms in clinic referred children and adolescents: Developmental differences and model specificity. *Journal of Abnormal Psychology, 110*, 97–109.

Werry, J. S. (1991). Overanxious disorder: A review of its taxonomic properties. *Journal of the American Academy of Child and Adolescent Psychiatry, 30*, 533–544.

Wood, J., Mathews, A., & Dalgleish, T. (2001). *Anxiety and cognitive inhibition. Emotion, 1*, 166–181.

World Health Organization (1992). *The ICD-10 classification of mental and behavioral disorders: Diagnostic criteria for research*. Geneva Switzerland: World Health Organization.

17

Cognitive Disorders of Childhood and Adolescence: Specific Learning Disabilities and Mental Retardation

Jack Naglieri
Claudia Salter
Johannes Rojahn
George Mason University

WHAT IS A LEARNING DISABILITY?

The term *learning disability* (LD) generally refers to a disorder where a child's achievement is substantially lower than what is expected based on intelligence. Simply stated, it means a person's level of achievement is inconsistent with his or her ability when measured using an achievement and IQ test. According to the U.S. Department of Education, up to 11% of school-aged children qualify as having a disability under the Individuals with Disabilities Education Act (IDEA), and approximately half of these children have a specific type of learning disability (U.S. Department of Education, 2000). Although the concept seems simple (ability versus achievement discrepancy), it has proven to be confusing because of a lack of consensus over how to operationalize it and a variety of definitions proposed by professional organizations and government officials. There is also great variability in the way that a learning disability has been assessed, including varying tests, methods, state and federal definitions, and in ways of using these definitions in professional practice. This variability of definition and method is also a problem because it makes it difficult for professionals to determine whether a child qualifies for special services and receives additional instruction. To better understand the current issues in the field of LD, it is first important to understand the history of the diagnosis.

Historical Definitions of Learning Disabilities

1910–1930s: Early Period.   During the early 1900s, it was first recognized that some children who were intelligent could not learn to read. At that time it was thought that brain damage caused problems that disrupted learning in a specific domain such as reading or writing.

Preparation of this manuscript was supported in part by Grant R215K010121 from the U.S. Department of Education.

Children thought to have such damage were considered intelligent in all areas except in reading or writing. In 1917, James Hinshelwood, a Scottish ophthalmologist, reported case studies of children who had difficulty acquiring reading skills. He attributed their problem to a condition that he called "congenital word blindness," which he thought resulted from damage to an area of the brain that stored visual memories for words and letters (Torgesen, 1998). In 1937, Samuel Orton, a child neurologist, published his influential work on children with reading disabilities; his explanations differed from those of Hinshelwood. Orton used the term "strephosymbolia" or twisted symbols to describe the condition, because these children often reversed words or letters when reading. He attributed the cause to a lack of hemispheric dominance in the brain, which caused visual images to be confused when transferred from one hemisphere to the other (Torgesen, 1998). Their initial concept that brain dysfunction contributes to a learning disability continues to influence the field of learning disabilities today.

Recent studies have evaluated brain functioning in children and adults with learning disabilities. The view that learning can be disrupted in a single area of the brain and influence a specific type of achievement, such as reading, is the basis for the diagnosis of a reading disorder in some current identification systems (see discussion of DSM–IV–TR that follows). In addition, Orton's work continues to influence the field of reading intervention: his multisensory educational approach for children with reading disabilities is incorporated into the Orton–Gillingham reading method.

1940s–1950s: Werner and Strauss.

1940s–1950s: *Werner and Strauss.*   Heinz Werner and Alfred Strauss at the Wayne County Training School in Michigan described a subset of children, presumed to have brain damage, who had problems working with certain kinds of information and who displayed behavioral and cognitive problems similar to those of head-injured soldiers described by Kirk Goldstein. For example, these children had problems inhibiting their responses and they seemed hyperactive. Importantly, these children had difficulties that were distinct from and not as broad as those found for persons with mental retardation (Torgesen, 1998). Werner and Strauss' work also differed from that of Orton and Hinshelwood in that they described problems in general learning areas rather than in specific academic skills. Since these children had difficulties similar to the head-injured soldiers, Werner and Strauss concluded that the children must have had brain damage.

Furthermore, Werner and Strauss concluded that these brain-damaged children needed special educational interventions to overcome their weaknesses. This work by Werner and Strauss suggested that children with learning problems were not all alike in their behavior profiles and that educational programming should be individualized. Since then, millions of dollars have been spent in diagnosing LD and developing special education programs in schools across the United States. The concept of individualized instructional plans (IEPs) was then initiated and remains in many rules and regulations to this day (Hallahan & Keogh, 2001).

1960s: Origins of the Concept of Learning Disabilities.

1960s: *Origins of the Concept of Learning Disabilities.*   By the 1960s, evidence had accumulated that children with learning problems often had histories of head injury, infections, or difficulties during pregnancy or labor. The U.S. Public Health Service Task Force I defined the term "minimal brain dysfunction" be used to describe these children (Clements, 1966). The suggested definition was broad and included diverse symptoms and etiology. This was not the only suggested label. In fact, numerous terms were used in the 1960s to describe children who were not achieving at the level expected based on their intelligence, including *dyslexic* and *perceptually handicapped.* Support organizations as well as the scientific community began to recognize the growing need for a unified term.

In 1963, Samuel Kirk introduced the term *learning disability* at a conference for parents exploring the problems of children who had specific learning problems and did not have mental retardation. One of the important issues addressed at the meeting was what to call these children. Parents were interested in not only a better label for their children, but also a term that would bring together the many small organizations into a more powerful group (Hallahan & Cruickshank, 1973). Kirk was cautious about the use of labels. In his speech he indicated that he preferred descriptions of the problem rather than technical terms such as *strephosymbolia*. However, he said that he recently started to use the term "learning disabilities" to describe children who have "disorders in development in language, speech, reading, and associated communication skills needed for social interaction" (Kirk, 1963). He excluded from this group children who have sensory handicaps such as deafness or blindness and children who have mental retardation. The response to his suggestion was mostly positive, and those at the convention voted the following day to organize under the title Association for Children with Learning Disabilities (Hallahan & Cruickshank, 1973).

Kirk's initiation of the term *learning disabled* was not as much an endorsement of labeling children, as it was a way of getting help for these individuals. He preferred that a child's behavior be analyzed to determine appropriate remediation and training (Kirk, 1972). He also later developed an approach to identifying specific learning disabilities, which was formalized into the Illinois Test of Psycholinguistic Abilities. Although the value of this test would eventually prove to be very limited, it did much to signify the need for a test that would identify the particular problems of children with learning disabilities.

1960s–1970s: Federal Legislation.

In 1967, the term *minimal brain dysfunction* was replaced by *learning disability* in U.S. federal legislation. The National Advisory Committee on Handicapped Children (NAHC) proposed a definition for learning disabilities that became the basis for the Education for All Handicapped Children Act (PL 94-142). This is the definition that remains in federal policy at this time:

> *"Specific learning disability" means a disorder in one or more of the basic psychological processes involved in understanding or in using language, spoken or written, which may manifest itself in an imperfect ability to listen, think, speak, read, write, spell, or to do mathematical calculations. The term includes such conditions as perceptual handicaps, brain injury, minimal brain dysfunction, dyslexia, and developmental aphasia. The term does not include children who have learning problems, which are primarily the result of visual, hearing, or motor handicaps, of mental retardation, of emotional disturbance, or of environmental, cultural, or economic disadvantage.*

The word "specific" was added to the term *learning disabilities* to avoid confusion with the learning problems of children with mental retardation. Children with mental retardation have a general difficulty in learning, whereas children with learning disabilities have difficulty in a more limited area (Kirk, 1972).

The Education for All Handicapped Children Act of 1975 (PL 94-142) retained the definition and added criteria for identifying children with learning disabilities. The law provided a guarantee that children would receive an appropriate public education in "the least restrictive environment." Each individual was entitled to publicly funded special education and special services and protected from discrimination. These laws have had extraordinary influence on public school practices of assessment, diagnosis, and instruction for children identified as having special educational needs.

1980s: National Joint Committee for Learning Disabilities (NJCLD).

In 1981, The National Joint Committee for Learning Disabilities (NJCLD) provided a modified definition of learning disabilities to address areas of confusion with the federal definition. This included recognizing that learning disabilities are a "heterogeneous group of disorders" and that they often co-occur with other disorders (NJCLD, 1991).

Around this time, learning disabilities were also included in the third version of the *Diagnostic and Statistical Manual of Mental Disorders*, published in 1980 (DSM–III, American Psychiatric Association [APA], 1980). Under the category Specific Delays in Development, the DSM–III listed diagnoses of specific reading retardation, specific arithmetical retardation, and other specific learning difficulties. Specific reading retardation was described as a "serious impairment in the development of reading or spelling skills not explicable in terms of general intellectual retardation or of inadequate schooling" (APA, 1980, p. 444). The revised version, DSM–III–R (APA, 1987), replaced the language of specific retardation with developmental disorders and listed them under the category of Academic Skills Disorders. Diagnoses included developmental arithmetic disorder, developmental expressive writing disorder, and developmental reading disorder. These are the three main areas of learning disabilities that remain in DSM–IV–TR.

1990s: DSM–IV; Individuals With Disabilities Act '97.   The DSM–IV was published in 1994 and a revision, which is the current version in use today, was published in 2000 (DSM–IV–TR). The diagnoses in the DSM–IV–TR remain the same as in DSM–IV. The DSM–IV–TR (APA, 2000) uses the term learning disorders rather than academic skills disorders. Learning disorders are classified into three main types: reading disorder, mathematics disorder, and disorder of written expression. This classification is similar to that of Hinshelwood and Orton from many years before. The DSM–IV–TR diagnoses apply to individuals who have a significant discrepancy between their achievement in one of the named areas and the achievement that might be expected according to their level of intelligence. Their academic achievement score must be substantially lower than their intellectual ability score, which according to DSM–IV–TR, is usually a score two standard deviations below the score on a measure of intelligence (APA, 2000).

The most current legislation regarding children with disabilities is the Amendments of the Individuals with Disabilities Education Act (IDEA '97), which reauthorized PL 94-142, also known as the Education for All Handicapped Children Act of 1975. The 1975 act was reauthorized as the Individuals with Disabilities Education Act (IDEA) in 1990. No changes were made to the definition or identification of a specific learning disability throughout these reauthorizations of the law. This law had significant influence on the field of learning disabilities because funding for special educational programs are tied directly to the number of children identified with a disability in each school district.

2000s: Ability/Achievement Discrepancy Under Fire.   In recent years there has been growing concern that the intelligence/achievement discrepancy approach is not effective for identification of learning disabilities and that it does not help professionals devise appropriate interventions. For example, in 2002, Robert Pasternack, the assistant secretary to the Office of Special Education and Rehabilitative Services, spoke about the "demise of IQ testing" at the National Association of School Psychologists conference. He concluded that IQ testing is not an appropriate way to diagnose LD and that the discrepancy approach should be eliminated. One of his most significant criticisms was that the intelligence/achievement discrepancy approach emphasizes eligibility issues more than the selection of academic interventions. Although the Assistant Secretary supported the definition of LD as a disorder in one or more of the basic psychological processes required for academic performance, the method of using a discrepancy to find these children was deemed ineffective and expensive.

The Commission on Excellence in Special Education also supports the elimination of the ability/achievement discrepancy approach for the purpose of diagnosing learning disorders (2002 report). The Commission was created by President Bush in 2001 to improve the special education system. In the report, concerns are raised that the vague federal definition of LD and the lack of consistency in diagnostic criteria leads to unreliable methods of diagnosis. Another concern is that children are often inappropriately identified as LD and placed in special education because they have not learned, in some cases because they were not taught, how to read. The Commission recommended early screening of children for LD and placing more focus on assessing the child's response to instruction.

Assessment and Diagnosis

The designation of a clear and objective system for identifying children with learning disabilities has turned out to be as elusive as developing a widely accepted way to define children with this disorder. Federal and state definitions provide guidelines, but these guidelines lack the precision necessary for identifying children with learning disorders. The result is that professionals have identified children with learning disorders using many different tests and methods in an attempt to follow the intelligence/achievement discrepancy model, which is the most widely used. Alternatively, some have attempted to identify children who have a disorder in one or more of the basic psychological processes involved in reading. Some issues surrounding each of these approaches will be more fully examined.

In the IQ/achievement discrepancy approach, a child is typically administered a test of intelligence, and this score is compared to a measure of achievement (e.g., score on a standardized test of achievement or performance in school). The most commonly used measure of intelligence for children is the Wechsler Intelligence Scale for Children (WISC–III; Wechsler, 1991), although there are problems with this test for the purpose of identifying LD (discussed later).

The advantage of the IQ/achievement discrepancy approach is that it helps differentiate between learning disorders and mental retardation (i.e., low achievement and low IQ, respectively) and can be used to identify a specific academic problem (not all achievement is low). There are at least two problems with this approach. First, there are several IQ tests available to psychologists and each one has many scores that could be used. Some state regulations allow the use of only a single total IQ score to determine if there is a discrepancy. Federal and state regulators cannot direct practitioners to use a particular IQ or achievement test, which has resulted in considerable variability in the way the IQ/achievement discrepancy is calculated. In fact, different states and school districts mandate different sizes of discrepancy (e.g., a difference of one or two standard deviations between IQ and achievement). State and county criteria also vary in how a discrepancy is operationalized, including deviation from grade level, expectancy formulas, regression analysis, and standard score comparisons (Mercer, Jordan, Allsopp, & Mercer, 1996).

The second major problem with the IQ/achievement discrepancy is that in order for a discrepancy to occur, the child has to have time to fall behind in an academic area. This means that a child will likely be in second or third grade before the discrepancy becomes obvious. By that time, however, the child is so far behind in acquiring academic skills that catching up may take many years. Some researchers have argued that not only is the IQ/achievement discrepancy ineffective for identification of children with learning disabilities but also that intelligence tests themselves are irrelevant to the diagnosis of learning disabilities (Siegel, 1989). In fact, after careful review of the research, Kaufman and Lichtenberger (2000) concluded that WISC–III subtest profiles "do not have adequate power on which to base differential diagnosis" (p. 205) for LD. This conclusion is reasonable considering that Wechsler's test was not designed to identify children with LD. Scores on verbal/nonverbal tests of intelligence have not been especially helpful for diagnosis of LD or attention deficit hyperactivity disorder (ADHD; Kavale & Forness, 1984; Kaufman & Lichtenberger, 2000). These problems and others with using the IQ/achievement discrepancy have led many in the field to recognize that an alternative should be considered.

The processing disorder method (cognitive processing disorder model) is an alternative to the IQ/achievement discrepancy model and traditional IQ tests. Recall that a specific learning disability means a disorder in one or more of the basic psychological processes involved in understanding or in using language, spoken or written, which may manifest itself in an imperfect ability to listen, think, speak, read, write, spell, or to do mathematical calculations. If a processing disorder is detected and the child has academic failure, then eligibility could be made. Historically, identification based on a disorder in one or more of the "basic psychological processes" has been limited because there is no definition of basic psychological processes in state and federal regulations. Practitioners have also been reluctant to use this approach to identification because of the limited availability of reliable and valid tests of basic cognitive processes. During the last 15 years, however, two methods have been published that offer psychologists well-validated tests to assess cognitive processes: the Kaufman Assessment Battery for Children (Kaufman & Kaufman, 1983) and the Cognitive Assessment System (Naglieri & Das, 1997). Both of these tests are nationally normed instruments with excellent reliability that provide a means to identify a disorder in one or more of the basic psychological (cognitive) processes (Naglieri, 1999). Additionally, researchers have found that the cognitive processing approach can provide measures of processes that are relevant to diagnosis and treatment (Naglieri, 1999). The use of these methods, however, has been limited because of the dominance of the IQ/achievement method and the relatively recent availability of well-standardized tests of cognitive processing.

Epidemiology

The prevalence of learning disabilities depends, of course, on how they are defined and identified, which is why prevalence rates have varied widely from study to study. According to the DSM–IV–TR, estimates of the prevalence of learning disorders range from 2% to 10% (APA, 2000). In the public schools, 4.5% of students are classified as having a specific learning disability (U.S. Department of Education, 2000). Students in this category comprise half of the approximately six million students served under IDEA, Part B (U.S. Department of Education, 2000). The next largest groups are students with speech and language impairments (1.7%) and mental retardation (0.95%). Since 1976, following the implementation of PL 94-142, the number of children in the specific learning disability group has grown considerably. Of the children identified, the great majority of children with learning disabilities have difficulties with reading. It is estimated that 4% of school-age children can be classified as having a reading disorder (APA, 2000).

Etiology of Learning Disabilities

Professionals in the field of learning disabilities have been more focused on describing the disability and developing interventions than on understanding the etiology (Torgesen, 1998). The etiology of learning disabilities is unclear, although most researchers think that they result from neurological impairment. There is a broad range or spectrum of learning disabilities, and there are likely many mechanisms involved, each contributing to particular learning disabilities. Studies have provided evidence that both genetic and environmental factors contribute to the development of some learning disabilities.

Neuroimaging studies have provided evidence for both functional and structural abnormalities associated with learning disabilities, adding further support for a biological basis. Functional abnormalities refer to differences in activation of brain regions (assessed by blood flow, oxygen uptake, or cellular metabolism), whereas structural abnormalities refer to differences in volume or shape. Filipek recently reviewed neuroimaging findings in children with developmental disorders and found structural and functional differences in some studies of individuals with reading disorders (Filipek, 1999). Results suggested that children with reading disorder have abnormalities in regions associated with receptive language (Hynd et al., 1995; Filipek, 1999).

There is also some evidence that genetic factors contribute to the development of learning disabilities. Family studies have shown a high prevalence rate of LD in first-degree relatives of children with LD. Twin studies have shown greater concordance of LD for monozygotic twins than for dizygotic twins. Together, these studies suggest a hereditary component for learning disabilities of approximately 50% (Ingalls & Goldstein, 1999). Work by Bishop has suggested that genetic factors are most substantial for severe literacy problems, which includes children with specific language impairment and specific reading disability (Bishop, 2001). In some families, reading disability has been linked to a region of chromosome 6 (Cardon et al. 1994).

Many factors may negatively affect the developing fetal brain, potentially causing neurological impairment and resulting in learning disabilities. Prenatal and postnatal factors are both important. Prenatal factors include hypoxia, maternal infection, maternal cigarette smoking, and maternal alcohol and drug use. Postnatal factors include infection, injury, and exposure to toxins such as lead. Lead toxicity has been associated with cognitive impairments ranging from subtle cognitive impairment to LD to mental retardation (Ingalls & Goldstein, 1999). Traumatic brain injury has also been shown to cause cognitive deficits and learning problems that may present months to years after injury (Yeates, 2000; Fay et al., 1994).

Summary of Learning Disabilities

Like other fields in psychology, the field of learning disabilities is evolving in an erratic and nonlinear manner as the various forces of science, practice, and state and federal legislation all converge to address the needs of children with learning problems. Although much progress has been made, considerably more research will be needed to resolve the many longstanding issues in this field.

MENTAL RETARDATION

Definition of Mental Retardation

Mental retardation is defined by three sine qua non criteria: (a) significant limitations in intellectual functioning, (b) significant limitations in adaptive behavior, and (c) the manifestation of these limitations before the age of 18. These basic criteria are shared by all major diagnostic classification systems, such as the *Diagnostic and Statistical Manual of Mental Disorders* (DSM–IV–TR; APA, 2000), the *International Classification of Diseases, 10th revision* (ICD–10; World Health Organization, 1993), and the *Mental Retardation—Definition, Classification and Supports* of the American Association on Mental Retardation (AAMR, 2002).

Intellectual functioning is operationalized by performance on intelligence tests. A significant limitation in intellectual functioning is characterized by scores of approximately two standard deviations below the mean or lower on a standardized, individually administered intelligence test, considering the standard error of measurement and the type of test used. The construct of adaptive behavior, which is not independent of intelligence, is less well defined, and there is no single instrument that is unanimously accepted to measure all domains of adaptive behavior. The latest rendition of AAMR's definition of adaptive behavior proposes three domains of adaptive skills: conceptual, social, and practical (AAMR, 2002). Deficits in adaptive behavior must be relative to standards of personal independence and social responsibility for the same age group within a culture. Depending on the person's age, different standards apply in assessing adaptive behavior. For example, during infancy and early childhood, sensory motor skills, communication skills, self-help skills, and socialization are emphasized. During childhood and early adolescence, basic academic skills, appropriate reasoning and judgment, and social skills are stressed; and during late adolescence and adult life, vocational and social responsibilities are most important. The third criterion for an individual to be diagnosed as mentally retarded is that the deficits must be manifested during the developmental period, which has been set between birth and 18 years of age. If the intellectual and adaptive deficits appear after the developmental period, then the condition is typically designated as dementia. It is important to note that this three-part definition does not make any assumption about the etiology of the condition and is based solely on the individual's current behavior.

Individuals with mental retardation can be classified by their level of cognitive functioning or by the intensity of supports needed. Levels of intellectual functioning are determined by standard deviations below the mean. For example, using the Wechsler scales with a standard deviation of 15, we speak of mild mental retardation if the IQ falls between 55 and 69, of moderate mental retardation for IQ scores between 40 and 54, severe mental retardation for IQs between 25 and 39, and profound mental retardation for IQ scores below 25. As mentioned, individuals with mental retardation can also be classified in terms of intensity of supports needed. This classification system follows a shift in definition by the AAMR in 1992. The definition placed greater emphasis on environmental interactions that influence an individual's level of functioning. Support intensities can be classified as intermittent (as-needed basis), limited (e.g., time-limited employment training), extensive (e.g., long-term home living support), and pervasive (e.g., life-sustaining technology). Typical areas of support are human development, teaching and education, home living, employment, health and safety, protection and advocacy, and social and behavioral (AAMR, 2002). Each of these areas may be difficult to define and assess.

A variety of factors can complicate a diagnosis of mental retardation. For example, the presence of a severe sensory impairment, such as blindness or deafness, can complicate the process of obtaining a legitimate estimate of IQ performance. Likewise, severe emotional and behavioral disturbance may confound attempts to obtain a reliable estimate of IQ level. In addition, medication may interfere with cognitive neurological functioning (including anticonvulsant drugs). Such effects may or may not be reversible, and they are particularly problematic in the case of individuals with mental retardation, because the signs and symptoms of drug intoxication (e.g., ataxia, confusion, and slurred speech) may be confused with symptoms of mental retardation commonly encountered in this population.

Prevalence of Mental Retardation

Prevalence estimates of mental retardation vary considerably from survey to survey because of differences in the definition of mental retardation, case finding conditions, sampling procedures, and survey methods. For instance, Larsen et al. (2000) analyzed the National Health Interview Survey data (National Center for Health Statistics, 1997, 1998) and state agency statistics (Prouty & Lakin, 1999) and concluded that the prevalence of mental retardation and/or developmental disabilities in the U.S. population was approximately 1.6%, while the prevalence of mental retardation was 0.78%. The prevalence of mental retardation among children and adolescents between the ages of 6 and 21 years of age who received special education services under IDEA, Part B, during the 1998–99 school year was 1.03% (U.S. Department of Education, 2000). These data also revealed significant over- and underrepresentations of

TABLE 17.1

The Percentage of Children Between 6 and 21
Years of Age Served Under the Individuals With
Disabilities Education Act (IDEA), Part B,
During the 1998–99 School Year

	Prevalence in %
American Indians/Alaskan	1.03
Asians/Pacific Islanders	0.43
African American	2.23
Hispanic	0.60
Caucasian	0.79

certain ethnic groups, ranging from a low of 0.4% of the Asian and Pacific Islanders population to 2.2% of the population of African Americans (see Table 17.1).

Etiology

The causes of mental retardation are typically complex interactions of biological, behavioral/psychological, and sociocultural factors. Figure 17.1, which is an adaptation and generalization of a model proposed by Baumeister (1988), delineates the interdependent factors that contribute to a person's psychosocial adaptation. It indicates that genetic endowment, behavioral and mental health characteristics, and demographic parameters (e.g., level of socioeconomic status) in a family tend to be associated with material resources, which in turn influence access to health services, resources, and supports. These factors also influence the quality of a nurturing and safe environment.

A simplified etiological classification of mental retardation is presented in Table 17.2, organized by known causes and outcomes. There are many inherited conditions due to single gene defects that are associated with mental retardation, including dominant disorders (e.g., tuberous sclerosis and neurofibromatosis), recessive disorders (e.g., phenylketonuria [PKU], microcephaly), and sex-linked disorders (e.g., fragile X syndrome and Lesch-Nyhan syndrome). Tuberous sclerosis is a multisystem disease that can affect the brain, kidneys, heart, eyes, lungs, and other organs and is characterized by seizures, mental retardation, and skin and eye lesions. Neurofibromatosis (von Recklinghausen's disease) causes nerve sheath tumors and can affect the development of non-nervous tissues such as bones and skin. It can also lead to developmental abnormalities, including a slight increase in frequency of mental retardation. PKU is caused by deficiency of the enzyme phenylalanine hydroxylase, resulting in a marked elevation of phenylalanine and its metabolites. These are toxic to the central nervous system (CNS), and, if the person is not maintained on a low-phenylalanine diet, they can produce brain damage resulting in severe mental retardation, often in combination with seizures and eczema. Lesch-Nyhan syndrome is a rare disorder of purine metabolism. Its most prominent features are mental retardation, often in association with cerebral palsy, and the presence of self-mutilating behavior and other behavior problems. Fragile X syndrome, which is named after an abnormality in the long arm of the X chromosome, usually affects only males. Its most prominent symptoms include long thin faces, prominent jaws, long ears and hands, and large testes after puberty. There are also likely many cases of mental retardation where more than one gene is involved. Understanding of polygenetic determination, which is only in its infancy at this time, holds great promise for our knowledge about the causation of mental retardation, particularly milder forms of mental retardation.

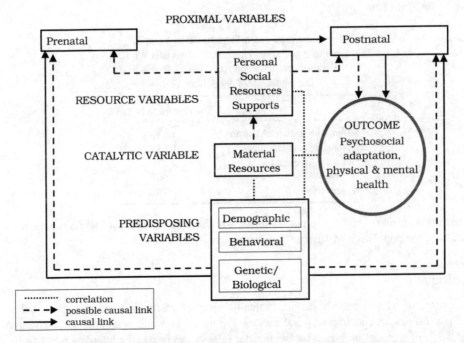

FIG. 17.1.   Generalized model of dynamic influences on individual health, adaptation, and development.
Adapted from The New Morbidity and the Prevention of Mental Retardation. Research Progress, by A. A.
Baumeister, 1988. Nashville, TN: Vanderbilt University. Adapted with permission.

There are also many chromosomal abnormalities that can cause mental retardation. Down syndrome, the most commonly diagnosed form of mental retardation (occurring in about one out of every seven hundred live births) is typically caused by the trisomy 21 variant, which has an extra chromosome 21. Other forms of Down syndrome are caused by translocation, when a major portion of chromosome 21 is translocated onto another chromosome, usually chromosome 14, and thus three copies of this portion of chromosome 21 are inherited. In mosaicism, some cells have a normal complement of forty-six chromosomes, whereas others have forty-seven, and such individuals may vary from apparently being unaffected to having the typical physical presentation of Down syndrome. Other examples of conditions caused by chromosomal abnormalities are Prader-Willi syndrome and Smith-Magenis syndrome. X-Linked anomalies include Klinefelter syndrome and Turner syndrome.

Congenital malformations are also associated with mental retardation. Such developmental defects include anencephaly, a fatal defect in brain development resulting in small or missing brain hemispheres, and hydrocephaly, an accumulation of cerebrospinal fluid (CSF) in the cranium that causes the ventricles and head to enlarge.

Certain maternal diseases can be transmitted to the fetus either in utero (i.e., prenatally) or during delivery. These include rubella (German measles), cytomegaly virus (the most common viral cause of mental retardation), and mumps. If contracted during the first trimester of pregnancy, the effects of rubella can be devastating to the fetus, with severe mental retardation and a variety of physical disorders ensuing. Other maternal infections that can permanently adversely affect the offspring include toxoplasmosis, herpes, human immunodeficiency virus (HIV), and syphilis. Maternal diabetes, especially if uncontrolled, can cause excessive or retarded growth, which may be associated with congenital abnormalities. Blood group incompatibility between the mother and fetus can also lead to mental retardation. Finally, toxemia is a metabolic disorder

TABLE 17.2

Classification of Causes of Mental Retardation

	Causation		*Outcome*
Single gene anomaly	Inherited chromosomal conditions	Dominant autosomal	Tuberous sclerosis, neurofibromatosis
		Recessive autosomal	Phenylketonuria (PKU), microcephaly, galactosemia, Tay-Sachs disease
		X-Linked	Fragile X, Lesch-Nyhan syndrome
	Noninherited chromosomal conditions	Autosomal	Down syndrome, Prader-Willi syndrome, Smith-Magenis Syndrome
		X-Linked	Klinefelter syndrome, Turner syndrome
Polygenetic anomalies			?
Other congenital conditions		Cranial malformations	Anencephaly, hydrocephaly
		Maternal disease (rubella, AIDS, venereal diseases, and blood group incompatibility, maternal diabetes); substance exposure	Mental retardation, fetal alcohol effects and syndrome
Environmental factors	Prenatal causes	*Biological:* neurotoxins (alcohol, lead, mercury, radiation, some illicit drugs) *Psychosocial:* poverty (maternal malnutrition, lack of prenatal care)	Mental retardation, prematurity
	Perinatal causes	*Biological:* trauma during birth, oxygen deprivation, brain hemorrhage, acute maternal herpes	Cerebral palsy, mental retardation, deafness
	Postnatal causes	*Biological:* infections (encephalitis, meningitis), head trauma, toxemia, poisons and toxins (lead and carbon monoxide), malnutrition, cerebrovascular accidents, degenerative diseases *Psychosocial:* secondary effects of poverty, deprivation, neglect, abuse	Mental retardation

of unknown origin that occurs during pregnancy and is characterized by hypertension, edema, and albuminuria (protein in the urine). It can affect the fetus' brain, heart, kidney, and liver.

Other prenatal causes of mental retardation include exposure to a variety of substances or conditions, including toxins such as lead, mercury, radiation, and some illicit drugs. Mothers who consumed alcohol during pregnancy can pose a threat to the fetus of developing fetal alcohol syndrome. The greatest risk for developing fetal alcohol syndrome appears to be during the first 6 weeks of pregnancy, when the mother may not even realize she is pregnant.

Perinatal (i.e., at the time of birth) insults can result in neurological injury, which may later be manifested as cerebral palsy, deafness, or mental retardation. The two most common perinatal causes of mental retardation are prematurity and low birth weight. Traditionally, prematurity is defined as birth before 38 weeks of gestation; low birth weight is defined as having a birth weight less than 2,500 grams (5 1/2 pounds). The major causes of prematurity include maternal health problems, dietary insufficiency, heavy cigarette smoking, and maternal age less than 18 or more than 35 years.

Because the premature neonate enters the world with an underdeveloped organ system, it is more susceptible to a variety of problems, such as oxygen deprivation and brain hemorrhage due to structural weakness of the blood vessels (Baroff & Olley, 1999). Low birth weight is also associated with prematurity, but the full-term infant who is born small for gestational age is also at risk for a variety of problems. Trauma caused by malpresentation of the fetus or disproportion between the infant's head and the pelvis of the mother can result in physical trauma and intracranial hemorrhage, which in turn can cause motor abnormalities, seizures, and mental retardation. Asphyxia is another perinatal factor sometimes associated with subsequent mental retardation, and it may be due to premature separation of the placenta, prolapse of the umbilical cord, anesthesia, or obstruction of the airways (Baroff & Olley, 1999; Kolb & Brodie, 1982). Finally, large birth weight (often associated with maternal diabetes) and herpes transmitted from mother to infant at the time of birth are further complications that can lead to mental retardation.

Of all the postnatal causes of mental retardation, encephalitis (inflammation of the brain) and meningitis (inflammation of the brain's covering membranes) are the most common. Other physical causes include head trauma (from automobile and other accidents), toxemia, poisons and toxins such as lead and carbon monoxide, malnutrition, cerebrovascular accidents or strokes, and degenerative diseases. Another extremely important postnatal cause is psychosocial deprivation. Psychosocial deprivation tends to occur under conditions of poverty, a chaotic living environment, family instability, child abuse and neglect, inadequate caregiving, and an emphasis on day-to-day survival rather than on developmentally appropriate intellectual, social, academic, and cultural stimulation.

Assessment

Intelligence.   To properly establish a diagnosis of mental retardation, the levels of intelligence and adaptive behavior have to be determined. Although this seems like a straightforward task, it is complicated by issues such as the definitions of intelligence used by authors of these tests. Tests such as the Wechsler Intelligence Scale for Children–Third Edition (WISC–III; Wechsler, 1991) and the Stanford-Binet Intelligence Scales: Fourth Edition (SB:FE; Thorndike, Hagen, & Sattler, 1986) are the typical instruments used to assess intelligence. These two tests have some similarities that are especially important given the special demands involved with the assessment of persons with mental retardation.

Wechsler's test and the Stanford-Binet are both based on a view of general intelligence that puts emphasis on the total IQ score. Although these tests comprise smaller subtests that are organized into three main types—verbal, nonverbal (also called performance), and quantitative—the tests measure what is called general ability that has a vague definition (Naglieri, 1999). The verbal tests measure general ability using questions that require the subject to define words or describe how two words are alike. Similarly, the nonverbal subtests measure general ability by tests that involve building a geometric design using blocks or combining parts of an object into a whole (like a child's puzzle). Quantitative subtests measure general ability by questions that involve solving arithmetic word problems or working with numbers. These three types of tests of general intelligence have formed the basic ingredients of intelligence tests since the early 1900s (Naglieri, 1999). For persons with mental retardation, however, the verbal and quantitative tests pose a particular challenge because of their resemblance to achievement tests.

The principal weakness of traditional IQ tests is that they require the examinee to demonstrate knowledge of English and skills at completing math word problems. These skills, also included in many tests of achievement, are particularly difficult for those with a history of school failure and cultural and linguistic differences. The effect that the content of an IQ test has on rates of identification of mental retardation for groups of Caucasian and African American children was illustrated by Naglieri and Rojahn (2000). They found that African American children who were tested with Wechsler's test (which includes verbal and nonverbal tests) were more likely to earn IQ scores that indicated mental retardation than when assessed using the Cognitive Assessment System, which measures basic psychological, or cognitive, processes such as planning and attention rather than verbal and arithmetic skills.

The assessment of persons for mental retardation also can be complicated by hearing impairment, visual impairment, motor problems (e.g., cerebral palsy), and speech problems. Additionally, the need to assess children at a very young age may pose problems with the tests discussed so far, particularly with the Wechsler scales. In the case of persons with visual impairments, Sattler (1988) suggests that the Wechsler scales and the Stanford-Binet (Thorndike et al., 1986), especially the verbal items, can be used so long as the visual handicap is not too severe. For individuals with mental retardation and hearing impairments, verbally based items should be avoided. Suitable nonverbal tests such as the Universal Nonverbal Intelligence Test (UNIT; Bracken & McCallum, 1998) or the Naglieri Nonverbal Ability Test–Individual Form (NNAT–I; Naglieri, 2003) offer well-standardized measures of ability that do not involve language tests. Persons with motor problems may be at a particular disadvantage with timed performance tests (Sattler, 1988), making tests like the NNAT-I and UNIT particularly suitable.

Adaptive Behavior Scales.   The assessment of adaptive behavior plays an important role in both the diagnosis of mental retardation and its ongoing habilitation process. As noted earlier in the chapter, a significant deficit in the ability of a person to behave in such a way as to meet the natural and social demands of his or her environment is one of the defining criteria for the diagnosis of mental retardation. The adaptive behavior assessment also can assist the clinician and other professionals in identifying a person's behavioral strengths and weaknesses, providing for a comparison of the person's behavior across different environments or stimulus conditions (e.g., home vs. school), and providing a relatively uniform and objective method of evaluation for ongoing educational and intervention programs. Sattler (1988) cautions that adaptive behavior scores typically reflect a complex interaction of factors related to the scale itself, the person being rated, the informant who is providing the information for the rating, the examiner who is taking that information, the setting in which the behavior is being observed and reported, and the reasons for the evaluation. Such influences should be kept in mind when interpreting the adaptive behavior scores, and prudent clinical judgment should be applied. Most adaptive behavior scales require an informant such as a parent, teacher, mental health worker, or other direct care staff person (usually relatively naive to the assessment procedures and their standards) to provide detailed information regarding an individual's behavior. Such reports are often subjective and open to potential bias and distortions. For instance, it is relatively common to find that parents rate the overall adaptive behavior of their child higher than the teachers do. The most commonly used instruments for estimating the level of adaptive behavior are the American Association on Mental Retardation (AAMR) Adaptive Behavior Scales (ABS; the School and Community version ABS–S:2 [Lambert, Nihira, & Leland, 1993] and the Residential and Community version ABS–RC:2 [Nihira, Leland, & Lambert, 1993]) and the *Vineland Adaptive Behavior Scales* (Sparrow, Balla, & Cicchetti, 1984).

Assessment of Psychopathology. Individuals with mental retardation often experience mental health and behavior problems, including difficulties with learning, adjustment, integration, and social acceptance. Epidemiological studies have produced variable prevalence rates, but the firm consensus among experts is that people with mental retardation are actually more vulnerable to mental illness than the general population (Nezu, Nezu, & Gill-Weiss, 1992; Rojahn & Tassé, 1996). Unfortunately, providing treatment to persons with a dual diagnosis of mental health problems and mental retardation continues to be hampered by the difficulty of rendering reliable psychiatric diagnoses, particularly in individuals with more severe intellectual disabilities (e.g., Rush & Frances, 2000). Nevertheless, management and treatment of mental health and behavior problems has been a priority for day-to-day care as well as for clinical research, and therefore, assessment and progress monitoring are key issues.

Two kinds of scales can be used for assessment and monitoring of persons with dual diagnosis: generalized and specialized behavior scales. Generalized scales cover a broad band of different conditions, including heterogeneous disorders, such as mood disorders and schizophrenia. Some of these generalized scales were developed deductively to reflect the structure of the DSM (e.g., Reiss Screen for Maladaptive Behavior, Reiss, 1988, Diagnostic Assessment for the Severely Handicapped–II, Matson, 1998), whereas others were developed inductively in an empirical fashion (e.g., Aberrant Behavior Checklist, Aman & Singh, 1986). Specialized behavior rating scales, on the other hand focus on specific, narrowly defined conditions such as specific behavior problems (e.g., Behavior Problems Inventory, Rojahn, et al.).

Functional Assessment and Analysis. Challenging behaviors such as self-injurious behavior (SIB), aggression, and property destruction are common and pose serious problems in persons with mental retardation. They interfere with learning, threaten, the individual and others, reduce the chances for successful community integration, and diminish the person's quality of life (Repp & Karsh, 1990). The functional-behavioral properties of problem behaviors are an important indicator for behavioral treatment selection. To determine functional properties of a target behavior such as gaining attention from others or avoiding unwanted activities, a variety of methods have been devised, ranging from informal and formal observations to interviews, behavior rating scales, and experimental analysis (or functional analysis). Several functional assessment rating scales have been developed. Arguably the most widely used and best-known is the Motivation Assessment System (MAS; Durand & Crimmins, 1988). Like other behavior rating scales, functional assessment rating systems have varying psychometric qualities. Typically the greatest shortcoming of functional assessment rating instruments has been interrater agreement.

In this chapter we have presented a summary of the history of and important considerations regarding learning disabilities and mental retardation. Although these two areas are quite different in their characteristics, both are dominated by controversies over definition and assessment. The very definition of children with learning disabilities is closely tied to how diagnosis is made (intelligence/achievement discrepancy or processing disorder, traditional IQ tests or processing tests, etc.). Although the essential definition of mental retardation seems obvious, it has been difficult to operationalize, especially because the type of intelligence test used can influence the results and definitions of adaptive behavior have been varied. Solutions to these complex problems will depend on the years of research and development to come from future generations of professionals.

REFERENCES

Aman, M. G., & Singh, N. N. (1986). *Aberrant Behavior Checklist: Manual*. East Aurora, NY: Slosson Educational Publications.

American Association on Mental Retardation. (2002). *Mental retardation: Definition, classification, and systems of supports* (10th ed.). Washington, DC: Author.

American Psychiatric Association. (1980). *Diagnostic and statistical manual of mental disorders* (3rd ed.). Washington, DC: Author.

American Psychiatric Association. (1987). *Diagnostic and statistical manual of mental disorders* (3rd ed., rev.). Washington, DC: Author.

American Psychiatric Association. (2000). *Diagnostic and statistical manual of mental disorders* (4th ed., text rev.). Washington, DC: Author.

Baroff, G. S., & Olley, J. G. (1999). *Mental retardation: Nature, cause, and management* (3rd ed.). Philadelphia: Brunner/Mazel.

Baumeister, A. A. (1988, August). *The new morbidity and the prevention of mental retardation. Research Progress*. Nashville, TN: John F. Kennedy Center for Research on Education and Human Development, George Peabody College, Vanderbilt University.

Bishop, D. V. M. (2001). Genetic influences on language impairment and literacy problems in children: Same or different? *Journal of Child Psychology and Psychiatry, 42*, 189–198.

Bracken, B. A., & McCallum, R. S. (1998). *Universal Nonverbal Intelligence Test*. Itasca, IL: Riverside.

Cardon, L. R., Smith, S. D., Fulker, D. W., Kimberling, W. J., Pennington, B. F., & DeFries, J. C. (1994). Quantitative trait locus for reading disability on chromosome 6, *Science, 266*, 276–279.

Clements, S. D. (1966). *Minimal brain dysfunction in children* (NINDS Monograph No. 3, U.S. Public Health Services Publication No. 1415). Washington, DC: U.S. Government Printing Office.

Durand, M. V., & Crimmins, D. B. (1988). Indentifying the variables maintaining self-injurious behavior. *Journal of Autism and Developmental Disorders, 18*, 99–117.

Fay, G. C., Jaffe, K. M., Polissar, N. L., Liao, S., Rivara, J. B., Martin, K. M. (1994). Outcome of pediatric traumatic brain injury at three years: A cohort study. *Archives of Physical Medicine Rehabilitation, 75*, 733–741.

Filipek, P. A. (1999). Neuroimaging in the developmental disorders: The state of the science. *Journal of Child Psychology and Psychiatry, 40*, 113–128.

Hallahan, D. P., & Cruickshank, W. M. (1973). Psychoeducational foundations of learning disabilities. Englewood Cliffs, NJ: Prentice-Hall.

Hallahan, D. P., & Keogh, B. K. (2001). *Research and global perspectives in learning disabilities*. Mahwah, NJ: Lawrence Erlbaum Associates.

Hynd, G. W., Hall, J., Novey, E., Eliopolus, D., Black, K., Gonzales, J., Edmonds, J. E., Riccio, C., & Cohen, M. (1995). Dylsexia and corpus callosum morphology. *Archives of Neurology, 52*, 32–38.

Ingalls, S., & Goldstein, S. (1999). Learning disabilities. In S. Goldstein & C. R. Reynolds (Eds.), *Handbook of neurodevelopmental and genetic disorders in children* (pp. 101–153). New York: Guilford.

Kaufman, A. S., & Kaufman, N. L. (1983). *Kaufman Assessment Battery for Children*. Circle Pines, MN: American Guidance Service.

Kaufman, A. S., & Lichtenberger, E. O. (2000). *Essentials of WISC-III and WPPSI-R Assessment*. New York: John Wiley & Sons.

Kavale, K. A., & Forness, S. R. (1984). A meta-analysis of the validity of the Wechsler Scale profiles and recategorizations: Patterns of parodies? *Learning Disability Quarterly, 7*, 136–151.

Kirk, S. A. (1963). Behavioral diagnosis and remediation of learning disabilities. In *Proceedings of the first annual meeting of the ACLD Conference on Exploration Into the Problems of the Perceptually Handicapped Child* (pp. 1–7). Chicago, Ill: Fund for the Perceptually Handicapped Child.

Kirk, S. A. (1972). *Educating exceptional children* (2nd ed.). Boston: Houghton Mifflin.

Kolb, L. C., & Brodie, H. K. H. (1982). Mental retardation. In L. C. Kolb & H. K. H. Brodie, *Modern Clinical Psychiatry* (10th ed., pp. 715–744). Philadelphia: W. B. Saunders.

Lambert, N., Nihira, K., & Leland, H. (1993). *AAMR Adaptive Behavior Scale—School and Community*. Austin, TX: Pro-Ed.

Larsen, S., Lakin, C., Andersen, L., Kwak, N., Lee, J. H., & Andersen, D. (2000, April). *MR/DD Data Brief*, 2, No. 1. Minneapolis: The College of Education and Human Development, University of Minnesota.

Matson, J. L. (1998). *Diagnostic Assessment for the Severely Handicapped II—Manual*. Baton Rouge, LA: Scientific Publishers Incorporated.

Mercer, C. D., Jordan, L., Allsopp, D. H., & Mercer, A. R. (1996). Learning disabilities definitions and criteria used by state education departments. *Learning Disability Quarterly, 19*, 217–232.

Naglieri, J. A. (1999). *Essentials of CAS assessment*. New York: Wiley.

Naglieri, J. A. (2003). *Naglieri Nonverbal Ability Test—Individual Form*. San Antonio, TX: The Psychological Corporation.

Naglieri, J. A., & Das, J. P. (1997). *Cognitive Assessment System*. Itasca, IL: Riverside.

Naglieri, J. A., & Rojahn, J. (2001). Intellectual classification of black and white children in special education programs using the WISC-III and the Cognitive Assessment System. *American Journal of Mental Retardation, 106*, 359–367.

National Center for Health Statistics. (1997, 1998). 1994, 1995 National Health Interview Survey [database on CD-ROM]. CD-ROM Series 10, Nos. 9 and 10c. SETS version 1.21a. Washington: U.S. Government Printing Office.

National Joint Committee on Learning Disabilities. (1991). Learning disabilities: Issues on definition. *ASHA, 33*, 18–20.

Nezu, M. N., Nezu, A. M., & Gill-Weiss, M. J. (1992). *Psychopathology in persons with mental retardation*. Champaign, IL: Research Press.

Nihira, N., Leland, H., & Lambert, N. (1993). *AAMR Adaptive Behavior Scale—Residential and Community* (2nd ed.). Austin, TX: Pro-Ed.

Pasternack, R. H. (2002, March). *The Demise of IQ testing for children with learning disabilities*. Paper presented at the meeting of the National Association of School Psychologists, Chicago, Illinois.

Public Law 94-142, *Education for All Handicapped Children Act of 1975*. (1977, August). 10. U.S. C. 1401 et seq. Federal Register, 42(163), 42, 474–518.

Prouty, R. W. & Lakin, C. (1999). *Residential services for persons with developmental disabilities: Status and trends through 1998*. Minneapolis: University of Minnesota, Research and Training Center on Community Living, Institute on Community Integration.

Reiss, S. (1988). The Reiss Screen for maladaptive behavior test manual. Worthington, OH: IDS.

Repp, A. C., & Karsh, K. G. (1990). A taxonomic approach to the nonaversive treatment of maladaptive behavior of persons with developmental disabilities. In A. C. Repp & N. N. Singh (Eds.), *Perspectives on the use of nonaversive and aversive interventions for persons with developmental disabilities* (pp. 331–347). Sycamore, IL: Sycamore.

Rojahn, J., Matson, J. L., Lott, D., Esbensen, A. J., & Smalls, Y. (2001). *The Behavior Problems Inventory*: An instrument for the assessment of self-injury, stereotyped behavior and aggression/destruction in individuals with developmental disabilities. *Journal of Autism and Developmental Disorders, 31*, 577–588.

Rojahn, J., & Tassé, M. J. (1996). Psychopathology in mental retardation. In J. W. Jacobson, & J. A. Mulick (Eds.), *Manual on mental retardation and professional practice* (pp. 147–156). Washington, DC: American Psychological Association.

Rush, A. J., & Frances, A. (Eds.). (2000). Treatment of psychiatric and behavioral problems in mental retardation [Special Issue]. *American Journal on Mental Retardation, 105*(3), 159–228.

Sattler, J. M. (1988). *Assessment of Children* (3rd ed.). San Diego: Jerome M. Sattler.

Siegel, L. S. (1989). IQ is irrelevant to the definition of learnig disabilities. *Journal of Learning Disabilities, 22*, 469–479.

Sparrow, S. S., Balla, D. A., & Cicchetti, D. V. (1984). *Vineland Adaptive Behavior Scales*. Circle Pines, MN: American Guidance Service.

Thorndike, R. L., Hagen, E. P., & Sattler, J. M. (1986). *Stanford-Binet Intelligence Scale* (4th ed.). Chicago: Riverside.

Torgesen, J. K. (1998). Learning disabilities: an historical and conceptual overview. In B. Y. L. Wong (Ed.), *Learning about learning disabilities* (pp. 3–28). San Diego: Academic Press.

U.S. Department of Education. (2000). *Twenty-first annual report to Congress on the implementation of the Individuals with Disabilities Education Act*. Washington, DC: U.S. Government Printing Office.

U.S. Department of Education Office of Special Education and Rehabilitative Services. (2002). *A New Era: Revitalizing Special Education for Children and Their Families*. Washington, DC: Author.

Wechsler, D. (1991). *Wechsler Intelligence Scale for Children—Third Edition* (WISC-III). San Antonio, TX: The Psychological Corporation.

World Health Organization. (1993). *International statistical classification of diseases and related health problems* (10th ed.). Geneva, Switzerland: Author.

Yeates, K. O. (2000). Closed-head injury. In K. O. Yeates, M. D. Ris, & H. G. Taylor (Eds.), *Pediatric neuropsychology: Research, theory, and practice* (pp. 92–116). New York: Guilford.

18

Mental Health and Aging: Current Trends and Future Directions

Kristen H. Sorocco
University of Oklahoma Health Sciences Center

Lisa M. Kinoshita and Dolores Gallagher-Thompson
Stanford University School of Medicine

WHO ARE OLDER ADULTS?

The population of older adults is growing at a rapid rate. In 1999, the older adult population (65 years and older) reached 34.5 million (Administration on Aging; AOA, 2000), of whom 20.2 million (56%) are older women. These numbers can be translated into one in every eight Americans being an older person, representing 12.7% of the U.S. population. By 2030, the older adult population will grow to 20%, totaling 70 million older persons (AOA, 2000; Siegel, 1999). The growth of the population of ethnic minority older adults will be one of the reasons for this significant increase: It will increase by 219% overall by the year 2030. The number of older adult Hispanics is expected to increase by 328%; Asian and Pacific Islanders by 285%; Indians, Eskimos, and Aleuts by 147%; African Americans by 131%; followed by European Americans by 81% (AOA, 2000). This rapid increase in the population of ethnic minority older adults has instigated a mental health initiative to examine the impact of culture on mental health issues in general (U.S. Department of Health and Human Services, 2001).

According to a 1999 study of the lifestyles of older adults, 77% of older men were married compared to 43% of women (AOA, 2000). However, this ratio is expected to change, reflecting the rates of separation and divorce in the younger population as they age. The AOA (2000) also reported that in 1998, 67% of older adults lived in a family setting and only a small proportion lived in a nursing home (4.3%). Geographically, about half of the older adult population lived in one of nine states (California, Florida, New York, Texas, Pennsylvania Ohio, Illinois, Michigan, and New Jersey). In regard to health and health care, only 27% of older adults assessed their health as fair or poor according to 1996 statistics (AOA, 2000). There were minimal differences between the sexes in self-reported health, but African American older adults (41.6%) and Hispanic older adults (35.1%) were much more likely to rate their health as fair or poor than were European Americans (26%; AOA, 2000). Given the rapid growth of the older adult population, both the physical and mental health needs of older adults will demand future attention.

The purpose of this chapter is threefold: (a) to discuss the risks and prevalence rates of several common mental health disorders among older adults, (b) to inform readers of the effective and culturally appropriate assessment and treatment interventions for older adults when possible, and (c) to discuss briefly how to meet the future needs of this growing population. Given that space is limited, we chose to focus on those disorders that are either the most prevalent or have been receiving recent research attention, namely: (a) anxiety, (b) depression, (c) dementia, and (d) alcohol abuse. Other disorders, such as late-life schizophrenia, personality disorders, bereavement and adjustment disorders, and more general substance abuse issues, are not included. Interested readers are referred to the suggested readings at the end of the chapter. Before we examine specific mental health issues, we will first examine the process of normal aging.

NORMAL AGING

There are a number of myths concerning aging in our society. Dychtwald and Flower (1990) discussed six of these: (a) people over 65 are old, (b) most older people are in poor health, (c) older minds are not as bright as young minds, (d) older people are unproductive, (e) older people are unattractive and sexless, and (f) all older people are pretty much the same. As a result of these myths (and that is exactly what they are because once they are examined, they are dispelled), many individuals spend an enormous amount of time and money fighting the aging process. For example, women and men buy antiaging products and even undergo painful, expensive surgical procedures to look younger. We also very seldom see the portrayal of older adult role models or positive images of the aging process. Have you ever seen a birthday card that truly celebrates aging? This lack is not surprising, given that our society equates beauty with youth. However, as the population of older adults continues to grow, there will be a need to re-examine these negative stereotypes associated with aging and determine how they influence the mental well-being of older adults.

Clinicians working with older adults need to be aware of these myths and also of normal age-related changes. All individuals do experience some physical, cognitive, and psychosocial changes as they age, but they are often not as severe as the myths of aging suggest. When working with older adults, it is important for therapists to be able to normalize age-related changes. Physically, for example, as individuals age, their risk for disease increases for several reasons. First, many body organs lose strength, and as a result, they do not function as efficiently. For example, changes in the immune system put older adults at increased risk of getting sick. Once ill, they also often take longer to heal in comparison to younger adults. Second, modest increases in blood pressure, blood sugar, and body weight occur with normal aging, thus placing an older adult at risk for cardiovascular disease and stroke.

Cognitive changes include an increase in reaction time and decrease in working memory function. Salthouse (1996) proposed a general slowing hypothesis, positing that the increases in reaction time are due to a general decline of information-processing speed within the aging nervous system (Whitbourne, 2000). Working memory is also affected: It does not function as efficiently with age because of reduced processing speed. Processing speed is slowed by the cognitive difficulty older adults experience when they are required to hold information in storage while simultaneously processing new information. These normal cognitive changes do not mean that older adults are incapable of learning new information, just that they have to use different strategies to learn effectively (Zeiss & Steffen, 1996).

Physical and cognitive decline can directly impact the psychosocial functioning of older adults. For example, physical illness can prevent older adults from engaging in activities that they enjoy, which can be detrimental to their mental health if they do not adapt by identifying new activities in which they can participate. Older adults also are often forced to examine issues related to their own mortality as they experience the deaths of their friends and family members. Those who are caregivers often experience anticipatory grief before the death of their care recipient, due to the strains of caregiving and the role loss they are witnessing (Lindgren, Connelly, & Gaspar, 1999). As with any age, these are common life experiences that might serve as a risk factor for the development of a mental health disorder, but many older adults adapt to these life challenges and experience them successfully.

Whether we are discussing physiological changes associated with aging or psychosocial issues among older adults, it is important not to overgeneralize commonalities among "normal" older adults. In fact, variability among individuals tends to increase with age (Knight, 1986). This variability is due to a wide range of cohort differences among the older adult population in addition to other diversity factors, such as ethnicity. In order to better understand the heterogeneity of the older adult population, Knight (1986) proposed that the older adult population should be divided into subgroups based on age cohorts: young-old (65 to 74 years), old (75 to 84 years), and old-old (85 years and older). As we begin to focus our discussion more on mental health issues among older adults, remember that although some risk factors for mental health problems increase with age, the majority of older adults are able to cope with late life stressors without developing significant mental health problems.

THEORIES OF ADJUSTMENT IN AGING

Henry and Cumming (1959) proposed the *disengagement theory* of aging, which states that there is a gradual withdrawal from life's activities in preparation for death. A contrasting view is *activity theory* (Havighurst, 1961), which proposes that normal aging involves the maintenance of activities and attitudes engaged in during middle age. Activity theory advocates that, to age successfully, people must make adaptations in activities to accommodate any physical, sensory, and or cognitive deficits as they age. A primary criticism of both of these theories is that they are too simplistic, leading later theorists to study human development writers, such as Sigmund Freud and Erik Erikson, who believed that later life adjustment can be understood only by examining earlier life development. Together, these aging theories illustrate the great debate concerning whether human development is continuous (gradual, cumulative from conception to death) or discontinuous (involving distinct changes in the life span) (Halonen & Santrock, 1996). The continuity–discontinuity debate also attempts to answer whether or not our behaviors are stable as we age or if behaviorally individuals can accommodate and make appropriate changes in their behavior depending on life circumstances (Lerner, 1986).

Recently, aging theorists and health professionals have begun to examine the concept of *successful aging* to understand optimal adjustment in later life. Successful aging is a key factor involved in the prevention of physical and mental health disorders in older adults. Successful aging, as defined by the MacArthur Foundation study (Rowe & Kahn, 1998), is the ability of an individual to maintain the following three behaviors: (a) low risk of disease and disease-related disability, (b) high mental and physical function, and (c) active engagement in life. Each of these three behaviors to some extent is independent from the others, but they are not mutually exclusive. In fact, Rowe and Kahn (1998) suggest that there is a hierarchical organization to these three behaviors. Specifically, the absence of disease and disability makes it easier to maintain high mental and physical function, which are the characteristics that enable us to engage in life as we age. Unfortunately, health care continues to focus on providing medical interventions only when necessary and places less emphasis on prevention. In our opinion, prevention is a key to successful aging. Theories of aging highlight the point that although there are some similarities among all older adults, there are also enormous individual differences to consider. Environmental, biological, and psychological factors all affect how an older adult will adjust to normative life events and changes.

Stress and Coping Model

Coping refers to "engaging in behavioral and cognitive efforts to deal with environmental and internal demands and with conflicts between the two" (p. 80, Rice, 1999). Life events may be stressful when the individual perceives them as threatening (either physically or psychologically) and when the individual perceives the demands of the event as exceeding his/her coping resources and skills (Lazarus & Launier, 1978). As individuals evolve and experience their world, they learn ways of coping with stressful life events that help get them through these events with little or no problem. They have the resources and skills needed to cope. As individuals age, however, multiple stressors begin to emerge (including death of spouse, relatives, friends; changes in family roles due to illness; increased demands of caregiving), such that old ways of coping that typically worked in the past are no longer effective in coping with these new situations. This situation in turn may lead to increased psychological distress and mental illness in later life.

COMMON MENTAL HEALTH PROBLEMS OF LATER LIFE

Anxiety Disorders in Older Adults

Given the number of psychosocial losses that an older adult is likely to experience, one might assume that depression is the most common psychological disorder among older adults; however, recent research has shown that anxiety disorders are actually more prevalent (Stanley & Beck, 1998). The Epidemiological Catchment Area (ECA) study found that with the exception of cognitive impairment, anxiety disorders were the most prevalent problem among older adults (Regier et al., 1988). Anxiety symptoms occur in 10% to 20% of the older adult population (Banazak, 1997; Beekman et al., 1998). Little information is available on the specific etiology of anxiety in older adults. Even though the onset of anxiety symptoms in general tends to occur earlier in life (Blazer, George & Hughes, 1991), some observations suggest that some conditions, such as generalized anxiety disorder (GAD), also occur for the first time in later life (Zarit & Zarit, 1998).

Assessment

Because anxiety disorders are difficult to diagnose in older adults, they are often present but go undiagnosed (Scogin, Floyd, & Forde, 2000). The assessment of anxiety disorders among older adults is difficult because of a number of challenges. The first challenge is the association between anxiety symptoms and other psychiatric disorders, particularly depression, because symptoms of anxiety and depression frequently occur simultaneously (Blazer, 2002). Second, anxiety disorders also co-occur with a number of medical diagnoses (Raj and Sheehan,1988), including cardiovascular/respiratory disorders (e.g., asthma, hypertension, chronic obstructive pulmonary disease), endocrine disorders (e.g., hyperthyroidism, hypothyroidism, menopause), neurological disorders (e.g., multiple sclerosis, dementia, Huntington's disease), or substance-related disorders (e.g., drug intoxication and withdrawal symptoms). As we will discuss later, a third challenge is selecting an assessment measure that is reliable and valid for older adult clients.

There is a paucity of research on how ethnic minority older adults conceptualize mental health issues, such as GAD, so it is no surprise that limited research has been conducted examining the cultural appropriateness of anxiety measures for ethnic minority older adults. To our knowledge, there is only one anxiety measure, the Beck Anxiety Inventory (BAI; Beck, Epstein, Brown, & Steer, 1988), for which reliability and validity have been assessed specifically with a population of ethnic minority older adults. Hilliard and Iwamasa (2001) conducted a study to determine if a Western measure of anxiety (BAI) was psychometrically sound to use with Japanese American older adults and whether they conceptualize anxiety in the same way as Western diagnostic criteria. Findings indicated that the BAI was a reliable and valid measure to use with Japanese American older adults, but future research with larger samples including other ethnic groups was recommended. However, Hilliard and Iwamasa's (2001) study found that conceptually, Japanese American older adults tended to use both anxiety and depressive symptoms to describe an anxious Japanese American older adult. Therefore, it might be important to assess for subsyndromal levels of both anxiety and depression with this population.

Generalized Anxiety Disorder

GAD is one of the most common anxiety disorders among older adults (Blazer et al., 1991). Even though GAD was not a DSM (see later) diagnosis at the time of the ECA study, researchers have since established its high prevalence rate among older adults. Blazer et al. (1991) found that 39% of older adults who were surveyed had experienced GAD onset before late adulthood; however, 50% who had a diagnosis of GAD had experienced their symptoms for 5 years or less. According to DSM–IV–TR (American Psychiatric Association [APA], 2000), the primary symptom of GAD is unrealistic or excessive worry about two or more life circumstances for a period of at least 6 months. In addition, individuals need to experience at least three of the following symptoms: restlessness, being keyed up or on edge, being easily fatigued, difficulty concentrating or mind going blank, irritability, muscle tension, or sleep disturbance. The final criterion for this diagnosis is that the symptoms need to cause the older adult significant distress or impairment. A diagnosis of GAD in an older adult is an example of a mental health disorder that must take into account age-related factors. Given the number of physiological symptoms associated with GAD there is the possibility for misdiagnosis if physical health factors are not adequately evaluated.

Behavioral Interventions.   Limited research has been conducted examining the effectiveness of treatment interventions for older adults suffering from anxiety disorders. Furthermore, most of the research has been conducted with older adults with general symptoms of anxiety rather than specific disorders such as GAD (Wetherell, 2002). These studies have found that behavioral interventions (relaxation, exposure therapy, and imaginal exposure) are effective with older adults with symptoms of anxiety (DeBerry, Davis, & Reinhard, 1989; Scogin, Rickard, Keith, Wilson, & McElreath, 1992). In comparison to progressive muscle relaxation, imaginal relaxation techniques (visualizing peaceful nature scenes) are more appropriate than progressive muscle relaxation to use with older adults. Progressive muscle relaxation, which involves the actual tensing and relaxing of muscles, might be ineffective and even painful to older adults with particular medical problems, such as arthritis.

Even though relatively few studies have examined the effectiveness of Cognitive-behavioral therapy (CBT) for GAD among older adults, CBT appears to be a potentially useful intervention, although modifications in format might need to be made for older adult clients (Beck & Stanley, 1997; Wetherell, 1998). CBT teaches clients to identify and modify unhealthy patterns in their thoughts, emotions, and behavioral responses. Stanley, Beck, and Glassco (1996) found that both CBT and a supportive therapy control group were effective interventions for older adults with GAD and that gains were maintained at 6 months follow-up. Suggested modifications when using CBT with older adults clients suffering with GAD include using a group format to increase social support networks, teaching at a slower pace, providing multiple examples when teaching the intervention, using handouts, and repeating information (Wetherell, 2002).

Pharmacological Interventions.   Antianxiety medications are frequently used among the older adult population (Graham & Vidal-Zeballos, 1998). This approach is not surprising, given that many older adults seek treatment for mental health problems from their primary care doctors. Because of space, we are unable to discuss specific drugs for the treatment of GAD among older adults, but would like to present a few cautions. First, normal age-related physiological changes that older adults experience impact drug absorption, distribution, metabolism, and sensitivity to side effects (Scogin et al., 2000). Generally, older adults are more susceptible to side effects of medication and are at a greater risk of drug interactions. Second, older adults are often taking several medications, which also puts them at a greater risk for a drug interaction. Even though for some older adults medication is necessary for successful treatment, many older adults would benefit from nonpharmacological interventions.

Posttraumatic Stress Disorder in Older Adults

Posttraumatic stress disorder (PTSD) in older adults has recently received attention in the research literature. Much of the available research related to PTSD in older adults focuses on veteran populations (namely World War II and Korean War veterans), Holocaust survivors, and to some extent on victims of assault in later life.

One of the issues to consider when examining PTSD in older adults is the nosology used to describe the psychological phenomenon. According to the *Diagnostic and Statistical Manual of Mental Disorders*, fourth edition, text revision (DSM–IV–TR; APA, 2000), PTSD is characterized by the following: (a) presence of a recognizable stressor that would evoke significant symptoms of distress in most individuals, (b) re-experiencing of the trauma, (c) hyperarousal symptoms, and (d) avoidance of stimuli that remind the individual of the traumatic event. However, this nosology was developed largely according to responses from younger individuals rather than from older adults. Moreover, PTSD was not considered a formal diagnosis until 1980 (DSM–III, 1980). Before this time, PTSD symptoms were often referred to as shell shock, combat fatigue, war neurosis, transient situational disturbance, or survivor's syndrome (Averill & Beck, 2000). Furthermore, accurate prevalence rates are nonexistent because no prevalence studies were conducted immediately following potentially traumatic historical experiences (e.g., World War I, World War II, Korean War). When PTSD became an official diagnosis in 1980, a number of individuals who experienced traumatic events earlier in their lifetime had died.

Thus, the question remains: is PTSD in older adults the same psychological phenomenon as PTSD in younger adults? Specific symptom profiles are not the same in older adults compared to younger adults, especially in those individuals who experience chronic PTSD (Averill & Beck, 2000). Such discrepancies impact accurate prevalence rates and accurate reporting of comorbid diagnoses.

Specific patterns of PTSD symptoms have been found in some older adult veterans (McLeod, 1994). For example, McLeod found that World War II veterans initially coped well in the immediate years following their wartime period. Then, they experienced an exacerbation of symptoms that lasted for approximately 5 years, followed by a time in middle age when their symptoms were masked as they excelled in their careers and family life. As these veterans grew older, their PTSD symptoms again were exacerbated. Thus, another complicating issue related to the investigation of PTSD in later life is the time of the assessment or study. Furthermore, late-onset PTSD (meaning no PTSD symptoms until old age) also has been documented in some older combat veterans (Spiro, Schnurr, & Aldwin, 1994).

In other studies of World War II veterans, it was found that intrusive symptoms decreased over time, whereas avoidance symptoms and isolation from others increased as the veterans grew older (McFarlane, 1990). World War II veterans who were treated in an outpatient mental health clinic commonly complained of insomnia, nightmares, irritability, social isolation, and flashbacks (Kaup, Ruskin, & Nyman, 1994). A 45-year retrospective study of surviving Pearl Harbor veterans found that roughly two thirds of them experience intrusive memories, approximately one half report survivor guilt, and one third report avoidance and hyperarousal symptoms and emotional numbing (Wilson, Harel, & Kahana, 1989). Thus, these PTSD symptoms remained with the veterans even decades after their initial traumatic experience. Overall, however, most studies have found that veterans report a decrease in PTSD symptoms over time, with the most reduction experienced in intrusive thoughts and survivor guilt.

Assessment of PTSD in Older Adults

Accurate assessment of PTSD in older adults is difficult because only a handful of PTSD assessment measures and semistructured interviews have been validated with this population. First, the combat and civilian forms of the *Mississippi PTSD Scales* (MISS) (Watson, 1990), thirty-five-item self-report measures, were found to be highly correlated with other diagnostic measures of PTSD (McFall, Smith, Mackay, & Tarver, 1990). Moreover, the combat form of the MISS was found to be the most accurate measure of PTSD severity in older adults who were former prisoners of war (Neal, Hill, Hughes, Middleton, & Busuttil, 1995). *The Clinician Administered PTSD Scale* (CAPS) (Blake et al., 1990) is a semistructured clinical interview used to assess core and associated symptoms of PTSD based on DSM diagnostic criteria. The CAPS has been used with older adults who experienced trauma during wartime events. It was found to have good discriminatory power, with a 93% accuracy rate (Hyer, Summers, Boyd, & Litaker, 1996).

Other validation studies have shown inconsistent results. Investigations of the *Impact of Events Scale* (IES) (Horowitz, Wilner, & Alvarez, 1979), a fifteen-item, self-report questionnaire used to assess intrusion and avoidance symptoms, suggests equivocal data for its use with older adults. Such inconsistent results suggest that the type of traumatic event is important when assessing PTSD in older adults (Neal et al., 1995). Thus, future research is needed to validate existing PTSD measures for older adults or researchers will need to develop specific measures to assess PTSD in older adults.

Treatment for PTSD in Later Life

There is evidence to suggest that psychotherapy, specifically CBT (Gillespie, Duffy, Hackmann, & Clark, 2002) and eye movement desensitization and reprocessing (EMDR) (Hyer, 1999), as well as certain psychopharmacological interventions, such as paroxetine/Paxil (Tucker et al., 2001; Wagstaff, Cheer, Matheson, Ormrod, & Goa, 2002), fluvoxamine/Luvox

(Martenyi, Brown, Zhang, Prakah, & Koke, 2002), and gabapentin/Neurontin (Hammer, Brodrick, & Labbbate, 2001) are effective in treating PTSD in young adults. However, models of PTSD in older adults have not been well formulated; therefore, the treatments for PTSD in older adults are not well studied.

Initial reports of common psychotherapeutic treatments, such as CBT, for older adults who have PTSD are promising. Hyer et al. (1990) evaluated a 12-session CBT protocol with older patients who had chronic PTSD or acute stress reactions related to loss. The CBT protocol included exploration of irrational beliefs as well as anxiety management training (AMT) that included relaxation. Although objective measures showed no difference between the CBT group and control group, participants reported that they benefited from the cognitive therapy, AMT, and relaxation training (Hyer et al., 1990).

Similarly, preliminary results related to the efficacy of eye movement desensitization and reprocessing (EMDR) treatment for PTSD in older adults are available (Hyer, 1995). EMDR is a type of psychotherapy that integrates successful elements from other therapeutic approaches and combines them with eye movements or other forms of rhythmical stimulation in ways that stimulate the brain's information processing system. Furthermore, EMDR involves limited exposure to specific information related to the trauma (Boudewyns & Hyer, 1997). This type of treatment uses emotions, sensations, cognitions, and images to uncover the traumatic event(s) at a pace set by the client. EMDR is different from CBT treatment in that it is more active and guides the client to uncover the trauma when this information is not readily available and allows for positive patient change (Hyer & Brandsma, 1997). In recent years, however, EMDR has received divergent reactions from researchers and clinicians alike. The confusion in the EMDR literature is based on the following five issues: (a) the lack of an empirically validated model to explain the effects of EMDR, (b) inaccurate and selective reporting of research, (c) poorly designed empirical studies, (d) outcome research with flawed treatment fidelity, and (e) a number of biased or inaccurate literature reviews (Perkins & Rouanzoin, 2002). Thus, sound outcome studies that investigate the efficacy of EMDR with older adults are needed in the future.

Depression in Later Life

Clinically significant depression is one of the most common psychiatric disorders reported by older adults with a prevalence of 4.4%, second only to anxiety disorders in prevalence (11.4%; U.S. Department of Health and Human Services, 1999). Although research suggests that the prevalence of major depressive disorder is relatively rare in community-dwelling older adults (Judd & Kunovac, 1998; Weissman, Bruce, Leaf, Florio, Holzer, 1991), epidemiological studies suggest that 10% to 25% of community-dwelling older adults over the age of 65 years report depressive symptoms that do not meet a clinically significant diagnosis of major depression (Blazer, 2002).

According to the DSM–IV–TR (APA, 2000), the diagnostic criteria for major depressive disorder include the following: depressed mood and/or diminished interest or pleasure in daily activities, weight loss or weight gain, sleep difficulty, psychomotor agitation or retardation, loss of energy, feelings of worthlessness or excessive guilt, decreased ability to concentrate or difficulty making decisions, recurrent thoughts of suicide or death (APA, 2000). Bereavement, adjustment disorder, or dysthymia make up the rest of the depressive symptoms. However, the first onset of dysthymia in later life appears to be rare (Blazer, 1986), suggesting that those suffering from chronic depression developed symptoms in middle age or young adulthood.

Four older adult populations have higher levels of depression than community-dwelling individuals: nursing home patients (Parmelee, Katz, & Lawton, 1989), recently bereaved individuals (Gallagher, Breckenridge, Thompson, & Peterson, 1983; Thompson, Tang, Kaye, &

TABLE 18.1

Adaptations in Treatment With Older Adults

- Discuss age difference between therapist and client
- Foster independence
- Use slower pace
- Make modifications for sensory and/or cognitive deficits
- Address common later life themes

Gallagher-Thompson, 2004), family caregivers (Gallagher, Rose, Rivera, Lovett, & Thompson, 1989), and individuals who are cognitively impaired (Teri & Gallagher-Thompson, 1991; Teri & Logsdon, 1991). In physically impaired, cognitively intact nursing home patients, the prevalence of late-life depression increases, ranging from 20% of new admissions to 42% of nursing home residents (Parmelee, Katz, & Lawton, 1989). This high number likely reflects the many losses (e.g., loss related to physical decline, loss of control and independence) that older adults experience when they are institutionalized in long-term care settings. Similarly, in recently bereaved individuals and cognitively impaired patients, 20% to 30% report significant depression. However, close to 50% of family caregivers are at least mildly depressed, with approximately 25% reaching criteria for major depression.

Assessment of Late Life Depression

Prevalence rates for depression in older adults vary widely because of differences in diagnostic systems, assessment measures, and assessment procedures. In particular, there are difficulties due to the nature of depression measures for older adults. Most commonly used depression inventories for younger adults—for example, Beck Depression Inventory–II (BDI–II; Beck, Steer, & Brown, 1996) and the Center for Epidemiologic Studies Depression Scale (CES–D; Radloff, 1977)—include items that assess somatic symptoms that are typically more prevalent in older adults. Therefore, these items may artificially increase so they can artificially increase the total score for depression. Yesavage et al. (1983) created a thirty-item depression measure, Geriatric Depression Scale (GDS), that is specifically designed to assess depression in older adults (see Table 18.2 for additional information). The GDS assesses psychological aspects of depression (e.g., pessimism about the future) rather than physical symptoms. Furthermore, because of the likely presence of concurrent health problems, clinicians should consult with medical professionals to rule out a medical basis for the observed depression. In addition, cognitive dysfunction can cloud the diagnostic picture: Decreased ability to concentrate and make decisions are common among people with cognitive impairments (e.g., Alzheimer's disease, vascular dementia) as well, which unfortunately are also common in later life. (For a detailed review of the issues involved in assessing depression among older adults, see Lichtenberg [1996]; Mui, Burnette, and Chen [2001]; and Powers, Thompson, and Gallagher-Thompson [2002]).

One primary question of interest for researchers and clinicians alike is the following: Is depression experienced differently by older adults than by younger adults? Preliminary research in the area suggests that both the type and severity of depression may be different. Two qualitatively different syndromes, the depressive syndrome and the depletion syndrome, were found through factor analysis (Newmann, Engel, & Jensen, 1991a, 1991b) and help illustrate these differences. The *depressive syndrome* is characterized by the emotional and cognitive features of depression, whereas the *depletion syndrome* is characterized by decreased appetite, lack of interest, feelings of hopelessness, and thoughts of death. Younger adults more readily report

TABLE 18.2

Summary of Geriatric Measures

Name of Scale	Key Citations
Beck Anxiety Inventory (BAI)	Beck, Epstein, Brown, & Steer, 1988
Beck Depression Inventory (BDI)	Gallagher, Nies, & Thompson, 1982
CES-D	Radloff, 1977
Geriatric Depression Scale (GDS)	Yesavage, Brink, Rose, Lum, Huang, Adey, & Leirer, 1983
Mini-Mental State Examination (MMSE)	Folstein, Folstein, & McHugh, 1975
Alzheimer's Disease Assessment Scale (ADAS)	Rosen, Mohs, & Davis, 1984
The Clinical Dementia Rating Scale (CDR)	Hughes, Berg, Danziger, Cohen, & Martin, 1982
Dementia Rating Scale (DRS)	Mattis, 1976
Mississippi PTSD Scales	Neal, Hill, Hughes, Middleton, & Busuttil, 1995
Clinician Administered PTSD Schedule (CAPS)	Hyer, Summers, Boyd, & Litaker, 1996
Michigan Alcoholism Screening Test–Geriatric Version (MAST–G)	Blow et al., 1992
CAGE	Ewing, 1984
	Fleming, 1995

features related to the former whereas older adults are more likely to report aspects of the latter (Newman, Engel, & Jensen, 1991a, 1991b). However, in actual practice, most older adults who seek treatment for depression do so because of losses that have overwhelmed their capacity to cope. These common losses include those related to social support network, health problems, and control and independence. Working successfully with older adults requires professionals to receive geropsychology training so that they can accurately assess the most common subtypes of geriatric depressive symptoms (Powers et al., 2002).

Treatment of Depression in Late Life

Many clinicians believe that psychotherapy is essential in the treatment of depression in older adults. Still others posit that psychotherapy in conjunction with psychopharmacologic interventions is beneficial to older adults who are acutely suffering from severe depression or who have recovered from a depressive episode and are now in the maintenance phase of treatment (National Institutes of Health Consensus Development Conference Consensus Statement, 1991). Empirical evidence suggests that both cognitive-behavioral therapy (Fry, 1984; Gallagher-Thompson & Steffen, 1994; Gatz et al., 1998; Thompson, 1996; Thompson, Coon, Gallagher-Thompson, Sommer, & Koin, 2001; Thompson, Gallagher, & Breckenridge, 1987) and interpersonal psychotherapy (Klerman, Weissman, Rounsaville, & Chevron, 1984) are effective in decreasing depressive symptoms in older adults. Moreover, advances in psychopharmacologic treatments have made additional effective interventions available to older adults diagnosed with depression.

Cognitive-Behavioral Psychotherapy. CBT is a structured, short-term psychotherapy in which the client learns new skills (e.g., initiating adaptive behaviors, challenging unhelpful thoughts) to cope with and overcome his/her depressive symptoms. The CBT model focuses on the interconnection of behavior, cognitions, emotions, and physiologic factors within the individual. The trained CBT therapist works with the individual to change unhelpful behaviors and cognitions to improve general mood state. The goal of CBT is to provide the individual with new, more adaptive skills that enable him/her to initiate specific activities and to challenge and replace distorted thought patterns with more rational ones (Beck, 1976; Lewinsohn, Munoz, & Youngren, & Zeiss, 1978).

Considerable evidence demonstrates that CBT is effective in the treatment of depression in older adults (see the comprehensive review article by Gatz et al., 1998, which contains data on a number of key studies on depression in later life), including individuals with dementia (Teri & Gallagher-Thompson, 1991; Teri & Logsdon, 1991). Moreover, cognitive therapy for older adults with severe depressive symptoms was found to be more accepted and preferred by these individuals than was cognitive bibliotherapy or antidepressant medication (Landreville, Laundry, Baillargeon, Guerette, & Matteau, 2001).

Manualized CBT treatments have been used for treating late-life depression in outpatients (Thompson, Gallagher-Thompson, & Dick, 1996), in family caregivers (Gallagher-Thompson, Ossinalde, & Thompson, 1996) and in Latina family caregivers (Gallagher-Thompson, Ossinalde, Menendez et al., 1996). Studies suggest that this form of therapy is effective with Latina and Caucasian caregivers (Gallagher-Thompson, Arean, Rivera, &Thompson, 2001; Gallagher-Thompson, Lovett et al., 2000). The latter investigation involved almost 200 caregivers and found that participants in the cognitive-behavioral psychoeducational group showed significant reductions in their depression and increased use of adaptive coping behavior compared to those in the wait-list control group (Gallagher-Thompson, Lovett et al., 2000). Other studies have found similar positive results, suggesting that CBT is an effective treatment for many common problems in later life.

Interpersonal Psychotherapy.   Interpersonal psychotherapy (IPT) is a type of therapy that was designed to treat depressed patients. IPT is a focused, time-limited therapy that focuses on the current interpersonal relationships of the depressed patient. Throughout treatment, the role of genetic, biochemical, developmental, and personality factors are also examined as they are believed to relate to the patient's vulnerability to depression (Klerman, Weissman, Rounsaville, & Chevron, 1984). IPT focuses on past and current interpersonally relevant issues that are related to the current depression. IPT is well established as a successful treatment for depression in younger adult populations (Klerman et al., 1984). (See also chapter 16 in this book.) Moreover, evidence suggests that interpersonal psychotherapy is effective in reducing depressive symptoms in older adults (Hinrichsen, 1999). Older adults commonly experience interpersonal changes such as loss of close friends or family members, transitions in social roles, conflicts with others, and the need to acquire new skills to adapt to changes in life that often makes IPT ideal for older adults (Hinrichsen, 1999). Moreover, the combination of nortriptyline, a tricyclic antidepressant, and weekly sessions of ITP in the initial and continuation phases of treatment for depression in late life was shown to benefit older adults (Reynolds et al., 1992).

More than 20 years of research suggests that psychopharmacological treatments can be beneficial for depressed older adults (Bell, 1999; Powers et al., 2002). Moreover, there is evidence to suggest that antidepressants are just as effective in older adult patients as they are in younger adults (Katona, 2000). (See also chapter 16 in this volume.) However, both the safety and efficacy of psychopharmacological treatment for older adults are complicated by pharmacokinetic changes associated with aging, the increased potential for adverse drug interactions and polypharmacy issues, the effect of psychotropic medications on certain concomitant illnesses, and difficulties in the management of common side effects.

In the past, tricyclic antidepressant (TCA) medications were commonly prescribed for depression in older adults. However, adverse side effects related to the anticholinergic effects of the TCAs (e.g., exacerbation of glaucoma, blurry vision, increased confusion, increased risk of urinary tract infection) were found to be intolerable by many older adult patients (Katona, 2000).

TCAs are also associated with postural hypotension and dizziness, so older adults are at higher risk of falling when taking TCAs to treat their depression. Moreover, TCAs are potentially fatal at high dosages. Thus, there is increased concern when an older adult is depressed that he or she may attempt suicide via overdose using TCAs (Kasper, Lepine, Mendlewicz, Montgomery, & Rush, 1995).

In recent years, a newer class of antidepressants called selective serotonin reuptake inhibitors (SRRIs) have been found to be effective in treating depression in older adults and have a safer side-effect profile compared to TCAs (Montgomery, 1998). For instance, SSRIs do not have the same anticholinergic effects of TCAs, and SSRIs have a lower potential for adverse drug interaction compared to TCAs (Katona, 2000). Moreover, in a meta-analysis of studies in which older adult patients took either SSRIs or TCAs to treat their depression, more individuals receiving an SSRI remained in the studies as they reported fewer adverse events related to the medication (Montgomery & Kasper, 1995). SSRIs were found to be as effective as TCAs in the treatment of late-life depression with better tolerability (Altamura et al., 1989). Thus, SSRIs rather than TCAs are often the current treatment of choice when treating an older adult suffering from depression. (See also chapter 16 in this volume.)

Suicide in Older Adults

The severe reality of suicide is an important issue to consider when an older adult is depressed. Given the multiple losses that older adults experience, suicide in later life has come to the forefront of attention in the last decade (Gallagher-Thompson & Osgood, 1997; McIntoch, Santos, Hubbard, & Overholser, 1994; Osgood, 1985; Richman, 1999). Older adults commit suicide at a higher rate than any other age group. Specifically, the highest rate of suicide (24.9 cases per 100,000 of the population) was in the 75 to 84-year-old age range (Hoyert, Kochanek, & Murphy, 1999). Furthermore, in the last 5 years, data suggest that older adults made up 13% of the U.S. population but committed 19% of all suicides (Kochanek & Murphy, 1999). In comparison, younger adults composed 14% of the U.S. population and committed 14% of all suicides. According to Zarit and Zarit (1998), the increase seen in suicide rates in older adults is due to high rates among older men. The ratio of suicide rates of men versus women was 4.2 to 1 in 1990 (Moscicki, 1995). Research shows that suicide rates in men dramatically increase at age 60 and peak in men over the age of 85. Moreover, older men compared to younger men tend to make suicide attempts with more lethal means (e.g., firearms, hanging) and with the serious intent to end their lives compared to women. Differences in suicide rates are related not only to gender but also to ethnicity. Specifically, suicide rates tend to increase over time for Caucasian, Japanese, Chinese, and Filipino American males, whereas in African American and Native American individuals, the suicide rate tends to peak at age 35 and then steadily decline in older age (Zarit & Zarit, 1998).

Researchers have found numerous risk factors related to suicide in older adults. The two most important risk factors are depression and physical illness, especially when the physical illness involves pain, discomfort, and poor prognosis (Zarit & Zarit, 1998). In some cases, the physical illness is not life threatening but causes a decrease in quality of life for the older adult. Furthermore, widows, widowers, and divorced men are more likely to commit suicide than married individuals, particularly if they also have poor social support overall. Additional risk factors include alcoholism, recent losses, and history of prior suicide attempts. Furthermore, although it is not common, some suicides occur in institutional settings, such as nursing homes. Individuals who commit suicide in nursing homes tend to have intact cognitive functioning and no diagnosis of dementia. Similarly, increases in suicide risk in older adults may be higher in those individuals who are anticipating nursing home placement.

Dementing Disorders

As the population of older adults exponentially increases in the United States, age-related diseases will inevitably increase. For example, dementia has an enormous impact on the patient, his/her family, and the health care system in general. According to Fields (1998), *dementia* is defined as "a deterioration in mental capacities that goes beyond the changes expected to occur with the normal aging process" (p. 211). According to the DSM–IV (APA, 1994), dementia syndromes are characterized by the "development of multiple cognitive deficits (including memory impairment) that are due to the direct physiological effects of a general medical condition, to the persisting effects of a substance, or to multiple etiologies" (p. 133). Moreover, dementia is an all-encompassing term used to refer to cognitive decline and impairment, especially in memory function and learning.

Prevalence of Common Dementing Disorders

Over the past several years, research has revealed the complexity and heterogeneity of dementia. Thus research provides evidence for several variants of the disease (e.g., Alzheimer's disease, vascular dementia, Lewy body dementia, frontotemporal dementia), all with different prevalences and etiologies. Postmortem studies of Alzheimer's disease (AD) patients suggest that AD is the most common form of dementia, accounting for 80% of cases (Luis, Mittenberg, Gass, Duara, 1999). The second most prevalent subtype is vascular dementia, which accounts for 7% to 18% of all cases (Luis et al., 1999). For discussions of other types of dementia, see Grossman, 2002; Lezak, 1995; Simard, van Reekum, and Cohen, 2000.

Alzheimer's Disease (AD)

AD is a progressive neurodegenerative disease in which neurons are lost and abnormalities develop in the neocortical areas of the brain (Kolb & Whishaw, 1996). It has specific neuropathological characteristics, including global neuronal loss, beta-amyloid deposits in cerebral blood vessels, and the development of neuritic plaques and neurofibrillary tangles (U.S. Department of Health and Human Services, 2000). These structural changes in the brain affect the association areas of the cerebral cortex, the hippocampus, and the middle and temporal lobes. Another significant neurological change that occurs in AD is a decrease in the concentration of the neurotransmitter acetylcholine that is related to the severity of the disease (O'Hara, Mumenthaler, Yesavage, 2000; U.S. Department of Health and Human Services, 2000).

According to the DSM–IV–TR (APA, 2000), a diagnosis of dementia is given when the following cognitive deficits are present: (a) memory impairment and (b) one or more of the following cognitive impairments: aphasia (language disturbance), apraxia (impaired ability to do motor tasks given intact motor function), agnosia (inability to recognize or identify objects given intact sensory function), or disturbance of executive function (i.e., planning, organizing, sequencing, abstraction skills).

The first signs of AD include subtle decline in memory functions when the individual is in a clear state of consciousness. This condition leads to impairment in daily functioning (e.g., increased problems handling finances, difficulty participating in conversations) (Braak et al., 1999; O'Hara et al., 2000). As the disease progresses, additional cognitive changes occur (e.g., deterioration in language function, impairment in ability to care for oneself) and quality of life of both the patient and caregiver often deteriorates. Personality changes and behavioral disturbances (e.g., agitation, physical aggression, hallucinations, delusions, sleep disturbance, wandering) may also occur as the disease progresses (O'Hara et al., 2000). In the final stages, the motor system deteriorates, motor reaction to stimuli decreases (often related to muscle spasms), and the individual becomes fully dependent on others for self-care. He or she may require nursing home placement at this point, when the burdens of care overwhelm the caregiver's capacity to respond. On average, an individual lives with AD for approximately 8 to 10 years after the initial diagnosis (U.S. Department of Health and Human Services, 2000).

Vascular Dementia (VaD)

VaD is defined by DSM–IV–TR (APA, 2000) as described previously for AD, but also includes the presence of focal neurologic signs and symptoms or laboratory evidence that is indicative of cerebrovascular disease (CVD; U.S. Department of Veterans Affairs, 1997). CVD is defined by the presence of focal signs on neurological examination, such as hemiparesis (weakness on one side of the body) and evidence of relevant CVD via brain imaging (e.g., multiple large vessel strokes, or a single major stroke placed in an area where multiple cognitive areas are disrupted). In brief, VaD occurs after an individual has experienced either a large stroke that in turn affects multiple cognitive functions or a series of small strokes. When an individual is diagnosed with VaD, it is difficult to know what cognitive deficits to expect because they vary from one individual to the next, depending on the location of the stroke in the brain. Moreover, a definitive diagnosis of VaD is complicated because an individual may have a mixed vascular degenerative dementia in which the symptoms of a progressive dementia, like AD (e.g., presence of neurofibrillary tangles and neuritic plaques), is accompanied or complicated by a cerebrovascular accident.

Risk Factors for AD and VaD

Researchers have identified a number of risk factors related to AD including the following: genetic predisposition, advanced age, ethnicity, a history of head trauma, and Down's syndrome (O'Hara, Mumenthaler, Yesavage, 2000; Petronis, 1999; Teng et al., 1998). In recent years, researchers have linked a specific gene to Alzheimer's disease, called apolipoprotein E4 (ApoE4), which can be inherited from the paternal and/or maternal sides. Thus, individuals who test positive for one or both of these ApoE4 alleles are at greater risk for eventually developing AD later in life than are those who do not have ApoE4 alleles. Individuals who inherited one ApoE4 allele have twice the risk, and individuals with two ApoE4s are ten times more likely to develop AD (O'Hara, Mumenthaler, Yesavage, 2000). Furthermore, the prevalence and incidence of AD increases as one advances in age. Estimates suggest that the incidence of AD doubles every 5 years after age 60 (Cummings, Vinters, Cole, Khachaturian, 1998).

Ethnicity is another possible risk factor, although research on ethnicity has been inconsistent (Fillenbaum, Heyman, et al., 1998). African Americans and Latino Americans may have a higher risk of AD than white Americans (Teng et al., 1998). Risk factors for VaD include health problems related to CVD, such as high blood pressure, diabetes, abnormally high fatty content of the blood, and cigarette smoking (Lezak, 1995).

Assessment of Dementia

The goals of the assessment process are fourfold: (a) to provide an accurate diagnosis, (b) to provide the patient and family with prognosis information, (c) to review treatment options with the patient and family, and (d) to assist the patient and family in planning for the management of the disease (Riley & Carr, 1989). A diagnosis of AD is typically made within the context of an interdisciplinary team that includes physicians, psychologists, nurses, and other health care professionals who have specialty training in geriatrics or geropsychology. In an attempt to make an accurate diagnosis, the diagnostic team gathers a combination of data such as neuroimaging results from computed tomography (CT) or magnetic resonance imaging (MRI) scans, neuropsychological test results, patient's medical records, and caregiver/informant observations (U.S. Department of Veterans Affairs, 1997). Several assessment measures are commonly administered. The Mini-Mental State Examination (MMSE) (Folstein, Folstein, & McHugh, 1975) is typically given to assess global cognitive functioning (see Table 18.2). The Alzheimer's Disease Assessment Scale (ADAS) (Rosen, Mohs, & Davis, 1984) assesses both cognitive and noncognitive symptoms related to AD (e.g., memory, language, constructions, ideational praxis, mood and behavioral disturbances) (see Table 18.2). The Clinical Dementia Rating Scale (CDR) (Hughes, Berg, Danziger, Cohen, & Martin, 1982) is administered to quantify a large number of functional impairments in dementia. The Dementia Rating Scale (DRS) (Mattis, 1976) is used to identify dementia and differentiate among the subtypes of dementia (e.g., AD, VaD).

Treatment of Dementia

Currently, there is no known cure for AD. Researchers continue to make advances in understanding the etiology and neuropathology of the disease. Thus, the available treatments only slow the progression of the disease and improve the quality of life for both the AD patient and his/her caregivers.

Behavioral Treatment With Dementia Patients. Dementia patients often suffer from concurrent depressive symptoms. Roughly 30% of patients with AD also have symptoms of depression that meet diagnostic criteria for major depressive disorder (Teri & Reifler, 1987; Teri & Wagner, 1992). These depressed dementia patients are prone to higher rates of behavioral and functional problems (e.g., increased irritability, agitation, and aggressive behavior), and their caregivers report higher levels of distress (Pearson, Teri, Wagner, Truax, & Logsdon, 1993). In recent years, research has focused on cognitive and behavioral treatments for depressed dementia patients and their family caregivers (Teri, 1994) as well as on training of health care staff in long-term care settings to treat depressed dementia patients (Teri & McCurry, 1994). Teri (1994) developed a 9-week treatment for both the dementia patient and caregiver in which they are provided with (a) education about AD and behavioral interventions, (b) methods of behavior change, (c) strategies for identifying and increasing patient pleasant events, (d) methods to maximize the patient's cognitive and functional abilities, (e) problem solving related to patient care, including depression behavior, (f) aid for caregiving responsibilities, and (g) plans for maintaining treatment gains. Investigations have shown somewhat promising results of this behavioral treatment (Teri et al., 2000; Teri, Logsdon, Uomoto, & McCurry, 1997).

Treatment for Distress in Family Caregivers. Caregivers of individuals with dementia experience extensive caregiver stress and often feel progressively overwhelmed as their loved one continues to deteriorate (Coon, Thompson, Gallagher-Thompson, 2002; Martin-Cook, Trimmer, Svetlik, & Weiner, 2000). Furthermore, the stress of caregiving often has negative effects on the psychological and physical health of the caregiver (Bauer et al., 2000; Schulz, O'Brien, Bookwala, Fleissner; 1995; Vedhara, Shanks, Anderson, & Lightman, 2000). A variety of caregiver interventions have been developed and have been empirically validated (Coon, Thompson, Gallagher-Thompson, 2002; Gallagher-Thompson, Coon, Rivera, Powers, & Zeiss, 1998; Gallagher-Thompson, McKibbin, et al., 2000). For example, Gallagher-Thompson,

Lovett et al. (2000) found that a cognitive-behavioral psychoeducational coping-with-caregiving group reduced caregiver affective distress and increased coping behavior more than a problem-solving psychoeducational class or a wait-list control condition in white participants. Similar results were found with a Latina sample of dementia caregivers in a smaller pilot study (Gallagher-Thompson et al., 2001). In the Resources for Enhancing Alzheimer's Caregiver Health (REACH) project, a multisite study that sought to examine culturally sensitive interventions for dementia caregivers, participants were randomized to a CBT-oriented coping-with-caregiving group, an enhanced support group, or a minimal support condition (Coon, Schulz, & Ory, 1999). Consistent with previous studies, preliminary results at the Palo Alto, California, site suggested that the CBT-oriented coping-with-caregiving group reduced caregiver distress and increased coping more than the other two treatment conditions.

Training families to cope with the burdens of caregiving has become increasingly necessary and increases the family caregiver's effectiveness (Teri, 1999). Thus, the individual living with dementia receives better care from his or her caregivers. Furthermore, providing both the individual with dementia and his or her caregivers with information about local community resources and social services can reduce caregiver stress (Thompson & Thompson, 1999).

Medication Interventions. In recent years, there have been important developments in medication treatment for dementia, such as the introduction of cholinesterase inhibitors that help slow the progression of brain atrophy. These medications act by inhibiting the enzyme acetylcholinesterase, which slows down the metabolic breakdown of acetylcholine. Unfortunately, the medications do not alter the underlying course of the disease (U.S. Department of Health and Human Services, 2000).

In 1993, tacrine (Cognex) was the first medication approved by the Food and Drug Administration in the United States for treatment of dementia. Efficacy studies of tacrine found only modest improvement in cognitive function (Sirvio, 1999). Furthermore, tacrine had serious side effects including liver toxicity (Nordberg & Swensson, 1998). Thus, the costs of taking tacrine often outweighed the benefits.

With the advent of newer acetylcholinesterase inhibitors with less serious side effects, tacrine is used less frequently. The newer medications, donepezil hydrochloride (Aricept), rivastigmine (Exelon), and galantamine (Reminyl), are now more widely used. Clinical trials have found these second-generation cholinesterase inhibitors to be efficacious. Specifically, 5 or 10 mg of donepezil hydrochloride daily was associated with some improvement in cognitive function after 12 or 24 weeks of treatment. Moreover, significant improvements were found in global function and activities of daily living after 24 weeks of treatment (compared with placebo) in patients with mild to moderate AD (Wilkinson, 1999).

In addition, in recent years researchers have found other medications that may delay the progression of dementia symptoms. Women who are taking estrogen hormone replacement therapy (HRT) may significantly delay the onset of AD and lower their risk for developing the disease (Kawas et al., 1997). HRT may also improve cognition in female patients who are already diagnosed with AD (Asthana et al., 1999). However, taking hormones is not without specific risks, including coronary heart disease (CHD), stroke, and breast cancer (Writing Group for the Women's Health Initiative Investigators, 2002).

Furthermore, researchers have hypothesized that anti-inflammatory drugs may help reduce the risk of developing AD (Kawas, 1999). However, few randomized controlled clinical trials have examined the effectiveness of anti-inflammatory drugs with AD, and results from existing studies are mixed. In one study, investigators found that prednisone had adverse effects on memory and cognition (Aisen et al., 1996). Thus, research on the effect of anti-inflammatory drugs with AD patients is inconclusive to date. Finally, the use of antioxidants (e.g., vitamin E and Gingko biloba) have been investigated with AD patients to determine if they are effective in slowing the progression of cognitive impairment. Initial results suggested that Gingko biloba showed modest improvements in cognition with AD patients (Le Bars et al., 1997). However, this study had some methodological flaws, so results need to be interpreted cautiously. Furthermore, in patients with moderate to severe symptoms of AD, a selective monoamine oxidase inhibitor (selegiline) or vitamin E slowed the progression of AD (Sano et al., 1997).

Alcohol Use Disorders Among Older Adults

A majority of research on alcohol abuse/dependence has focused on younger populations (Wechsler, Kuo, Lee, & Dowdall, 2000; Weitzman & Wechsler, 2000). Despite the fact that limited research has been conducted examining alcohol abuse/dependence in older adults, estimates of alcohol use among older adults warrants research attention. Gomberg (1980) estimated that anywhere from 2% to 10% of community-based elders have an alcohol problem. Estimated rates are even higher for older adults who have health problems. Among primary care patients, 4% to 10% have alcohol problems and the prevalence increases to 14% for emergency room patients (Adams, Ockene, Wheller, Hurley, 1998). Despite the high prevalence rates of alcohol use among older adults, older adults are less likely than younger adults to receive treatment for substance use disorders (Moos, Mertens, & Nrennan, 1993).

There are many risk factors for alcohol use among older adults. As noted earlier, older adults face a number of psychosocial stressors, such as physical decline, loneliness, bereavement, and so on. These stressful events, in addition to particular environmental factors (e.g., limited social support), can put older adults at greater risk for abusing alcohol. Similar to younger adults, older adults who are withdrawn, isolated, impulsive, and hypersensitive are more likely to abuse substances. Additionally, those with comorbid anxiety and depression are more likely to have substance use disorders.

Assessment

There are a number of barriers to early detection of alcohol use among older adults. First, older adults are less likely to seek out and use mental health or substance abuse services. When alcohol abuse is identified, it is often found as a secondary condition within primary care settings. A second barrier is that too few elders are screened for alcohol abuse or depression by physicians, nurses, and social workers so that problems might be detected and treated in their early stages. Third, older drinkers tend to have fewer social indicators, such as family complaints, DUIs, and work impairment. Older adults with substance use diagnoses also have significant physiological difficulties as a result of use. First, smaller amounts of alcohol have a stronger net affect in older adults because of physiological changes that occur as the body ages. Second, there is significant risk for malnutrition in that excess amounts of alcohol decrease the ability of the stomach to absorb food and thus increase the risk for malnutrition. Third, there is a risk of negative interaction between alcohol and other regularly prescribed medications. This risk is of particular concern because of the high prevalence of substance use problems among older adults with health problems. Finally, substance use also has a significant impact on the cognitive functioning of older adults, affecting memory performance on tasks involving frontal lobe activity (e.g., flexibility of thinking) and perceptual-motor deficits (e.g. they perform poorly on speed-dependent and visual spatial tasks).

There are also a number of indicators of substance abuse among older adults (Egbert, 1993). One such indicator is when a therapy for a normally treatable medical illness (e.g., hypertension) is not working for an older patient. Second, there are certain physical problems associated with alcohol use in older adults including insomnia, diarrhea, urinary incontinence, weight loss, and malnutrition. Third, older adults who complain of anxiety, experience unexplained postoperative agitation, or those who frequently ask for prescriptions of anxiolytics, sedative, or hypnotics might be suffering from a substance use disorder.

According to the Treatment Impairment Protocol Series #26 (TIPS; Substance Abuse and Mental Health Services Administration [SAMHSA], 1998), four main assessment measures have been found to be reliable and valid for assessing alcohol use among older adults (refer to Table 18.2). After an older adult has been appropriately assessed for alcohol use, he or she is categorized by drinking onset. Those who have had alcohol-related problems over several decades are diagnosed with early-onset alcohol abuse (about two thirds of older adults who are diagnosed with alcohol use disorder are classified as early onset) or late-onset alcohol abuse (referring to older adults whose alcohol problems began in their 50s or 60s, often as a reaction to losses experienced in later life).

Treatment

Even though older adults are less likely than younger adults to receive substance abuse treatment, a number of effective treatment interventions have been identified for those fortunate enough to get into these programs. The Gerontology Alcohol Project (GAP, 1979–1981; Dupree, Broskowski, & Schonfeld, 1984) used a treatment that included a CBT-based analysis of drinking behavior (ABCs of drinking) and self-management groups. Of those who completed the program, 75% maintained abstinence or limited drinking at 1-year follow-up and reported increased social support networks at discharge and at 1-year follow-up.

Brief interventions also can be effective in treating substance abuse among older adults. TIPS #26 (SAMHSA, 1998), focusing on substance abuse among older adults, found that 10% to 30% of problem drinkers, who did not meet criteria for a DMS–IV (APA, 1994) diagnosis of substance dependence, reduced their drinking to moderate levels following a brief intervention. The brief intervention consisted of one or more counseling sessions that included motivations for change strategies, patient education, assessment and direct feedback, contracting and goal setting, behavioral modification techniques, and the use of written material. One approach designed to facilitate effective brief interventions with older adults is known by the acronym FRAMES (feedback, responsibility, advice, menu, empathetic, self-efficacy; SAMHSA, 1998). The FRAMES approach emphasizes providing feedback on personal risk or impairment, personal responsibility for change, clear advice to change, a menu of ways to change, an empathetic counseling style, and enhancing a client's self-efficacy (SAMHSA, 1998).

The Substance Abuse Mental Health Service Administration has developed practice guidelines for treating older adults with substance abuse problems (SAMHSA TIPS #26, 1998; Schonfeld & Dupree, 1998). When working with older adults receiving treatment for alcohol use:

- Emphasize age-specific group treatment that is supportive rather than confrontational in nature.
- Treatment facilities should employ staff experienced in working with elders.
- The overall treatment approach should be broad and holistic, recognizing the age-specific psychological, social, and health factors related to substance use.
- The pace of treatment should be slowed and the content should be sure to attend to negative emotions, such as depression, loneliness, overcoming losses, and so on.
- Treatment should also teach skills to rebuild social support networks.

- Substance abuse treatment centers for older adults should be linked with aging services to address other needs of older adults that might potentially put them at an increased chance of relapse.

Other mental health disorders that were omitted due to space constraints include schizophrenia, bipolar disorder, personality disorders, substance abuse problems (other than alcohol), family stress and dysfunction, and sexual dysfunction. Interested readers are encouraged to read selected works under Suggested Readings.

PSYCHOLOGICAL ASSESSMENT OF OLDER ADULTS

Selecting an assessment instrument for an older individual is a challenge because there are few assessment measures designed specifically for older adults. More research needs to be done in this area, particularly to determine if current assessment measures are culturally appropriate for ethnic minority older adults. As we discussed some of the diagnostic criteria for particular disorders are not always applicable to older adults and could result in an inaccurate diagnosis.

Once an appropriate assessment measure has been selected, modifications in the assessment procedure must be made, beginning with slowing the pace of testing (Zarit & Haynie, 2000). Older adults tire more easily, so assessment procedures need to be accommodating. Test sessions might need to be spread across several days and frequent breaks taken to ensure more accurate results. Instructions and testing materials also should be presented at a slower pace and in multiple modalities if possible. Second, the mental health professional needs to be aware of any sensory deficits. As with any client, it is important to ensure that the testing environment is quiet with minimal distractions, but it is also important to have older adults actually use any sensory aids they may require, such as glasses or hearing aids. Third, it is important for clinicians working with older adults to collaborate with other health professionals. Ideally, physicians should be involved in the assessment process to rule out any physical health problem that might be associated with the presenting mental health problem, thus leading to more accurate treatment recommendations.

TREATMENT ISSUES WITH OLDER ADULTS

The actual treatment interventions used with older adults who are suffering from mental health problems are not all that different from those used with younger or middle-aged adults. What differs is the *process* and *content* of therapy. The *process* of therapy differs in three main ways: (a) There is often a need to directly address the age difference between therapist and client, (b) it is necessary to conduct therapy in a way as to foster independence in older clients, and (c) it is usually necessary to use a slower pace of treatment and to make appropriate modifications due to cognitive and/or sensory deficits (Zeiss & Steffen, 1996), see Table 18.1.

Regarding the first point, there is a good chance that you, the therapist, will be considerably younger than your client. Therefore, it is necessary to openly address any concerns your client has related to your age at the onset of therapy. This can be achieved by treating clients with respect and explaining how specific training in geropsychology helps therapists to understand age-related problems and needs (Zarit and Zarit, 1998). The second component, the need to foster independence, can be done primarily through a collaborative relationship, which encourages the older adults' involvement in therapy decisions, such as frequency and time of visits and between-session interventions for the client to do independently. Regarding the third point, the pace of therapy is usually slower with older adult clients, who generally benefit from repetition of information. Reviewing and summarizing what has been discussed in a session helps the older clients to learn and remember new information more easily. It is important for therapists to be patient with the pace of treatment and not to get discouraged. Change in older adults is possible, but usually occurs in smaller increments (Zeiss and Steffen, 1996).

Another factor influencing the pace of therapy is the need to accommodate sensory deficits. Older adults are able to hear better when they are spoken to in a voice that is louder, slower, and at a lower pitch (Zarit & Zarit, 1998). Presenting information in multiple modalities, such as in verbal and written formats, also assists older adult's ability to maintain information. All written material should be presented in a large, easy-to-read font. Daily log books are also useful to help older adults record observations related to treatment between sessions and to take notes during therapy sessions. Some clients also find it helpful to audiotape or videotape sessions for further review.

Zeiss and Steffen (1996) have summarized the basic adaptations needed when treating older adults into five components using the mnemonic MICKS (*m*ultimodal, *i*nterdisciplinary *a*wareness, *c*learer *k*nowledge of aging challenges and strengths, and *S*lower). Using the strengths of older clients is a concept that fits well with the notion of successful aging. Zeiss and Steffen (1996) suggest that during the process of therapy, clinicians can foster older adults' strengths by demonstrating respect for the role of the elder, having the older adult identify their personal strengths and how they can be used to alleviate the presenting problem, discussing past experiences in which they handled similar problems, and considering the client's wisdom.

The content of therapy differs because of the particular life experiences of older adults, including chronic illness and disability, concerns with death and dying, and interpreting the aging process (Thompson, 1996). Knight (1986) also suggests that the content of therapy should include themes such as empowerment in later life, how to cope with losses and maintain independence, the importance of everyday pleasant activities, and life review.

MEETING THE FUTURE NEEDS OF OLDER ADULTS

Although there is not a direct causal relationship between growing old and developing psychological disorders, a significant number of older adults do suffer with mental health disorders in later life. Appropriate assessment and treatment of mental health disorders among older adults are going to be a growing concern as the population of older adults continues to grow. Given the future increase in the older adult population in the coming years, a future mental health need of older adults is access and use of mental health services. Relatively few older adults seek treatment for mental health problems (Scogin, Floyd, and Forde, 2000). Service use is even lower among ethnic minority older adults (U.S. Department of Health and Human Services, 2001). Furthermore, when an older adult does receive treatment for a mental health problem, services are often obtained via a primary care physician (Robinson, 1998) rather than a trained mental health professional.

A second way to address the future mental health needs of older adults is to foster interdisciplinary collaboration and to encourage health care to move toward an interdisciplinary treatment team model. Given the physiological changes associated with normal aging and the related possible psychosocial stressors, both the mental and physical health needs of older adults would be better met with an interdisciplinary treatment team approach. As the population of older adults continues to grow, health professionals are going to be asked how we can foster well-being and enhance the quality of life of older adults. We have some answers, but many more to discover.

DISCUSSION QUESTIONS

1. To get a better understanding of your stereotypes of aging, create a list of positive and negative images of aging in our society.

2. What do we know about other cultures' views of aging and how can these values be applied to the development of treatment interventions in the United States? How do these views change the way we conceptualize or define mental health problems?

3. Create a senior outreach program designed to reduce mental health problems among older adults. Address the following issues: prevalent mental health issues, ethnic minority older adults, interdisciplinary health teams, and successful aging.

4. Discuss ways to create a paradigm shift in the current health care system for older adults—government policies, community programs, and so on.

SUGGESTED READINGS

Duffy, M. (Ed.). (1999). *Handbook of counseling and psychotherapy with older Adults.* New York: Wiley.
Whitbourne, S. K. (Ed.). (2000). *Psychopathology in later adulthood.* New York: Wiley.
Zarit, S. H., & Zarit, J. M. (1998). *Mental disorders in older adults.* New York: Guilford.

ACKNOWLEDGMENT

This work is supported by grants AG18784 and AG17824 from the National Institute on Aging, grant AA07222 from the NIAAA, grant IIRG-01-3157 from the National Office of the Alzheimer's Association, and by the Department of Veterans Affairs Sierra-Pacific Mental Illness Research, Education, and Clinical Center (MIRECC).

REFERENCES

Adams, A. Ockene, J. K., Wheller, E. V., & Hurley, T. G. (1998). Alcohol counseling: Physicians will do it. *Journal of General Internal Medicine, 13,* 692–698.
Administration on Aging. (2000). *A Profile of Older Americans.* Washington, DC: Author.
Aisen, P. S., Marin, D., Altstiel., L., Goodwin, C., Baruch, B., Jacobson, R., Ryan, T., & Daviski (1996). A pilot study of prednisone in Alzheimer's disease. *Dementia, 7,* 201–206.
Altamura, A. C., De Novellis, F., Guercetti, G., Invernizzi, G., Percudano, M., & Montgomery, S. A. (1989). Fluoxetine compared with amitriptyline in elderly depression: A controlled clinical trial. *International Journal of Clinical Pharmacological Research, 9,* 391–396.
American Psychiatric Association. (1980). *Diagnostic and Statistical Manual of Mental Disorders* (3rd ed.). Washington, DC: Author.
American Psychiatric Association. (1994). *Diagnostic and Statistical Manual of Mental Disorders* (4th ed.). Washington, DC: Author.
American Psychiatric Association. (2000). *Diagnostic and Statistical Manual of Mental Disorders* (4th ed., text rev.). Washington, DC: Author.
Asthana, S., Craft, S., Baker, L. D., Raskind, M. A., Zimbaum, R. S., Lofgreen, C. P., Veith, R. C., & Plymate, S. R. (1999). Cognitive and neuroendocrine response to transdermal estrogen in postmenopausal women with

Alzheimer's disease: Results of a placebo-controlled, double-blind pilot study. *Psychoneuroendocrinology*, *24*, 657–677.

Averill, P. M., & Beck, J. G. (2000). Posttraumatic stress disorder in older adults: A conceptual review. *Journal of Anxiety Disorders*, *14*(2), 133–156.

Banazak, D. A. (1997). Anxiety disorders in elderly patients. *Journal of the American Board of Family Practice*, *10*, 280–289.

Bauer, M. E., Vedhara, K., Perks, P., Wilcock, G. K., Lightman, S. L., Shanks, N. (2000). Chronic stress in caregivers of dementia patients is associated with reduced lymphocyte sensitivity to glucocorticoids. *Journal of Neuroimmunology*, *103*(1), 84–92.

Beck, A. T. (1976). Cognitive therapy and the emotional disorders. New York: International Universities Press.

Beck, A., Epstein, N., Brown, G., & Steer, R. (1988). An inventory for measuring clinical anxiety: Psychometric properties. *Journal of Consulting and Clinical Psychology*, *56*, 893–897.

Beck, J. G., & Stanley, M. A. (1997). Anxiety disorders in the elderly: The emerging role of behavior therapy. *Behavior Therapy*, *28*, 83–100.

Beck, A. T., Steer, R. A., & Brown, G. K. (1996). BDI-II Manual. San Antonio, TX: The Psychological Corporation.

Beekman, A. T. F., Bremmer, M. A., Deeg, D. J. H., Van Balkom, A. J. L. M., Smit, J. H., De Beurs, E., Van Dyck, R., & Tilburg, W. V. (1998). Anxiety disorders in later life: A report from the longitudinal aging study, Amsterdam. *International Journal of Geriatric Psychiatry*, *13*, 717–726.

Bell, I. (1999). A guide to current psychopharmacological treatments for affective disorders in older adults : Anxiety, agitation, and depression. In M. Duffy (Ed.), *Handbook of counseling and psychotherapy with older adults* (pp. 561–576). New York: Wiley.

Blazer, D. (1986). Depression. *Generations*, *10*, 21–23.

Blazer, D. (2002). *Depression in late life.* New York: Springer.

Blazer, D., George, L. K., Hughes, D. (1991). The epidemiology of anxiety disorders: An age comparison. In C. Salzman & B. Lebowitz (Eds.), *Anxiety in the elderly* (pp. 17–30). New York: Springer.

Blake, D. D., Weathers, F. W., Nagy, L. M., Kaloupek, D. G., Klauminzer, G., Charney, D. S., & Keane, T. M. (1990). A clinician rating scale for assessing current and lifetime PTSD: The CAPS-1. *Behavioral Therapist*, *13*, 187–188.

Blow, F. C., Brower, K. J., Schulenberg, J. E., Demo-Dananberg, L. M., Young, J. P., & Beresford, T. P. (1992). The Michigan Alcoholism Screening Test—Geriatric Version (MAST-G): A new elderly-specific screening instrument. *Alcoholism: Clinical and Experimental Research*, *16*, 372.

Boudewyns, P., & Hyer, L. (1997). Changes in psychophysiological response to war memories among Vietnam veteran PTSD patients treated with directed therapeutic exposure. *Behavior Therapy*, *21*, 63–87.

Braak, E., Griffing, K., Arai, K., Bohl, J., Bratzke, H., & Braak, H. (1999). Neuropathology of Alzheimer's disease: What is new since A. Alzheimer? *European Archives of Psychiatry and Clinical Neuroscience*, *249*(Suppl. 3), 14–22.

Coon, D., Schulz, R., & Ory, M.G. (1999). Innovative intervention approaches for Alzheimer's disease caregivers. In D.E. Biegel & A.B. Blum (Eds.), *Innovations in practice and service delivery across the lifespan* (pp. 295–325). New York: Oxford University Press.

Coon, D., Thompson, L. W., & Gallagher-Thompson, D. G. (Eds.). (2002). *Innovative interventions to reduce dementia caregivers' distress: A sourcebook and clinical guide.* New York: Springer.

Cummings, J. L., Vinters, H. V., Cole, G. M., & Khachaturian, Z. S. (1998). Alzheimer's disease: Etiologies, pathophysiology, cognitive reserve, and treatment opportunities. *Neurology*, *51*(Suppl. 1), S2–17.

Deberry, S., Davis, S., & Reinhard, K. E. (1989). A comparison of meditation-relaxation and cognitive-behavioral techniques for reducing anxiety and depression in a geriatric population. *Journal of Geriatric Psychiatry*, *22*, 231–247.

Dupree, L. W., Broskowski, H., & Schonfeld, L. (1984). The gerontology alcohol project: A behavioral treatment program for elderly alcohol abusers. *Gerontologist*, *24*, 510–516.

Dychtwald, K., & Flower, J. (1990). *Age wave: How the most important trend of our time will change your future.* New York: Bantam Books.

Egbert, A. M. (1993). The older alcoholic: Recognizing the subtle clinical clues. *Geriatrics*, *48*(7), 63–6, 69.

Ewing, J. A. (1984). Detecting alcoholism: CAGE Questionnaire. *Journal of the American Medical Association*, *252*, 1905–1907.

Fields, R. B. (1998). The dementias. In P. J. Snyder & P. D. Nussbaum (Eds.), *Clinical neuropsychology: A pocket handbook for assessment* (pp. 211–239). Washington, DC: American Psychological Association.

Fillenbaum, G. G., Heyman, A., Huber, M. S., Woodbury, M. A., Leiss, J., Schmader, K. E., Bohannon, A., Trapp-Moen, B. (1998). The prevalence and 3-year incidence of dementia in older black and white community residents. *Journal of Clinical Epidemiology*, *51*(7), 587–595.

Fleming, K. C., Evans, J. M., Weber, D. C., & Chutka, D. S. (1995). Practical functional assessment of elderly persons: A primary care approach. *Mayo Clinic Proceedings, 70,* 890–911.

Folstein, M. F., Folstein, S. E., & McHugh, P. R. (1975). "Mini-mental state." A practical method for grading the cognitive state of patients for the clinician. *Journal of Psychiatric Research, 12,* 189–198.

Fry, P. S. (1984). Cognitive training and cognitive-behavioral variables in the treatment of depression in the elderly. *Clinical Gerontologist, 3,* 25–45.

Gallagher, D., Breckenridge, J., Thompson, L. W., & Peterson, J. (1983). Effects of bereavement on indicators of mental health in elderly widows and widowers. *Journal of Gerontology, 38,* 565–571.

Gallagher, D., Nies, G., & Thompson, L. W. (1982). Reliability of the Beck Depression Inventory with older adults. *Journal of Consulting and Clinical Psychology, 50,* 152–153.

Gallagher, D., Rose, J., Rivera, P., Lovett, S., & Thompson, L. W. (1989). Prevalence of depression in family caregivers. *The Gerontologist, 29,* 449–456.

Gallagher-Thompson, D., Arean, P., Rivera, P., Thompson, L. W. (2001). A psychoeducational intervention to reduce distress in Hispanic family caregivers: Results of a pilot study. *Clinical Gerontologist, 23,* 17–32.

Gallagher-Thompson, D., Coon, D., Rivera, P., Powers, D., & Zeiss, A. (1998). Family caregiving: Stress, coping, and intervention. In M. Hersen & V. B. Van Hasselt (Eds.), *Handbook of clinical geropsychology* (pp. 469–494). New York: Plenum.

Gallagher-Thompson, D., Lovett, S., Rose, J., McKibbin, C., Coon, D., Futterman, A., Thompson, L.W. (2000). Impact of psychoeducational interventions on distressed family caregivers. *Journal of Clinical Geropsychology, 6*(2), 91–110.

Gallagher-Thompson, D., McKibbin, C., Koonce-Volwiler, D., Menendez, A., Stewart, D., & Thompson, L. W. (2000). Psychotherapy with older adults. In C. R. Snyder & R. Ingram (Eds.), *Handbook of psychological change: Psychotherapy processes and practices for the 21st century* (pp. 614–637). New York: Wiley.

Gallagher-Thompson, D., & Osgood, N. (1997). Suicide in later life. *Behavior Therapy, 28,* 23–41.

Gallagher-Thompson, D., Ossinalde, C., Menendez, A., Fernandez, E., Romero, J., Valverde, I., & Thompson, L.W. (1996). Como mantener su bienestar. Una clase para cuidadores. Palo Alto, CA: VA Palo Alto Health Care System.

Gallagher-Thompson, D., Ossinalde, C., & Thompson, L.W. (1996). Coping with caregiving: A class for family caregivers. Palo Alto, CA: VA Palo Alto Health Care System.

Gallagher-Thompson, D., & Steffen, A. M. (1994). Comparative effects of cognitive behavioral and brief psychodynamic psychotherapies for depressed family caregivers. *Journal of Consulting and Clinical Psychology, 62,* 543–549.

Gatz, M., Fiske, A., Fox, L. S., Kaskie, B., Kasl-Godley, J. E., McCallum, T. J., & Wetherell, J. L. (1998). Empirically validated psychological treatments for older adults. *Journal of Mental Health and Aging, 4*(1), 9–46.

Gillespie, K., Duffy, M., Hackmann, A., & Clark, D. M. (2002). Community based cognitive therapy in the treatment of posttraumatic stress disorder following the Omagh bomb. *Behavior Research and Therapy, 40,* 345–357.

Gomberg, E. S. (1980). *Drinking and problem drinking among the elderly.* Ann Arbor, MI: Institute of Gerontology, University of Michigan.

Graham, K., & Vidal-Zeballos, D. (1998). Analysis of the use of tranquilizers and sleeping pills across five surveys of the same population (1985–1991): The relationship with gender, age, and use of other substances. *Social Science and Medicine, 46,* 381–395.

Grossman, M. (2002). Frontotemporal dementia: A review. *Journal of the International Neuropsychological Society, 8,* 566–583.

Halonen, J. S., & Santrock, J. W. (1996). *Psychology: Contexts of behavior.* Chicago: Brown & Benchmark.

Hammer, M. B., Brodrick, P. S., & Labbbate, L. A. (2001). Gabapentin in PTSD: A retrospective, clinical series of adjunctive therapy. *Annals of Clinical Psychiatry, 13*(3), 141–146.

Havighurst, R. J. (1961). Successful aging. *Gerontologist, 1,* 8–13.

Henry, W. E., & Cumming, E. (1959). Personality development in adulthood and old age. *Journal of Projective Techniques and Personality Assessment, 34,* 384–390.

Hilliard, K. M., & Iwamasa, G. Y., (2001). The conceptualization of anxiety: An exploratory study of Japanese American older adults. *Journal of Clinical Geropsychology, 7*(1), 53–65.

Hinrichsen, G. A. (1999). Interpersonal psychotherapy for late-life depression. In M. Duffy (Ed.), *Handbook of counseling and psychotherapy with older adults* (pp. 470–486). New York: Wiley.

Horowitz, M. J., Wilner, N., & Alvarez, W. (1979). Impact of Event Scale: A measure of subjective stress. *Psychosomatic Medicine, 41*(3), 209–218.

Hoyert, D. L., Kochanek, K. D., & Murphy, S. L. (1999). *Deaths: Final data for 1997.* National vital statistics report, 47(19). Hyattsville, MD: National Center for Health Statistics. DHHS Publication No. PHS 99-1120 (p. 85, Table 26).

Hughes, C. P., Berg, L., Danziger, W. L., Cohen, L. A., & Martin, R. L. (1982). A new clinical scale for the staging of dementia. *British Journal of Psychiatry, 140*, 566–72.

Hyer, L. (1995). Use of EMDR in a "dementing" PTSD survivor. *Clinical Gerontologist, 16*, 70–74.

Hyer, L. (1999). The effects of trauma: Dynamics and treatment of PTSD in the elderly. In M. Duffy (Ed.), *Handbook of counseling and psychotherapy with older adults* (pp. 539–560). New York: Wiley.

Hyer, L., & Brandsma, J. M. (1997). EMDR minus eye movements equals good psychotherapy. *Journal of Traumatic Stress, 10*, 515–522.

Hyer, L., Summers, M. N., Boyd, S., & Litaker, M. (1996). Assessment of older combat veterans with the Clinician-Administered PTSD Scale. *Journal of Traumatic Stress, 9*, 587–594.

Hyer, L., Swanson, G., Lefkowitz, R., Hillesland, D., Davis, H., & Woods, M. (1990). The application of the cognitive behavioral model to two older stressor groups. *Clinical Gerontologist, 9*(3/4), 145–190.

Judd, L. L., & Kunovac, J. L. (1998). Bipolar and unipolar depressive disorders in geriatric patients. *International Academy of Biomedical Drug Research, 13*, 1–10.

Kasper, S., Lepine, J. P., Mendlewicz, J., Montgomery, S. A., & Rush, J. A. (1995). Efficacy, safety, and indications for tricyclic and newer antidepressants. *Depression, 2*, 127–137.

Katona, C. (2000). Managing depression and anxiety in the elderly patient. *European Neuropsychopharmacology, 10*(Suppl. 4), S427–S432.

Kaup, B., Ruskin, P., & Nyman, G. (1994). Significant life events and PTSD in elderly World War II veterans. *American Journal of Geriatric Psychiatry, 2*, 239–243.

Kawas, C. H. (1999). Inflammation, anti-inflammatory drugs and Alzheimer's disease. In R. Mayeaux & Y. Christen (Eds.). *Epidemiology of Alzheimer's disease: From gene to prevention* (pp. 65–72). New York: Springer-Verlag.

Kawas, C., Resnick, S., Morrison, A., Brookmeyer, R., Canada, M., Zonderman, A., Bacal, C., Lingle, D. D., Metter, E. (1997). A prospective study of estrogen replacement therapy and the risk of developing Alzheimer's disease: The Baltimore longitudinal study of aging. *Neurology, 48*, 1517–1521.

Klerman, G. L., Weissman, M. M., Rounsaville, B. J., & Chevron, E. S. (1984). *Interpersonal psychotherapy of depression*. New York: Basic Books.

Knight, B. (1986). Psychotherapy with older adults. Newbury Park, CA: Sage.

Kochanek, K. D., & Murphy, S. L. (1999). *Deaths: Final data for 1997*. National vital statistics report, 47(19). Hyattsville, MD: National Center for Health Statistics. DHHS Publication No. (PHS) 99-1120.

Kolb, B., & Whishaw, I. Q. (1996). *Fundamentals of human neuropsychology* (4th ed.). New York: W. H. Freeman.

Landreville, P., Laundry, J., Baillargeon, L., Guerette, A., & Matteau, E. (2001). Older adults' acceptance of psychological and pharmacological treatments for depression. *Journal of Gerontology: Psychological Sciences, 56B*(5), P285–P291.

Lazarus, R. S., & Launier, R. (1978). Stress-related transactions between person and environment. In L. A. Pervin & M. Lewis (Eds.), Perspectives in interactional psychology (pp. 287–327). New York: Plenum.

Le Bars, P. L., Katz, M. M., Berman, N., Itil, T. M., Freedman, A. M., & Schatzberg, A. F. (1997). A placebo-controlled, double-blind randomized trial of an extract of Gingko biloba for dementia. *Journal of the American Medical Association, 278*, 1327–1332.

Lerner, R. M. (1986). *Concepts and theories of human development* (2nd ed.). New York: Random House.

Lewinsohn, P. M., Munoz, R. F., Youngren, M. A., & Zeiss, A. M. (1978). *Controlling your depression*. Englewood Cliffs, NJ: Prentice Hall.

Lezak, M. D. (1995). Neuropsychological Assessment (3rd ed.). New York: Oxford University Press.

Lichtenberg, P. A. (Ed.). (1996). *Handbook of assessment in clinical gerontology*. New York: Wiley.

Lindgren, C. L., Connelly, C. T., & Gaspar, H. L. (1999). Grief in spouse and children caregivers of dementia patients. *Western Journal of Nursing Research, 21*, 521–537.

Luis, C. A., Mittenberg, W., Gass, C. S., & Duara, R. (1999). Diffuse Lewy body disease: Clinical, pathological and neuropsychological review. *Neuropsychology Review, 9*(3), 137–150.

Martenyi, F., Brown, E. B., Zhang, H., Prakah, A., & Koke, S. C. (2002). Fluoxetine versus placebo in posttraumatic stress disorder. *Journal of Clinical Psychiatry, 63*(3), 199–206.

Martin-Cook, K., Trimmer, C., Svetlik, D., & Weiner, M. F. (2000). Caregiver burden in Alzheimer's disease: Case studies. *American Journal of Alzheimer's Disease, 15*(1), 47–52.

Mattis, S. (1976). Mental Status examination for organic mental syndrome in the elderly patient. In L. Bellack & T. Karasu (eds.), Geriatric psychiatry (pp. 77–120). New York: Grune & Stratton.

McFall, M. E., Smith, D. E., Mackay, P. W., & Tarver, D. J. (1990). Reliability and validity of the Mississippi scale for combat related PTSD. *Psychological Assessment, 2*, 114–121.

McFarlane, A. (1990). Posttraumatic stress disorder. *International Review of Psychiatry, 3*, 203–213.

McIntoch, J. L., Santos, J. F., Hubbard, R. W., & Overholser, J. C. (1994). *Elder suicide research, theory and treatment*. Washington, DC: American Psychological Association.

McLeod, A. (1994). The reactivation of posttraumatic stress disorder in later life. *Australian and New Zealand Journal of Psychiatry, 28*, 625–634.

Montgomery, S. A. (1998). Efficacy and safety of the selective serotonin reuptake inhibitors in treating depression in elderly patients. *International Clinical Psychopharmacology, 13*(Suppl. 5), S49–S54.

Montgomery, S. A., & Kasper, S. (1995). Comparison of compliance between serotonin reuptake inhibitors and tricyclic antidepressants: A meta-analysis. *International Clinical Psychopharmacology, 9*(Suppl. 4), 33–40.

Moos, R. M., Mertens, J. R., & Nrennan, P. L. (1993). Patterns of diagnosis and treatment among late-middle aged and older substance abuser patients. *Journal of studies on Alcohol, 54*, 479–487.

Moscicki, E. K. (1995). Epidemiology of suicide. *International Psychogeriatrics, 7*, 137–148.

Mui, A. C., Burnette, D., & Chen, L. M. (2001). Cross-cultural assessment of geriatric depression: A review of the CES-D and GDS. *Journal of Mental Health and Aging, 7*(1), 137–164.

National Institutes of Health Consensus Development Conference Consensus Statement (1991). *Diagnosis and treatment of depression in late life, 9*(3), 1–27.

Neal, L. A., Hill, N., Hughes, J., Middleton, A., & Busuttil, W. (1995). Convergent validity of measures of PTSD in an elderly population of former prisoners of war. *International Journal of Geriatric Psychiatry, 10*, 617–622.

Newmann, J. P., Engel, R. J., & Jensen, J. (1991a). Age differences in depressive symptom experiences. *Journals of Gerontology, 46*(5), P224–P235.

Newmann, J. P., Engel, R. J., & Jensen, J. (1991b). Changes in depressive symptom experiences among older women. *Psychology and Aging, 6*(2), 212–222.

Nordberg, A., & Swensson, A. L. (1998). Cholinesterase inhibitors in the treatment of Alzheimer's disease: A comparison of tolerability and pharmacology. *Drug Safety, 19*, 465–480.

O'Hara, R., Mumenthaler, M. S., & Yesavage, J. A. (2000). Update on Alzheimer's disease: Recent findings and treatments. *Western Journal of Medicine, 172*, 115–120.

Osgood, N. J. (1985). *Suicide in the elderly: A practitioner's guide to diagnosis and mental health intervention.* Richmond, VA: Aspen.

Parmelee, P. A., Katz, I. R., & Lawton, M. P. (1989). Depression among institutionalized aged: Assessment and prevalence estimation. *Journal of Gerontology, 44*, M22–M29.

Pearson, J. L., Teri, L., Wagner, A., Truax, P., & Logsdon, R. (1993). The relationship of problem behaviors in dementia patients to the depression and burden of caregiving spouses. *American Journal of Alzheimer's Disease and Related Disorders Research, 8*, 15–22.

Perkins, B. R., & Rouanzoin, C. C. (2002). A critical evaluation of current views regarding eye movement desensitization and reprocessing (EMDR): Clarifying points of confusion. *Journal of Clinical Psychology, 58*(1), 77–97.

Petronis, A. (1999). Alzheimer's disease and down syndrome: From meiosis to dementia. *Experimental Neurology, 158*(2):403–413.

Powers, D. V., Thompson, L., & Gallagher-Thompson, D. (2002). Depression in later life: Epidemiology, assessment, impact and treatment. In I. Gotlib & C. Hammen (Eds.), *The handbook of depression* (3rd ed.). New York: Guildford.

Radloff, L. (1977). A self-report depression scale for research in the general population. *Applied Psychological Measurement, 1*, 385–401.

Raj, B. A., & Sheehan, D. V. (1988). Medical evaluation of the anxious patient. *Psychiatric Annals, 18*, 176–181.

Regier, D. A., Boyd, J. H., Burke, J. D., Rae, D. S., Myers, J. K., Kramer, M., Robins, L. N., George, L. K., Karno, M., & Locke, B. Z. (1988). One-month prevalence of mental disorders in the United States: Based on five Epidemiologic Catchment Area sites. *Archives of General Psychiatry, 45*, 977–986.

Reynolds, C. F., Frank, E., Perel, J. M., Imber, S. D., Cornes, C., Morycz, R., Mazumdar, S., Miller, M., Pollock, B., Rifai, A. H., Stack, J. A., George, C. J., Houck, P. R., & Kupfer, D. (1992). Combined pharmacotherapy and psychotherapy in the acute and continuation treatment with recurrent major depression: A preliminary report. *American Journal of Psychiatry, 149*, 1687–1692.

Richman, J. (1999). Psychotherapy with the suicidal elderly: A family-oriented approach. In M. Duffy (Ed.), *Handbook of counseling and psychotherapy with older Adults* (pp. 650–661). New York: Wiley.

Rice, P. L. (1999). *Stress and health* (3rd ed.). Pacific Grove, CA: Brooks/Cole.

Riley, K. P., & Carr, M. (1989). Group psychotherapy with older adults: The value of an expressive approach. *Psychotherapy: Theory, Research, and Practice, 26*, 366–371.

Robinson, P. (1998). Behavioral health services in primary care: A new perspective for treating depression. *Clinical Psychology: Science and Practice, 51*(1), 77–93.

Rosen, W. G., Mohs, R. C., & Davis, K. L. (1984). A new rating scale for Alzheimer's disease. *American Journal of Psychiatry, 141*, 1356–1364.

Rowe, J. W., & Kahn, R. L. (1998). *Successful Aging.* New York: Pantheon Books.

Salthouse, T. A. (1996). The processing-speed theory of adult age differences in cognition. *Psychological Review, 103*, 403–428.

Sano, M., Ernesto, C., Thomas, R. G., Klauber, M. R., Schafer, K., Grundman, M., Woodbury, P., Growdon, J., Cotman, C. W., Pfeiffer, E., Schneider, L. S., & Thal, L. J. (1997). A controlled trial of selegiline, Alpha-tocopherol, or both as treatment for Alzheimer's disease: The Alzheimer's Disease Cooperative Study. *New England Journal of Medicine, 336*(17), 1216–1222.

Schonfeld, L., & Dupree, L. W. (1998). Relapse prevention approaches with the older problem drinker. *Southwest Journal on Aging, 14,* 43–50.

Schulz, R., O'Brien, A. T., Bookwala, J., & Fleissner, K. (1995). Psychiatric and physical morbidity effects of dementia caregiving: Prevalence, correlates, and causes. *Gerontologist, 35,* 771–791.

Scogin, F., Floyd, M., & Forde, J. (2000). Anxiety in older adults. In S. K. Whitbourne (Ed.), *Psychopathology in later adulthood* (pp. 117–140). New York: Wiley.

Scogin, F., Rickard, H. C., Keith, S., Wilson, J., & McElreath, L. (1992). Progressive and imaginal relaxation training for elderly persons with subjective anxiety. *Psychology and Aging, 7,* 419–424.

Siegel, J. S. (1999). Demographic introduction to racial/Hispanic elderly populations. In T. P. Miles (Ed.), *Full-color aging: Facts, goals, and recommendations for America's diverse elders* (pp. 1–19). Washington, DC: The Gerontological Society of America.

Simard, M., van Reekum, R., & Cohen, T. (2000). A review of the cognitive and behavioral symptoms in dementia with Lewy bodies. *Journal of Neuropsychiatry and Clinical Neuroscience, 12,* 425–450.

Sirvio, J. (1999). Strategies that support declining cholinergic neurotransmission in Alzheimer's disease patients. *Gerontology, 45,* 3–14.

Spiro, A., Schnurr, P. P., & Aldwin, C. M. (1994). Combat-related posttraumatic stress disorder symptoms in older men. *Psychology and Aging, 9*(1), 17–26.

Stanley, M. A., & Beck, J. G. (1998). Anxiety disorders. In M. Hersen & V. B. Van Hasselt (Eds.), *Handbook of Clinical Geropsychology* (pp. 217–238). New York: Plenum.

Stanley, M. A., Beck, J. G., & Glassco, J. D. (1996). Treatment of generalized anxiety in older adults: A preliminary comparison of cognitive-behavioral and supportive approaches. *Behavior Therapy, 27,* 565–581.

Substance Abuse and Mental Health Services Administration (SAMHSA) (1998). *Substance abuse among older adults: Treatment Improvement Protocol (TIP) Series #26.* Rockville, MD: U.S. Department of Health and Human Services.

Teng, M. X., Stern, Y., Marder, K., Bell, K., Gurland, B., Lantigua, R., Andrews, H., Feng, L., Tycko, B., & Mayeux, R. (1998). The APOE-epsilon4 allele and the risk of Alzheimer's disease among African Americans, Whites, and Hispanics. *Journal of the American Medical Association, 279,* 751–755.

Teri, L. (1994). Behavioral treatment of depression in patients with dementia. *Alzheimer's disease and associated disorders, 8*(Suppl. 3), 66–74.

Teri, L. (1999). Training families to provide care: Effects on people with dementia. *International Journal of Geriatric Psychiatry, 14*(2), 110–116.

Teri, L., & Gallagher-Thompson, D. (1991). Cognitive-behavioral interventions for treatment of depression in Alzheimer's patients. *Gerontologist, 31,* 413–416.

Teri, L., & Logsdon, R. (1991). Identifying pleasant activities for Alzheimer's disease patients: The Pleasant Events Schedule-AD. *Gerontologist, 31,* 124–127.

Teri, L., Logsdon, R. G., Peskind, E., Raskind, M., Weiner, M. F., Tractenberg, R. E., Foster, N. L., Schneider, L. S., Sano, M., Whitehouse, P., Tariot, P., Mellow, A. M., Auchus, A. P., Grundman, M., Thomas, R. G., Schafer, K., & Thal, L. J. (2000). Treatment of agitation in AD: A randomized, placebo-controlled clinical trial. *Neurology, 55*(9), 1271–1278.

Teri, L., Logsdon, R. G., Uomoto, J., & McCurry, S. M. (1997). Behavioral treatment of depression in dementia patients: A controlled clinical trial. *Journal of Gerontology: Psychological Sciences, 52B*(4), P159–P166.

Teri, L., & McCurry, S. M. (1994). Psychosocial therapies. In C. E. Coffey & J. L. Cummings (Eds.), The American Psychiatric Press textbook of geriatric neuropsychiatry (pp. 662–682). Washington, DC: American Psychiatric Press.

Teri, L., & Reifler, B. V. (1987). Depression and dementia. In L. Carstensen & B. Edelstein (Eds.), *Handbook of clinical gerontology* (pp. 112–119). New York: Pergamon.

Teri, L., & Wagner, A. (1992). Alzheimer's disease and depression. *Journal of Consulting and Clinical Psychology, 3,* 379–391.

Thompson, C., & Thompson, G. (1999). Support for carers of people with Alzheimer's type dementia. *Cochrane Library, Issue 4.* Oxford: Update Software.

Thompson, L. W. (1996). Cognitive-behavioral therapy and treatment for late-life depression. *Journal of Clinical Psychiatry, 57*(Suppl. 5), 29–37.

Thompson, L. W., Coon, D., Gallagher-Thompson, D., Sommer, B., & Koin, D. (2001). Comparison of desipramine and cognitive/behavioral therapy in the treatment of elderly outpatients with mild to moderate depression. *American Journal of Geriatric Psychiatry, 9,* 225–240.

Thompson, L., Gallagher, D., & Breckenridge, J. S. (1987). Comparative effectiveness of psychotherapies for depressed elders. *Journal of Consulting and Clinical Psychology, 55*, 385–390.

Thompson, L., Gallagher-Thompson, D., & Dick, L. (1996). *Cognitive-behavioral therapy for late-life depression: A therapist manual.* Palo Alto, CA: Veterans Affairs Palo Alto Health Care System.

Thompson, L. W., Tang, P., Kaye, J., & Gallagher-Thompson, D. (2004). Bereavement and adjustment disorders in later life. In D. Blazer, D. Steffens, & E. Busse (Eds.), *Textbook of geriatric psychiatry* (3rd ed.). Washington, DC: American Psychiatric Press.

Tucker, P., Zaninelli, R., Yehuda, R., Ruggiero, L., Dillingham, K., & Pitts, C. D. (2001). Paroxetine in the treatment of chronic posttraumatic stress disorder: Results of a placebo-controlled, flexible-dosage trial. *Journal of Clinical Psychiatry, 62*(11), 860–868.

U. S. Department of Health and Human Services. (2001). *Mental health: Culture, race, and ethnicity—A supplement to mental health: A report of the Surgeon General—Executive summary.* Rockville, MD: Author, Public Health Service, Office of the Surgeon General.

U. S. Department of Health and Human Services. (2000). *Progress report on Alzheimer's disease: Taking the next steps.* Rockville, MD: Author, Public Health Service, National Institutes of Health, National Institute on Aging.

U. S. Department of Health and Human Services. (1999). *Mental Health: A Report of the Surgeon General.* Rockville, MD: Author, Substance Abuse and Mental Health Services Administration, Center for Mental Health Services, National Institutes of Health, National Institute of Mental Health.

U. S. Department of Veterans Affairs. (1997). *Dementia identification and assessment: Guidelines for primary care practitioners.* Washington, DC: Author and the University Health System Consortium.

Vedhara, K., Shanks, N., Anderson, S., & Lightman, S. (2000). The role of stressors and psychosocial variables in the stress process. A study of chronic caregiver stress. *Psychosomatic Medicine, 62*(3), 374–385.

Wagstaff, A. J., Cheer, S. M., Matheson, A. J., Ormrod, D., & Goa, K. L. (2002). Paroxetine: An update of its use in psychiatric disorders in adults, *Drugs, 62*(4), 655–703.

Watson, C. G. (1990). Psychometric PTSD Measuring techniques: A review. *Psychological Assessment, 2*, 460–469.

Wechsler, H., Kuo, M., Lee, H., & Dowdall, G.W. (2000). Environmental correlates of underage alcohol use and related problems in college drinkers. *American Journal of Preventative Medicine, 19*(1), 24–29.

Weissman, M. M., Bruce, M. L., Leaf, P. J., Florio, L. P., & Holzer, C. (1991). Affective disorders. In L. N. Robins & D. A. Regier (Eds.), *Psychiatric disorders in America* (pp. 53–80). New York: Free Press.

Weitzman, E. A., & Wechsler, H. (2000). Alcohol use, abuse and related problems among children of problem drinkers: Findings from a national survey of college alcohol use. *Journal of Nervous & Mental Disease, 188*(3), 148–154.

Wetherell, J. L. (1998). Treatment of anxiety in older adults. *Psychotherapy, 35*, 444–458.

Wetherell, J. L. (2002). Behavior therapy for anxious older adults. *The Behavior Therapist, 25*(1), 16–17.

Whitbourne, S. K. (2000). The normal aging process. In S. K. Whitbourne (Ed.), *Psychopathology in later adulthood* (pp. 27–60). New York: Wiley.

Wilkinson, D. G. (1999). The pharmacology of donepezil: a new treatment of Alzheimer's disease. *Expert Opinions in Pharmacotherapy, 1*(1), 121–135.

Wilson, J., Harel, Z., & Kahana, B. (1989). The Day of Infamy: The legacy of Pearl Harbor. In J. Wilson (Ed.), *Trauma, transformation, and healing* (pp. 129–156). New York: Brunner/Mazel.

Writing Group for the Women's Health Initiative Investigators. (2002). Risks and benefits of estrogen plus progestin in healthy postmenopausal women: Principal results from the Women's Health Initiative randomized controlled trial. *Journal of the American Medical Association, 288*, 321–333.

Yesavage, J. A., Brink, T. L., Rose, T. L., Lum, O., Huang, V., Adey, M. B., & Leirer, V. O. (1983). Development and validation of a geriatric depression screening scale: A preliminary report. *Journal of Psychiatric Research, 17*, 37–49.

Zarit, S. H., & Haynie, D. A. (2000). Introduction to clinical issues. In S. K. Whitbourne (Ed.), *Psychopathology in later adulthood* (pp. 1–26). New York: Wiley.

Zarit, S. H., & Zarit, J. M. (1998). Mental disorders in older adults: Fundamentals of assessment and treatment. New York: Guilford.

Zeiss, A. M., & Steffen, A. (1996). Treatment issues with elderly clients. *Cognitive and Behavioral Practice, 3*(2), 371–390.

Author Index

Note: Numbers in italics indicate pages with complete bibliographic information; *n* indicates footnote; *f* indicates figure; *t* indicates table.

A

Abbot, E. S., 64*n*, 79, *82*
Abed, R. T., 234, *249*
Abi-Dargham, A., 189, *196*
Abikoff, H., 326, 328, 332, 333, *345, 348, 349, 351*
Abikoff, H. B., 332, 333, 334, *350, 351*
Ablon, J. S., 334, *338*
Abramowitz, A., 332, 333, *351*
Abramowitz, A. J., 341, *345*
Abramowitz, J. S., 146, *149*
Abramson, L. Y., 166, 168, 169, *175*
Abukmeil, S. S., 188, *198*
Achenbach, T. M., 28, 29, *33, 37,* 325, *345,* 356, 362, 369, *371*
Ackerman, R. F., 117, *119*
Acklin, M. W., 94, 95, *102*
Adams, A., 409, *413*
Adams, E. H., 302, *321*
Ad-Dab'bagh, Y., 213, *221*
Adey, M. B., 401, 402, *419*
Adler, D., 44, *58*
Adler, D. A., 99, *102, 205t, 223*
Ageton, S. S., 271, *277*
Aghajanian, G. K., 110, *123*
Agras, W. S., 92, *105,* 129, 133, 136, 146, *149, 152, 153,* 246, 248, *249, 250*
Aguilar-Gaxiola, S., 30, *37*
Ahadi, S. A., 206, 211, 218, 219, *225*
Ahern, G. L., 115, *122*
Aikins, D. E., 139, 145, *149*
Aikins, J. E., 296, *297*
Aisen, P. S., 408, *413*

Akamatsu, T. J., 97, *102*
Alanen, Y. O., 73, *81*
Alarcon, A. D., 71
Alarcon, R. D., 11, *17,* 22, *33,* 68, 75, 76, 77, 78, *79, 82,* 219, *221*
Albano, A. M., 360, 362, *371, 376*
Albee, G. W., 170, *175*
Albert, S., 93, 97, *102*
Albo, M., 258, *280*
Alborzian, S., *120*
Albrecht, B., 215, 220, *224*
Aldrete, E., 30, *37*
Aldwin, C. M., 399, *418*
Alegria, M., 30, *36*
Alexopoulos, G. S., 68, 71, *81*
Alford, B. A., 368, *372*
Ali, A., 235, *253*
Allain, A. N., 206, 207, 209, *226*
Allan, C. A., 307, *319*
Allbeck, P., 186, *197*
Allen, J. P., 315, 316, *322*
Allen, L. A., 285, 289, *298*
Allen, N. B., 367, *371*
Allen-Burge, R., 51, *58*
Alloy, L. B., 166, 168, 169, *175*
Allsopp, D. H., 381, *392*
Alpert, M., 183, *196*
Alreja, M., 110, *123*
Altamura, A. C., 404, *413*
Altemus, M., 114, *120*
Alterman, A., 207, 210, *223, 226*
Alterman, A. I., 48, 50, *58,* 91, *102,* 310, 314, *319, 324*
Alterman, M., 209

421

Subject Index

Note: *n* indicates footnote; *f* indicates figure; *t* indicates table.